MUNICIPAL AND RURAL SANITATION

MUNICIPAL AND RURAL SANITATION

Sixth Edition

Victor M. Ehlers, C.E.
Late Director, Division of Sanitary Engineering,
Texas State Department of Health

Ernest W. Steel, C.E.
Late Professor of Civil Engineering,
University of Texas

McGraw-Hill Book Company

New York   St. Louis   San Francisco   Toronto   London

Municipal and Rural Sanitation

ISBN 07-0019089-5

14 15 16 17 18 19 20 - MAMM - 7 6 5 4 3

PREFACE

The protection of health and the promotion of human comfort and well-being through control of man's environment are responsibilities which modern conditions have forced upon us. The population increase and the diversity of human activities which have accompanied that increase have made control more difficult. This book defines the field of environmental control or sanitation, sets forth the important problems which confront workers in that field, and suggests solutions to those problems.

Environmental control, or sanitation, is particularly the field of the engineer and sanitarian, although a knowledge of its principles is essential to all workers in public health. This book should be helpful as a reference to workers already in the field since it contains material dealing with the newer problems now confronting them. It will also serve as a textbook in general sanitation for engineering students and for sanitarians and others who are enrolled in schools of public health.

A chapter on air pollution and its control has been added since, in recent years, this has become an important activity in many health departments. In addition, the chapter on radiological health has been rewritten and expanded. The community approach to the solution of environmental problems has been stressed, and this has been emphasized further by the addition of a chapter on environmental engineering planning. A discussion of accident control has been added, and much new material has been included throughout the book and particularly in the chapters on water, treatment and disposal of human wastes, milk sanitation, food sanitation, and vector control.

The death of the senior author, Victor M. Ehlers, has unfortunately ended his wise counsel and contributions to the book, but the general plan which he favored was followed in this edition.

Thanks are due to numerous friends for helpful suggestions: Clayton H. Billings, Associate Editor of *Public Works*, assumed responsibility for Chap. 1, Communicable Diseases; Chap. 2, Water: General Characteristics, Treatment, and Protection; and Chap. 12, Bathing-place Sanitation. Others who contributed with advice and suggestions are: C. H. Atkins; Malcolm C. Hope; Dr. H. D. Pratt; James G. Terrill, Jr.; Dr. R. D. Grove;

Arthur C. Stone; R. S. Mark; Dr. K. Sikes; A. H. Neill; Dr. W. Clark Cooper; Dr. H. G. Scott; Edwin L. Ruppert; W. H. Felsing, Jr.; Dr. E. F. Gloyna; Dr. J. O. Ledbetter; H. E. Hargis; H. D. McGaw; M. C. Wukasch; J. E. Cowen; D. Decker; R. G. Waggener; G. R. Herzik, Jr.; F. J. Von Zuben, Jr.; and H. L. Dabney.

While names of individuals have been given in the above list, mention should be made of organizations to which they, and perhaps some others who contributed, belong. They are the Public Health Service of the U.S. Department of Health, Education, and Welfare; the Texas State Department of Health; and the Environmental Engineering Division of the Department of Civil Engineering of the University of Texas.

For preparation of the manuscript, proofreading, and indexing, thanks are due to M. C. Steel; and for typing, to Johanne H. Turner.

Ernest W. Steel

The death of Ernest W. Steel shortly after completing the manuscript of this sixth edition of *Municipal and Rural Sanitation* brought to an end his many contributions to the instruction of workers in public health. He was a pioneer in a not too well understood area of endeavor, when he began teaching the first course in sanitary engineering to be offered in the Southwest and one of the first anywhere. From the outset, as reflected in the many editions of this text, he was one who appreciated the broader scope of sanitary science in relation to man's environment. By sharing this viewpoint with those he taught in his 43 years of practice, he had an important influence in shaping the modern dimensions of the profession.

Clayton H. Billings

CONTENTS

Milking. Milking Machines. Straining. Cooling. Bottling, Capping, and Delivery. Pasteurization. Pasteurization Methods. Sanitary Control of Pasteurization. The Pasteurization Plant. Operation of the Plant. Municipal Regulation of Milk Supplies. The Milk Ordinance and Code. Inspection and Sampling. The Laboratory and Testing. Collection and Delivery of Milk. Rating of Cities. Interstate Milk Shipments. Certified Milk. Milk Products. Dry Milk and Dry-milk Products. Butter. Cheese. Frozen Desserts.

for Children. Water Supply. Excreta Disposal. Prevention of Vermin. Food Storage. Provision of Sufficient Space in Sleeping Rooms. Materials and Construction. Fire Protection. Accident Prevention. Satisfaction of Fundamental Psychological Needs. Privacy. Provision for Normal Family and Community Life. Provision for Cleanliness and Convenience. Housing and Government. Housing Regulation. Enforcement of Housing Regulations. Zoning and Housing. Municipal Housing Programs. Federal Government and Housing.

Schools. School Health Program. Location. Building. Interior Finish. Light and Color. Heating and Ventilation. Noise Control. Furnishings. Plumbing. Water Supply and Sewage Disposal. Cleaning and Maintenance. Hospitals. Physical Structure and Maintenance. Central Supply and Sterilizing Areas. Hospital Plumbing. Operating and Delivery Rooms and Nurseries. Isolation Areas. Refuse Disposal. Nursing Homes and Related Institutions. Nursing Homes. Jails. Physical Structure. Cleanliness and Maintenance. Examination of Inmates and Inspections. Lighting and Ventilation. Water Supply and Sewerage. Pest Control. Food Service. Cell Furnishings.

Health Work in Industry. Programs for Small Plants. Governmental Control. Organization for Occupational Health. Occupational Hazards. Industrial Poisons. Threshold-limit Values. The Dust Hazard. Radiation Hazards. Industrial Noise. Light as a Hazard. Heat. Compressed Air. Repeated Motion, Vibration, Pressure, and Shock. Infections. Plant Sanitation. Ventilation. Illumination. Water Supply. Toilet Facilities.

Atomic Structure. Radioactivity. Half-life of Radioisotopes. Ionization. Units of Radiation and Radioactivity. Radiation Dosage. Instruments Used for Detection and Measurement of Radiation. Maximum Permissible Radiation Exposures. Harmful Effects of Radiation. Radiological Sanitation. Monitoring of Air, Milk and Other Foods, and Water. Environmental Protection from Nuclear Power Reactors. Disposal of Radioactive Wastes. Health Departments and Radiological Health.

Magnitude of the Problem. Epidemiology of Accidents. Accident Prevention. Organization for Accident Prevention. Sanitation of Public Conveyances. Railways. Vessels. Airplanes. Buses. Community Noise Abatement. Sources of Noise. Noise Prevention. Motels, Trailer Parks, Camps, and Migratory Labor Camps. Motels and Tourist Courts. Summer Camps. Migratory Labor Camps. Mobile Home Parks. Disaster Sanitation.

INTRODUCTION

In the preamble to the constitution of the World Health Organization, health is defined as "a state of complete physical, mental and social well-being and not merely the absence of disease or infirmity." This considerably broadens the field of public health work, which formerly was considered to be concerned primarily with preventive medicine, or the application of measures to prevent disease. Preventive medicine must be clearly differentiated from the older science, curative medicine, the object of which is to cure the person already attacked by disease. Preventive medicine is still, however, an important concept in public health work since the bulk of such work is disease prevention.

While the individual may take advantage of preventive medicine by his own efforts, for example, by having his family physician vaccinate him against such diseases as smallpox and typhoid fever, in the main, prevention must be applied through community efforts.

Public Health Work. Obviously, preventive medicine would be limited in value if it were practiced only by the individual. An epidemic, for example, requires the efforts of all the skilled persons and facilities available for investigation of the source and prevention of further spread. Nor could one person conduct a campaign to eradicate mosquitoes, improve the milk supply of a city, or reduce infant mortality by establishing maternity and child welfare clinics. Such efforts, which are carried out by an organization for the benefit of a community or certain classes of the community, are known as public health work. Mostly they are carried on at public expense, but note that the definition does not exclude work done by charitable organizations. Curative activities that are carried on at public expense, while generally considered charity or welfare work rather than preventive medicine, are not excluded entirely from public health work. Tuberculosis and the venereal diseases, for example, are prevented to a considerable degree by prompt cure, in the case of the former, and quick cure at public expense, in the case of the latter.

Public health work includes the following activities: control of communicable diseases by means of immunization, isolation, etc.; maternity, infant, and preschool hygiene; school hygiene; control of the venereal diseases; mental health work; control of tuberculosis; environmental

1

sanitation; and recording of vital statistics. Sanitation is the principal subject of this book, but the other activities are briefly discussed in Chap. 20.

Sanitation. This activity, sometimes called environmental sanitation or environmental health work, is defined by the World Health Organization as "the control of all those factors in man's physical environment which exercise or may exercise a deleterious effect on his physical development, health, and survival." The definition becomes comprehensive when the definition of health given above is recalled. An outline of this field of public health work follows:

1. Water supply
2. Wastes
   a. Excreta disposal, without water carriage
   b. Sewerage
   c. Collection and disposal of solid wastes
3. Insect control
   a. Mosquitoes
   b. Flies
   c. Other
4. Rodent control
5. Food sanitation
   a. Milk
   b. Meat
   c. Other foods
   d. Food-processing and food-handling establishments
6. Plumbing
7. Prevention of atmospheric pollution
8. Heating, ventilation, and air conditioning
9. Lighting
10. Housing
11. Institutional sanitation
12. Occupational health work
13. Sanitation of swimming pools and bathing places
14. Eradication of nuisances
15. Radiological protection
16. Accident prevention

Some of the above activities also have value in producing comfort, for example, eradication of non-disease-bearing mosquitoes, air conditioning of buildings, improvement of housing, and elimination of some types of noise and atmospheric pollution.

Sanitation is practiced by the sanitary inspector, the sanitarian, and the sanitary engineer or environmental engineer. The sanitary inspector makes inspections as a means of enforcing sanitary regulations and works under the supervision of a sanitarian or engineer. The sanitarian is a person who has had formal training in the fundamental sciences that apply to sanitation, such as biology, bacteriology, chemistry, and vital statistics. He should be able to translate the sanitary needs of a community into terms of sanitary regulations and procedures and train and supervise inspectors. The sanitary or environmental engineer[1] has received engineering training which he applies to the field of sanitation or control of the environment. He should be able to head a division of sanitation in industry and in a health department and to apply the principles of sanitary engineering to such diverse activities as air-, water-, and insect-control measures, waste disposal, and the planning of community improvements, including housing.

The Changing Environment. Sanitation is necessary to overcome the effects of man's activities on his environment. The increase in population and the movement of population into urban and metropolitan areas (Art. 21-2) have intensified environmental-control difficulties in those areas. The provision of safe water; the collection and disposal of human, domestic, and industrial wastes; the prevention of atmospheric pollution and stream pollution; and the control of ionizing radiation are becoming more difficult from year to year. Unfortunately the response of governmental agencies in meeting some of these problems has been rather slow. Mention should also be made of the hazards presented by the use of pesticides for agricultural purposes. These are at present under governmental control and do not appear to be an important danger to human life or wildlife.

---

[1] The title "sanitary engineer" is not looked upon with favor by some since it is frequently misunderstood by the public and has been appropriated by some persons who are not engineers. "Public health engineer" has been used, but it is not considered completely satisfactory. "Environmental engineer" is rising in favor and may supplement or replace "sanitary engineer." In this book, the terms "sanitary engineer" and "environmental engineer" are used interchangeably.

1

COMMUNICABLE DISEASES

1-1. Definitions. Health officials prefer to apply the term "communicable disease" to all ailments which may be transmitted by any means from person to person or from animal to person. Such terms as "contagious disease," implying communication by direct contact, and "infectious disease," indicating transmission of an infection, are not in favor because of vagueness. A communicable disease may result from the direct or indirect transmission of an infectious agent or its products.

Reportable diseases are those which state laws, rules, or regulations, supplemented by municipal ordinances, require that the attending physician report to the health officer. Practice varies in different cities and states regarding which diseases are to be reported. In practically

4

all of them, the major communicable diseases, such as tuberculosis, plague, typhoid fever, yellow fever, diphtheria, scarlet fever, smallpox, measles, and the venereal diseases, are reportable. A few considered of international significance statistically are reportable by the Public Health Service to the World Health Organization. The other diseases may or may not be reportable. The classification systems established by the American Public Health Association [1] on reporting of diseases is an excellent guide.

An *epidemic* is the incidence of a communicable disease among a number of people to an extent that is recognized statistically as being well beyond the normal expectancy for the disease in a community in a definite period of time. Usually large groups are affected, but only a few persons might be. For example, a few cases of smallpox, where the disease has been absent for years, might be termed an epidemic. A disease is *endemic* in an area if it is constantly present in some degree. An endemic disease may flare up at times and become epidemic. An *epizootic* is an epidemic among animals. A *zoonosis* is an infection or an infectious disease of animals transmissible under natural conditions to man.

A *sporadic* disease is one that occurs in occasional scattered cases. A *pandemic* affects large numbers of people at the same time and transcends community boundaries. For instance, the influenza of 1918–1919 was pandemic.

Epidemiology has been defined as the study of the distribution of a disease or condition in a population, and the factors that influence that distribution [4]. Note that the definition applies not only to communicable diseases but also to those which are noncommunicable and to accidental deaths and injuries. An important epidemiological study of noncommunicable disease is the investigation of the physiological effects ascribed to cigarette smoking. An *epidemiologist* is a person versed in epidemiology who may also direct measures to control or prevent epidemics.

Channels of infection are the means through which the body becomes infected by disease-producing agents. The channels may be the respiratory tract, the digestive tract, or the exterior surfaces of the body. Of these, the mouth is the portal of entry for the majority of infections.

An *infectious agent* is a microorganism capable of producing infectious disease under circumstances of host and environment favoring transmission.

Vehicles of infection are the means by which infectious agents are transported in causing disease. Water, food, insects, and inanimate objects may be vehicles of infection. Insect or rodent vehicles are sometimes called "vectors."

Carriers are persons who harbor specific infectious agents without discernible clinical disease but who can be reservoirs or sources of infection. They may be "healthy carriers," without clinical manifestations throughout the course of disease, or they may be "incubatory" or "convalescent" carriers, meaning that the carrier state is a feature of the incubation or convalescent stage of a disease having a clinical stage. In either case, the carrier state may be short, or temporary, or long (chronic). Some of the diseases that produce carriers are typhoid, diphtheria, cholera, hookworm, scarlet fever, and cerebrospinal fever. The release of infectious agents may be continuous or intermittent, but carriers can often be identified by laboratory examinations. The best public health practice requires the examination of the feces of all convalescents from typhoid fever to establish that the patient will not continue to harbor the infectious agent after recovery. A small percentage of typhoid patients are likely to become carriers. The danger of their being employed in occupations connected with the preparation of food is apparent, and many epidemics have been traceable to this cause. Known carriers of typhoid fever are listed by many health departments and are not permitted to work in food-handling establishments.

The *incubation period* is the time elapsing between the entrance of an infectious agent into the body and the appearance of signs or symptoms of the disease.

1-2. Microorganisms. These are forms of life which generally cannot be seen without the aid of a microscope. The term includes bacteria, protozoa, rickettsia, viruses, and fungi. Simply stated, bacteria are typically single-celled vegetative organisms; protozoa are single-celled animals; rickettsia are similar to both bacteria and protozoa but are classified under a single genus; viruses are ultramicroscopic, considered by some to be proteins capable of multiplication; and fungi are microscopic plants devoid of chlorophyll. All microorganisms are not infectious, though all known viruses are.

1-3. Methods of Communication. It was formerly supposed that the atmosphere was an important vehicle of infection and that diseases were due to miasmas floating about, particularly in damp or foggy night air. It is now known, however, that the atmosphere is relatively free from bacteria, particularly in unconfined areas, and that its importance in the communication of disease has been greatly overestimated. Humanly exhaled air, even in cases of diseases of the respiratory tract, is free from bacteria during quiet breathing. Sneezing, coughing, or forcible speaking, however, permits the entrainment of droplets of moisture which may be infectious. Droplets usually do not travel more than a few feet, and droplet infection is a recognized method of communication of such diseases as common colds, tuberculosis, poliomyelitis, and influenza, although there are other methods of spread.

Sunlight and dryness tend to kill some bacteria which have been discharged into the air. However, sunlight will not kill spores. Bacteria and other organisms may be carried on dust particles.

Water and food are involved in disease communication where the channel of infection is the mouth and intestinal tract. Water may contain infectious agents of typhoid and paratyphoid fever, dysentery, infectious hepatitis, and cholera. Infectious agents from the intestinal discharges of sick persons or carriers are responsible for unsafe water. Milk-borne epidemics of typhoid fever and scarlet fever were frequent in the past. They resulted from infectious agents entering the milk during handling and in the absence of pasteurization. Diphtheria has been occasionally disseminated in this manner. Foods have often been involved in the communication of typhoid and paratyphoid fever and dysentery. Foods are usually contaminated by the hands of carriers or persons in the early stages of disease or by flies and other insects.

Fomites[1] (inanimate objects that have come in contact with a sick person) also undoubtedly enter into the communication of disease to some extent. Not all fomites, however, are equally dangerous. Books, coins, and similar objects are of little importance in spreading disease, but eating utensils, pencils which have been placed in the mouth, and fragments of food which have been nibbled upon are of great importance, particularly among children, where close contact with such fomites is very likely. The common towel and drinking cup are also in this category. The transmission of disease through fomites may be considered an indirect-contact transmission. Another example of this type of transmission is putting the hand to the mouth after shaking hands with an infected person.

Animals are involved in the communication of certain diseases. Rabies is transmitted from dogs or other animals by bites. Tularemia is contracted by contact with infected rabbits. Brucellosis, or undulant fever, is carried from infected cows or goats by milk and is also transmitted through direct contact with diseased cattle, goats, and hogs, slaughtered or alive. Cattle, sheep, and goats are reservoirs of Q fever, commonly involved in airborne transmission.

Insects are the vectors of infection of several diseases. Malaria, yellow fever, dengue, arthropod-borne viral encephalitis, and filariasis are carried by mosquitoes. Plague and endemic typhus are carried from rats and other rodents by fleas. Epidemic typhus fever is carried by the human-body louse.

Diseases Communicated by Intestinal Discharges

1-4. The diseases of the gastrointestinal tract, because of their usual methods of communication, are important to the sanitarian. They include typhoid fever, the paratyphoids, cholera, dysentery, poliomyelitis, in-

---

[1] Pronounced fo'-mi-tees.

fectious hepatitis, hookworm disease, and a few other parasitic infections. Cholera has not been epidemic in this country for many years, but it is endemic in India and southwest Asia. Infectious hepatitis, although possibly transmissible by nose and throat discharges, can also be communicated by fecal contamination of water or milk.

1-5. Typhoid Fever. Before the application of sanitary measures, the annual typhoid death rate in cities was likely to be from 50 to 80 deaths per 100,000 population. At present it is less than one death per 1,000 population in the large cities. The major part of this reduction was caused by water purification, later followed by improvement of milk supplies, detection of carriers, and immunization against the disease. However, it is still common in some parts of the world and is endemic in small rural portions of the United States. There is a growing complacency, particularly among Americans, with regard to this disease. This is unwarranted, for periodic typhoid epidemics occur because of careless sanitation practices.

Typhoid is transmitted as a result of some serious sanitary defect, and it is still more prevalent than necessary, considering that the methods of communication are fully understood and subject to easy control. Carriers play a large part in the transmission of this disease. (See Fig. 1-1.) Female carriers are especially dangerous since they are more likely to be engaged in the preparation of food. The typhoid epidemics that are not traceable to water are usually due to carriers infecting milk or other foods. Shellfish may also be involved, but they are usually contaminated by the water in which they grow. The control of typhoid fever will include the following expedients: disinfection of the discharges of patients, examination of convalescents to discover carriers, obtaining histories of carriers and eliminating them from public food handling, boiling or purification of water, boiling or pasteurization of milk, and proper disposal of sewage.

Vaccination, which confers a degree of immunity from the disease, is another important preventive measure. Typhoid fever was formerly prevalent in armies, but vaccination has virtually eliminated it from modern wars. In civil life all persons who have come in contact with a patient are usually vaccinated by the attending physician. The vaccina-

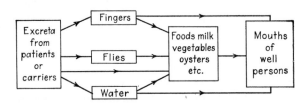

FIGURE 1-1 How typhoid fever is spread. (*After Lumsden, Public Health Service.*)

tion of everyone would have the effect of not only raising the resistance to typhoid fever but also lessening the chances of susceptible persons' coming into contact with cases, thus working two ways. The requirement of vaccination for all food handlers is an improvement that may be applied in the future.

1-6. Typhoid Epidemics. Investigation of epidemics of typhoid fever is a classic example of the functioning of a public health team. If possible, the investigation should be made by a group which would include a physician, a sanitary engineer, a nurse, and other professional workers whose techniques are adaptable to field investigations. The procedure includes obtaining full histories of the cases and tracing the movements of each patient previous to his illness so that the sources of his food, milk, and water may be identified. Thus it may be learned that the parties involved used the same milk, attended the same banquet, or consumed food or ice cream prepared at the same place. A spot map is of great value and can easily be prepared by marking on a map of the city the location of the houses in which the infected persons live. If no points of contact are found, a spot map showing a wide distribution of the cases would possibly indicate water carriage of the disease. Cases occurring in the neighborhood of an industrial plant may mean pollution of the water supply by a cross-connection (see Art. 2-34).

Typhoid epidemics have been traced to water contaminated by the discharges of patients or carriers. Milk-borne epidemics are usually due to milkers or other dairy attendants being carriers of the disease. One typhoid epidemic observed by the authors was apparently due to contamination of the teats and udders of cattle by sewage. Food contamination by carriers during preparation, food contamination by flies, the eating of vegetables fertilized with human excreta, and consumption of contaminated oysters have all been responsible for typhoid epidemics. Sporadic cases of typhoid fever are exceedingly difficult to trace. Usually they may be considered to be due to food contamination by a carrier or by flies.

1-7. Paratyphoid Fever. There are three varieties of paratyphoid, known as the A, B, and C types according to the causative organism (*Salmonella paratyphi*, *S. schottmuelleri*, and *S. hirschfeldi*, respectively), all resembling typhoid fever in their symptoms although much milder in their effects. Epidemics occur because of infected water, milk, and other foods, and carriers are also involved. Preventive and investigative methods are similar to those of typhoid. Type B is the only one common in the United States, often as transient diarrhea.

1-8. Dysentery. There are several kinds of dysentery. The bacillary type is, as its name indicates, caused by bacilli of the *Shigella* genus. Amoebic dysentery is due to an amoeba, a protozoon or single-celled animal, known as *Entamoeba histolytica*.

Bacillary dysentery has occurred very widely in armies and is often epidemic among civilians. The bacilli can appear in the excreta for several weeks after apparent recovery, but there appear to be no permanent carriers, and there is no immunization, either by an attack of the disease or by vaccination. The methods of transmission and control are similar to those of typhoid fever.

An outbreak of amoebic dysentery originating in Chicago in 1933 and involving 1,049 known cases with 98 deaths served to focus attention upon this dangerous disease. It was formerly considered that the infection was spread through food by food-handler carriers. Facts uncovered by a study of the Chicago epidemic indicate that water carriage is more important than food contamination. The outbreak was caused by sewage entering the ice-water systems of two hotels. *Entamoeba histolytica* forms cysts, which are present in human excreta. In the cyst form, the amoeba exists outside the body until it dies or is swallowed by a susceptible animal or person. The cysts are particularly resistant, emphasizing the importance of sanitary measures in preventing the spread of this disease: adequate sewage disposal, water treatment, fly control, and personal hygiene of food handlers. The cysts are removed from water by the standard treatment, coagulation, filtration, and disinfection. There is no immunization.

1-9. Ancylostomiasis (Hookworm Disease). There are several species of hookworm which infect man. The two most important are *Ancylostoma duodenale* and *Necator americanus*. The latter is the prevailing species in the southeastern United States and tropical West Africa; *A. duodenale* is common in the Mediterranean countries. Both species are found in Asia, Central and South America, and the West Indies. Other types confine their activities to dogs, cats, and other animals but can infest man, causing a dermatitis called creeping eruption. The adult hookworm is about the thickness of hairpin wire and is $3/8$ to $1/2$ in. long. The adults live in the intestines, fastening themselves to the walls by means of their strong mouth parts. The biting injures the walls and causes loss of blood. In addition, there are toxins liberated which are responsible for anemia. The adult worm is supposed to live for 6 to 8 years, spending all its adult life in the intestines. The female worms are constantly producing large numbers of eggs, which leave the host in the feces. Examination of feces under the microscope for the presence of eggs is the usual method of determining infection. The eggs hatch within 24 hr if temperature and moisture conditions are favorable. The larva is able to move about to a limited extent and feeds on the excrement. It molts once, and 4 to 5 days after hatching it molts for the second time but remains within the loose skin from which it has detached itself. During this period the larva becomes infective and is able to enter a victim at the first opportunity. It may exist in this stage for as long as 6 weeks, although in general its life is not so long. Should a barefooted person step on soil in which the larva is present, the larva clings to the skin and starts to bore its way in. The larva makes its way into the lymph vessels and veins and is carried with the blood to the heart and finally to the lungs. It leaves the blood vessels of the lungs and penetrates the air passages, thus obtaining a clear route up the bronchial tubes and windpipe to the throat. From the throat it is swallowed, going to the stomach and intestines. This journey requires about 10 days, and during the process the worm becomes sexually mature.

While the great majority of infestations are obtained through the bare feet, the worms may also enter through other parts of the body. In the mines, infestation is frequently obtained through contact of the hands with infected soil or with ladders which have received infective material from shoes. It also is possible to become infected through the mouth by eating vegetables which have been grown in fields fertilized by human excreta and possibly by drinking infected water.

The disease was formerly highly prevalent in the southeastern United States, with more than 50 per cent of rural schoolchildren infected. Education of the public, reduction of soil pollution, and wearing of shoes have reduced its incidence.

The most important factor in control of the disease is elimination of soil pollution by provision of toilet facilities. Where water carriage cannot be employed, chemical toilets or pit privies are essential. Hookworm eggs may survive as long as 5 months in the soil. Apparently they hatch only in the presence of oxygen, which suggests the possible danger in the use of sludge from septic and sewage treatment plants for fertilizer. It is known that the eggs may come unharmed through septic tanks with the effluent. Disinfectants appear to have no effect upon them.

Favorable temperature, favorable soil, and favorable rainfall characteristics are necessary to maintain a high rate of infestation in a population. A heavy clay soil is unfavorable because it quickly dries and becomes hard. A sandy soil that is continuously dry is also unfavorable. A sandy soil or a sandy loam combined with a well-distributed rainfall is most favorable. This permits the larval worms to retreat downward when the soil surface becomes too dry and to return to the surface when a rain wets the topsoil.

The inability of the worm to travel horizontally indicates that unless it is transported by animals or insects, the danger occurs where fecal matter is indiscriminately scattered on the ground where the bare feet of children or adults may come in contact with the polluted soil.

1-10. Infectious Hepatitis. This disease, also known as jaundice, is caused by a virus, its linkage with the gastrointestinal route of transmission being of fairly recent history. The virus is present in the blood and feces of an infected person. Infectious hepatitis is clinically indistinguishable from serum hepatitis, which is transmitted by the inoculation of infected human blood plasma, serum, or thrombin or by use of syringes contaminated with the blood of an infected person. Infectious hepatitis is worldwide in distribution, appearing sporadically and in epidemics. It is most common in rural areas and among children and young adults. Lifetime immunity is believed to be conferred. The gastrointestinal route of infection and that by blood contamination have been proved, and epidemics have been related to contaminated water, milk, and food, including shellfish. The presence of the virus in nose and throat discharges is possible. Control measures call for proper sewage disposal and water treatment to destroy the virus.

Diseases Communicated by Nose and Throat Discharges

1-11. The diseases communicated by discharges from the mouth and respiratory system are numerous and important. As their communication is dependent upon personal contact and personal habits rather than upon environmental factors, they are the most difficult to control. The diseases of this category are listed below:

Poliomyelitis	Whooping cough	Pneumonia
Tuberculosis	Cerebrospinal fever	Influenza
Diphtheria	Smallpox	Common colds
Measles	Chicken pox	Septic sore throat
Scarlet fever		

Of these diseases, smallpox and chicken pox may also be transmitted through material from pustules or lesions of the skin. The infection may be transmitted by direct contact, by droplets, by fomites, or from hand to mouth. Scarlet fever, diphtheria, and septic sore throat may also be carried by milk.

Poliomyelitis and tuberculosis are discussed below in greater detail. Control of the other diseases is frequently directed toward isolation of the patient, disinfection of discharges, and perhaps quarantine and observation of persons who have come in contact with the patient. In smallpox and diphtheria epidemics, artificial immunity is given to contacts and is required for, or recommended to, all persons as a preventive measure. Artificial immunity is now available for measles. Influenza has proved difficult to control, partly because the virus which causes it can withstand drying for days and even weeks on clothing, bedding, and dust.

1-12. Poliomyelitis. The virus of poliomyelitis has been found in the pharyngeal passages and the intestinal tract of human beings and has been isolated from the secretions and excretions of these areas. It is quite apparent that control measures should be directed toward preventing the spread of the virus from these sources. Such control measures as isolation and vaccination are indicated. Under epidemic conditions, mass vaccination is advisable. While the virus persists in feces longer than in the throat, there is no reliable evidence that it is spread by insects, food, or sewage. Milk has been responsible on rare occasions, but water is not likely to be involved. Recent widespread vaccination programs have been responsible for greatly reducing the incidence of this disease.

In epidemics, urban schools should not be closed, but unnecessary close contact of children with persons outside the family should be avoided. However, intensive athletic programs should be postponed. Where children attend school from considerable distance and have to be transported by bus, school closing is desirable.

1-13. Tuberculosis. With the advent of mass X-ray surveys, the increasing availability of hospital beds, and the growing use of major chest surgery and antimicrobial drugs, the tuberculosis death rate has been declining, although this disease is still one of fairly high mortality, varying in different countries from 5 to 100 deaths per 100,000 population annually. In the great majority of instances, however, recovery is possible. Since poor housing, overwork, worry, and insufficient and poor food diminish resistance, tuberculosis is particularly prevalent among the poor.

There are three distinct types of tuberculosis bacilli: human, avian, and bovine. The human type is pathogenic to man and also to cows and guinea pigs. The avian type affects birds and rabbits, but not man.

In man, bovine tuberculosis does not affect the lungs, but usually only the lymph glands or bones. In the United States and some other countries, it has become rare. It can be found in children as a result of drinking contaminated cow's milk. The milk becomes contaminated either directly from a diseased udder or, more frequently, from the manure, which, in the case of infected animals, often contains tuberculosis bacilli.

Human tuberculosis is mainly transmitted through the sputum, although any or all of the body discharges may be infective. There are several theories as to the means by which the infectious material reaches a second person. The sputum may dry and pulverize, liberating the bacilli in dust which may be stirred up by sweeping or walking over floors. Crawling infants and playing children are likely to get such infectious material on their hands and, by placing their hands in their mouths, to become infected.

Droplets from sneezing, coughing, etc., contain fresh and virile bacilli which may be inhaled or may fall upon food, hands, or other objects that may be placed in the mouth. Drinking cups and other utensils may also be involved. Direct and indirect contact are important. It appears that ingestion of bacilli, whether in food, droplets, or dust, will allow infection through the intestines in addition to direct infection of the lungs. However, infection through the alimentary canal is of less importance than contact.

The abrasive dust produced in many of the industries, when breathed for any length of time, appears to be conducive to tuberculosis. This is accounted for by the fact that such dust causes irritation of the lungs, creating a favorable place for the development of the chance infections mentioned previously.

The prevention of tuberculosis is a vast undertaking, involving such diverse matters as the education of the infected persons themselves and their families; the elimination of tuberculous workers from food-handling occupations; the safe disposal of infectious material; the proper treatment of patients and, where possible, their segregation; the improvement of housing and industrial conditions; the tuberculin testing of cattle and the removal of tuberculous animals from dairy herds; and the pasteurization of milk.

Other Communicable Diseases

1-14. Arthropod-borne Diseases. The arthropods, which are animals having jointed limbs, include the insects and arachnids, some of which are important in disease transmission. They may become vectors—agents of infection—by inoculating infectious material into or through the skin or mucous membrane of the victim or by depositing such material on fomites, food, or the skin. Insects such as houseflies and cockroaches may become mechanical carriers of pathogenic organisms by breeding or feeding in excrement and also by gaining access to food or milk. Examples of diseases transmitted in this manner are typhoid fever, paratyphoid fever, cholera, dysentery, and others already discussed.

The arthropod vector may be infected with microorganisms which undergo a cyclical change and multiplication within the body of the arthropod. Also, the pathogenic organism may undergo cyclical change within the vector but not multiply, or it may undergo no cyclical change but still multiply. In other cases, the arthropod may be said to be hereditarily infective, having acquired the pathogenic organism from infected parents.

While houseflies and cockroaches may also harbor certain pathogens of gastroenteric infections, many diseases important in America are primarily transmitted by arthropods capable of inoculating human beings and other vertebrate animals by virtue of their skin-piercing mouth parts. Included in this category are typhus fever, plague, relapsing fever, malaria, yellow fever, dengue, filariasis, tularemia, Rocky Mountain spotted fever, and arthropod-borne viral encephalitis.

There are three types of *typhus fever*. Epidemic, or classical, typhus is carried by the body louse, which in feeding upon the infected person takes into its body with the blood some of the organisms of the disease. However, it does not inject the microorganism directly into the blood of the second host; instead, infection results from the crushed body or feces of the louse being rubbed into a skin abrasion. Control of epidemic typhus includes bodily cleanliness and delousing of clothing and bedding. In Italy and elsewhere during World War II, epidemics were prevented by using dust guns to blow 10 per cent DDT powder into sleeves and other openings of clothing while it was being worn. Another method used during the war was to moisten the clothing in a 1.5 to 2 per cent water emulsion of DDT. The DDT will usually retain its efficiency even after six launderings of the clothing. The eggs of the lice are not killed, and the adults may live for as long as 24 hr.

Endemic, or murine, typhus occurs in temperate, semitropical, and tropical areas. It is harbored by rats and transmitted to man and from rat to rat by the bites of rat fleas and rat mites. Rodent control will reduce this disease; this is discussed in Chap. 9.

Scrub typhus occurs in parts of Asia and Australia. It is transmitted by the bite of infected larval mites. Mites and wild rodents provide the reservoir, and a mite–wild rodent–mite cycle maintains infection.

Plague, primarily a disease of rats and wild rodents, with the latter constituting the natural reservoir, is transmitted to man by the bite of the rat's fleas, which, upon the death of the original host, will feed upon man. Plague is of several types. As transmitted by fleas it is of the bubonic variety, which causes swelling of various glands. Should the lungs become infected, however, the pneumonic type results; this type may be transmitted directly to the lungs of others in a manner similar to the manner of transmission of pneumonia and pulmonary tuberculosis.

Relapsing fever, the tick-borne variety, is found in the western United States and other parts of the American continents. Wild rodents are reservoirs, and ticks are responsible for transmission. In other parts of the world, the louse-borne variety may result when an infected louse is crushed into a bite wound or an abrasion of the skin.

Malaria, yellow fever, dengue, and *filariasis* are carried by mosquitoes and are discussed in Chap. 9. Of these, malaria is of primary importance on a worldwide basis, but it has been eradicated for all practical purposes from the United States. However, even in this country two generations prior to the present it presented one of the most serious problems in the history of public health practice. The infectious agents are *Plasmodium vivax, P. malariae, P. falciparum,* and *P. ovale.* These are protozoons present in the blood of an infected person. Certain species of the *Anopheles* mosquito ingest blood containing the parasite in a specific stage of its life cycle, known as the gametocyte stage. The parasite further develops in the mosquito into sporozoites in from 8 to 35 days.

Sporozoites are concentrated in the salivary glands of the mosquito and infect man when the insect obtains a blood meal.

Tularemia (see Art. 1-15) is sometimes transmitted by ticks and bloodsucking flies.

Rocky Mountain spotted fever occurs throughout most of the United States but is most prevalent in the Rocky Mountains and along the Middle Atlantic seaboard. It is also found in Canada, Mexico, Colombia, and Brazil. Infected ticks are responsible for transmission, the variety depending upon the endemic location. Animal reservoirs are dogs, rabbits, and field mice.

Birds are suspected of being the principal reservoirs of infection from *arthropod-borne viral encephalitis*. It is transmitted by mosquitoes, which acquire the infection from birds. There have been occasional epidemics of this disease in man in the United States.

1-15. Diseases of Animals Transmissible to Man. The diseases mentioned in Art. 1-14, particularly murine typhus, plague, Rocky Mountain spotted fever, tularemia, and arthropod-borne viral encephalitis, include some in which vertebrate animals are reservoirs and share the transmission cycle with arthropods. With the exception of tularemia and arthropod-borne viral encephalitis, the diseases in the following discussion are those which have vertebrate animals as reservoirs and in which transmission is wholly or principally by means other than arthropods.

More than eighty diseases are known to involve vertebrate animals as reservoirs and are transmissible to humans. Bacterial and rickettsial diseases include brucellosis, bovine tuberculosis, Q fever, anthrax, leptospirosis, salmonellosis, tularemia, glanders, and tetanus. Among the more important infections caused by viruses are rabies, ornithosis, cat-scratch fever, Colorado tick fever, lymphocytic choriomeningitis, arthropod-borne viral encephalitis, and foot-and-mouth disease. Mycotic (*i.e.,* caused by fungi) infections include ringworm of cats and dogs (*Microsporum* species) and ringworm of cattle (*Trichophyton* species). Also of importance are such parasitic infestations of animals as trichinosis, pork tapeworm (*Taenia solium*), beef tapeworm (*T. saginata*), hydatidosis, and broad fish tapeworm of man (*Dibothriocephalus latus*).

Brucellosis, or undulant fever—formerly known as Malta fever in man and as infectious abortion or Bang's disease in cattle, goats, and swine—may be transmitted to man by the ingestion of raw milk from infected animals or by direct or indirect contact with aborted fetuses, afterbirths, and other discharges that are released during or following abortion in animals. Abattoir workers occasionally contract the disease while slaughtering infected animals. Control measures include (1) the compulsory pasteurization of all milk and milk products destined for human consumption, (2) the periodic testing and elimination of infected animals, (3) the establishment of resistant herds by vaccination of calves, and (4) the practice of sound sanitary husbandry. Cooking will eliminate the danger of contracting the disease through the consumption of meat. Nationwide calf immunization has greatly reduced the incidence of this disease.

Bovine tuberculosis has been virtually eliminated in this country; nevertheless, it still exists and serves as a potential threat. In other parts of the world it remains a serious economic and public health problem. It was discussed in greater detail in Art. 1-13.

Q fever is a disease of recent discovery, having been first recognized during the mid-thirties in Australia. Of the domestic animals, cattle, sheep, and goats are the principal reservoirs. The infection in domestic animals is entirely asymptomatic. The organism is discharged in the milk and also with the birth fluids and membranes during parturition. Human infection occurs primarily from the inhalation of rickettsia-laden particles that contaminate the environment of cattle lots, meat-packing and meat-rendering plants, and wool-processing factories. Raw milk likewise may serve as a mode of transmission. Although several species of ticks have been found naturally infected, they are not considered important in the transmission of this disease. A control measure is pasteurization of milk products. Vaccination measures are available for persons in hazardous occupations and for controlling the disease in animals.

Anthrax, the so-called "wool sorter's disease," occurs among textile- and wool-factory workers and among agricultural people. It is primarily a disease of cattle and horses. Man may be infected through skin abrasions, the lungs, or the intestinal tract. Control measures consist of isolation and treatment of infected animals. Carcasses of infected animals should be incinerated or buried deeply with quicklime. The control of waste effluents from industries concerned with processing animals or animal products and the education of the employees of these establishments are also indicated. The disinfection, by steaming, of animal hair used for brushes—particularly shaving brushes—is required by the Public Health Service. The individual may disinfect his own brush by soaking it, with frequent agitation, for a period of 4 hr in a 10 per cent solution of formalin at 110°F.

Leptospirosis, also known as Weil's disease or hemorrhagic jaundice, occurs among rats, other rodents, dogs, swine, cattle, and occasionally other animals. Presumably, human cases result from penetration of abraded skin or mucous membrane or possibly through the ingestion of water which has been contaminated with urine of animals. Avoidance of swimming or wading in water holes to which animals have access is an indicated preventive measure.

Salmonellosis is caused by the *Salmonella* group of bacteria. Poultry and meat products frequently become contaminated with *Salmonella* organisms from the contents of the intestinal tracts of the birds and animals when the processing or slaughtering operations are done in a careless or an insanitary manner. Pastries contaminated by rodent feces or possibly through the medium of cockroaches are also implicated. Such *Salmonella*-contaminated products can cause a serious form of food poisoning or diarrhea if they are not adequately cooked. Control measures include prevention of contamination of the carcass by fecal material, protection of prepared foods from insects and rodents, and education of the public in the hygienic values of cooking poultry and meat products thoroughly.

Tularemia is usually contracted by man from rabbits, opossums, rodents, quail, and other game animals. The infection occurs during skinning or dressing and enters through a skin abrasion. The disease, though of long duration, is rarely fatal. Sick or sluggish animals, since they may be infected, should be avoided by hunters. This disease is also transmitted by certain biting insects and ticks and by ingesting insufficiently cooked rabbit and drinking contaminated water.

Rabies is an acute fatal encephalitis caused by a specific virus. Reservoirs of this virus include any of a large group of wild and domestic mammals. The incubation period of rabies in man varies from 2 to 6 weeks or longer, and this variation depends on the severity of the laceration, the relationship of the bite wound to richly supplied nerve areas, and the length of the nerve path from the bite wound to the brain. Bites on the head and face are particularly dangerous because of the richness of the nerve supply to these areas and the short distance from them to the brain. Rabies is most frequently observed in dogs; however, infections in cats, cattle, horses, other domestic animals, and many species of wild animals, such as skunks and foxes, are also very common. Rabid dogs are the source of most human infection. Transmission occurs through the entrance of virus-laden saliva into lesions or open wounds, which are generally caused by the bite of the rabid animal.

When there is ample evidence to suspect that a person has been bitten by a rabid animal, the Pasteur treatment is indicated. This consists of a regimen of 14 consecutive daily doses of the rabies vaccine. There is a slight chance that postvaccinal encephalitis may occur when using this nerve-tissue vaccine, and consequently the need for vaccination must be critically evaluated.

Maximum protection is probably not imparted with this vaccine until 3 to 4 weeks after treatment is begun. For this reason, in the case of short-incubation face and head bites, it is imperative that the treatment be started as soon as possible after exposure. Hyperimmune antirabies serum can be used to supplement the vaccine. Immediate protection is provided by serum; however, it is of short duration. Antirabies serum in conjunction with vaccination is of particular value in severe exposures such as occur in head and face bites.

Infected bats have been found in certain locations. These include yellow bats (insectivorous) in Florida, Mexican freetail bats in Texas (also insectivorous), and vampire bats in Mexico and Venezuela. The vampire bats are not likely to be found north of the 30° parallel of latitude, and no instances of transmission of rabies from bats to humans are known.

An animal that has bitten a person should be caught, if possible, and confined for observation by a veterinarian for 10 days. If at the end of this interval the animal has shown no signs or symptoms of rabies and is still alive, there is no reason to suspect that the bitten individual has been exposed to rabies virus. Should the animal show signs or symptoms of rabies or die during this interval, vaccination of the bitten person should be initiated, and laboratory confirmation of rabies in the animal should be sought. Other animals known to be exposed to rabies should be either treated and held in quarantine for not less than 60 days, and preferably longer, or destroyed. When laboratory confirmation is desired, the head should be removed, packed in a watertight container, iced, and expressed to the laboratory. Pertinent information relative to the reason for shipping the specimen should accompany the specimen to the laboratory.

The successful control of rabies is based upon the application of three essential principles:

1. Impoundage and disposal of all stray and ownerless dogs.
2. Annual antirabies vaccination of all claimed dogs. However, if phenolized vaccine (an attenuated live rabies as grown in chick embryos) is used, an immunity for 3 years is secured.
3. Reduction of a wildlife population, i.e., foxes, skunks, etc., when that population is serving as a reservoir of rabies.

Rabies is best controlled at the local health levels because it is here that the enforcement of a program is carried out. The adoption of local ordinances which in some way encompass the three broad principles stated above is the key to effective rabies control. It must be remembered that no matter how well a program of control is drafted, it does not have its desired effect unless a well-planned educational program goes along with it.

Ornithosis (psittacosis), also called "parrot fever," is a virus disease of parrots, parakeets, canaries, pigeons, and numerous other species of birds, including some of our domestic fowl—chickens, ducks, and turkeys. The disease is transmitted to man through direct contact with infected birds. Several outbreaks of ornithosis have occurred among poultry-plant workers who had processed infected turkeys. The inhalation of dispersed infectious particles appears to be the principal method of transmission. Man-to-man transmission is rare. Antibiotics are highly effective in the treatment of ornithosis, but prior to their use the mortality rate was fairly high. Control is directed primarily at strict regulation of import of, or traffic in, birds of the parrot family, based on quarantine and laboratory examination. Contact with visibly sick birds should be avoided. Apparently healthy birds have occasionally spread the disease. Banding of psittacine birds should be encouraged so that birds suspected as a source of human ornithosis may be traced to their origin. Large doses of antibiotics will suppress but will not eliminate aviary infection.

Arthropod-borne viral II encephalitis is recognized in three distinct types of mosquito-borne disease in the United States. These are Western and Eastern equine encephalomyelitis and St. Louis encephalitis. Various species of wild and domestic birds have been identified as the basic reservoirs of these viruses. Certain species of mosquitoes are responsible for transmitting the disease from birds to horses and to man. Horses are not considered to be natural reservoirs of the Western and Eastern viruses but are merely terminal, end-chain victims to these agents, as man is. Control is achieved by continuous, effective mosquito-abatement programs. Vaccines are being used with success in preventing the disease in horses.

Foot-and-mouth disease is caused by a virus to which all cloven-hoofed animals are susceptible, although cattle are more commonly infected. The disease is transmitted to man through milk or milk products and possibly by the hands. It is rarely fatal to man. It is controlled through quarantine, isolation, and the slaughtering and burning of infected animals

Ringworm is a general term used to describe mycotic or fungal infection of keratinized parts of the body (skin, hair, and nails). Children of prepuberty age are highly susceptible to the ringworm (*Microsporum canis*) of cats and dogs. Adults are highly resistant to *Microsporum* species, but all ages are susceptible to *Trichophyton mentagrophytes* and *T. verrueosum*, which commonly infect cattle and horses. Control primarily involves public education, pointing out the danger of permitting ringworm infection in pets and domestic animals to continue untreated. When animals are suspected as the source of human infection, they should be located and subjected to treatment. Ringworm infections are a serious problem in that they are exceedingly difficult to treat.

Trichinosis is caused by the larva of a parasitic nematode infecting man and animal hosts. The principal source of infection among humans is the meat of infected animals, particularly pork and occasionally wild game. Swine and many wild animals, including rats, are reservoirs of infection. Trichinosis occurs throughout the world except among the native populations of the tropics, where swine are fed on root vegetables and ordinarily do not gain access to the flesh of animals. Control involves meat inspection, education of raisers in methods of hog production that minimize trichinosis infection, elimination of feeding uncooked garbage and offal to swine, and thorough cooking of fresh pork and pork products. See Art. 7-3.

Taeniasis, or beef- or pork-tapeworm infection, involves various animal hosts. The common varieties that occur in man result from ingestion of infected beef, pork, and fish. See Art. 7-3. Eggs of the worm are discharged in the feces of the infected person. Transmission also occurs through direct hand-to-mouth transfer of the eggs and feces. The disease is prevalent wherever beef or pork is eaten raw or only slightly cooked. Control consists in proper sewage disposal, thorough cooking of beef and pork, and immediate treatment of human beings. Meat inspection is of little value.

Diphyllobothriasis, or fish-tapeworm infection, has as its source the flesh of infected freshwater fish. See Art. 7-3. The feces of infected persons contain eggs, and the eggs must reach bodies of fresh water in order to hatch and infect the first intermediate host, copepods, which are small crustacea. The latter are eaten by susceptible fish, which in turn become the second intermediate hosts. This disease is endemic in many parts of Europe and Asia; in the Great Lakes region, eastern Canada, Alaska, and Florida in North America; and in Argentina and Chile in South America. Prevention and control are accomplished by adequate sewage treatment and by thoroughly cooking fish or freezing it for 24 hr at minus 10°C.

Echinococcosis, or the dog-tapeworm infection, is relatively common in South America, Alaska, eastern Australia, New Zealand, and the Middle East. Infection exists to some extent in Central Europe and parts of Asia. A source of infection is feces containing eggs of the adult worm from dogs and some wild animals. The disease is transmitted through ingestion of contaminated food and water as well as through hand-to-mouth transfer of eggs. Prevention lies in the control of slaughtering processes so that dogs do not have access to meat, the licensing and periodic examination of dogs, the incineration of dead animals, and the education of the public in the possibility of infection through close association with dogs.

1-16. Miscellaneous Diseases. Venereal diseases are transmitted by direct contact. Blindness in newborn infants may be due to gonorrheal infection, and many states require preventive treatment against this variety of blindness by the attending physician. Proper treatment is always successful.

Trachoma is a communicable disease of the eyes which may be transmitted by towels, handkerchiefs, or fingers.

Leprosy, called Hansen's disease, is caused by a bacillus, *Mycobacterium leprae*. It affects chiefly the skin, mucous membrane, and peripheral nerves. Comparatively little is known about transmission of the disease. Direct personal contact, with invasion by the bacillus of the skin or of the mucous membrane of the upper respiratory tract, is likely to be the usual route. The disease occurs predominantly in the warm climates of China, India, central Africa, Indonesia, Japan, and some Latin-American republics. Though a far less important problem in the United States, the disease has been reported in Southern California, Florida, Louisiana, and southern Texas. Treatment with sulfone drugs arrests the disease much more rapidly and in a larger proportion of patients than older forms of treatment do, but it is still a process which requires many years. The patient is considered infectious until the arrested stage is achieved. Adequate housing and cleanliness can greatly hamper the spread of this particular disease. In the United States the disease is controlled by treating volunteer patients at the Carville Sanitorium in Carville, La.

General Methods of Communicable Disease Control

1-17. Immunization. Immunity is the power of living beings to resist infection. It varies in degree not only among persons but also in the same person from time to time, depending upon his physical condition. It may be natural or acquired. Certain diseases give immunity against a second attack, and immunity can also be artificially obtained by the introduction of a serum, toxin, vaccine, or virus. An outstanding example of the conferring of artificial immunity is the vaccination for smallpox. In this connection it should be noted that smallpox, as the result of virtually complete vaccination a generation ago, is showing a very low incidence rate. The absence of smallpox epidemics, however, has sometimes had the unfortunate effect of breeding contempt for the disease, with the result that vaccination may be neglected. Other diseases for which artificial immunization may be given are typhoid, paratyphoid, diphtheria, measles, rabies, polio, influenza, and tetanus.

Prompt immunization of contacts is required by active city and county health departments in all cases of communicable diseases where immunization treatment is available. This is an important epidemic measure.

1-18. Quarantine and Isolation. Quarantine has been applied since medieval times in Venice and elsewhere. It gets its name from the Italian word *quaranta*, meaning "forty," the number of days that suspected vessels were held in quarantine before being allowed to land goods or passengers. Maritime quarantine at ports of the United States is always administered by the Public Health Service. It applies to cholera, plague, louse-borne relapsing fever, smallpox, louse-borne typhus fever, yellow fever, and ornithosis. Upon arrival in United States ports, lepers who are United States citizens are sent to the leprosarium in Carville, La. Persons with diseases other than those named are allowed to enter, and the regulations of the local authorities are applied to them. Quarantine in areas other than ports is no longer considered effective, and in the United

States it is applied only to smallpox by state, city, and county authorities. Contacts may be released from quarantine after their immunity has been established.

Isolation, as the term implies, involves the segregation of the patient. The degree of isolation depends upon the nature of the disease. For the most readily communicable diseases, such as smallpox and measles, strict isolation should be applied. This requires separate rooms for patients. In some cases of scarlet fever and diphtheria, strict isolation is indicated. For yellow fever and dengue, covering the bed of the patient with a mosquito netting is sufficient isolation. In general, isolation is most easily obtained in hospitals. For safety in homes, careful and, preferably, trained attendants are required.

1-19. Control of Epidemics. This is one of the most important functions of health departments. Investigations and epidemic measures are carried out by the division of communicable disease, in some cases with the cooperation of the division of sanitation. In any event, for effective work a responsible head must be provided, with undivided authority and legal backing.

The essentials in the prevention and control of epidemics may be summarized as follows:

1. Prompt notification to the health department of all communicable disease by the attending physician.

2. Analysis and investigation of reports by the health officials. This may include the preparation of graphs and spot maps showing where cases occurred and the time of occurrence and the compilation of concise epidemiological histories.

3. Prompt hospitalization and isolation where necessary. Public health nurses should be available to give instructions as to isolation and disinfection in the home.

4. Immunization of contacts where practical and effective.

5. Laboratory work directed toward verification of diagnosis, establishment of cure for release from isolation, detection of carriers, and tests of suspected water or milk, especially in gastroenteric diseases.

6. Special investigations by the division of sanitation in regard to food and water supplies and the application of emergency measures.

Bibliography

1. "The Control of Communicable Disease," 9th ed., American Public Health Association, New York, 1960.
2. Herms, William B.: "Medical Entomology," The Macmillan Company, New York, 1939.
3. Rosenau, M. J.: "Preventive Medicine and Hygiene," 8th ed., by Kenneth F. Maxcy, Appleton-Century-Crofts, Inc., New York, 1956.
4. Hilleboe, H. E., and G. W. Larimore (eds.): "Preventive Medicine," W. B. Saunders Company, Philadelphia, 1959.

2

WATER: GENERAL CHARACTERISTICS, TREATMENT, AND PROTECTION

2-1. Practically all the water that appears in public or private supplies has been exposed to pollution while falling as rain, running over the ground surface or in streams, or percolating through the soil. The growth of population in most areas of the United States and the increasing use of streams and other bodies of surface water for the disposal of wastes have been detrimental to water supplies, particularly to surface supplies and to a lesser extent to ground waters. There is increasing concern about water supplies since the amount available in any area is fixed by rainfall, geology, topography, and geographical boundaries. In some areas the demand for unpolluted sources has become competitive, and the problems have been intensified by the use of synthetic organic chemicals in household cleansers and in agriculture.

2-2. **Underground Water.** The hydrologic cycle has three phases: precipitation, runoff, and evapotranspiration. Precipitation includes rain, hail, and snow and is the primary source of water. Of the precipitation, some evaporates, and some percolates into the soil immediately or after a snow melt or after running some distance on the ground surface. Most of the runoff becomes surface water in streams or lakes, finally to enter the ocean. Somewhere in its passage, evaporation will replace some of it in the atmosphere, from which it will again be precipitated.

The water which percolates into the soil passes through a zone of aeration to a zone of saturation and then somewhat laterally to a discharge point or outlet. From the zone of aeration, plants absorb water which they use and thereafter discharge most of it into the air by the process known as transpiration. The upper surface of the zone of saturation if unconfined by an impervious formation becomes the "water table" and can be referred to in terms of elevation. In the zone of saturation, movement is controlled by gravity and will usually be toward a valley bottom, following roughly the ground surface, with the outlet being the stream in the valley or springs on the hillside. Wherever the water table outcrops at the ground surface, water will appear as a spring, pond, swamp, or stream. Flow from springs or from the banks or bottom of the river into the river itself is the dry-weather flow of that stream. If the riverbed is of sand or gravel, there may be a well-defined water flow beneath the surface stream and in the same direction. In many cases the undersurface flow is present after a stream has dried. These conditions are shown in Fig. 2-1. When a well is drilled into such a formation, the water will rise into it to the elevation of the water table. Such a well is sometimes called a water-table or shallow well.

The water table tends to fluctuate with rainfall or recharge and with water withdrawal from wells and springs or otherwise. Water tables usually assume a slope or grade. Normally this shallow water has traveled a relatively short distance.

In some areas there are strata of pervious materials which outcrop at the ground surface or just under the surface soil and then dip at some angle below the surface, becoming deeper with distance from the outcrop. Where such a geologic formation, or stratum, has other strata above and below it which are impervious, a water-carrying formation, or aquifer, results. It might be considered an underground reservoir through

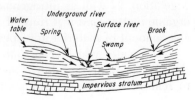

FIGURE 2-1   How the ground-water surface or water table follows the contour of the land.

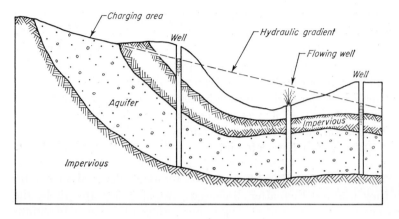

FIGURE 2-2   Flowing and nonflowing artesian wells.

which water slowly moves toward some outlet, which might be at a great distance, possibly even under the sea. When a well is drilled into such a stratum, the water rises above the top of the aquifer; this is known as an artesian well. If the water rises above the ground surface, it is a flowing artesian well. (See Fig. 2-2.)

If a number of wells are drilled into an artesian aquifer, it will be noted that the rise of water in them will be to variable heights. If a line is drawn through the water heights as shown in Fig. 2-2, the hydraulic gradient will be established, and flow in the aquifer will be down the slope of the gradient. In water-table wells the slope of the water table is the hydraulic gradient. Waters of artesian wells have traveled long distances and have had more opportunity to dissolve mineral impurities. Movement of water through soils is rather slow. In sand with a hydraulic gradient or water-table slope of a few feet per mile, the rate of movement might be only a few inches per day. This will vary directly with the degree of slope. In gravels, velocities of 30 to 400 ft/day have been noted depending upon their permeability and the slope of the hydraulic gradient.

2-3. Impurities of Water. Pure water is not found in nature. As rain or snow falls toward the earth, it absorbs dust and such gases as carbon dioxide and oxygen. After reaching the ground surface, it is exposed to pollution by organic matter, including human excreta in populated areas. At the ground surface the water absorbs more carbon dioxide from vegetation, as well as nitrogenous and other material from decomposed organic matter, and if it runs off into a stream it takes with it a considerable amount of material in suspension, such as silt, clay, and sand.

The water which seeps into the ground is filtered as it proceeds to the zone of saturation, but it may or may not receive sufficient filtration to remove impurities. As it percolates through soil or rock, it dissolves

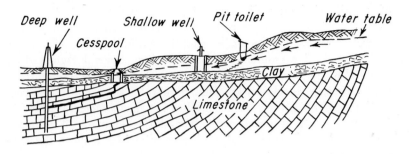

FIGURE 2-3   How pollution may enter wells through soil pollution and by means of fissures in limestone.

and carries with it various minerals, the amount depending upon the distance of percolation and the mineral composition of its environment. As percolation continues, the original suspended impurities, including microorganisms, tend to disappear, until the water which is obtained from deep wells may be expected to be free from all impurities except those dissolved.

To summarize, the common impurities of water can be listed as follows:

1. Entrained gases: carbon dioxide, hydrogen sulfide, methane, oxygen, and nitrogenous and organic compounds

2. Dissolved minerals: calcium, magnesium, sodium, iron, and manganese and their carbonates, bicarbonates, hydroxides, chlorides, sulfates, fluorides, nitrates, and silicates; alkyl benzene sulfonate from detergents; and synthetic organics from insecticides and pesticides

3. Suspended and colloidal materials: bacteria, algae, fungi, protozoa, silt, and colloidal matter causing water to be acid or have color

4. Radioactive materials: radioactivity imparted by contact with radiation sources, by entrainment of radioactive substances from mining or processing of ores, or by wastes from industrial use of radioactivity

The type of treatment facilities needed to render water palatable and satisfactory for its intended uses is determined by the types of impurities present and their concentrations.

2-4. Water and Disease. The most important of the waterborne diseases are those of the intestinal tract; they include typhoid fever, the paratyphoids, dysentery, infectious hepatitis, and cholera. A few parasitic worms may also be disseminated by water. All are due to organisms which are found in the intestinal discharges of patients or carriers and which have found their way into water by some means.

Public health literature records many waterborne typhoid fever epidemics caused by the entrance of intestinal discharges from persons having typhoid fever or from carriers of the disease into surface sources of supply, shallow wells, or springs and wells penetrating limestone formations. This disease was once common, particularly in urban areas where untreated surface-water supplies or individual wells were used without regard to sources of contamination. Several factors have contributed to the decline in the incidence of typhoid fever and other waterborne diseases. Increased knowledge of water treatment and recognition of the need for protection of supplies are major factors. Others include improved waste disposal methods and development of immunization techniques and their application during epidemics or when the sources of water become suspect.

Sanitation of water supplies can never be neglected without unfortunate consequences. Waterborne epidemics of typhoid fever and, more commonly, of dysentery and gastroenteritis are still occasionally reported. The recognition of waterborne cases of infectious hepatitis in recent years may imply that there are many unrecognized cases.

Certain minerals in drinking water, because of their known hazardous properties, are considered undesirable if present beyond prescribed limits of concentration. Among these are arsenic, barium, cadmium, chromium, lead, selenium, and silver. Anionic constituents in the same category include fluoride, chloride, sulfate, cyanide, and nitrate. Of course, there are other harmful inorganic chemicals, but the foregoing include only those having any likelihood of being present in water either naturally or through artificial measures. Article 2-9 discusses limiting concentrations.

Among minerals not naturally occurring in water and likely to be present through artificial means is lead. Lead pipe is still in use to some extent. It should not be used for the distribution of soft, acid water or for water having a high concentration of dissolved oxygen or chlorides. The solution of lead in a water with such characteristics may cause lead poisoning. Copper and iron are also used in water systems, and some dissolving of the metals occurs, the degree of solution depending on the concentrations of free or dissolved oxygen or carbon dioxide, the concentrations of free mineral acids and acid salts such as alum, and also water temperature and velocity of flow. They are not considered hazardous.

In many areas, ground water contains fluorides in concentrations sufficient to cause dental fluorosis, or mottled enamel, which affects only children up to eight or nine years of age, after which little or no damage is done. Paradoxically, the presence of some fluorides in drinking water is beneficial to teeth, not only during the period of tooth formation but to some extent afterward. The optimum fluoride level varies because the amount of water drunk by children depends mostly on air temperature. The recommended limits are given in Art. 2-9.

To avoid fluorosis in areas with excessive fluorides, children within susceptible age limits should be given bottled water of low fluoride content or water from the household supply diluted to the proper fluoride concentration with fluoride-free bottled water. This water should also be used in preparing their food.

Individual household units for fluoride removal are available. These involve contact media, such as bone char, tricalcium phosphate, or activated alumina, which are replaced with new media when the unit is no longer effective in the removal of fluorides. Removal of fluorides or controlled defluoridation to optimal concentration has been demonstrated as practical on a municipal treatment-plant scale. The defluoridating agent is activated alumina.

The consumption of water having a high nitrate-nitrogen content or of milk formulas using such water is reported to be the cause of "blue babies," a condition known as "idiopathic" methemoglobinemia and sometimes causing death of infants. The nitrates are reduced to nitrites in the digestive system, and these enter the bloodstream to unite with the red blood cells, resulting in interference with the oxygen-carrying capacity of the blood. The disease is restricted to infants because their stomach pH is higher than that of adults, thus permitting the growth of nitrate-reducing bacteria in the upper gastrointestinal tract. A nitrate-nitrogen concentration of 10 mg/l (milligrams per liter), or 45 mg/l as nitrate, has been suggested as a safe upper limit.

Highly mineralized water, especially that which has a high sulfate content (in excess of 250 mg/l theoretically combined with magnesium ions), may cause temporary diarrhea or other disorders of the alimentary tract in persons not accustomed to the water.

The increasing use of synthetic organic compounds for household and agricultural purposes—compounds not found in nature and employed as insecticides, herbicides, and detergents—is a matter of concern with respect to water quality. Little is known regarding the possible toxic effects of ingestion of small amounts of these substances over prolonged periods. Minimizing their entry into water supplies, however, appears to be a desirable public health measure.

With respect to detergents, most research has been concentrated on the removal of an ingredient present in most of the household detergents in current use, alkyl benzene sulfonate (ABS). This is one of the "wetting" or "surface-active" agents, often termed "surfactants." ABS is not considered to be toxic in the concentrations likely to be found in contaminated water or even sewage. However, 1.0 mg/l or more will cause foaming and may impart undesirable tastes. The taste problem is not considered to be from the ABS itself, but from the degradation of products of other wastes which may be present with the surfactant. The importance of ABS as a contaminant is that it is remarkably stable and is not readily broken down chemically by biological agents that carry out the nitrogen and carbon cycles of decay (Art. 4-4). Thus the presence of ABS in water is an indication of contamination by wastes, and as an indicator it is readily discernible. Whether the water contains microorganisms or biodegradable waste products depends on how recently the contamination occurred.

It was feared by some that the presence of a wetting agent in sewage might allow bacteria to move through sand formations more freely, thus destroying this natural barrier to ground-water contamination or reducing the efficiency of filtration in water treatment plants. A study made by the Robert A. Taft Sanitary Engineering Center of the Public Health Service, however, showed that the rate of migration of bacteria when mixed with 10 mg/l ABS solution through a water-saturated sand column was no greater than the rate of migration through a similar sand column containing no ABS.

2-5. Chemical Examination of Water. A chemical analysis of water indicates its history from its origin as rainfall to the point of collection. In its travels through the atmosphere, on the ground surface, and underground, it will have the opportunity to dissolve or otherwise acquire the dissolved-mineral impurities mentioned in Art. 2-3.

During the early stages of water-supply development, considerable attention was directed to the collection of chemical data, such as the chloride concentration and the presence of the nitrogen-cycle products cited in the preceding article. Analysis for these constituents was classified as a "sanitary chemical analysis" to obtain an indication of the sanitary quality of the water. Today this type of analysis is used primarily to appraise the efficiency of waste treatment facilities and is made in conjunction with routine sewage or industrial-waste analysis. It also includes tests for suspended solids, biochemical oxygen demand, oxygen consumed, ABS, nitrates, and hydrogen sulfide. In some instances, however, these data together with quantitative bacteriological examinations (most probable number) are used in appraising the sanitary aspects of surface-water sources subject to development for potable water supplies.

The routine chemical analysis made on developed water sources is usually to determine the acceptability of the water for drinking and household purposes, boiler use, manufacture of ice, preparation of beverages and foodstuffs, manufacture of paper, dyeing of textiles, and other industrial usages. The results of these analyses also show what corrective treatment should be considered to reduce soap consumption, improve boiler operation, minimize corrosion, prevent "red-water" troubles, adjust treatment processes at the plant, and solve special problems. All analysis results are expressed in terms of milligrams of indicated substance per liter of water,[1] with the exception of pH, which

---

[1] The term "parts per million by weight" has been used, but "milligrams per liter" (which, as far as water and sewage is concerned, also means parts per million) is considered a more desirable term. This is because some industrial wastes have specific gravities considerably greater than that of water.

is given as a number between 1 and 14 with a decimal fraction thereof. For example, water having a pH of 7.0 is neutral, neither acid nor basic, whereas a pH of less than 7.0 shows water to be acid, and a pH of more than 7.0 shows water to be basic or alkaline.

In collecting samples of water for chemical analysis, of either the routine or the sanitary type, a clean gallon glass container should be used. The cap or stopper should not be subject to corrosion. After thorough cleaning, the container should be rinsed with the water to be analyzed, and the water collected should be representative of the water normally available, unless special considerations are involved. All samples should be identified to show location of water-sample source, name of person collecting, purpose of the analysis, source of supply (well, spring, lake, stream, pond, etc.), point in system from which sample was collected (at well-pump discharge, prior to treatment, distribution-system tap, etc.), date of sample collection, and name and address of individual to whom the report is to be sent. If the sample is collected from a well, the type and depth of the well should be given, and the water level, whether low, normal, or high, should be stated. A comment might also be made as to the physical appearance of the water during normal conditions.

2-6. **Bacteriological Examinations.** Several types of determinations are available to the bacteriologist in evaluating the sanitary status of a water. From a public health standpoint, it is necessary to determine whether the water for drinking and household purposes is contaminated or safe. If only such information is desired, the routine examination is made to learn whether the laboratory test shows the presence or absence of *coliform organisms,* harmless bacteria which are used as indicator organisms.[1] The coliform organisms are found in sewage since they have their origin in the intestinal tract of humans and other warm-blooded animals. See Art. 4-4. They are also found in soil and in water which has been subjected to pollution by dust, insects, birds, small animals, or surface drainage or which has been contaminated during construction of new, or rehabilitation of old, water facilities. Since the primary purpose of the "qualitative test" is to prove the effects of past contamination and the effects of pollutional hazards, the general opinion is that water samples for this examination should be secured only from supplies which are protected adequately from contamination. Also, since the water is exposed to contamination during the construction or rehabilitation program, samples from new or repaired wells should not be submitted for bacteriological examination until the wells have been fully developed and disinfected with chlorine in an approved manner. Likewise, when new pumping equipment is installed or the existing equipment is withdrawn from the well for repairs, a similar procedure should be followed.

[1] There is no easily applicable method of demonstrating the presence or absence of pathogenic microorganisms in water.

Quantitative tests estimating the density of coliform organisms may be made. These are useful in determining the extent of water treatment facilities necessary to render unprotected ground water and surface water safe for human consumption, in establishing the sanitary status of water for oyster production and recreational purposes, and in measuring the effects of the discharge of putrescible wastes into streams, lakes, or coastal waters. By applying the test for coliform organisms to quantities of the sample varying in geometric series (0.01, 0.1, 1.0, 10.0, and 100 ml), it is possible to make a statistical estimate—the "most probable number" (MPN)—of coliform organisms per 100 ml of water from tables or from calculations [3].

2-7. Methods of Bacteriological Examination. An understanding of the method of bacteriological examination of water is of value to the sanitarian, although he may not be required to do more than interpret the reports of the tests. Methods and interpretations are given in "Standard Methods for the Examination of Water and Wastewater" [3].

A test which is made at many water treatment plants but which is not considered in the Public Health Service Drinking Water Standards [1] is that for determining the "total count," or "plate count," of bacteria per milliliter. Actually, this test determines merely the increase in number of bacteria under the test conditions. It consists in placing a small amount of the sample, 1 ml or less, in a sterilized petri dish containing a film of agar and incubating it at 20 or 35°C for 24 hr. Individual bacteria will increase in numbers to form visible colonies on the agar, and counting the colonies gives the total count. It will differ for 20 and 35°C. Total counts are usually reduced as water passes through the treatment processes.

Two methods are used for determining the presence of coliform organisms: the multiple-tube fermentation technique and the membrane-filter technique. In the fermentation technique, advantage is taken of the faculty of coliform organisms of fermenting lactose, the fermentation being indicated by formation of gas trapped in small inverted tubes placed in larger test tubes. A mixture of lactose broth and beef broth is placed in the larger tube, which contains the smaller tube, and this is placed in an autoclave for sterilization. After sterilization and cooling of the tubes and liquid media, 10 ml of the water sample is placed, by means of sterilized pipettes, into each of the five tubes containing the media. In some instances, 100-ml samples of water are treated in lieu of 10-ml samples. The tubes containing the desired portions of the sample are placed in an incubator for 24 hr at 35°C. At the end of the 24-hr period of incubation, the number of tubes showing the presence of gas is recorded, and a loopful of the media in one of the tubes showing gas is transferred to a sterilized tube containing 2 per cent brilliant green bile lactose broth to determine whether the gas production was due to coliform organisms or to certain sporeformers, which also have the ability to ferment lactose.

The lactose tubes which did not show production of gas at the end of 24 hr are left in the incubator for an additional 24 hr to allow more time for the slow lactose fermenters to grow and produce gas. If, at the end of 48 hr, gas is present in the tubes which did not show gas at the end of 24 hr, transfers are made from them to a brilliant green bile liquid confirmation medium, as was done at the end of the first 24-hr period of incubation. After 24 and 48 hr of incubation, results of the tests with the brilliant green bile lactose are recorded. The formation of gas under these conditions constitutes a "confirmed test." A few nonfecal organisms will show positive in the confirmed tests, and accordingly techniques are available for a "completed test" for absolute evidence of the presence of coliform organisms. They are elaborate and are not used in routine bacterial analyses of drinking water.

In the membrane-filter technique, definite quantities of water (50, 100, 200, or 500 ml) are filtered through a thin cellulose sheet of uniform porosity, impregnated with endo broth. Coliform organisms develop as colonies, as on agar plates, within 18 to 20 hr of incubation. This technique produces results in a much shorter time than the multiple-tube fermentation test, which requires 2 to 4 days. It is also adapted to field testing with the use of portable kits that are commercially available. It

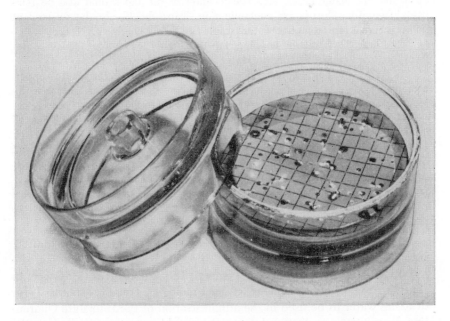

FIGURE 2-4 Membrane-filter technique. Coliform colonies are shown on the filter surface. Top of dish is removed. (*Courtesy of Millipore Filter Corp.*)

is of special value in disaster sanitation measures where large numbers of samples and prompt results may be required.

The number of tubes showing positive results in the multiple-tube fermentation test or the number of colonies in the membrane-filter test and the presence of coliform organisms are indicated on the analysis report. This information is used in computing compliance or noncompliance with the Public Health Service Drinking Water Standards, as outlined in Art. 2-9. A sample-analysis report card may show the absence of coliform organisms, or it may show that coliform organisms were found in one to five of the 10-ml portions tested for each sample. From a public health standpoint, however, any indication of contamination or the presence of coliform organisms should be sufficient to warrant immediate correction to remove existing sources of contamination and to safeguard the water from subsequent contamination.

2-8. Collection of Samples for Bacteriological Analyses. Unless the sample is collected in a sterile bottle and every precaution is taken to prevent accidental contamination of the sample during its collection, the results of the bacteriological examination are meaningless. The following procedures should be meticulously observed:

1. Select a sampling tap which is in such a condition that leaking of water around the turn key does not occur. The sampling tap should preferably be one of the nonwasher type, and the outlet should not have threads for connection of water hoses, etc. The location of the tap should also be relatively free from dust-borne contamination. Taps should also be selected at points where a representative water sample can be obtained.

2. Flush the faucet or sampling tap thoroughly to remove stagnant water from the supply line, allowing the water to run for at least ½ min.

3. While the bottle is being filled, hold the cap through the hood wrapper, usually provided by the laboratory. Do not allow the fingers or any other object to come in contact with either the cap or the lip of the bottle.

4. Complete the sample-identification-analysis report card, giving all information requested by the laboratory performing the examination.

5. Examine samples as soon as possible after collection. If possible and practicable, keep the samples at 0 to 10°C until they are examined. Any deviation from the temperature requirement should be stated in the record of examination. If the water to be tested has a chlorine or chloramine residual present, sterilized bottles containing sodium thiosulfate should be used to neutralize it at the time of collection.

2-9. Public Health Service Drinking Water Standards. On Jan. 22, 1913, the Secretary of the Treasury appointed a commission upon the recommendation of the Surgeon General, U.S. Public Health Service, to consider the establishment of a bacteriological quality standard for drinking water to be used in the administration of the Interstate Quarantine Regulations as they relate to the drinking water supplied to the public by common carriers operating in interstate commerce. On Oct. 21, 1914, the Treasury Department adopted the standards recommended by the commission. The original standards were revised in 1925, 1942, 1946, 1956, and 1962. They have been accepted by the American Water Works Association and also by the state departments of health.

The laboratory procedures to be followed in making the analyses for contaminants listed in the standards are those prescribed in the latest edition of "Standard Methods for the Examination of Water and Wastewater" [3].

The 1962 standards of water quality, in terms of bacteriological and chemical analysis, are as follows:

BACTERIOLOGICAL QUALITY

3.2. *Limits.* The presence of organisms of the coliform group as indicated by samples examined shall not exceed the following limits:

3.21. When 10-ml. standard portions are examined, not more than 10 per cent in any month shall show the presence of the coliform group. The presence of the coliform group in three or more 10-ml. portions of a standard sample shall not be allowable if this occurs:

(*a*) In two consecutive samples;

(*b*) In more than one sample per month when less than 20 are examined per month; or

(*c*) In more than five per cent of the samples when 20 or more are examined per month.

When organisms of the coliform group occur in three or more of the 10-ml. portions of a single standard sample, daily samples from the same sampling point shall be collected promptly and examined until the results obtained from at least two consecutive samples show the water to be of satisfactory quality.

3.22. When 100-ml. standard portions are examined, not more than 60 per cent in any month shall show the presence of the coliform group. The presence of the coliform group in all five of the 100-ml. portions of a standard sample shall not be allowable if this occurs:

(*a*) In two consecutive samples;

(*b*) In more than one sample per month when less than five are examined per month; or

(*c*) In more than 20 per cent of the samples when five or more are examined per month.

When organisms of the coliform group occur in all five of the 100-ml. portions of a single standard sample, daily samples from the same sampling point shall be collected promptly and examined until the results obtained from at least two consecutive samples show the water to be of satisfactory quality.

3.23. When the membrane filter technique is used, the arithmetic mean coliform density of all standard samples examined per month shall not exceed one per 100 ml. Coliform colonies per standard sample shall not exceed 3/50 ml., 4/100 ml., 7/200 ml., or 13/500 ml., in:

(*a*) Two consecutive samples;

(*b*) More than one standard sample when less than 20 are examined per month; or (*c*) More than five per cent of the standard samples when 20 or more are examined per month.

When coliform colonies in a single standard sample exceed the above values, daily samples from the same sampling point shall be collected promptly and examined until the results obtained from at least two consecutive samples show the water to be of satisfactory quality.

PHYSICAL CHARACTERISTICS

4.2. *Limits.* Drinking water should contain no impurity which would cause offense to the sense of sight, taste, or smell. Under general use, the following limits should not be exceeded:

Turbidity	5 units
Color	15 units
Threshold Odor Number	3

CHEMICAL CHARACTERISTICS

5.2. *Limits.* Drinking water shall not contain impurities in concentrations which may be hazardous to the health of the consumers. It should not be excessively corrosive to the water system. Substances used in its treatment shall not remain in the water in concentrations greater than required by good practice. Substances which may have deleterious physiological effect, or for which physiological effects are not known, shall not be introduced into the system in a manner which would permit them to reach the consumer.

5.21. The following chemical substances should not be present in a water supply in excess of the listed concentrations where, in the judgment of the Reporting Agency and the Certifying Authority, other more suitable supplies are or can be made available.

Substance	*Concentration in mg/l*
Alkyl Benzene Sulfonate (ABS)	0.5
Arsenic (As).	0.01
Chloride (Cl)	250.
Copper (Cu)	1.
Carbon Chloroform Extract (CCE)	0.2
Cyanide (CN)	0.01
Fluoride (F).	(See 5.23)
Iron (Fe)	0.3
Manganese (Mn)	0.05
Nitrate[1] (NO_3)	45.
Phenols	0.001
Sulfate (SO_4)	250.
Total Dissolved Solids.	500.
Zinc (Zn)	5.

[1] In areas in which the nitrate content of water is in excess of the listed concentration, the public should be warned of the potential dangers of using the water for infant feeding.

5.22. The presence of the following substances in excess of the concentrations listed shall constitute grounds for rejection of the supply:

Substance	Concentration in mg/l
Arsenic (As)	0.05
Barium (Ba)	1.0
Cadmium (Cd)	0.01
Chromium (Hexavalent) (Cr^{+6})	0.05
Cyanide (CN)	0.2
Fluoride (F)	(See 5.23)
Lead (Pb)	0.05
Selenium (Se)	0.01
Silver (Ag)	0.05

5.23. *Fluoride.* When fluoride is naturally present in drinking water, the concentration should not average more than the appropriate upper limit in the table below. Presence of fluoride in average concentrations greater than two times the optimum values in the table shall constitute grounds for rejection of the supply.

Where fluoridation (supplementation of fluoride in drinking water) is practiced, the average fluoride concentration shall be kept within the upper and lower control limits in the table below:

Annual average of maximum daily air temperatures[1]	Recommended control limits— Fluoride concentrations in mg/l		
	Lower	Optimum	Upper
50.0–53.7	0.9	1.2	1.7
53.8–58.3	0.8	1.1	1.5
58.4–63.8	0.8	1.0	1.3
63.9–70.6	0.7	0.9	1.2
70.7–79.2	0.7	0.8	1.0
79.3–90.5	0.6	0.7	0.8

[1] Based on temperature data obtained for a minimum of five years.

6.2. *Radioactivity Limits*

6.21. The effects of human radiation exposure are viewed as harmful and any unnecessary exposure to ionizing radiation should be avoided. Approval of water supplies containing radioactive materials shall be based upon the judgment that the radioactivity intake from such water when added to that from all other sources is not likely to result in an intake greater than the radiation protection guidance recommended by the Federal Radiation Council and approved by the President. Water supplies shall be approved with further consideration of other sources of radioactivity intake of Radium-226 and Strontium-90 when the water contains these substances in amounts not exceeding 3 and 10 $\mu\mu$c/liter,[1] respectively. When these concentrations are exceeded, a water supply shall be approved by the certifying authority if surveillance of total intakes of radioactivity from all sources indicates that such intakes are within the limits recommended by the Federal Radiation Council for control action.

[1] See Art. 17-6 for the definition of this unit.

6.22. In the known absence of Strontium-90 and alpha emitters, the water supply is acceptable when the gross beta concentrations do not exceed 1,000 $\mu\mu$c/liter. Gross beta concentration in excess of 1,000 $\mu\mu$c/liter shall be grounds for rejection of supply except when more complete analyses indicate that concentrations of nuclides are not likely to cause exposure greater than the Radiation Protection Guides as approved by the President on recommendation of the Federal Radiation Council.

2-10. Application of Drinking Water Standards. The Drinking Water Standards have been widely adopted by the states, cities, and other suppliers of water to the public, and time and use have demonstrated the practicability and value of the bacterial requirements.

Strict application of some of the criteria for chemical quality is somewhat difficult in certain areas since water of the recommended mineral content may not be available and the development of more remote sources of water supply or the application of a desalination process may not be practicable from the standpoint of economy.

The standards should be regarded as generally attainable by good water-quality-control practices. In all instances, water made available for public use should not contain toxic materials, and it should be of such chemical quality as to be suitable for the intended beneficial usages.

2-11. Treatment of Water. The development of plant facilities for making contaminated surface water or ground water safe and palatable for municipal and domestic purposes requires the application of the basic sanitary sciences, such as chemistry, bacteriology, biology, limnology, rheology, and sanitary engineering. Preliminary planning of water-treatment-plant works should include a comprehensive study of the catchment area in terms of (1) size, topography, population density, and surface geology; (2) sources of pollution; (3) sewage treatment facilities; (4) raw-water characteristics, including physical, radiological, chemical, bacteriological, and biological characteristics; (5) rainfall and runoff data; (6) evaporation data; (7) anticipated water-supply requirements, minimum, maximum, and average; and (8) other items of importance in providing a safe water supply, adequate in amount for the community in question.

For the purpose of classifying and evaluating raw-water quality with respect to its treatment requirements, the Public Health Service [2] has offered the following criteria:

Group I. *Water Requiring No Treatment:* Underground water without any possibility of contamination.

Group II. *Water Requiring Disinfection Only:* Water from underground and surface sources subject to a low degree of contamination, clear (without turbidity), and having an MPN of coliform organisms not exceeding 50 per 100 ml. in any one month.

Group III. Water Requiring Complete Rapid Sand Filtration Treatment or Its Equivalent, Together With Continuous Chlorination by Pre- and/or Post-chlorination: All waters requiring filtration for turbidity and color removal, having a high or variable chlorine demand, or polluted by sewage so as not to be admissible to Groups I and II; and having an MPN of coliform organisms not more than 5,000 per 100 ml. in 20 per cent of samples examined in any one month.

Group IV. Water Requiring Auxiliary Treatment in Addition to Complete Filtration Treatment and Post-Chlorination: Waters which might require pre-sedimentation or long term storage of 30 days or more with pre-chlorination, and having an MPN more than 5,000 per 100 ml. in more than 20 per cent of samples collected but not more than 20,000 per 100 ml. in more than 5 per cent of samples collected.

Group V. Water Requiring Unusual Treatment Measures: Waters requiring treatment by multiple chlorination or other provisions and not falling into Groups I to IV, but having to be used because of unusual circumstances; and having in no case an MPN exceeding 250,000 per 100 ml.

2-12. Storage and Plain Sedimentation. When surface water is confined in impounding reservoirs or natural lakes, the water undergoes purification by the action of sedimentation, sunlight, and oxidation. As a result of these natural means of purification, suspended matter, or turbidity, is considerably reduced, color is reduced by sunlight, putrescible matter is decomposed and oxidized by biological activity, and bacterial content is reduced. In view of the beneficial results obtained by long-time storage of water, it is advantageous to withdraw water directly from lakes instead of streams, which may receive contamination from the immediate watershed or from the local sources of pollution. Artificial reservoirs will make available raw water of more uniform quality and reduced turbidity, which will facilitate treatment. Presettling tanks or basins, if required or deemed advantageous, should be located or operated so that they will not receive flood waters. There should be at least two, in order to permit continuous operation under all circumstances, and they should be of sufficient capacity to afford a nominal retention period of at least 1 day and preferably 2 or 3 days. Provision should be made for rapid and convenient removal of sludge from the tanks. In the treatment of highly polluted water of variable quality, provision should be made for coagulation at the inlet or the outlet of the tanks whenever measures may be necessary.

2-13. Aeration. Aeration is a process whereby the water is brought into intimate contact with air to improve the quality of potable water. This process is used in an effort to accomplish the following:

1. Removal or reduction of tastes and odors
2. Removal or reduction of gases such as carbon dioxide, methane, and hydrogen sulfide

3. Increase in the pH of water by the removal of carbon dioxide
4. Addition of gases
    a. Oxygen in the removal of iron and manganese
    b. Carbon dioxide after excess lime treatment used to soften water
5. Removal of heat from deep well waters, which are at a higher temperature than desired upon their discharge at the earth's surface

It has been shown by various investigators that the rate of gas absorption by water is influenced most by the films of the gas at the water-gas interface, and it seems reasonable to assume that the greatest influence on the release of gases from water is also affected by these films, especially by the liquid film. The thickness of the films varies under different conditions. They are very thin when first formed and become considerably thicker shortly after formation. Other factors determining efficiency of aeration are the amount of agitation of the water and the agitation within the droplet, which affect film thickness; the maximum agitation being produced by the creation of falling droplets; temperature; solubility and concentration of the gas; vapor pressure of the gas; and barometric pressure.

Aerators may be classified as (1) injection aerators (perforated pipes, diffusers, air-lift pumps, mechanical patented devices), which permit the bubbling of air through water; (2) gravity aerators (inclined planes, cascades, perforated traps); and (3) pressure sprays or fountain aerators (orifices, nozzles).

2-14. Slow Sand Filter. Filtration of water through sand as a means of improving its quality has been used since 1829, when the first filter was built at London to treat Thames River water. This filter was the forerunner of the slow sand type, which was developed in England and was used very largely in the United States until the early part of the twentieth century. While a few cities in the northeastern part of the United States still use slow sand filters, they are gradually being replaced by more modern facilities. The slow sand filter is well adapted for the treatment of slightly turbid water without preliminary coagulation and sedimentation. It does not completely clarify water with a turbidity higher than 50 units except for a very short period of time.

The filters consist of a layer of sand, 2 to 5 ft in depth and of 0.25 to 0.35 ml effective size (Art. 2-17), underlain by gravel. In the gravel are open-jointed pipes to carry off the filtered water to the clear-water reservoir. The water flows through the bed by gravity. The bulk of the suspended matter is caught on the surface and in the first few inches of the bed, and the resulting layer of slimy silt or mud acts as an efficient strainer. Impurities are also removed by what might be considered sedimentation in the minute openings that occur between the grains of sand as the water moves very slowly through the sand bed, the matter taken out being held as a film on the surfaces of the grains. In addition to the physical process of sedimentation and straining, there appear to be other influences at work aiding in the purification process. This is evidenced by the fact that filters which have been in use for a considerable time give much better results than new filters, possibly because of the accumulation of slimy film, which is organic and contains many living organisms, on the sand grains.

This type of filter is operated at the rate of about 2.5 million gal per acre of filter area per day, with the higher rates being used where some preliminary treatment, such as sedimentation, is given to the water.

After a period of operation, which depends upon the nature of the water treated, the upper layers of the sand become so clogged that cleaning is necessary. The filter bed is then thrown out of operation, the water is allowed to drain out, and the clogged layer of sand is scraped off.

While the bacterial efficiency of the slow sand filter is high, the land areas and manpower requirements have been responsible for favoring the rapid sand filter (discussed in Art. 2-17).

2-15. Coagulation. The purpose of coagulation is to get the impurities of water into such a condition that they will settle out or be removed by rapid sand filters. Colloids, suspended material, and some dissolved solids may be removed by this method. By coagulation is meant the clumping together of colloidal particles to such an extent that they settle readily. The various methods of coagulation that may be applied are as follows:

1. Aging the colloidal matter. (This method is too slow for modern water-treatment-plant operation.)
2. Applying heat.
3. Providing an antagonistic colloid.
4. Altering pH.
5. Adding an electrolyte or coagulant.
6. Flocculating (slow stirring).

Of these methods, only the last three are used in water treatment.

Upon the addition of certain electrolytes, which are defined as coagulants, gelatinous flocs are formed which collect and/or absorb colloidal particles. As the weight of the floc is gradually increased by agglomeration and adsorption, settling takes place. In waterworks practice, the coagulants used are aluminum sulfate (alum), ferric chloride, ferric sulfate, ferrous sulfate (copperas), and sodium aluminate.

Where a water is difficult to coagulate or if the coagulation and sedimentation time is shortened by overloaded facilities, a coagulant aid may be employed. Coagulant aids include activated silica, activated carbon, bentonite, pulverized limestone, and synthetic polyelectrolytes. Most of the synthetic polyelectrolytes are proprietary formulas not revealed to the user. However, those sold for municipal water treatment

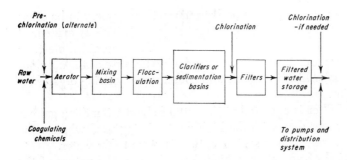

FIGURE 2-5   Flow diagram of a modern water treatment plant employing coagulation, sedimentation, rapid sand filtration, and chlorination.

are tested for toxicity by the Public Health Service, which in turn issues public notices of those approved, giving the name of the compound and of the manufacturer and the recommended dosage.

Good coagulation requires a proper amount of the coagulant, an optimum pH value, efficient mixing of the coagulant with the water, and, after the rapid mix, a slow mix, sometimes called "flocculation," which encourages formation of floc masses and their adsorption and absorption of colloids and suspended particles. Mixing is done rapidly by mechanical agitation, usually provided by turbine mixers, or by vertical rotating shafts with one or more pairs of blades. Flocculation is accomplished by slow-moving paddle wheels operating in a tank having a detention period of 20 to 40 min.

2-16. Sedimentation or Clarification. Sedimentation or clarification basins may be rectangular with flat, sloping, or hopper bottoms; circular with flat or hopper bottoms; rectangular with multiple bottoms; or of the upflow-suspended-solids-contact type. The basins may or may not be equipped with facilities for continuous or intermittent sludge removal. From the flocculation tank to the clarification basin, the water should move at a velocity great enough to prevent settling and low enough to prevent breaking up of the floc. The sedimentation basins are provided with inlet and outlet connections arranged in a manner that will prevent short-circuiting of water flow, and the path of water should be long enough to permit settling of the floc and suspended particles prior to reaching the outlet weir. Usually when rectangular or circular basins without facilities for continuous sludge removal are provided, the theoretical retention period of the water is from 6 to 8 hr, which also includes the retention period within flocculation units. The theoretical retention period for basins provided with facilities for mechanical continuous sludge-removal facilities may be reduced to 4 or 4.5 hr, including flocculation time.

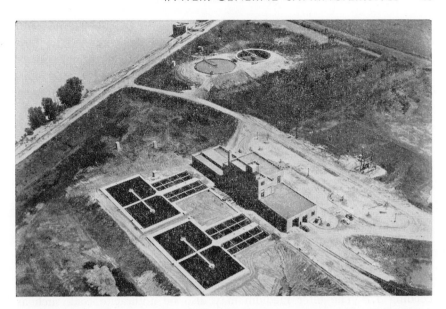

FIGURE 2-6 Water treatment plant, Council Bluffs, Iowa. This plant treats water from the Missouri River. Its high turbidity requires presedimentation tanks, shown near the top of the figure. The water then flows to four flash mixers mixing and coagulation tanks operating in parallel, each serving one of four square clarifiers. The filters are housed in the building. (*Courtesy of the Dorr Company and Public Works Magazine.*)

The path of flow of the water in a basin may be horizontal, *i.e.,* introduced at one end of a rectangular basin and removed at the other, or introduced at the center of a circular basin and removed at the periphery. The path may also be vertical—introduced at the bottom and removed at the top. In this type, the retention period is shortened, clarification being aided by passage of the water upward through a "sludge blanket," or mass of suspended matter. The blanket is continuously losing sludge masses which settle from its lower surface. Designs vary, depending on the equipment manufacturer, and patents are involved. Concerning the upflow-suspended-solids-contact clarification units, it may be pointed out that the various state agencies charged with the responsibility of reviewing plans and specifications for water treatment plants have adopted varying policies as to design practices to be met by the equipment manufacturers and suppliers.

2-17. Rapid Sand Filter. Rapid sand filters were developed in the United States about 1893. With this development in water filtration, there began a new era in water treatment. It was determined by the first experimenters that the optimum filtration rate was 125 million gal of water per acre of filter surface per day [2 gal/(sq ft)(min)] and that water to be filtered at these high rates, in comparison with slow-sand-filter rates, would require pretreatment with coagulants and sedimentation. The rapid sand filter is composed of the tank, or filter box; the inlet; the effluent, or underdrain, system; the filtering medium, usually sand underlain by gravel or anthracite coal graded in particle size; rate-of-flow controllers; loss-of-head gages; and operating tables. In recent years, many filters of this type have also been provided with surface-wash systems. In most municipal water plants, the flow of water through the filter is by gravity. Some filters operate entirely enclosed in a steel shell, under the pressure within the water system. They are much used in the industrial treatment of water and also at swimming pools (Chap. 12).

The coagulated water, having a turbidity of about 10 units upon leaving the clarification basin, flows through pipe or channels to the filter gullet, to which are attached the filter wash-water troughs. (See Fig. 2-7.) The coagulated water is distributed uniformly over the filter bed, which consists of 20 to 30 in. of filter sand having an effective size ranging between 0.4 and 0.8 ml and a uniformity coefficient not exceeding 1.7[1] The filter medium may also be anthracite coal, such as Anthrafilt, supplied commercially at the desired size and uniformity. When sand is used, it is supported by 16 to 24 in. of gravel, ranging in size from $\frac{1}{8}$ to $2\frac{1}{2}$ in. in diameter, which is usually arranged in three to five layers with each layer containing material about twice the size of the material above it.

After passing through the filter medium, the water enters the underdrain system. Such systems are of various designs, but all are intended to collect the filtered water as well as distribute the wash water. A frequently used underdrain system consists of a central manifold to which perforated collecting pipes discharge. Other types of systems are also used.

As filtration proceeds, the flocculant material remaining after clarification, containing suspended matter, silt, clay, algae, bacteria, and other impurities, causes clogging of the filter. When the loss of hydraulic head through the bed approaches 7 to 8 ft, backwashing of the filter is indicated. In this operation the influent valve is closed, and the water level in the filter unit is allowed to drop to the top of the wash-water troughs. The effluent valve is then closed, and the waste valve is opened. The wash-water valve is then opened gradually until it is fully open or to the point that the filter sand has been expanded to the point of complete suspension, by the supply of 15 to 20 gal of treated water per sq ft of filter surface per min from wash-water pumps or a wash-water tank. After the filter has been washed a sufficient time to

[1] The effective size of a sand is the size than which 90 per cent by weight is smaller. The uniformity coefficient is the ratio of the size than which 60 per cent is smaller to the effective size.

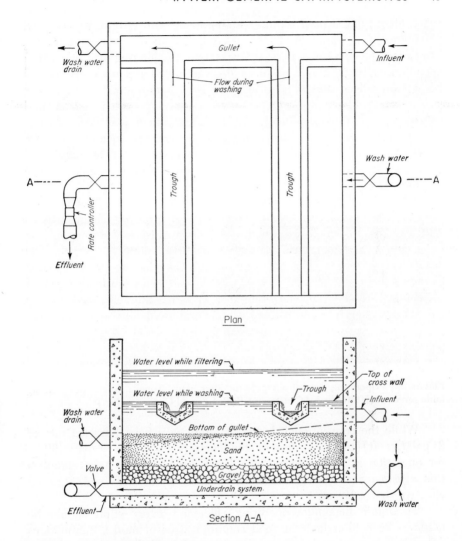

FIGURE 2-7   Rapid-sand-filter bed.

clean the sand, the wash-water valve is closed; the waste-water drain valve is closed after draining out the dirty water from the filter wash-water troughs and gullet; and the influent and effluent valves are opened to place the filter unit back into service.

It is important that the rate of filtration not exceed the rate for which the filter units were designed and that rate-of-flow controllers located in the filter effluent line from each filter be employed. A rate-of-flow controller may also be placed in the line carrying water for back-washing of filters.

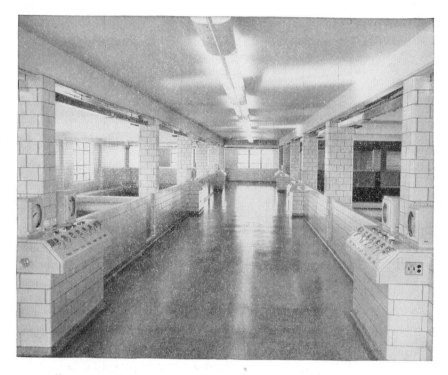

FIGURE 2-8   Operating floor of a rapid-sand-filter plant, Topeka, Kans. An operating table serves each filter bed. (*Courtesy of F. B. Leopold Company, Inc.*)

While the conventional design of filters calls for a filtration rate of 2 gal/(sq ft)(min), a present tendency is to design gravity filters for operation at higher rates, 3 or 4 gal/(sq ft)(min). To accomplish this satisfactorily and economically, coarser sands are used, 0.50 ml effective size or larger.

To obtain maximum operating efficiency, every effort should be made to keep filter beds in good condition, free of mud accumulations (mud balls), crevicing of the sand surface while filtering, algae growths, unusual flow patterns, etc. Surface wash, which applies water to the sand surface before or during backwashing, is used in some plants to prevent mud accumulations. At intervals, bacterial plate counts may be made on water samples secured before and after filtration for each unit to determine the cleanliness of the medium.

2-18. Chlorination. Even though surface water is coagulated, settled, and filtered, the bacteria and microorganisms responsible for waterborne diseases are likely to be present in the treated water unless it is disinfected. In many instances water from protected wells is disinfected with chlorine gas or chlorine compounds. This maintains a chlorine residual in the water throughout the distribution system and thus acts as a safeguard against contamination which might occur during main repairs or through faulty plumbing installations. Continuous disinfection of the water, however, should not be used as a substitute for plumbing inspection and control. All new and repaired sections of a water distribution system as well as water-storage reservoirs and new pump-station facilities should be disinfected to eliminate the contamination which may have entered the water system during the construction or rehabilitation program. Disinfection procedures should be checked by bacteriological examinations to be sure that the procedure followed has been effective. Disinfection means killing of the pathogens, the disease-producing organisms. Coliforms will also be killed in the process. Chlorine or its compounds are generally used for both purposes in water treatment.

Factors affecting disinfection are the concentration of the agent and the period of contact; however, temperature and pH also play important roles. The disinfection powers of the various chlorine compounds used depend upon their content of chlorine (Cl_2), or "available chlorine."

In disinfection of water, a number of chlorine compounds are used, namely, chlorinated lime or bleaching powder, $CaOCl_2$, having an available chlorine content of 33.5 to 39 per cent; calcium hypochlorite $Ca(OCl)_2$, sold under such trade names as HTH, Pittchlor, Perchloron, etc., and having an available chlorine content of 70 per cent; sodium hypochlorite solutions, $NaOCl$, containing 3 to 5 per cent or 10 to 16 per cent by weight of available chlorine and sold under such trade names as Clorox and Purex; and liquid chlorine, sold in cylinders of 10, 15, 25, 100, and 150 lb capacity; in 2,000-lb drums; and in railroad single-unit tank cars having capacities of 32,000, 60,000, or 110,000 lb.

In the use of the powdered chlorine compounds, with various concentrations of available chlorine, a solution containing 1 per cent chlorine is made and applied to the water at a constant rate by means of mechanical devices known as hypochlorinators. The required dosage of chlorine varies with the degree of organic pollution and the minerals or gases present which are subject to oxidation. The dosage should be sufficient not only to meet the "chlorine demand" of the water but also to maintain a detectable chlorine residual in the water at distant points of the water distribution system.

The effectiveness of chlorine as a disinfectant decreases with an increase of pH above 8.0. When applied to alkaline waters, the chlorine dosage should be increased to provide at least 0.4 mg/l residual at pH 8.0 to 10.0 and 0.8 mg/l above pH 10.0. At times of threatened or prevalent outbreaks of waterborne disease, the residual free chlorine should be increased regardless of tastes and odors which may be present in the water. In many water systems, residuals of 1.0 mg/l or greater are routinely maintained. Frequent tests should be made on water samples collected at the plant discharge sampling tap and at taps at representative points within the distribution system to determine residual chlorine content.

2-19. The Orthotolidine Test. This simple color test is made by using orthotolidine solution, which is obtainable from laboratory supply firms. Add 10 drops of orthotolidine solution to 1 oz of water. If the water sample changes to a canary yellow, sufficient chlorine has been applied to overcome the "chlorine demand" of the water, and an excess or residual chlorine content of 0.2 to 0.3 mg/l exists. Should a deep-orange color be developed, too much chlorine has been applied. A blue color denotes excessive alkalinity in the water, and the water sample should be acidified prior to adding the orthotolidine solution; or additional drops of orthotolidine solution, which is acid, may be added to neutralize the alkalinity. Chlorine comparators can be obtained from chemical supply houses; these have containers and droppers for making the orthotolidine test, and they also provide colored glass disks so that residuals can be accurately determined.

2-20. Chlorine Dosage and Application. To prepare 50 gal of a 1 per cent available chlorine solution, the following calculations are used:

1. 50 gal of water $\times$ 8.34 lb/gal = 417 lb.
2. 1 per cent of this weight = 4.17 lb of chlorine gas.
3. If 70 per cent available chlorine compound is used, 4.17 $\div$ 0.70 = 6.0 lb of 70 per cent available chlorine compound required to produce 4.17 lb of chlorine.
4. Therefore, if 6.0 lb of the chlorine compound is added to 50 gal to secure a chlorine content of 4.17 lb, each gallon of the chlorine solution will contain 4.17 lb $\div$ 50, or 0.083 lb of equivalent chlorine gas.

Now assume that 250 gal of water per min is to be treated at a dosage rate of 2.0 mg/l so as to meet the chlorine demand and allow for a chlorine residual of 0.3 mg/l and that it is desired to know the amount of 1 per cent solution which will be required per 10 hr of water plant operation at this rate of continuous treatment.

1. 250 gpm $\times$ 10 hr $\times$ 60 min/hr = 150,000 gal of water to be treated during period of operation.
2. 150,000 gal $\times$ 8.34 lb/gal = 1,251,000 lb of water.
3. $\dfrac{1,251,000 \text{ lb}}{1,000,000 \text{ lb}} \times 2.0 = 2.5$ lb of equivalent chlorine gas.
4. 2.5 lb of equivalent chlorine gas $\div$ 0.70 = 3.6 lb of 70 per cent calcium hypochlorite.
5. Since 6.0 lb of 70 per cent calcium hypochlorite is required to prepare 50 gal of 1 per cent solution, then $\dfrac{3.6}{6.0} \times 50$, or 30 gal of this solution would be required to disinfect the water as specified by the example given above.

In the preparation of hypochlorite solutions, a sludge of calcium carbonate and inert materials will be deposited in the container in which the hypochlorite is mixed with water. Therefore, it is advisable to carry out the mixing in an earthenware crock or rubber-lined barrel and to decant the chlorine solution into another container of similar materials. Since calcium carbonate will deposit on orifices and the valves of hypochlorinators, it is recommended that soda ash (sodium carbonate) be added to the water used in making the chlorine solution so as to soften the water by precipitation of the calcium carbonate.

2-21. Chlorinators. At the larger water plants, disinfection of the water is accomplished by the use of liquid chlorine, purchased in 150- or 2,000-lb-capacity cylinders under pressure, which, when pressure is released, becomes gaseous chlorine. The gaseous chlorine is either fed directly into the water through a porous diffuser or mixed with water by means of a chlorinator and fed as a water solution. Direct-feed chlorinators find application chiefly as emergency equipment and on small installations where it is not possible to obtain a suitable water supply to operate solution-feed apparatus. Solution-feed chlorinators are much more widely used and are preferable because of greater capacity, greater flexibility of control and installation, and greater adaptability to widely varying requirements. Chlorinators, ranging in feed capacity from 0.1 lb per 24 hr to thousands of pounds per 24 hr, may be

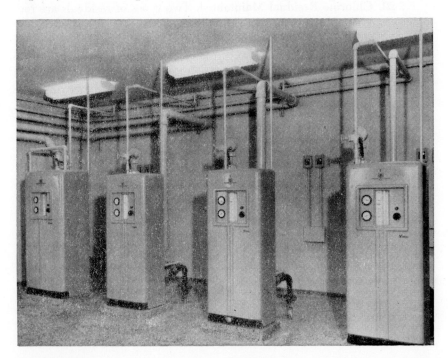

FIGURE 2-9   High-capacity solution-feed chlorinators, Metropolitan Water District Purification Plant, Salt Lake City, Utah. (*Courtesy of Wallace and Tiernan, Inc.*)

operated by manual or automatic controls. They may be "programmed" to be turned on or off as water is pumped, or they may be "paced" to vary dosage with rate of flow of the water. Instruments are available which will vary dosage with chlorine demand or which will automatically maintain a preestablished residual, the apparatus performing the analysis required. If direct-feed chlorinators are to be used, the pressure at the point of application must be below 20 psi (pounds per square inch). If solution-type chlorinators are used, they require either an auxiliary water supply of city-water quality at a pressure between 25 and 75 psi or an injector water supply with an approximate minimum quantity of 35 gal per lb of chlorinator capacity at a pressure at least three times the pressure at the point of chlorine-solution application.

The simplest type of hypochlorinator is a device which feeds the solution of hypochlorite at a constant rate to the water to be treated. This may be a small tank or head box in which a float-controlled valve maintains a constant head over an adjustable orifice. The constant-head tank is fed through the float valve from the solution tank. Hypochlorinators that include pumps which can be adjusted to feed chlorine solution at any desired rate are obtainable. They can inject the solution against pressure.

2-22. Chlorine Residual Maintained. Two types of residuals are recognized. A *combined available residual* is likely to be obtained if just sufficient chlorine is added to the filtered water to obtain a residual of 0.2 or 0.3 mg/l as the water leaves the plant. This will usually require a dose of 0.5 to 1.5 mg/l of chlorine. Such a residual will be a combined available residual because the chlorine is probably combined in large part with nitrogenous compounds to form chloramine. It is available

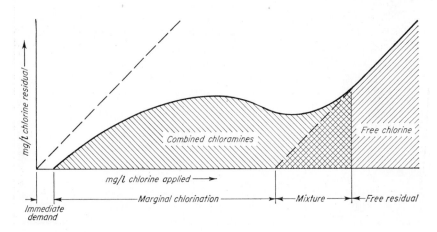

FIGURE 2-10 Curve showing formation of combined available residuals or combined chloramines, the break point, and free chlorine residual.

for disinfective action but may cause a noticeably chlorinous odor. Chlorination in this range is sometimes called marginal.

If the chlorine dose is continuously increased until there is a consistent increase of the residual, a *free available residual* can be obtained. In this procedure, at some point there is a noticeable decrease of the residual. This is known as the *break point*. Beyond the break point, the chlorine residual increases in direct proportion to the additional chlorine. It is not known exactly what occurs at the break point, but it is supposed that oxidation of nitrogenous and possibly other matters has been completed. Usually no chlorinous odors are noticeable beyond the break point, and the free chlorine which results destroys bacteria more rapidly than the combined chlorine. Free residuals are desirable particularly for highly polluted and odorous waters but will require relatively large doses of chlorine.

Water is sometimes treated with ammonia and chlorine. This combination is known as chloramine. The combined available residual which results is long-lasting but less rapid in action than a free residual and is not effective above pH 9.0. It sometimes prevents formation of chlorinous odors.

2-23. Iron and Manganese Removal. In the development of water resources for public or individual water systems, it may be necessary to remove iron naturally present in the water. Iron or manganese, if in excess of 0.3 mg/l, may form a colored precipitate which interferes with laundering and preparation of foods and drinks and which causes staining of plumbing fixtures. It may also cause the water to have a chalybeate taste and may foster the growth of "iron bacteria," which impart undesirable tastes and odors to the water. Iron-bearing water when first withdrawn from the ground may be clear, but contact of the air with soluble ferrous bicarbonate in the water rapidly oxidizes it to insoluble iron oxide or rust, which is the colored precipitate. To reduce excessive iron content, the following methods of treatment are used: (1) oxidation by aeration, followed by sedimentation and filtration to remove the precipitated iron; (2) use of ordinary zeolites, zeolites treated with pyrolusite, or beds composed entirely of pyrolusite; (3) use of lime or chlorine in a closed system ahead of pressure filters; (4) coagulation at pH values above 9.0; (5) oxidation by potassium permanganate ahead of a sand or manganese filter; (6) use of limestone filters in conjunction with aeration units to remove carbon dioxide; (7) special iron-removal units using induced vacuum and anthracite coal beds; and (8) use of slow sand filters. The most effective form of treatment for a water is usually determined by trial.

2-24. Softening of Water. "Hard water" is the classification ordinarily given to a water that has a high soap-consuming power, or water in which a lather cannot be produced without the use of an excessive quantity of soap. Hardness is caused by metallic ions which will form insoluble metal soaps. The principal hardness-producing ions are calcium and magnesium, but the presence of iron, manganese, copper, barium, zinc, and lead ions may cause slight increases in hardness. The adverse effects of hard water are many. However, the principal effects are that it (1) consumes or neutralizes soap; (2) clogs skin, discolors porcelain, stains and shortens life of fabrics, and toughens and discolors vegetables; (3) causes difficulty in textile and paper manufacture, canning, and other industrial processes; and (4) forms scale in boilers, resulting in great heat-transfer losses and danger of boiler failures.

Hardness is a relative term and often is defined by local custom. In the East, for example, a hardness of 75 mg/l may be considered "hard water," while in some parts of the Great Plains it would be "soft water." Hardness is expressed as milligrams per liter of calcium carbonate, though it may be caused by the presence of other compounds.

Water softening is the process of removing totally, or in part, the hardness-producing ions. Two methods are used: the lime-soda process, whereby calcium and magnesium ions are precipitated as calcium carbonate and magnesium hydroxide, respectively, to be removed by sedimentation and filtration; and the zeolite, or base-exchange, process, whereby calcium and magnesium ions are replaced by sodium ions from the zeolite. Zeolites are compounds which have the faculty of exchanging ions as solutions are passed over them. In water softening, the calcium and magnesium ions of the water are taken from the water in exchange for sodium ions, which do not cause hardness. When the sodium ions are exhausted, the zeolite is "rejuvenated" by passing a strong solution of sodium chloride over it. It then gives up the calcium and magnesium ions to the solution and takes sodium ions.

2-25. Stabilization of Water. A lime-softened water remains supersaturated with respect to calcium carbonate for some time after the initial softening reaction has taken place. In this event, calcium carbonate will come out of solution to encrust filter media, and some will pass into the distribution system and form deposits on the mains, meters, and service connections. The degree of supersaturation depends on a number of factors, the principal one being the characteristics of the water being treated. If the water is low in magnesium content, such that a satisfactory degree of softening can be achieved without removing magnesium, it is possible to undertreat slightly with lime and minimize calcium carbonate supersaturation. Where the water is being treated in the presence of a calcium carbonate sludge in suspension, as in an upflow-sludge-blanket type of clarifier, supersaturation may be avoided.

Lime-softened water may be "stabilized" to prevent deposition of calcium carbonate in the distribution system. This is done by adding carbon dioxide, produced at the treatment plant by burning gas or coke or purchased in cylinders in which it is stored under pressure. Another method of stabilization is known as "threshold treatment," which consists in adding sodium hexametaphosphate or other polyphosphates in dosages of around 2 mg/l.

2-26. Fluoridation. Minute concentrations of fluoride in water consumed by children during the period of tooth formation have been found to reduce dental caries as much as 60 to 65 per cent. Most of the urban population of the United States is now protected with a controlled or natural fluoride content in their water supplies. The concentration of fluoride that accomplishes this varies with the rate of water consumption, which in turn depends largely on air temperature. The range is 0.6 to 1.7 mg/l (see Art. 2-9). Since an excess of fluoride has the effect of damaging tooth enamel in children, and since most fluoride-bearing compounds employed in fluoridation are toxic, careful control of this process is indicated. However, with the precision available in feeding equipment and with care and vigilance in operating procedures, danger can be avoided. As with chlorinators, fluoride-feeding equipment can be automated with fail-safe provisions, so that unattended treatment stations are feasible.

Chemicals commonly added to water for controlled artificial fluoridation are sodium silicofluoride, sodium fluoride, hydrofluosilicic acid, ammonium silicofluoride, and calcium fluoride. All are powdered or crystalline, except hydrofluosilicic acid. Feeding equipment varies with the chemical being added. Hydrofluosilicic acid is always fed directly as a solution and is convenient for use by communities without treatment plants. The others may be fed as dry chemicals, though in some cases the chemical may be dissolved in water and fed as a solution. Calcium fluoride, as naturally mined fluorspar, can be dissolved in alum solution and added to water with the alum to effect simultaneous coagulation and fluoridation.

Where the dry chemicals are used in a treatment plant, special facilities should be provided to avoid a dust hazard. Trained operators should supervise the operation, and strict control is advisable.

Some devices are being marketed for home installation to fluoridate residential water systems. Some of these employ sodium or potassium fluoride or fluorspar. These are being installed under rental agreements similar to those available for home water-softening equipment, where the distributor makes the installation and periodically checks and services it. Any home facility employing the toxic fluorides should be installed by a competent person, and its operation should be periodically observed. Installations employing fluorspar have an inherent safety factor in the very low solubility of the chemical and hence are conducive to safe handling.

2-27. Corrosion Control. Corrosion of water pipes or other metal parts of a water system involves an electrochemical reaction. There are three forms of corrosion: (1) self-corrosion, exemplified by corrosion of iron in water, which is caused by the electrochemical tendency of metals to dissolve in water; (2) galvanic corrosion, exemplified by battery action between two dissimilar metals; and (3) electrolytic corrosion, brought about by stray electrical currents passing from water pipes into the ground, taking metal with them, and causing external pitting. Factors affecting rates of corrosion of the first type, which is the most important, are (1) dissolved oxygen—without oxygen there is no corrosion; (2) carbon dioxide—causes deposition of carbonate coatings and also causes acid waters; (3) free mineral acids—decrease pH, which is favorable to corrosion; alkalies increase pH and are unfavorable to corrosion; (4) acid salts—such salts as aluminum chloride and magnesium chloride increase corrosion; (5) temperature—an increase in temperature increases rate of corrosion; and (6) velocity of water flow—an increase in velocity accelerates corrosion since more oxygen or other impurities come in contact with the metal. To control corrosion, it may be necessary to consider the following: (1) use of nonmetallic pipes; (2) use of metals more resistant to corrosion; (3) use of protective coatings on ferrous pipe; (4) treatment of water to secure high caustic alkalinity—saturation with calcium carbonate to cause it to deposit in the piping system under controlled conditions; use of sodium silicate; or removal of dissolved gases by deactivation, deaeration, or degasification; and (5) cathodic protection, which sets up electrical currents that protect the metal tank, etc., at the expense of a metal anode.

2-28. **Algae Control.** Algae are a group of chlorophyll-bearing plants which occur as small microscopic individuals and may exist alone or in company with like individuals. Under favorable conditions, particularly in terms of sunlight and food, they may occur in such numbers as to make a water turbid or to give it an apparent color. They are undesirable because they impart odors and tastes to water. To control algal growths, attempts are made to reduce the available food supply, to destroy the organisms by the addition of chemicals, or to control some physical factors that affect microscopic growths. In practice, the food supply in a body of water, such as a reservoir, can be regulated by (1) conditioning of the watershed to prevent appreciable amounts of organic matter from reaching the reservoir; (2) clearing, grubbing, and burning of vegetation on the site before flooding; (3) preparation of shorelines to prevent water from coming in contact with vegetation; and (4) thorough cleaning of the reservoir bottom. When filtered or ground water is stored in clear wells or in storage tanks, these should be covered to exclude sunlight since darkness deprives the algae of energy for growth. Copper sulfate is widely used to destroy algae and other microscopic organisms in impounded waters. It has been demonstrated that the consumption of water containing the small amounts of copper sulfate required for destruction of algal growths and microscopic organisms is not dangerous to public health. The application of the copper sulfate, however, should be carried out under intelligent supervision. The upper limit of copper concentration that should be permitted is 3.0 mg/l, as prescribed by the Public Health Service Drinking Water Standards. It should also be realized that fish may be adversely affected, although the tolerance varies from 0.14 mg/l for trout to 2.1 mg/l for black bass. Copper sulfate dosages can be prescribed according to the species of alga, but ordinarily from 5 to 10 lb per million gal (0.6 to 1.2 mg/l) is used. Chlorine can be used effectively to control algal growths, the dosages varying according to the form of organism causing difficulty.

Copper sulfate and chlorine are applied by placing the crystals of the copper sulfate or the chlorine-compound powder in coarse bags, perforated buckets, or wire baskets and dragging these containers back and forth through the body of water to obtain a fairly uniform distribution of the chemicals in the impounded body of water. Powdered copper sulfate and solutions have also been sprayed on the water surface. If local conditions permit, copper sulfate and chlorine may be applied by dry-feed or solution-feed machines so that all water can be treated as it passes through a narrow conduit or opening. Open treated-water reservoirs or swimming pools are treated for algae control by emptying and then applying a 5 per cent solution of copper sulfate or chlorine to walls and floors by means of mops or brushes. When pipelines or other conduits contain troublesome growths, treatment with chlorine can be provided as the water leaves the water plant, and appropriate residuals can be maintained in the water throughout the distribution system.

Tastes and odors are also produced by a group of fungi, known as actinomycetes, which grow in water enriched in organic matter, principally aquatic vegetation. There is no additive known which may be applied to destroy actinomycetes.

2-29. Taste and Odor Control. Not only should every attempt be made to control algal growths in the impounded reservoir, flowing stream, or lake, but control should also be practiced at the water treatment plant. Should tastes and odors from algae be anticipated, the plant facilities might include those for aeration, which, however, is of only minor value in controlling algal tastes and odors; those for pre- as well as postchlorination; and those for application of activated carbon. Activated carbon is a specially treated charcoal and is generally used as a fine powder applied by a dry-feed machine to the water before it enters the sedimentation tank or as it goes to the filters. It is highly effective in adsorbing odor- and taste-producing compounds and is widely used. Potassium permanganate used alone or in combination with activated carbon is efficient and economical when the threshold odor is high, and it has advantages in ease of feeding and feed control. Routine limnological examinations of raw water in various sections of the impounded-water reservoir will be helpful in predicting the likely occurrence of the undesirable tastes and odors from algae growths present.

2-30. Demineralization of Saline Waters. Since 1952, the U.S. Department of the Interior has conducted extensive research into methods of removing minerals from sea water and other saline waters to make them suitable for domestic and industrial use. This program, under the administration of the Office of Saline Water, has as its objective not only developing methods of demineralization but making them economically feasible to operate on a municipal scale. Five municipal-scale demonstration plants have been built and are operating, employing flash distillation, vapor compression distillation, solar distillation, and electrodialysis. Twenty-two pilot plants have been built for investigating new methods. These include freezing, reverse osmosis, and variations of distillation and electrodialysis procedures.

It is claimed that it is now possible to produce fresh water from sea water at 30 cents per 1,000 gal if fuel can be obtained at 10 cents per million Btu and the plant can be constructed in the 25- to 30-million-gal/day range. The above cost, which is $300 per million gal, is treatment cost only. Most cities can produce, treat, pump, deliver, and care for administration costs and overhead charges for about $150 per million gal or less. Of this total, the treatment cost will be about $30 per million gal in a complete rapid-sand-filter plant. The present cost of desalting sea water makes the process economical only under very special conditions.

2-31. Development of Ground-water Sources of Supply for Public Use. In the development of ground-water sources of supply, such as wells, springs, and infiltration galleries, adequate protection of the available water from sources of pollution should be emphasized. If the well is not protected from bacterial contamination, it must be considered in the same category as a "protected surface source of water supply" and given such treatment as necessary, depending upon the density of coliform organisms found to be present and the frequency with which they are found by regular bacteriological examinations.

In practice, wells supplying water for public use are located so as to minimize the possibility of contamination. The principal location requirements are that the number of people residing within a 300-ft radius of the well be at a minimum; that all residents within this zone be provided with sanitary sewer service; that no tile or concrete sanitary sewers exist within 50 ft of the well; and that no outdoor privies, cesspools, septic-tank drain fields, or stock pens be located within 150 ft of the well. The area should be well drained to divert surface waters from the well and minimize the possibility of flooding. All abandoned wells near the site chosen for a new well should be plugged and properly sealed to prevent possible contamination of the ground-water formation.

Drilled wells are generally used for public supplies. The well should be cased with high-grade steel or wrought-iron pipe with screw-type or welded joints. The casing should extend from a point 18 in. above the elevation of the finished floor of the pump house down to the top of the shallowest water-producing formation to be developed. After the well casing has been suspended in the drill hole, the space between the casing and drill hole is sealed by portland cement grout. Sufficient grout should be used under pressure so that it is forced up around the annular space between the casing and the drill hole and appears at the surface. After the grouting has been completed and at least 24 hr has been allowed for the cement to set, the cement plug at the bottom of the casing is removed by drilling. The bottom of the well is then completed. If a gravel wall-type well is constructed, gravel, selected as to size, is placed in the cavity in the aquifer between the drill hole and the screen. The gravel is washed and disinfected by adding ½ to 1 lb of high-strength calcium hypochlorite per cu yd to it as it is placed in the well. After the well has been fully developed to remove silt, debris, drilling mud, and other undesirable material, it should be again disinfected with a chlorine solution containing 40 to 50 mg/l of chlorine residual. After the production tests are made, samples for chemical and bacteriological analysis are obtained. After the permanent well-pumping equipment has been installed, or at the time of installation, the completed well unit should be disinfected again, and the base of the well-pump motor should be sealed or grouted to the pump-foundation block. It is important that the opening between the well casing and the discharge pipe be closed. Figure 2-11 shows a method of doing this.

To ensure that intermittent contamination is not occurring, samples for bacteriological examination should be collected from an approved

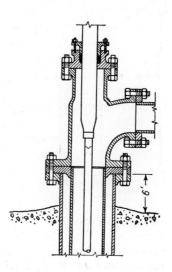

Figure 2-11   Detail of well-casing head protection. (*Courtesy of Minnesota State Board of Health.*)

nonwasher sampling tap located on the well-pump discharge main. The sampling should proceed for 5 consecutive days to determine whether the bacteriological quality of the sample conforms to the Drinking Water Standards or whether water treatment facilities are required.

In the development of springs and infiltration galleries, the existing pollutional hazards should be evaluated, and such treatment as deemed necessary should be provided to ensure the continuous delivery of water of safe quality.

2-32. Water-storage Reservoirs and Pump Houses. Clear wells and ground- or elevated-water-storage reservoirs should be constructed of nonleaking materials and provided with covers that afford protection against contamination, dust, insects, and rain. Vents and overflows should be protected as shown in Fig. 2-12. Manholes should be placed on a curb above the reservoir cover and should be provided with a bar and lock. The inlet and outlet connections can be arranged to prevent short-circuiting of water flow and water stagnation. Underground reservoirs are constructed to be thoroughly tight against leakage and situated above the ground-water table. If drains are provided, they should not be directly connected to any waste or sewage collection system. Also, no sanitary sewer lines should be located within 50 ft of the reservoir or clear well unless the sewer is of cast-iron pipe with leaded joints; if the sewer is of tile or concrete, it must be encased in concrete.

Pump pits or sub-ground-level pump rooms should be avoided. To facilitate the checking of water-system operation, meters and gages for measuring the amount of water pumped and the water pressure at the plant site should be provided. If direct-feed or solution-feed chlorinators

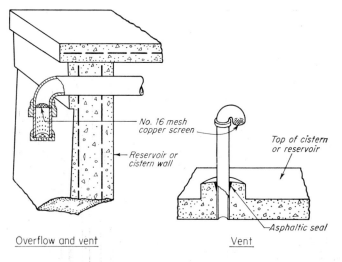

No. 16 mesh
copper screen

Reservoir or
cistern wall

Top of cistern
or reservoir

Asphaltic seal

Overflow and vent   Vent

Figure 2-12 Protection of overflows and vents of water reservoirs. (*From Public Health Service Bull.* 24.)

are installed, a separate well-ventilated room of the pump station should be provided where the cylinders can be handled without difficulty and where there is no danger of damage to electrical controls by leakage of chlorine gas.

2-33. Distribution of Water. Even though water leaving the water plant may be of satisfactory chemical and bacteriological quality, the provision of substandard facilities for water distribution may adversely affect the quality of the water being supplied and result in complaints concerning water service. For these reasons, the following features of water-distribution-system planning should be given consideration:

1. The system should be designed to provide an adequate supply of water at ample pressure to the extremities of the system.

2. The safety and palatability of the water should not be impaired by defects in the system.

3. Sufficient valves and blowoffs should be provided to permit repairs without undue interruption of service over any considerable area and to allow flushing of the system.

4. No unprotected open reservoir or physical cross-connection with inferior water systems, whereby unprotected water can enter the distribution system, should exist.

5. The system should be tight against excessive leakage, and its various mains and branches should not be submerged by surface water or subjected to any other source of contamination.

6. The system should be designed to afford effective circulation of water, and with a minimum number of dead-end mains.

7. The system should be maintained with due precautions against contamination of the water in any part of it as the result of repairs, replacements, or extension of mains.

8. When new mains are installed or old mains repaired, these mains should be filled with a strong chlorine solution (40 to 60 mg/l of chlorine) for at least 24 hr and then flushed with water to be supplied normally by the mains. Following this main-disinfection procedure, samples of water should be submitted for bacteriological examination, and the disinfection should be repeated, if necessary, until favorable laboratory results are obtained.

9. Water mains should be laid, insofar as possible, above the elevation of tile or concrete sanitary sewers at crossover points and at least 10 ft horizontally from such sanitary sewers when they are parallel. Where this recommended spacing is impossible because of local physical conditions, extra precautions should be taken to secure absolute and permanent tightness of water-pipe joints and to safeguard the water from contamination by sewage. In practice this usually is attempted by encasing the sewer mains with concrete or replacing the tile or concrete sewer with cast-iron pipe having leaded joints within the suggested spacing distances.

2-34. Cross-connections. The distribution systems of many public water supplies are connected with other sources of water which are used only in emergencies [5]. The emergency supplies may be of a public nature also but used only when the regular supply fails or is inadequate to furnish all the water needed, say, for a large fire. The emergency supply may be a river or lake from which the water is obtained without purification. Many industrial plants, in addition to the public supply, have a private source of water for fire protection or other use, and in many cases the two supplies are connected. These connections between the public water supply and emergency or private supplies are known as cross-connections. They should receive very close attention on the part of the sanitarian as they are responsible for waterborne epidemics. If the unsafe supply permanently or at times is under higher pressure than the public supply, unsafe water may enter through leaky valves or other connections between the two supplies, or valves may be opened by unauthorized persons.

There are methods by which such supplies may be safely connected. One of these is by means of a "reduced-pressure backflow preventer." This consists of two loaded pressure-reducing check valves separated by a pressure-regulated relief valve. Another is the "factory-mutual assembly," involving two gate valves with two check valves between them. An additional factor of safety may be provided in the factory-mutual assembly by installing valved nipples between each gate valve and check valve and a union between the two check valves, the union and valves on the nipples to remain open except when the connection is to be made operable. Neither of these, however, can offer positive protection unless maintained and inspected, and some state health departments do not permit them. The most positive protection against accidental backflow is to provide a surge tank and air gap, with the line carrying the potable supply terminating at least two pipe diameters above the rim of the tank. Figure 2-13 illustrates this method.

Faulty plumbing and other hazards can provide cross-connections between the sewer system and the water system. See Table 11-8 for a list of such hazards. The danger results from possible back siphonage of dirty water from toilets, washbowls, tanks, etc., into the water-supply pipes when a vacuum or negative pressure occurs in the water system. The last is particularly likely in hotels, hospitals, and other large buildings having very complicated plumbing systems. The amoebic dysentery outbreak in Chicago in 1933 was caused by sewage from poor plumbing entering the refrigerated water system which served two hotels.

Other types of cross-connections which occur are found in swimming pools having freshwater inlets so placed beneath the water surface that contaminated water may run back into the mains. At water treatment plants, bypass pipes are sometimes found running from the raw-water pump discharge around the plant to a filtered-water tank, or in some other fashion that permits untreated water to enter the water distribution system. Filtered-water basins and raw-water basins may be placed side by side with a single wall between them, and this may leak.

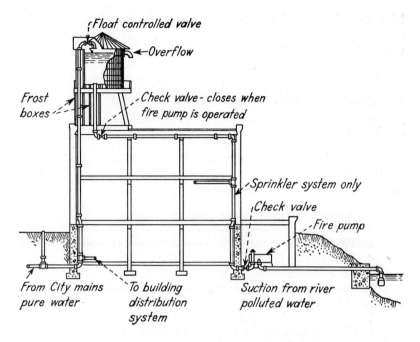

FIGURE 2-13 Safe method of obtaining dual water supplies. (*Courtesy of Minnesota State Board of Health.*)

At industrial plants and in commercial buildings, cross-connections other than to an auxiliary supply are all too common. Condenser water and cooling water may be returned to the building drinking-water system, which in turn is connected with the public supply. Pumps which handle polluted water may be primed with water from the public supply in such a manner that possible contamination will result. Many industries have underwater inlets in tanks used for various purposes. The remedy, as for swimming pools, is a complete break or gap between the inlet pipe and the highest possible water level in the tank. In some cases actual connections have been made between the discharge lines of sewage-sump pumps and water lines so that sewage has been pumped into a supply pipe, although an extreme situation such as this is soon noted. Such mistakes can be prevented by a system of painting water-supply and drainage pipes in different colors throughout a plant.

In many cities elaborate and thorough cross-connection surveys have been made. The number of unsafe conditions found is usually surprising to the health and water authorities. The survey is followed, of course, by efforts to have matters remedied, which is a time-consuming task.

2-35. Laboratory Practice for Waterworks Operators. When surface waters must be given complete treatment, including aeration, coagulation and mixing, sedimentation, filtration, and pre- and/or postchlorination, laboratory facilities for performing routine bacteriological and chemical control tests at the water treatment plant should be provided. The bacteriological examinations include:

1. Most probable numbers of coliform organisms in the raw water
2. Standard plate counts of bacteria at 20 or 35°C
3. Presumptive and confirmed tests for coliform organisms in the water sample collected from a tap located on the plant discharge main and on water samples collected from various points of the water distribution system

The specific chemical examinations considered at a particular location will vary with the type of treatment given to the raw water, but in general the following tests would be considered very useful:

1. "Jar tests" for determining coagulant dosages.
2. Alkalinity—raw, settled, filtered.
3. Total hardness—filtered, also raw if the water is softened.
4. Total solids—filtered.
5. Chlorides—filtered.
6. Fluorides—filtered, also raw and at points of distribution system if fluoridation is practiced.
7. Iron—raw and filtered.
8. Chlorine residual—at intermittent points of treatment, final, and at various points of the distribution system.
9. pH—raw, settled, filtered.
10. At periodic intervals, a complete chemical analysis should be made on the raw water, treated water, and water supplied at an active point of the distribution system. These complete analyses might include the following: total solids, silica residue, total alkalinity, total hardness, calcium, magnesium, iron, manganese, sodium (calculated), carbonate, bicarbonate, sulfate, chloride, fluoride, nitrate ABS, and pH. If there is reason to suspect the presence of such constituents, analysis should also be made for arsenic, barium, cadmium, hexavalent chromium, cyanide, lead, selenium, silver, copper, phenols, and unknown organics (carbon chloroform extract method). Continual monitoring of public water supplies for radioactivity is desirable.

For effective sanitary control of ground-water systems, bacteriological examinations may be made on water samples secured from the various wells and also on samples collected from representative points of the distribution system in the numbers recommended by the Public Health Service Drinking Water Standards, which approximate one sample per month per 1,000 population served by the facilities. If special treatment is given the well water, i.e., softening, iron removal, fluoridation, and chlorination, then appropriate chemical control tests, as outlined above for surface-water systems, may be considered desirable.

2-36. Sanitation and Development of Individual Water Facilities. Most of the water made available at farms, ranches, and residences in suburban or fringe areas of cities is derived from wells, springs, or cisterns; however, in some areas ground water is not available, or the available ground water is of undesirable chemical quality, and it has become necessary to develop surface sources of water supply. The water for the individual water-supply systems in many instances is not protected adequately from contamination, and proper sanitation and development of these small facilities should be emphasized to improve existing conditions. From a theoretical standpoint, these small water systems should be developed in a manner similar to that for water facilities for public use; however, because of the economic aspects, the provision of facilities to provide maximum protection of water quality may not be practical. Well drillers, water-system equipment suppliers, and plumbers, as well as local, state, and Federal agencies interested in water-supply development, should make every effort to acquaint the layman with the features of water-supply development, operation, and maintenance required to ensure adequate protection or treatment of water to render the water thus made available potable for domestic use. The significance of bacteriological-analysis results should be understood, and the possible causes of contamination evaluated. Disinfection of water systems with chlorine after their construction, rehabilitation, and repair should be practiced. A comprehensive educational program covering individual water supplies will no doubt result in many needed improvements.

2-37. Springs. Contrary to popular belief, spring water is not always of good bacteriological quality. In many instances, springs are nothing more than very shallow wells with water derived from a water stratum composed of creviced limestone, sand, or gravel lying only a few feet below the earth's surface. Since it is not always practicable to determine accurately the depth of the stratum from which the water is produced or whether the water is protected from surface-water contamination by impervious formations, extreme precautions should be exercised in developing springs for drinking and household use. Springs which produce turbid water after a rain are likely to be contaminated.

If the spring water is to be used for drinking and household purposes, the spring should be protected from surface or runoff water, dust, insects, wildlife, and stock. The fissure from which water is flowing should be completely enclosed with a reservoir of concrete, tile, steel, or other impervious material. The walls of the reservoir should be of such depth as to penetrate the impervious formation beneath the water-producing stratum; the reservoir cover should be insectproof, dustproof, and rainproof; and a manhole of the raised curbing type having an overlapping cover, the edges of which terminate in a downward direction, should be provided with facilities for locking. In constructing this, allowance should be made for concrete expansion and contraction. To prevent the intermittent contamination of the spring by dipping of utensils, a water-discharge pipe should be provided which will permit

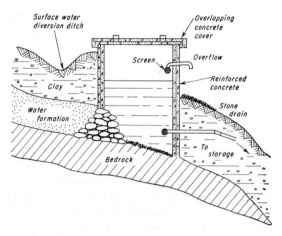

FIGURE 2-14   A protected spring. (*Drawing courtesy of Texas State Department of Health.*)

the water to flow from the enclosure by gravity. If the water is to be pumped from the spring to the point of use, it is preferable to allow the water to flow from the spring to a clear well reservoir where the pump is installed rather than to install the pump at the spring enclosure.

Spring water should not be used until bacteriological test results show that intermittent contamination is not occurring and that the water is of safe quality at all times. After a new or cleaned spring has been made ready for use, the entire spring enclosure should be disinfected with a chlorine solution and the installation flushed prior to submitting samples for laboratory examination. If satisfactory bacteriological examination results cannot be obtained, such treatment as filtration through sand and gravel and continuous disinfection may be considered. Also, should the spring water be considered too hard, too high in iron content, or otherwise objectionable, special treatment to reduce or remove the troublesome mineral may be provided.

2-38. Cisterns. Ground-water supplies may not always be available; production from a ground-water formation may be insufficient to meet domestic water demands; and the development of a surface-water system may be impossible in view of the large expenditure of funds required for such facilities. Under such local conditions, individuals find it necessary to use rainwater and to develop cistern supplies for household purposes. It should be realized, however, that cistern waters are subject to contamination if the following defects are not corrected in the provision of such facilities:

1. Possibility of entrance of such contaminants as dust, soot, bird droppings, vermin from the roof or other catchment areas, and trash or soil which has accumulated in the gutters

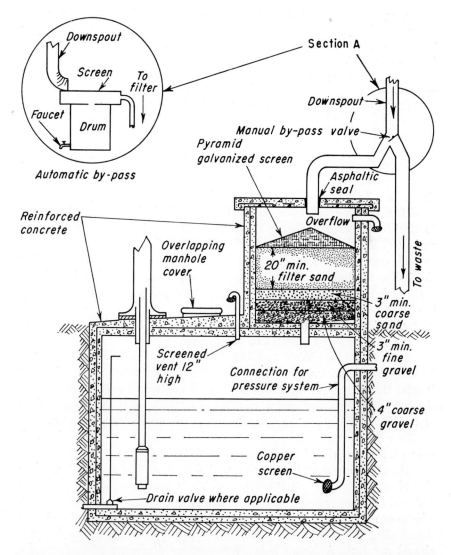

FIGURE 2-15 Cistern with sand filter. The filter sand should have an effective size of 0.3 ml. Size of the coarse sand should be to ⅛ in.; of the fine gravel, ⅛ to ⅜ in.; and of the coarse gravel, ¾ to 1¼ in. The automatic bypass may be used to replace the manual bypass valve. (*Drawing courtesy of Texas State Department of Health.*)

2. Uncovered cisterns or tanks, manhole covers which are not tight-fitting, or unscreened vents

3. No provision made for excluding from the cistern the first portion of each rainfall, until the roof or other collecting surface has become rinsed thoroughly

4. No provision made for a first-class filter of clean well-selected sand

5. Improper facilities for raising water from the cistern, such as rope and bucket, pumps which require priming, or pumping equipment which allows leakage water to drain into the cistern

6. Cracks in walls of underground cisterns permitting shallow ground water to enter

7. Existence of cesspools, septic-tank drain fields, privies, or other sources of contamination located close enough to cisterns to permit entrance of sewage wastes

Even though precaution is taken to correct these defects, cistern water should be checked frequently by bacteriological examination to determine its safety. If the water is found to be contaminated, water used for drinking purposes should be treated (1) by boiling the water to sterilize it or by bringing the water to the boiling point to kill any pathogens which may exist, or (2) by adding two drops of tincture of iodine to each quart of water to be treated and allowing the water containing the iodine to stand for 30 min after thorough mixing, or (3) by adding 1 tsp of 1 per cent hypochlorite solution to 2 gal of water and allowing the chlorinated water to stand for 20 min after thorough mixing. A 1 per cent chlorine solution is prepared by diluting household sodium hypochlorite bleach, 1 part bleach to 5 parts water.

2-39. Individual Well Supplies. Wells for the individual home may be dug, bored, driven, or drilled. If it is assumed that the ground water is safe, the principal consideration in well construction is prevention of the entrance of contaminating material directly from the ground surface or in water which has entered the well with insufficient filtration. Precautions are normally taken to ensure that no water can enter the well unless it has percolated through at least 10 ft of soil.

Hand pumps are frequently used for small water supplies. They should not be of the pitcher type, which is open around the pumping rod and requires priming and for which unsafe water is sometimes used. The pump cylinder should be in the well so that it is always primed, and the stuffing box where the pump rod emerges from the pump housing should not leak. A "weep hole" in the pump discharge pipe above the piston cylinder will allow water to drain between pumpings and thus prevent freezing. There should be no opening between the well casing and water-discharge pipe of drilled or driven wells by which contaminating matter can enter the well.

At the ground surface, a reinforced-concrete slab or cover is placed that extends at least 18 in. horizontally beyond the well curb or casing. The extension discourages seepage of water down the outside of the curbing or casing. The earth is sloped away from the top of the slab, and a lined gutter should be provided to carry away spilled water.

A well should be located in higher ground than, and at a distance from, such sources of pollution as a privy, septic tank, tile disposal field, or barnyard. The distance should be that specified by the health department, usually 50 to 100 ft.

A newly constructed well or one that has been repaired should be disinfected, including the pump and all piping. This is usually done with chlorine, using a solution that will provide about 50 mg/l (50 ppm) of available chlorine. For each 100 gal in the well to be disinfected, about 1 oz of hypochlorite containing 70 per cent available chlorine would be used. The hypochlorite is dissolved in 5 gal of water, and the solution is applied. At the end of a 12-hr contact period, there should be a chlorine residual of at least 0.5 mg/l in the well and at points in the water system. The water should be tested bacteriologically before it is used.

Dug wells are usually shallow. Some older types were open, and ropes and buckets were used for water withdrawal; these were obviously insanitary. Figure 2-16 shows a protected dug well. Note that the curbing is tight for a distance of 10 ft below the ground surface; that the sleeve through the well cover terminates well above the cover; and that the pump stand has a watertight joint with the cover. The pump cylinder should be placed where it will always be submerged. Figure 2-17 shows a reconstructed dug well.

Dug wells are sometimes lined with large-diameter concrete or clay pipe with joints filled with grout or asphalt to the water-bearing stratum. The pipe is also surrounded with 6 in. of concrete for at least 10 ft below the ground surface. With pipe linings, the water enters the well through the bottom, on which has been placed a 1-ft or thicker layer of coarse

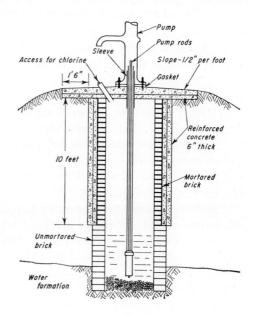

FIGURE 2-16 A protected dug well. (*Drawing courtesy of Texas State Department of Health.*)

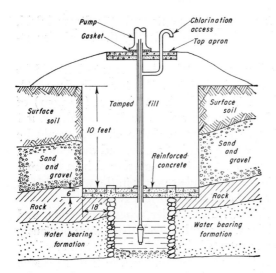

FIGURE 2-17   A reconstructed dug well. (*Drawing courtesy of Texas State Department of Health.*)

gravel or broken stone which allows water to enter and also serves to support the pipe.

Bored wells are dug with hand- or machine-operated earth augers and are of various diameters up to 36 in. They are lined and finished in the same manner as dug wells. If of small diameter, they may be lined with steel casing driven into the hole. In this case some type of screen will be needed at the bottom of the casing in the water-bearing formation.

Driven wells are constructed by driving a string of pipe into the ground. At the end of the pipe is the well point, which has openings through which water can enter the drive pipe when the well is completed. It then becomes the discharge or drop pipe. (See Fig. 2-18.) An outside casing is driven down for a distance of 10 ft or more below the ground surface to prevent the entrance of unfiltered water.

Drilled wells are of small diameter and usually of considerable depth. (See Fig. 2-19). Note that the casing has been grouted into the first rock formation encountered in order to prevent seepage down the outside of the casing. Power pumps are likely to be used with drilled wells. They will require some type of flange connection between casing and discharge pipe, as shown in Fig. 2-11.

2-40. Individual Surface-water Supplies. The provision of safe and otherwise satisfactory water from a surface source for a single home presents a difficult problem. Articles 2-12 to 2-18 describe the methods used for public supplies and also the expense, trouble, and technical knowledge involved. If at all possible, ground-water or rainwater cisterns should be used.

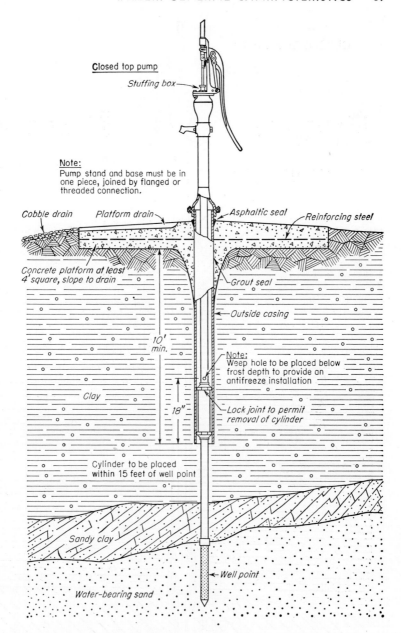

FIGURE 2-18   A driven well. (*From Public Health Service Bull. 24.*)

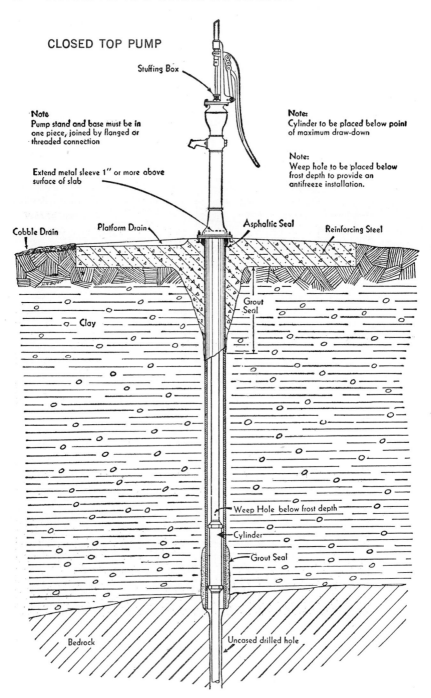

CLOSED TOP PUMP

Stuffing Box

Note
Pump stand and base must be in one piece, joined by flanged or threaded connection

Note:
Cylinder to be placed below point of maximum draw-down

Note:
Weep hole to be placed below frost depth to provide an antifreeze installation.

Extend metal sleeve 1" or more above surface of slab

Cobble Drain   Platform Drain   Asphaltic Seal   Reinforcing Steel

Grout Seal

Clay

Weep Hole below frost depth

Cylinder

Grout Seal

Bedrock   Uncased drilled hole

FIGURE 2-19   A drilled well. (*From Public Health Service Bull. 24.*)

If the surface water to be used is relatively clear, the water that is to be drunk or used for cooking may be run through one of the commercial stone filters and then boiled. Disinfection using chlorine (Arts. 2-18 and 2-20) or iodine may also be used. Two drops of tincture of iodine to 1 qt of water will disinfect it, but thorough mixing and at least a 10-min contact period should be provided. A dosage of 8 mg/l of elemental iodine will kill the pathogenic bacteria and also the cysts of *E. histolytica,* the organism which causes amoebic dysentery, in 10 min unless the temperature of the water is near zero or conditions of high iodine demand (as in colored water) exist. Then more time is required.

If the water is noticeably turbid at all times, the water may be pumped to a covered concrete tank that provides an average storage period of about 30 days. This is expensive and requires provision for emptying and cleaning the tank. The water to be drunk can then be treated as suggested in the preceding paragraph. An alternative is to apply the settled water to a small slow sand filter constructed and operated as indicated in Art. 2-14. The effluent should be disinfected by one of the methods mentioned.

Another alternative which requires skilled operation is to apply the water from the source, if it is very clear, or from the concrete tank mentioned above to one or more pressure filters, giving doses of a coagulant to the water as it enters the pressure filter. Pressure filters and their operation are described in Chap. 12. Such filters must be backwashed with filtered water. The filtered water to be drunk should be disinfected.

2-41. Drinking Fountains. The common drinking cup is implicated in the spread of tuberculosis, diphtheria, and other respiratory infections. Recognition of the dangers of the common drinking cup has resulted in drinking fountains of various sorts replacing it in schools, factories, and public buildings. All drinking fountains, however, cannot be considered satisfactory. Those in which the water rises vertically through a cup-shaped apparatus must be condemned because the cup quickly becomes dirty and the drain holes frequently clog. Those in which the water rises intermittently in a vertical jet are especially dangerous as the water which has been in contact with the drinker's lips falls back to the orifice after the water is turned off. If the vertical jet runs constantly, there are still grounds for suspicion as it has been found that bacteria may remain at the top of the jet. The safest drinking fountain provides a diagonal jet with guards so placed that the mouths of users cannot touch the orifice and the drippings from the mouth cannot possibly fall on it. A double diagonal jet with the two streams meeting beyond the guard is safe and also convenient to drink from as the velocity of the water is somewhat checked. The water outlet, or orifice, should be above the rim of the bowl so that a stoppage will not submerge it and thereby cause a cross-connection or contaminate the orifice edges. (See Fig. 2-20.)

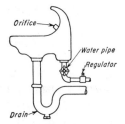

Orifice

Water pipe

Regulator

Drain

FIGURE 2-20.   A satisfactory type
of drinking fountain.

2-42. Bottled Water. The safety of bottled water should be the concern of the health department of the community in which it is sold. Some state departments of health have adopted regulations governing production and handling of bottled drinking water [6]. The principal features of the regulations are: (1) The source of the water must satisfy the standards of the Public Health Service for drinking water; (2) frequent bacteriological tests of the water as delivered must be made, and its bacteriological quality must at all times comply with those standards; (3) at least once a year a complete chemical analysis must be made of each type of water sold; (4) methods of handling the water, sanitizing the building, washing and disinfecting the containers, maintaining the cleanliness of employees, and taking precautions in delivery are all prescribed; (5) the water containers must be labeled as to type of water, such as distilled, demineralized, or spring water. Therapeutic or medicinal claims are not permitted on the label.

2-43. Manufacture of Ice. Ice frequently comes in contact with foods, beverages, and drinking water, and therefore it should be free from contamination. Regulations governing manufacture of ice have been adopted by some state health departments [7]. The principal features of the regulations are as follows: (1) The water used must comply with the Drinking Water Standards of the Public Health Service as to chemical and bacteriological quality; (2) bacteriological tests should be made of the ice to determine defects in freezing and handling; (3) ice containing foreign objects should not be sold for human consumption, and the plant should be so constructed and operated as to prevent entrance of foreign objects; (4) only authorized attendants should walk on the tank floor, and when on the floor they should wear shoes used for that area only; (5) similar precautions as given in (4) should apply to attendants who enter the storage rooms; (6) ice-storage rooms should be kept clean, and no ice should come into contact with meats or other foods; (7) chutes and loading platforms must be maintained in sanitary condition; (8) ice must be kept covered during delivery, and trucks must be so operated and maintained that contamination cannot occur; and (9) crushing or grinding of ice for human consumption should be done in a sanitary manner and permitted on trucks or other vehicles only on approval by the health authorities as to methods and safeguards.

Bibliography

1. Public Health Service Drinking Water Standards, *Public Health Service Pub.* 956, 1962.
2. Manual of Public Drinking Water Supply Evaluation, *Public Health Service Pub.* 296, rev. 1963.
3. "Standard Methods for the Examination of Water and Wastewater," 11th ed., American Public Health Association, New York, 1960.
4. Manual of Individual Water Supply Systems, *Public Health Service Pub.* 24, rev. 1962.
5. Water Supply and Plumbing Cross Connections, *Public Health Service Pub.* 957, 1963.
6. "Minimum Standards for Production, Processing and Distribution, Bottled Drinking Water," Texas State Department of Health, 1952.
7. "Minimum Standards Covering Manufacture, Storage, and Distribution of Ice Sold for Human Consumption, Including Ice Produced at Point of Use," Texas State Department of Health, 1954.
8. Steel, E. W.: "Water Supply and Sewerage," 4th ed., McGraw-Hill Book Company, New York, 1960.
9. Hardenbergh, W. A., and E. B. Rodie: "Water Supply and Waste-water Disposal," International Textbook Company, Scranton, Pa., 1961.
10. Fair, G. M., and J. C. Geyer: "Elements of Water Supply and Waste-water Disposal," John Wiley & Sons, Inc., New York, 1958.
11. Babbitt, Harold E., *et al.*: "Water Supply Engineering," 6th ed., McGraw-Hill Book Company, New York, 1962.
12. Salvato, Joseph A., Jr.: "Environmental Sanitation," John Wiley & Sons, Inc., New York, 1958.

3

AIR POLLUTION AND ITS CONTROL

3-1. Air pollution is defined by the Engineers' Joint Council [1] as follows:

> Air pollution means the presence in the outdoor atmosphere of one or more contaminants, such as dust, fumes, gas, mist, odor, smoke, or vapor, in quantities, of characteristics, and of duration such as to be injurious to human, plant, or animal life or to property, or which unreasonably interfere with the comfortable enjoyment of life and property.

It should be noted that the above definition applies to outdoor air and not to pollution which occurs in indoor working areas, where exposures occur under different conditions.

Air pollution is an increasing problem in the United States and in all countries where urban growth and population increase are accompanied by extensive industrial development and much use of automobiles. Obviously, air pollution generally increases with population, and cities not now experiencing troubles may expect them in the future. The increase of metropolitan areas in number, size, and population is recognized by health authorities as indicative that attention to the problem must be increased.

Air pollution also has economic effects. A cost estimate made in 1951 for the United States [2, p. 183] was 1.5 billion dollars per year, or about $10 per inhabitant. Later estimates [20] place the annual cost at 7.5 billion dollars. This included unburned fuel in smoke and also damage to property, repainting, excessive laundry and cleaning costs, and crop damage. For example, it is stated that in the Los Angeles area the damage to crops has amounted to 3 million dollars per year since 1953, and this covers only visible damage. No attempt has been made to compute the cost of sickness.

Radioactive air pollution is discussed in Chap. 17.

3-2. Classification of Pollutants. Pollutants may be classified as either (1) airborne particulates, also known as aerosols, or (2) gases or vapors, including the permanent gases and those compounds having a boiling point below about 200°C.

Another method of classification of pollutants is according to whether they are (1) those substances which arise directly from industrial, commercial, domestic, transport, or agricultural activities or (2) those which do not come ready-formed from primary sources but are products of interaction among primary pollutants under the influence of natural forces in the atmosphere [3, p. 34].

Tables 3-1 and 3-2 show the sources of air pollution and amounts that may be expected from each source.

3-3. Aerosols. The aerosols are air suspensions, including dusts, smokes, mists, and fumes. They differ widely in terms of particle size, particle density, and importance as pollutants. Their sizes generally range from 100 to 0.1 μ (micron) or less.[1] Sources and characteristics of aerosols are as follows.

DUST. These are generated by the crushing, grinding, etc., of organic and inorganic materials. They do not flocculate, except under electrostatic forces. They do not diffuse in the air but settle under the influence of gravity. Generally they are over 20 μ in diameter, although some are smaller. Fly ash from chimneys varies from 80 to 3 μ; bacteria, from 15 to 1.0 μ; cement, from 150 to 10 μ; plant spores, from 30 to 10 μ; foundry shakeout dust, from 200 to 1 μ; and plant pollens, from 60 to 20 μ. As indicated, most dusts will settle to the ground as dustfall, but particles 5 μ or smaller tend to form stable suspensions.

[1] The micron is 0.000,001 m, or 0.001 ml, or 0.000,039,37 in.

Table 3-1. SOURCES OF AIR POLLUTION

Class	Aerosols	Gases and vapors	Typical loss rates
Combustion processes .	Dust, fume	NO$_2$, SO$_2$, CO, organic acids	0.05–1.5% by weight of fuel (complete combustion)
Automotive engines. .	Fume	NO$_2$, CO, SO$_2$, acids, organics	4–7% by weight of fuel (hydrocarbons)
Petroleum operations .	Dust, mist	SO$_2$, H$_2$S, NH$_3$, CO, hydrocarbons, mercaptans	0.25–1.5% by weight of material processed
Chemical processes. .	Dust, mist, fume, spray	Process-dependent (SO$_2$, CO, NH$_3$, acids, organics, solvents, odors, sulfides)	0.5–2% by weight of material processed
Pyro- and electro- metallurgical processes	Dust, fume	SO$_2$, CO, fluorides, organics	0.5–2% by weight of material processed
Mineral processing . .	Dust, fume	Process-dependent (SO$_2$, CO, fluorides, organics)	1–3% by weight of material processed
Food and feed oper- ations	Dust, mist	Odorous materials	0.25–1% by weight of material processed

NOTE: Additional data may be found in "Health Officials' Guide to Air Pollution Control," American Public Health Association, New York, 1962.

SOURCE: "Air Pollution," World Health Organization, Columbia University Press, New York, 1961.

SMOKES. These are made up of carbon particles generally less than 1 μ in size. Oil-smoke particles range from 1.0 to 0.03 μ, and coal smoke from 0.2 to 0.01 μ. Particles smaller than 0.1 μ will not settle, and most smoke particles are in this range.

MISTS. These particles result from condensation of gases or vapors to the liquid state or from the breaking up of a liquid through splashing, spraying, or foaming. Natural mists forming from water vapor in the atmosphere are rather large, from 500 to 40 μ in size. In natural fog the size is 40 to 1.0 μ. Particles may coalesce.

FUMES. These are solid particles generated by condensation from the gaseous state, generally after volatilization of minerals being processed, or from chemical reactions. Fumes may flocculate or coalesce.

The concentration of suspended particulate matter is an index of air pollution caused by human activities as well as that from natural sources. Variations will result not only from human habits but also from meteorological conditions. In many cities a diurnal variation is noted, a maximum occurring at 8 to 9 A.M. and another in late afternoon or

Table 3-2. ESTIMATED RATES OF EMISSION OF CONTAMINANTS FROM FUELS—INTERNAL-COMBUSTION ENGINES AND INCINERATORS

| Contaminant | Pounds of contaminants per ton of fuel burned | | | | | | |
| | Coal | Oil | Gas | Engines | | Incinerators | |
				Auto-mobile (gaso-line)	Diesel (diesel fuel)	House-hold	Munici-pal
Solids (carbon and other particulates) . . .	200	5	.....	0.1	30	46.3	24
Carbon monoxide . .	...	....	.....	1,100	...	.....	....
Sulfur oxides, such as SO₂ .	80	60	.....	5.8	4	2	2
Nitrogen oxides, such as NO₂	8	27	12–18	9–18	20	10.6	2
Ammonia	...	....	.....	0.6	...	2.0	0.4
Acids, such as CH₃COOH .	30	27	2.6	0.6	10	27.4	0.6
Aldehydes, such as formaldehyde	...	2.6	2.0	6.2	8	5.1	1.4
Organic vapors, including hydrocarbons . . .	20	9.2	2.8	70–140*	†	274	1.2

NOTE: For additional information, see "Health Officials' Guide to Air Pollution Control," American Public Health Association, New York, 1962.

* These figures do not include losses from automobile tanks and carburetors, estimated at 2.5 to 5.0 per cent of the throughput, or losses by evaporation of gasoline during storage, handling, and marketing, estimated as 100 lb per 1,000 gal.

† Not available.

SOURCES: "Air Pollution," World Health Organization, Columbia University Press, New York, 1961; and H. H. Schrenck et al.: Air Pollution in Donora, Pennsylvania, Public Health Service Bull. 306, 1949.

evening. This variation is caused by air cooling, solar heating, and air turbulence.

Particulate loading of the atmosphere is indicated by the dustfall and concentration of particles in the air. Dustfall is reported in tons per square mile per month. Figures for some cities are: Detroit, 78.4; New York, 85.5; Los Angeles, 40.8; Chicago, 75.0; London, 97.1. Variations are found in different parts of cities. In Toronto the industrial area had 85.3 tons; an industrial-residential area, 43.7; and a residential-semirural area, only 21.5 [2, p. 129]. Dustfall particles will range in size from 20 to 40 μ.

Concentrations of airborne particulates are expressed in milligrams or micrograms per cubic meter. At urban sampling sites the National Air Sampling Network of the Public Health Service [21] found that from 1957 to 1961 concentrations varied from 6 to 1,706 micrograms/cu m, with an arithmetic mean of all observations of 118 micrograms. At non-urban sampling sites the minimum, maximum, and mean figures were 1, 461, and 36, respectively.

Particulate matter caught on filters is analyzed to determine its constituents. The organic fraction is usually reported as benzene-soluble matter. At urban sites it varied from 0.0 to 123.9 micrograms/cu m, with an arithmetic mean of all observations of 9.9 micrograms. At nonurban sites the benzene-soluble organics varied from 0.0 to 23.5 micrograms/ cu m, with a mean of 2.0.

Table 3-3 shows mean and maximum concentrations of selected particulate contaminants. The organic substances will include the benzo-pyrenes, which have been associated with increase in incidence of lung cancer. Another toxic ingredient is lead, which is derived from the anti-knock compounds used in gasoline. Its amount is apparently related to the density of vehicular traffic. So far no damage to health has been reported from the lead.

Table 3-3.   MEAN AND MAXIMUM CONCENTRATIONS OF SELECTED PARTICULATE CONTAMINANTS
(Micrograms per cubic meter)

Pollutant	Urban		Nonurban	
	Mean*	Maximum	Mean	Maximum
Suspended particulates	104	1706	27	461
Benzene-soluble organics.	7.6	123.9	1.5	23.5
Nitrates	1.7	24.8	....	.....
Sulfates	9.6	94.0	....	.....
Antimony	†	0.230	....	.....
Bismuth	†	0.032	....	.....
Cadmium	†	0.170	....	.....
Chromium	0.020	0.998	....	......
Cobalt	†	0.003	....	.....
Copper	0.04	2.50	....	.....
Iron	1.5	45.0	....	.....
Lead	0.6	6.3	....	.....
Manganese	0.04	2.60	....	.....
Molybdenum	†	0.34	....	.....
Nickel	0.028	0.830	....	.....
Tin	0.03	1.00	....	.....
Titanium	0.03	1.14	....	.....
Vanadium	†	1.200	....	.....
Zinc	0.01	8.40	....	.....

* Geometric means (see Art. 19-15) are given here.
† Indicates less than minimum detectable quantity.
SOURCE: Air Pollution Measurements of the National Air Sampling Network, *Public Health Service Bull.* 978, 1962.

3-4. Gaseous Materials. These are considered to include the vapors, which are gaseous materials derived from materials usually solid or liquid, such as gasoline. Gases and vapors will diffuse throughout the atmosphere. The more important gases will be discussed briefly.

SULFUR DIOXIDE. The principal source of sulfur dioxide is the combustion of fuels, especially coal. Therefore, its concentration in the atmosphere will depend upon the amount of sulfur content of the fuel used for heating and power generation. Since the former use is variable throughout the year, the sulfur dioxide content of the air will also vary. The increased use of natural gas for space heating has reduced the average air concentrations. Some cities, for example, St. Louis, prohibit the use of high-sulfur coal as a pollutant-control measure. Tables 3-1 and 3-2 indicate other sources of sulfur dioxide, including fuel oils and diesel oils. Some average concentrations [2, p. 138] reported in parts per million by volume are: Baltimore, 0.074; Cleveland, 0.042; St. Louis, cold months, 0.041, and warm months, 0.03; Chicago, manufacturing area, 0.50; and London, 0.14. Maximum concentrations may vary from two to ten times the average values given.

HYDROGEN SULFIDE AND ORGANIC SULFIDES. These gases cause odor nuisances in very small amounts. Concentrations of 1,000 to 3,000 ppm are fatal in a few minutes, and 100 to 150 ppm will cause discomfort in a few hours of exposure. Only by accident will such concentrations occur in the atmosphere. Hydrogen sulfide and the highly odorous mercaptans are produced in the manufacture of coke, tar distillation, refining of petroleum and natural gas, manufacture of viscose rayon, pulp mills, and various chemical processes.

HYDROGEN FLUORIDE AND CHLORIDE. The major sources of fluorides are the production of some types of steel, the manufacture of phosphate fertilizers, the production of aluminum, potteries, and brick-making plants. Some average concentrations in parts per million reported are: Baltimore, industrial area, 0.018; Los Angeles, 0.008; Cincinnati, 0.005; and Cleveland, 0.014. In the amounts produced, these contaminants are more important in terms of injury to vegetation and animals than in terms of injury to humans. The chlorides and chlorine are produced by various industries, and amounts of them reported in city air are greater than amounts of fluorides. In large amounts they are injurious to vegetation.

OXIDES OF NITROGEN. The oxides of nitrogen are important gaseous contaminants in polluted air. As Table 3-2 indicates, they are products of combustion, particularly of gasoline, oil, natural gas, and diesel fuel. Diesel engines, however, are comparatively few in number. The gasoline-driven vehicle is the important offender (Art. 3-16). Oxides of nitrogen are also produced in various chemical industries but are usually recovered as by-products. Maximum concentration in the Los Angeles area has been reported as 3.0 ppm. On days of good and poor visibility it has been reported as 0.08 and 0.4 ppm, respectively. Oxides of nitrogen are highly injurious to vegetation. They are also involved in important interactions in the air.

ALDEHYDES. These are oxidized alcohols produced by the combustion of gasoline, diesel oil, fuel oil, and natural gas. Incomplete oxidation of motor fuel and lubricating oils leads to the formation of aldehydes and also organic acids. Aldehydes may be present in concentrations equal to sulfur dioxide. Formaldehyde is irritating to the eyes.

CARBON MONOXIDE. The amount of this contaminant may show wide variations throughout the day and with the density of motor traffic. In the commercial and industrial districts of Cincinnati, concentrations ranged from 0 to 55 ppm, with an average of 9.5. In the residential districts the average was 4.0 ppm [2, p. 146]. In Los Angeles a mean peak of 8.8 ppm was found at 8:30 A.M. It dropped to 3.5 in the early afternoon and rose again to 7.0 at 5:30 P.M. The highest concentration reported was 72 ppm in November, 1959. Los Angeles (Art. 3-20) broadcasts a second alert when the concentration of carbon monoxide reaches 200 ppm. The California air-quality standards [5] place the level of carbon monoxide in air at which there will be alteration of bodily function or which is likely to lead to chronic disease at 30 ppm for 8 hr or 120 ppm for 1 hr.

ORGANIC VAPORS. These contaminants include a large number of chemical compounds, including paraffins, olefins, acetylenes, aromatic hydrocarbons, chlorinated hydrocarbons, and others reported in industrial areas. Tables 3-1 and 3-2 indicate that they are produced by combustion processes (particularly in automobiles), household incinerators, and petroleum processes. There is evidence that they undergo changes in the atmosphere which contribute to the formation of smog [4].

3-5. Interaction Products. Investigations made in the Los Angeles area indicate that chemical interactions of air contaminants occur. These interactions, which are influenced by the contaminant concentrations, solar radiation, and meteorological conditions, are complicated and not yet fully explained [3, p. 109; 5]. Vehicular contamination and its relation to smog formation are explained by the theory of Haagen-Smit [4]. During smogs in Los Angeles it was found that concentrations of ozone and other oxidants reached 0.20 to 0.65 ppm, whereas on nonsmoggy days the range was 0.05 to 0.30 ppm [5], much higher than in other atmospheres tested. The ozone is not found in appreciable amounts at night but begins to appear in the smoggy air shortly after dawn. This indicates that the photochemical action of sunlight is forming ozone or oxidants from the atmospheric impurities. Haagen-Smit's studies established that sulfur dioxide, nitrogen dioxide, and aldehydes may absorb ultraviolet radiation and react with molecular oxygen to produce atomic oxygen and then ozone (O_3). The reactions with aldehydes and sulfur dioxide are irreversible, but in the case of nitrogen dioxide (NO_2) the ultraviolet light forms atomic oxygen and NO, which first reacts with molecular oxygen (O_2) to form NO_3 and then with more oxygen to form NO_2 and O_3. The nitrogen dioxide is thus regenerated to continue the reaction. A somewhat similar but less effective reaction occurs as a result of ultraviolet irradiation of sulfur dioxide to form sulfur trioxide and ozone. In the presence of water vapor, sulfuric acid will result.

Relatively small amounts of nitrogen dioxide will produce large amounts of ozone. This reacts with organic pollutants to yield compounds that cause eye irritation, reduced visibility, crop damage, and accelerated cracking of rubber. Sulfur dioxide, through formation of sulfuric acid in a humid atmosphere, contributes a considerable amount of visibility-reducing aerosol [5, p. 421].

The aerosols resulting from the photochemical actions and following interactions, together with other small particulates from smoke and dusts, unite to form the "smog," which is common in the Los Angeles area and which is accompanied by decreased visibility and eye irritation. The term "smog" has also been applied to a combination of smoke and

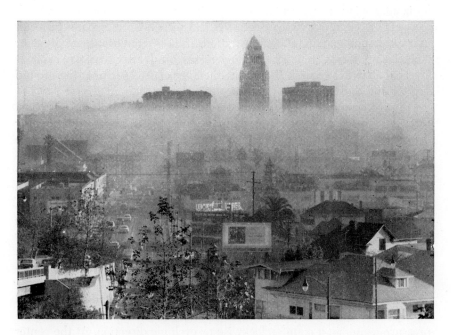

FIGURE 3-1 Los Angeles smog. Temperature-inversion layer with base 350 ft above the ground surface is holding pollution down upon city. (*Courtesy of Los Angeles County Air Pollution Control District.*)

fog, and there is also a tendency to apply it to all haze-producing and objectionable air pollution.

3-6. Meteorology and Air Pollution. Contaminants discharged into the air are diluted and their concentration is affected by air motion and turbulence. The larger particles will settle out, the location of the dust-fall areas being affected by wind direction and velocity. Turbulence, which is caused by wind gusts, convection currents, topographical irregularities, and high buildings, or the lack of turbulence, is important in affecting vertical dispersion and concentration of contaminants near the ground surface.

Precipitation, whether rain or snow, is only slightly effective in cleansing the atmosphere. Rain will remove some of the soluble contaminants, and snow removes some in removing aerosols. Fog has little or no cleaning effect since its evaporation will leave the contaminants in the air.

Horizontal dispersion is brought about by winds. Effectiveness depends upon velocity and also upon the turbulence of the air flow. When it is very smooth, the pollutant will be carried downstream in a narrow ribbon, resulting in concentrations which may be serious even at considerable distances. Vertical dispersion resulting from turbulence is important because the pollutants are carried upward and also because horizontal wind velocities are usually higher aloft than near the ground. Conversely, conditions adverse to vertical dispersion are likely to result in troublesome pollutant concentrations. These conditions are light or nonexistent winds, temperature inversions, and heavy smoke or haze layers that interfere with the normal heating of cold air near the ground surface and thus reduce vertical convection currents.

There are a number of causes of air motion and its direction. Cooling and warming of air at the poles and equator cause differing air densities. The rotation of the earth from west to east tends to move the atmosphere in that direction by friction, thus setting up the prevailing high-level winds, which begin at 2,500 ft or more above the earth. They move toward the east, deflecting toward the south in the Northern Hemisphere and toward the north in the Southern Hemisphere, because of the rise of heated air in the tropics. The local variations in wind direction are caused in part by local topography, such as mountains and valleys, presence of buildings, heating and cooling of air in contact with various types of surfaces, and differences in day and night temperatures.

Local wind velocities and directions are also affected by low- and high-pressure areas. In the former the air movement is toward the low-pressure center in a counterclockwise or cyclonic direction. At the center it rises, expands, and cools, and precipitation is likely to follow. In the high-pressure center the air movement is clockwise or anticyclonic, very light, and toward the ground. Barometric pressure is caused by the weight of the column of air above the earth. As altitude increases, the pressure decreases, and the density or concentration of molecules per unit volume becomes less. A gas of greater density and pressure free to expand will move toward a gas of lower pressure and will expand in doing so. In the process its temperature will decrease. In well-mixed air that is dry, or above the dew-point temperature, each 1,000-ft increase in altitude will result in a temperature decrease of about 5.4°F. This vertical temperature gradient is known as the lapse rate, and the decrease given is the normal lapse rate. When the reverse, or a negative lapse rate, occurs, and cool air is thus overlain by warmer air, an *inversion* exists, vertical air movement is stopped, and pollution will be concentrated beneath the inversion layer. This will occur only when horizontal air movement is very light. (See Fig. 3-2.) There are several types of inversions.

The *radiation inversion* usually occurs at night, when the earth loses heat by radiation and cools the air in contact with it. If the air is moist and its temperature is below the dew point, a fog will form. The cool-air stratum is overlain by warmer air, and vertical movement is stopped until the sun warms the lower air. This type of inversion is more common in winter than in summer because of the longer nights. Valley areas, because of the restriction of horizontal air movement by surrounding high ground, may frequently have such inversions.

The *subsidence inversion* is caused by a high-pressure area. The air circulating around the area descends, and as it does so it is compressed and heated to form a warm dense layer. This acts as a lid to

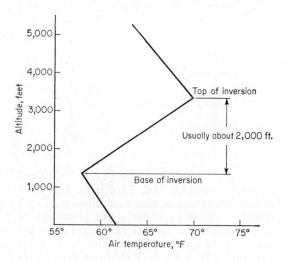

FIGURE 3-2   Subsidence inversion common in Los Angeles area.

prevent the upward movement of contaminants to the cooler air above. This is the type of inversion which is responsible for the air-pollution troubles of Los Angeles. It results from a more or less permanent high-pressure area over the Pacific Ocean which brings warm air over the land at low elevations. Horizontal air movement is restricted by the mountains around three sides of the area. The inversion height may vary from the ground surface to 4,800 ft. When it drops to less than 500 ft, extreme pollution is noted. Figure 3-2 illustrates the type of inversion common in the Los Angeles area, while Fig. 3-1 pictures an air inversion with its base only 350 ft above the ground.

Narrow valleys are favorable to inversions since horizontal air movement is restricted. There may be diurnal currents up the mountainsides as the sun warms the ground surface and downward again at night as radiation of heat from the ground causes air cooling at night. In more or less level areas as the sun warms the ground surface and convection currents are set up, downward countercurrents are established that may bring to the surface pollutants which have accumulated at higher levels during the night. This is known as "fumigation."

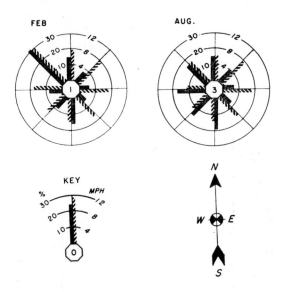

FIGURE 3-3 Surface wind roses for February and August, Washington, D.C. Solid radial bars show average percentage of time wind blows from each direction. Figure in center shows percentage of time of calm. The hatched radial bars show the average wind speed from each direction in miles per hour. (*From G. B. Welsh, Air Pollution in the National Capital Area, Public Health Service Pub. 955, 1962.*)

Cities located near the seashore experience daily exchanges in wind direction. During the day the sun warms the earth, which in turn warms the air. It rises, and a breeze blows in from the sea. During the night the earth loses heat by radiation, and the air cools and becomes denser. The surface temperature of the sea does not change during the night, and the overlying air may be warmer than that over the land, causing a movement of the cooler air from land to sea.

In many areas there are local prevailing winds, and if these are known as to directions and velocities the dissemination of pollutants can be predicted. Velocities of less than 6 mph are the most important. This information can be of value in city or regional planning in relation to the location of industrial areas. The wind rose (Fig. 3-3) is a means of showing pertinent information. The U.S. Weather Bureau will cooperate to make wind data available.

Effects of Atmospheric Pollution

3-7. Major Disasters. Public health history includes a number of air-pollution episodes which attracted attention because of much illness and loss of life.

MEUSE VALLEY. In December, 1930, an anticyclonic, or high-pressure, area blanketed Belgium, resulting in fog and a temperature inversion in the Meuse Valley. In a 15-mile length, with hills 250 to 350 ft high on each side, are many industrial plants, including steel mills, coke ovens, power plants, zinc reduction plants, glass factories, blast furnaces, a sulfuric acid plant, and an artificial-fertilizer plant [2, p. 163]. After 3 days of the abnormal weather many people became ill, although the exact number was never ascertained, and about sixty died. The illness, indicated by irritation of the membranes of the respiratory tract, affected all ages and sexes. The persons who died were the elderly and those with chronic disease of the heart or lungs. A pollutant in the air that irritated respiratory passages was believed to be the cause, and it was supposed to be a mixture of the sulfur oxides, such as sulfur dioxide gas and sulfur trioxide aerosol. Airborne oxides of nitrogen may also have been involved in the change from sulfur dioxide to the trioxide. It was also believed that aerosols, ordinarily inert physically, may have absorbed gases and that these were conveyed deeper into the lungs than they ordinarily would have penetrated.

DONORA. In October, 1948, a high-pressure area, characterized by little or no air movement and a temperature inversion, covered northwestern Pennsylvania, including the industrial city of Donora. It is located inside a horseshoe bend of the Monongahela River with steeply rising hills on each side of the river. A large steel mill and a large zinc reduction plant are located beside the river. A very still atmosphere, inversion, and fog occurred over a period of 4 days and were then terminated by a rain and change of weather. During the 4 days there was much respiratory illness and 17 deaths, although normally there would have been only two deaths during that time. Of the total population of 13,839 persons, there were 5,910 persons affected, of all ages, sexes, and occupations. The fatal cases were confined to elderly persons, 13 of whom had histories of heart or respiratory disease. The cause or causes of the deaths and illness are unknown. Various investigators [2, p. 171; 7] have suggested "metal" ammonium sulfates, oxides of nitrogen, and a combination of sulfur dioxide (estimated to have reached 0.5 to 2.0 ppm) with its oxidation products and particulate matter.

LONDON. From Dec. 5 to Dec. 9, 1952, a high-pressure area and temperature inversion, with heavy fog, occurred in many parts of the British Isles and particularly over London [2, p. 172]. Within 12 hr of the beginning of the fog, large numbers of people became ill with symptoms involving the respiratory tract. Mortality records showed a total of 4,000 deaths in excess of the normal number during the 2-week period beginning with the onset of the fog. All ages were affected, but the very young and persons over forty-five years of age showed the highest mortality. Most of the people who died had histories of chronic bronchitis, bronchopneumonia, and other lung or heart disease. A government report suggested that the excessive mortality and morbidity were caused by irritation of the respiratory tract by contaminants in the fog and that these contaminants were probably derived from coal and its products. It should be pointed out that the large amount of coal used in Great Britain has an average sulfur content of 1.5 per cent and that much of it is burned in relatively inefficient open grates.

3-8. Los Angeles. Meteorological conditions in Los Angeles were discussed in Art. 3-6. The only known physical difficulties caused by the smog are much eye irritation and some irritation of the nose and throat. Complaints cease when the smog disappears, and there are no apparent permanent effects [2, p. 176]. Preliminary results of an investigation of the hospitalization of elderly persons indicate no relationship to occurrence of smog. Many airborne substances have been studied in relation to the smog, including the sulfur oxides, oxides of nitrogen, aldehydes, various hydrocarbons, acids, acrolein, ozone, etc. It is supposed that oxides of nitrogen and hydrocarbons, both produced by combustion processes, particularly of petroleum products, are involved in photochemical changes that take place in the air. Some investigators [27] ascribe eye irritation to peroxyacetyl nitrite (PAN), which is found when oxides and certain hydrocarbons known as olefins are irradiated by sunlight in air. It is a strong eye irritant in the 1-ppm range and is therefore considered responsible, along with acrolein and formaldehyde, for the eye irritation in photochemical air pollution. At concentrations well below 1 ppm, PAN damages plants.

Much of the difficulty is ascribed to the products emitted by the nearly 3,600,000 automobiles which operate in the Los Angeles area. Reduction of air pollutants in industry under legal control and elimination of the backyard incinerators have reduced the air pollution somewhat, but Los Angeles control officials claim that motor vehicles are responsible for 75 to 80 per cent of the existing air-pollution problem, and there is reason to fear that the rapidly increasing population and growing number of automobiles will so augment air pollution that health effects will become more serious.

3-9. Atmospheric Pollution and Health. Mention has been made of causation of eye irritation and respiratory illness by various gases. Some of the aerosols may also enter the lungs and contribute to the effects of air pollution. More research is required, however, before the roles played by the various pollutants will be known.

Reduction of sunlight by pollutants may, in extreme cases, cause automobile accidents by lowering visibility. The reduction of ultraviolet rays and the effects upon bacteria and viruses require further investigation. The effect upon the antirachitic vitamin D is not considered to be of importance.

It has been recognized that some of the organic hydrocarbons occurring in the atmosphere are carcinogens, *i.e.*, causative agents of cancer. Aromatic compounds, particularly the benzopyrenes, have been associated with increases in lung cancer [2, pp. 134, 201], and they have been reported in city airs of the United States, Canada, Britain, and elsewhere. All the cancer increase cannot be accounted for by cigarette smoking. There is evidence also that carcinogenic agents inhaled may cause cancers in other parts of the body than the lungs.

Among the important causes of human disease are the pollens produced by various plants. Pollens cause hay fever in 2 to 4 per cent of the population living east of the Rocky Mountains, and hay fever, it is reported, is increasing.

3-10. Effects upon Animals. Little is known about the effects of atmospheric pollution on animals. During the disasters mentioned above, mortality was reported at London among show cattle, and 10 canine deaths were reported at Donora [2, p. 223]. Fluorosis has occurred among cattle consuming forage crops which had been contaminated by hydrogen fluoride or fluoride-containing dusts from various industries. Forage may be rendered unsafe if it contains more than 50 ppm dry-weight basis of fluorine [2, p. 274].

3-11. Effects upon Plants. Plant injury is an important economic effect of certain types of air pollution [2, p. 273]. Sulfur dioxide in concentrations from 0.1 to 0.2 ppm is toxic, depending upon length of exposure, although the injury is chronic rather than acute. Above 4 ppm, acute injury occurs more frequently. Hydrogen fluoride behaves somewhat similarly to sulfur dioxide, although with some plant species it is ten times as effective. The Los Angeles smog is known to be toxic to plants, particularly spinach, endive, romaine, Swiss chard, and celery [2, p. 265]. Visible damage to crops in California is established at nearly 10 million dollars.

3-12. Property Damage. Aside from injury to vegetation, property damage is most noticeable where smoke pollution exists. Property values decline. Buildings become grimy, requiring repainting or cleaning of stone, brick, and concrete surfaces. Fabrics affected include home drapes and goods stored on shelves or displayed. Clothing is soiled, and laundering is more expensive and more injurious to the fabric. Smog causes corrosion of metals and leads to short lives of metal roofs, eaves, and downspouts. Rubber in automobile tires and electrical insulation shows excessive cracking caused by ozone. Manufacturers add a special antiozone compound to rubber of tires sold in some areas, such as Los Angeles.

Prevention and Control of Air Pollution

3-13. Smoke. Smoke is the first air contaminant to provoke popular complaint and community control methods. Pittsburgh, St. Louis, and other cities of the United States have done notable work in reducing this type of pollution. As Table 3-2 indicates, the principal sources of solid contaminants are the burning of coal and the incineration of municipal or domestic wastes; oil burned in diesel engines or elsewhere is also a contributor.

The carbon particles which make smoke are unburned fuel. Therefore, smoking chimneys are indications of inefficiency in the process of converting fuel into useful energy. The offenders may be power plants, factories, locomotives, domestic heating appliances, open fires or fireplaces, backyard waste burners, municipal incinerators, and refuse dumps burning openly. Smokeless combustion of solid fuels requires an adequate air supply and proper stoking. Use of low-volatile fuels (such as anthracite), low-volatile bituminous coals, and coke will reduce the possibilities of smoke.

A grate on which solid fuel is burned receives air from below by stack draft alone or aided by forced draft. If a high-volatile fuel is fed from above to the bed of ignited fuel, the rising hot gases are cooled as they pass through it, and hydrocarbons and tars are distilled off to produce smoke unless air and heat are available to burn them. Hand stoking is now little used because of smoke production, which can be

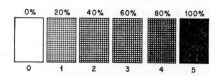

FIGURE 3-4 The Ringelmann smoke-inspection chart. Observe from a distance of 10 ft for smoke density.

reduced only by skillful methods. Mechanical stokers are used which will assure an even feeding of fuel and which allow hot gases to rise from some parts of the burning fuel to consume distilled material. Additional air inlets to assure oxygen above the fuel are also used. Upfeed of fuel requires mechanical stoking which pushes the fuel up from below. Hydrocarbons distilled from the new fuel are then consumed as they rise through the ignited fuel.

Smoke emission from stacks is checked by inspection, using the Ringelmann chart, Fig. 3-4. The smoke inspector checks the color or opacity of the stack emissions and notes its number and minutes of duration. The Los Angeles County Air Pollution Control District prohibits emissions of smokes with density greater than No. 2 on the Ringelmann chart for more than 3 min/hr [8]. More accurate smoke-measuring devices are also used [9].

Open fires, including fireplaces, backyard burning, and burning of leaves, cannot be done without production of smoke. In Los Angeles and other areas, the burning of domestic or other rubbish is prohibited except in multiple-chambered incinerators. Chapter 5 includes a discussion of public and private incinerators for refuse burning.

Smoke prevention does not eliminate air pollution. Sulfur dioxide and particulates in the form of grit or fly ash will be discharged in the stack. Their removal will be discussed in Arts. 3-14 and 3-15.

Stacks aid in the dilution and dispersion of pollutants but are not considered a positive means of pollution control. Two equations—the Bosanquet and Pearson and the Sutton—have been developed to establish stack heights or to determine pollutional effects at various points downwind [9, 10]. Examination of the two formulas indicates the following relationships between stacks and atmospheric pollution [9]:

1. Average concentrations of a contaminant downwind from a stack are directly proportional to the discharge rate.

2. In general, dilution of stack gases by excess air does not appreciably affect the ground-level concentration.

3. For equivalent effective stack heights, the average downwind concentrations are inversely proportional to wind speed. That is, an increase of wind speed by two will reduce ground-level concentration by one-half. Knowing wind direction and speed probabilities permits estimation of frequencies of different levels of pollution at various locations in the vicinity of the stack.

4. Average downwind concentrations are inversely proportional to the square of the effective stack height. Doubling the stack height, therefore, will

reduce the maximum ground-level concentration to one-fourth the previous value.

5. Effective stack height is the sum of three terms—actual height, the rise caused by the velocity of the stack gases, and the rise attributable to the density difference between the stack gases and the atmosphere.

6. The stack equations are based on smooth, level terrain. The effect of the topography can be estimated to some extent by correcting the effective stack height to account for differences in grade elevation.

7. The location of the maximum ground-level concentration is a function of atmospheric stability. During unstable atmospheric conditions, the maximum concentration occurs relatively close to the stack. As atmospheric conditions become increasingly stable, the location of the maximum ground-level concentration moves farther away from the stack.

3-14. Removal of Particulates. Some of the methods used for removing particulates to prevent air pollution will be described briefly [11].

SETTLING CHAMBERS. This is a simple form of collection that, where used, is a first stage to reduce the load of the larger particles on more elaborate methods. The most common form is a long boxlike structure, set horizontally and often on the ground. In it are installed wires and wide mesh screens to reduce eddy currents. Drags, screw conveyors, rapping devices, and scrapers are also provided to aid in removal of settled material. In general, settlers are not used to remove particles less than 40 to 50 μ in diameter.

CYCLONES. This device depends upon centrifugal force (Fig. 3-5). The particulate-laden air enters tangentially a vertically placed cylinder which has an inverted cone attached to its base. The air or gas spirals downward toward the apex of the cone. Centrifugal force moves the particles to the wall, and they fall into the cone and then to a collecting hopper. The clean air escapes through a tube set centrally and extending some distance into the cylinder. Cyclones are used for separation of many types of dusts but are not adapted to the collection of fine metallurgical fumes. They will clean large volumes of air, 30 to 25,000 cfm (cubic feet per minute), and at wide temperature ranges. For good efficiencies the dust loading must be high, generally over 10 g by weight per cu ft. Particle size should be 5 to 200 μ. Several modifications of the cyclone are used. One type uses water sprays radially directed, and the particles are caught on the wetted walls. Banks of cyclones operated in parallel are sometimes used in industry.

SCRUBBERS. Scrubbers, washers, and various modifications are widely used for cleaning and cooling air and other gases. Water is the liquid generally used, but detergents may be added or caustics for acid-mist collection. High cleaning efficiencies for particles less than 1 μ in size are not obtained by wet devices without high expenditure of energy. Several of the commonly used devices will be described.

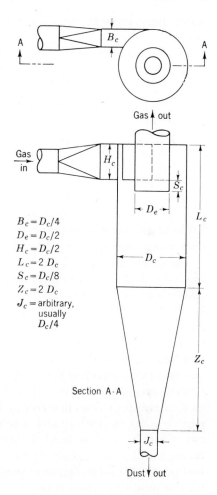

$B_c = D_c/4$
$D_e = D_c/2$
$H_c = D_c/2$
$L_c = 2\,D_c$
$S_c = D_c/8$
$Z_c = 2\,D_c$
J_c = arbitrary, usually $D_c/4$

Section A·A

FIGURE 3-5   Typical cyclone showing design proportions. (*From J. H. Perry (ed.), "Chemical Engineers' Handbook," 4th ed., McGraw-Hill Book Company, New York, 1963.*)

Air washers employ water sprays either with or against the air stream. Eliminators, usually zigzag plates at the outlet, remove water particles from the air. They are not very efficient as air cleaners but are widely used in air conditioning (Fig. 10-3). Water requirements are from 0.5 to 20 gal per 1,000 cu ft of gas.

Wet filters contain banks of cells having fine glass filaments, the banks being set at an angle to the gas flow. Nozzles placed above them spray water with or against the gas stream, and eliminators are used at the outlet. The coarse fiber pads (filaments 0.01 in. in diameter) generally used are not effective for removing insoluble particles less than 1 μ in size, and removal is about the same with wet or dry operation. High efficiencies are obtainable with wet operation in removing acid mists and vapors.

Spray towers are often plant-made by fitting a tower or a flue with water sprays along the wall or at the top. Continually wetted baffle plates are usually placed along the sides. The dusty gas is passed either up or down the tower. Spray towers are used as coolers and as cleaners in treating blast-furnace gas and for fly-ash and cinder removal.

A recent development is the venturi scrubber. In this the particulate-laden stream is directed through a venturi tube at a throat velocity of 200 to 300 fps. Water sprays are introduced just ahead of the venturi throat. The water and particles are then removed from the gas in a cyclone spray separator.

FILTERS. A commonly used filter employs tubular bags 5 to 18 in. in diameter, 2 to 30 ft long, and suspended with open ends attached to an inlet manifold at the top or bottom of the housing, or both. The lower manifold serves as a collector for the dust. The entering air strikes a baffle plate, which causes the larger particles to fall into a hopper. It then passes through the bags, leaving the dust on the interior surface of the cloth. Cleaning is generally done by shutting down and shaking the bags at the top. The material used for the filters depends upon the temperature of the gases and their corrosiveness. Cotton is much used and is satisfactory for cold noncorrosive gases. The efficiency of cloth filters is largely dependent upon the accumulated layer of dust. Therefore, they are most efficient at high dust loadings, and efficiencies of over 99.9 per cent have been obtained.

ELECTRIC PRECIPITATORS. This type of cleaner, frequently called the Cottrell precipitator, is suitable for gases that are wet or dry and hot or cold. It is expensive in first cost and upkeep. It is best adapted for small particles, less than 0.5 μ, and accordingly cyclones or settling chambers are generally used as precleaners. The Cottrell type has one chamber through which the gas or air passes between negatively charged wires and positively charged pipes or plates. The ionized particles are collected on the positively charged electrodes, which are cleaned by rapping or with water. Plates are used for dusts. High voltages are used, and there is some danger, but accidents from electric shock have been rare. Cottrell precipitators will remove 98 per cent or more of acid mist but only 95 per cent or less of fly ash and metallurgical fumes. They are also inefficient for removal of carbon black or any substance that readily loses its electric charge.

Two-stage precipitators are used to remove greasy suspensions, such as oil and tobacco smoke, foundry smoke, and miscellaneous dusts. Particles are ionized in the first chamber and collected in the second chamber. Efficiencies are higher than with the Cottrell type, and shock danger is less.

3-15. Gas Removal. Methods used are less standardized than for aerosols and present difficulties because of the widely differing properties and concentrations of the contaminants. Methods used include combustion, absorption, and adsorption.

Combustion is used where the gas or its undesirable or odorous components can be burned. It is accomplished in incineration chambers at temperatures over 1200°F, with an average retention time of 0.2 to 0.3 sec [2, p. 334]. Under certain conditions the use of catalysts will allow lower temperatures. Absorption is usually accomplished by transferring a soluble gas to water, sometimes other liquids, by means of sprays or other types of scrubbers described in Art. 3-14. Particulate matters will also be removed in the process. Adsorption requires a highly porous agent, such as activated carbon, which will require precooling of high-temperature gases. Adsorption is used successfully where the contaminant concentration is low and when other means are difficult or hazardous.

Sulfur dioxide may be recovered economically if its concentration in gases is over 5 to 10 per cent. Various processes for recovery from power plant stack gases have been proposed but have not been adopted. The "Battersea" process has been used in England [2, p. 357]. Control generally is exerted by use of low-sulfur fuels, high stacks, and scrubbers.

Other gases may be mentioned briefly. Hydrocarbons are burned, although vapor recovery methods are used in some plants. Carbon monoxide is usually burned. Nitrogen dioxide is absorbed by water, but nitric oxide must first be oxidized to the dioxide with air or oxygen before it is soluble in water. Halogenated hydrocarbons, such as carbon tetrachloride and other cleaning agents, are removed by adsorption on activated carbon. Soluble fluorides are removed by water scrubbing, but elemental fluorine is removed in a caustic solution. Hydrogen sulfide removal is accomplished by water-spray towers and packed towers for high gas volumes and by jet or cyclone scrubbers for small volumes.

3-16. Automobile Exhausts. The role of the automobile in pollution of the air of cities and metropolitan areas is so important that it merits special discussion. The gasoline-driven vehicles in Los Angeles County pollute the air daily with 1,180 tons of hydrocarbons, 330 tons of nitrogen oxides, and 8,950 tons of carbon monoxide. Of these, the nitrogen oxides and certain of the hydrocarbons are important contributors to the smog [5]. Automobiles contribute to air pollution from the carburetor, fuel tank, crankcase, and exhaust. Particulates are emitted in the exhaust, according to one observation [5, p. 302] at the rate of 358.5 mg per vehicle-mile, including organics, 158.5 mg; lead, 31.0 mg; and iron, 15.1 mg. Nitrogen oxides are emitted only in the exhaust at rates from 0.16 to 0.56 lb/hr, directly dependent upon cruising speed, with acceleration increasing the rate and deceleration decreasing it.

Expressed in proportional terms, the hydrocarbons are discharged by the present-day automobile in (1) crankcase blowby, which comes from the breather tube of the crankcase, 25 to 35 per cent; (2) fuel-tank evaporative losses, 2 to 5 per cent; (3) carburetor losses, 4 to 7 per cent; and (4) engine exhaust from the tail pipe, 70 per cent [5, p. 323]. Automobiles manufactured since 1963 are equipped with blowby controls,

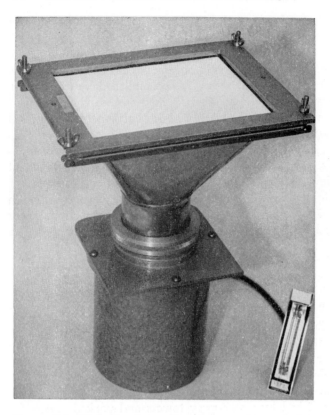

FIGURE 3-6 High-rate air-sampling apparatus for particulate determinations. Filter paper is removed from frame and sent to laboratory. (*Courtesy of Public Health Service, Robert A. Taft Sanitary Engineering Center.*)

which consist of a tube that returns crankcase vapors to the intake manifold. This will, of course, change the emission percentages for new cars. Blowby controls are required in California.

Various exhaust-control devices have been proposed, but only two have shown promise, a type of afterburner and a catalytic converter. These convert the exhaust hydrocarbons and carbon monoxide to carbon dioxide and water. Two devices are now under study by the Motor Vehicle Pollution Control Board of the California State Department of Health. When two or more devices are certified, they will be required on all new cars registered in that state.

No method has been devised to eliminate or reduce nitrogen oxides or particulates from automobile exhausts.

3-17. Legal Control of Air Pollution. Protection from the adverse effects of air pollution is a responsibility of government. Federal, state, and local agencies are concerned [13].

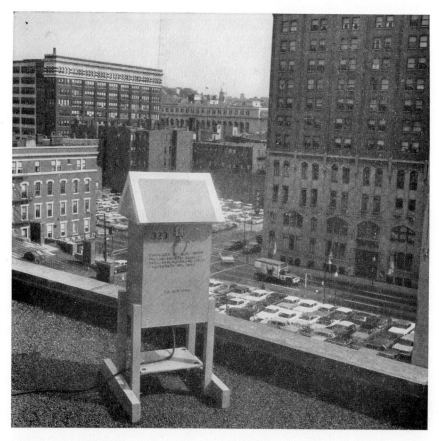

FIGURE 3-7   Air-sampling apparatus of Fig. 3-6 is installed in shelter for use. (*Courtesy of Public Health Service, Robert A. Taft Sanitary Engineering Center.*)

Federal agencies should perform services which can be done most efficiently by some central agency rather than by the states, counties, or cities.

The Public Health Service has a Division of Air Pollution which provides training of personnel and technical assistance in this area to states, local governments, and industry. Its Robert A. Taft Sanitary Engineering Center examines particulates of air samples collected at 250 sampling sites located in various parts of the country [21]. Of these, 213 are urban, and 37 nonurban. Of the urban stations, 73 sample biweekly every year, and 140 in alternate years. A sample is obtained by passing for 24 hr a known amount of air through an 8- by 10-in. glass-fiber filter that will remove particles 0.3 μ or larger. The filters are sent to the Center for analysis of the particulates per cubic meter and for benzene-soluble matter, beta radioactivity, and various metals. The nonurban sites are sampled each year. There are also a number of continuous monitoring stations that automatically measure and record the important gaseous pollutants. These stations are located in the larger cities [20].

The Public Health Service also conducts research and, through its National Institute of Health and Division of Air Pollution, sponsors research at the universities. It also acts as a coordinator and leader in the activities of other Federal agencies.

Other Federal agencies concerned include the Bureau of Mines, which is interested in air pollution by fuels and their combustion; the Department of Agriculture, which is concerned with damage by air pollution to livestock and crops; the Weather Bureau, which is interested in the measurement and prediction of the meteorological factors responsible for transport of pollutants; and the Bureau of Standards, which does basic research in chemistry and physics as it applies to air pollution. The Department of Defense needs information as to transport of pollutants in order to defend the country from chemical, biological, and radiological agents. This agency, and those which are concerned with civil aeronautics, is interested in visibility at airports and along airways. The Atomic Energy Commission is concerned with what happens to radioactive particles discharged into the air.

State agencies are important. The states have the power to pass laws regulating air pollution, and most state legislatures have delegated the authority of applying the laws to cities, to counties, or, in some states, to special districts. The state health department is usually the state agency having the major responsibility for administering the control program. Its laboratories, chemists, engineers, and epidemiologists may be used for investigations and for interpretation of the state's air-pollution-control program and also to function in emergencies. It may render important service to the local authorities and industry by providing technical assistance, giving demonstrations, training local workers, and studying special problems.

Local agencies for control of air pollution include cities, counties, or a group of such units to form an air-pollution-control district. Such districts may be desirable because of the cost of control and the necessity for unified control measures applied to a considerable area. State laws, the state permitting, may be supplemented by local ordinances or regulations. Such local legislation should center control authority in one agency, whose work should include (1) determination of the present and future quality of the community's air supply, considering effects of growth of population and industry; (2) relation of the air quality to health and other factors; (3) development of a program and implementation of rules and regulations; (4) planning of emergency procedures for acute pollutional episodes and for coordination with other agencies for major disasters; (5) investigation of existing problems; (6) obtaining the necessary degree of abatement by persuasion or legal means; (7) review of plans, establishment of equipment standards, and preventive maintenance of potential pollution sources, probably implemented by a permit system; (8) control of pollution by cooperation with community zoning and planning agencies; (9) coordination of the agencies which inspect private properties and which may have some effect upon air pollution; (10) provision of information to industry through consultative services to engineers and management and instruction of operating personnel; and (11) maintenance of a continuing program for informing the public as to the origin and control of air pollution.

3-18. Industry and Air Pollution. Industry is frequently an important contributor to air pollution. It should therefore assume responsibility for prevention. The public recognizes that a forest of chimneys emitting black smoke, while indicating prosperity, also signifies a largely preventable air pollution and assumes that industry should do something about it. Industry can contribute by (1) measuring and evaluating its emissions that contribute to air pollution; (2) providing means of eliminating or reducing them to acceptable levels; (3) engaging in or sponsoring research; and (4) supporting and participating in all phases of the air-pollution-control program.

Industry may contribute to the improvement program by location or relocation of plants so that meteorological conditions or population distribution is less likely to cause trouble. Industries which are particularly likely to produce troublesome air pollutants, including odorous materials, such as petroleum processing, rendering plants, and soap manufacturing, should place air-pollution-control activities under competent technical personnel who will make studies, recommend process changes, inspect operating procedures, and have complete responsibility for abatement or control of pollution [14]. Changes in fuel specifications may also be helpful.

3-19. Pollen Control. Hay fever is a widespread disease that affects a considerable number of the population of the United States. Hay fever caused by trees affects people in the early spring; that caused by the grasses, in the summer; and that caused by ragweed, in the autumn. Evidence indicates that ragweed is the principal offender.

Ragweed is able to establish itself in recently disturbed soils, and it is common in vacant city lots, in suburban areas, along highways, and in areas where certain crops are raised. In time the ragweed will be replaced by grasses and other vegetation, and this time can be shortened by ragweed control. Since it tends to concentrate in populous centers, ragweed control may become a part of the sanitary work of a city. Both varieties of ragweed, the giant and common, are annuals and produce one crop of seeds per year. If all plants are killed before the seed crop is produced, it would seem that ragweed would be eradicated, but some

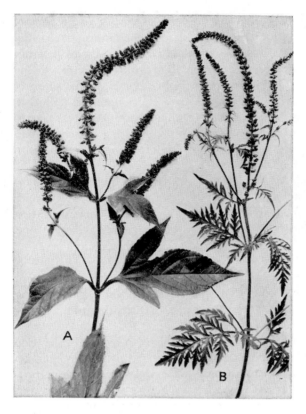

FIGURE 3-8   *A,* Giant ragweed; *B,* common ragweed.
(*Courtesy of U.S. Department of Agriculture.*)

seeds remain viable for 2 years or more before coming up. Therefore follow-up work may be necessary.

Campaigns against ragweed should be preceded by surveys to determine its presence and effect in the city and also in suburban areas since control may be necessary beyond the city limits. Studies of the pollen content of the air should also be made [6, pp. 39–50].

Weed killers must be applied by city forces, as control by notices to lot owners has not been successful [15]. The herbicide 2,4-D is an effective killer of ragweed. The sodium salt of this chemical was preferred in New York City, and 2½ lb dissolved in 250 gal of water will treat 1 acre. About 90 per cent of the plant foilage should be drenched. Treatment should be started as soon as the plants are up several inches and completed before pollination begins. In New York City, spraying continued from early May to early September. Spraying was found to have cumulative effects, and much of the ragweed area sprayed during the first year is converted to grasses and other plants. After 3 years of spraying only about one-third of the area each year, the ragweed area was reduced to about 40 per cent of the original.

3-20. Monitoring. Continuing or routine examinations of air samples to determine their quality are known as monitoring. In programs for reduction of air pollution, monitoring has four functions: (1) It may signal the existence, amount, and type of pollution; (2) it may identify the source of pollution; (3) it may indicate trends; and (4) it may serve to warn of air-pollution emergencies [3, p. 99].

Monitoring should be carefully planned and occasionally scrutinized to determine whether it is accomplishing its purposes without excessive costs. A series of routine measurements over a period may indicate base levels of pollution. One year of observations may suffice if the year chosen is representative in terms of meteorology and industrial activity. Thereafter, only spot measurements may be needed, at such intervals that pollution trends can be observed. They may be upward to a level where more active antipollution measures will be required, or downward, as an indication of successful control measures. Where disasters are to be expected, monitoring should be of such a character, at least for the pollutants considered dangerous, that warnings can be given to the industries concerned.

Los Angeles has an "alert system." See Table 3-4. The first alert indicates a close approach to the maximum allowable concentrations for the population at large—still safe, but approaching a point where preventive action is required. The following action is taken: (1) burning of combustible rubbish in open fires is forbidden, and (2) operators of plants or businesses—other than power or heating plants essential to health or safety—emitting hydrocarbons or pollutants named in Table 3-4 and any persons operating any private noncommercial vehicles must take necessary preliminary steps to action required by a second alert.

The second alert is considered a preliminary health-hazard alert. Under previously developed plans, the Air Pollution Control officer orders an immediate shutdown of polluting establishments and stopping

Table 3-4.   ALERT STAGES FOR TOXIC AIR POLLUTANTS,
LOS ANGELES COUNTY AIR-POLLUTION DISTRICT
(Parts per million)

Pollutant	First alert	Second alert	Third alert
Carbon monoxide . . .	100	200	300
Nitrogen oxides	3	5	10
Sulfur oxides	3	5	10
Ozone	0.5	1.0	1.5

SOURCE: Environmental Health Planning Guide, *Public Health Service Pub.* 823, 1962.

of all vehicular traffic, except vehicles used for emergency purposes or public transportation.

The third alert indicates a dangerous health hazard. If it appears that the steps taken by the Air Pollution Control officer under the first and second alerts are inadequate, the Air Pollution Control Board shall request the governor of the state to declare a state of emergency and to take appropriate action under the California Disaster Act.

3-21. Air-pollution Surveys. Air-pollution surveys are made to determine whether the need for a pollution-control program exists [22, 23] or to establish the details of a program preliminary to organization and prosecution of work. Information given in Art. 3-17 in connection with local agencies will be helpful in indicating survey activities. Briefly, they will include such matters as factors affecting air pollution, dispersion of pollutants, sources of pollution, existing air-pollution levels, and status of local activity in air-pollution control, and there will be a summary with recommendations [16, 22, 23]. The Public Health Service has prepared a guide for the purpose [17].

3-22. Sampling. Much information can be obtained by estimating contaminant emissions from available records. Tables 3-1 and 3-2 give useful information for this purpose, and additional data are given in "Health Officials' Guide to Air Pollution Control" [25]. Sample collection will be necessary, however, in making surveys and monitoring.

A sampling program may include (1) sampling of all types of impurities; (2) sampling under various conditions, such as stack or conduit emissions or from the open air; and (3) sampling according to the time factor, for example, continuous or intermittent sampling. Decisions will depend upon the purpose of the sampling. Statistical studies of the program are advisable so that there will be some assurance, in terms of probability, that the data obtained will be accurate within known limits.

Sample size should be such that analyses will be possible. Accordingly, there should be agreement with the analyst as to sample size and sampling methods.

Smoke sampling by the Ringelmann-chart method has been mentioned (Art. 3-13). The Public Health Service has devised a smoke inspector's guide, which is an improvement over the Ringelmann chart. Automatic smoke samplers which collect smoke and other suspended matter on a moving paper filter are also used.

Dustfall jars are used to collect and measure particulates that will settle. Quantities and characteristics are determined by weighing and chemical analyzing. The number and location of the jars are important in determining the accuracy of the data obtained. High-volume samplers pass a measured amount of air through a filter, and material caught is weighed and analyzed. This filter is pictured in Fig. 3-6 and mentioned in Art. 3-17. Electric precipitators (Art. 3-14) have also been used for sampling of particulates, and other methods have been used as well [26].

Gases in the atmosphere are difficult to collect and detect because of their highly diluted state. They may be collected by drawing known amounts of air through reagent solutions. Gas samples have also been collected in plastic bags. The Public Health Service has developed an air-pollution field-test apparatus that permits spot surveys of 18 pollutants in a short time. This is used for initial studies or to assist in planning a monitoring program. Automatic continuous sampling, analyzing, and recording devices have been developed for obtaining maximum and minimum concentrations (Art. 3-17).

Bibliography

1. Bishop, C. A.: Engineers' Joint Council Policy Statement, *Chem. Eng. Progr.*, vol. 53, no. 11, 1957.
2. "Air Pollution," World Health Organization, Columbia University Press, New York, 1961.
3. Domestic and Municipal Sources of Air Pollution, Proceedings of the National Conference on Air Pollution, 1958, *Public Health Service Pub.* 654.
4. Haagen-Smit, A. J.: Chemistry and Physiology of Los Angeles Smog, *Ind. Eng. Chem.*, vol. 44, pp. 1342–1346, 1952.
5. "Motor Vehicles, Air Pollution and Health," Report of the Surgeon General, Public Health Service, to Congress, 1962, U.S. Government Printing Office.
6. "Inservice Training Course in Air Pollution," The University of Michigan Press, Ann Arbor, Mich.
7. Schrenck, H. H., *et al.*: Air Pollution in Donora, Pennsylvania, *Public Health Service Bull.* 306, 1949.
8. "Rules and Regulations," Air Pollution Control District, Los Angeles, Calif., 1963.
9. Magill, P. L., *et al.* (eds.): "Air Pollution Handbook," McGraw-Hill Book Company, New York, 1956.
10. "Air Pollution Control Manual," Manufacturing Chemists' Association, Washington, D.C., 1953.
11. "Handbook on Air Cleaning: Particulate Removal," Department of Industrial Hygiene, Harvard University, and U.S. Atomic Energy Commission, U.S. Government Printing Office, 1952.
12. Perry, J. H. (ed.): "Chemical Engineers' Handbook," 3d ed., McGraw-Hill Book Company, New York, 1950.
13. Role of Public Health Agencies in Air Pollution Control, Report of the Air Hygiene Committee, American Public Health Association, *Am. J. Public Health*, vol. 50, no. 10, October, 1960.
14. Byrd, J. F.: Program for Surveying and Abating the Odor Nuisance from a Processing Plant, *Proc. 11th Ind. Waste Conf.*, Purdue University.

15. Weinstein, I., and A. H. Fletcher: Essentials for Ragweed Control, *Am. J. Public Health*, vol. 38, no. 5, May, 1948.
16. Welsh, G. B.: Air Pollution in the National Capital Area, *Public Health Service Pub.* 955, 1962.
17. Environmental Health Planning Guide, *Public Health Service Pub.* 823, 1962.
18. Faith, W. L.: "Air Pollution Control," John Wiley & Sons, Inc., New York, 1959.
19. Stern, A. C. (ed.): "Air Pollution," Academic Press, Inc., New York, 1962.
20. "Measuring Air Quality," Public Health Service, Robert A. Taft Sanitary Engineering Center, Cincinnati, Ohio, 1961.
21. Air Pollution Measurements of the National Air Sampling Network, *Public Health Service Bull.* 978, 1962.
22. Mees, Q. M., and R. L. Wortman: "Preliminary Report: Air Pollution Surveillance Study, Tucson, Ariz.," Bull. 13, Civil Engineering Series, no. 6, University of Arizona, Tucson, Ariz., 1960.
23. Bell, F. A.: Short Term Air Pollution Studies, *Civil Eng.*, vol. 33, no. 2, February, 1963.
24. "Continuous Air Monitoring Program," Public Health Service, Robert A. Taft Sanitary Engineering Center, Cincinnati, Ohio.
25. "Health Officials' Guide to Air Pollution Control," American Public Health Association, New York, 1962.
26. "Standards on Methods of Atmospheric Sampling and Analysis," American Society for Testing and Materials, Philadelphia, 1962.
27. Stephens, E. R., *et al.*: Photochemical Reaction Products in Air Pollution, *Intern. J. Air Water Pollution*, vol. 4, nos. 1 and 2, pp. 79–100, June, 1961.

4

TREATMENT AND DISPOSAL OF
HUMAN WASTES

4-1. The collection and safe disposal of human wastes are among the most important problems of environmental health. Articles 1-4 to 1-10 give the diseases which may be transmitted by organisms in human excreta. In this chapter, methods of treatment and disposal will be discussed from the standpoints of principles involved and, to some extent, methods of treatment-plant operation. Some attention is also given to liquid industrial wastes.

4-2. **Extent of the Problem.** Water-carried sewerage solves the excreta disposal problem of the city dweller. The dangerous materials are conveyed away, and he thinks no more of them. Since they are carried by water, they are usually discharged into a watercourse, lake, bay, or ocean. If the wastes are not properly treated their pathogenic organisms will present dangers to water supplies, bathers, and shellfish, and their putrescibility will result in killing of fish and nuisances from odors and unsightly conditions. Also dangerous is the indiscriminate discharge of untreated sewage in small or large amounts into roadside ditches, gullies, or ravines.

The increasing size of our cities and number of industries are causing an ever-rising level of pollution in the rivers and other bodies of water which are receiving their liquid wastes. Cities and industries have been concerned with the problem and have constructed new treatment plants and enlarged old ones, but they have not kept pace with pollution. The Federal government is concerned, and funds have been made available to assist cities in obtaining new treatment plants or rejuvenating old ones.

The rural dweller may also have water-carried methods of excreta disposal, and with them he has the problem of preventing water and soil pollution. If he does not have water carriage, the problem is to construct a privy that will prevent contamination of water, exclude access of flies, and be otherwise sanitary.

Fringe areas of cities or suburban communities that have water service and no sewers, or neither water nor sewers, present especially difficult problems to the environmental health engineer.

4-3. Characteristics of Excreta and Sewage. Human excreta are small in daily volume per capita, averaging about 83 g of feces and 970 g of urine. They include large amounts of water; some organic (putrescible) matter, amounting to about 20 per cent of the feces and 2.5 per cent of the urine; and small amounts of nitrogen, phosphoric acid, sulfur, and other inorganic compounds. When diluted with water to form sewage, at the rate of 30 to 100 gal or more of water per capita per day, the solid contents become a very small portion and are expressed in milligrams per liter, or parts per million by weight. Thus expressed, an average sewage may have about 800 mg/l of solids, so composed that 300 mg/l will be in suspension and 500 mg/l in solution. Of the total sewage solids, about 50 per cent will be organic and therefore putrescible. Small as the amount of organic matter is in the sewage, as decomposition progresses it becomes highly odorous and dark in color. Whether fresh or stale it will contain the organisms which cause disease.

4-4. Bacteriology of Sewage and Stabilization. Decomposition of organic matter derived from excreta is a bacteriological process which is carried on by aerobic, anaerobic, and facultative bacteria. The first-named carry on their life processes in the presence of free oxygen. The anaerobic bacteria function in the absence of free oxygen and obtain the oxygen they must have by splitting oxygen-containing compounds. Facultative bacteria can function with or without free oxygen available.

All these bacteria have no relation to disease; they occur naturally in sewage and excreta and will function when conditions are favorable in terms of food supply, temperature, and moisture and in the absence of antiseptics or disinfectants.

Decomposition proceeds until the organic matter is changed into material that can no longer be utilized by bacteria in their life processes. It is then said to be stabilized. Anaerobic decomposition, sometimes called putrefaction, is accompanied by unpleasant odors. It is slow and may require from several weeks to months for practical stabilization. A sewage which has become dark and evil-smelling as a result of anaerobic decomposition is frequently called "septic." Aerobic decomposition is not accompanied by disagreeable odors, and practical stabilization is accomplished in times which cannot be stated definitely but which will be within a matter of hours.

THE ANAEROBIC PROCESS. In this process the anaerobes and facultative anaerobes increase in numbers and produce, from the decomposition of carbonaceous matters, carbon dioxide, organic acids, and methane; from the proteins and other nitrogenous matters are produced ammonia, amino acids, amides, indole, and skatole; and the sulfur compounds are broken down into hydrogen sulfide and some other compounds, such as the mercaptans. Indole, skatole, hydrogen sulfide, and the mercaptans are unpleasantly odorous. Some of the products of anaerobic decomposition can be taken up by plants from air or water, and the plants will die and decay, or they may be eaten by animals, in which case their dead bodies or wastes again go through the cycle. Figure 4-1 illustrates the process. Solid stabilized material remaining after decomposition is dark, has little or no odor, and is known as humus.

THE AEROBIC PROCESS. Aerobic or aerobic facultative bacteria need oxygen from the air or from solution in water to carry on aerobic decomposition. Figure 4-2 illustrates this cycle. Frequently there is an initial breakdown of easily decomposable materials which is anaerobic decomposition. Thereafter direct oxidation takes place, with the formation of more carbon dioxide by respiration of the active organisms and also the formation of nitrite, nitrogen, and sulfur, which are later oxidized to nitrates and sulfates. These compounds are available for use by plants, and the cycle is repeated. Note the reversed curve called "reduction." This indicates that, should the supply of oxygen become insufficient, reduction or a retrogression back to anaerobic decomposition, with its odorous by-products, may occur. Stability is reached when the oxygen demand is nearly or completely satisfied.

IMPORTANCE OF THE CYCLES. The cycles are necessary for the existence of life on earth. To the engineer concerned with sewage treatment, they are important because sewage treatment plants are designed to employ under controlled conditions the anaerobic and aerobic cycles to bring

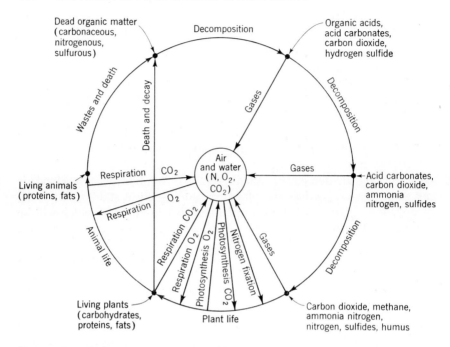

FIGURE 4-1   Carbon, nitrogen, and sulfur cycles in anaerobic decomposition. (*From E. W. Steel, "Water Supply and Sewerage," 4th ed., McGraw-Hill Book Company, New York, 1960.*)

the organic matters of sewage to a suitable degree of stability. Laboratory tests of sewage are designed to indicate the stability and the remaining oxygen demand of the organic matter.

The cycles will occur not only in sewage but also in any unstable organic matter. The type of cycle established will depend upon the oxygen supply. A mass of human feces, a pile of garbage, or a dead body, since free oxygen cannot penetrate the mass, will decompose anaerobically and with bad odors. On the other hand, a small amount of organic matter discharged into, and mixed with, a large volume of water that has a high content of dissolved oxygen will decompose aerobically.

THE COLIFORMS. Among the many bacteria found in sewage will be the coliforms (Art. 2-6). They include *Escherichia coli* (*E. coli*), which normally inhabits the intestines of man and animals and is excreted with the feces; *Aerobacter aerogenes*, which is normally found on plants and grains, in the soil, and to a varying degree in the feces of man and animals; and *A. cloacae*, which is found in soils and in the feces of man and animals. The coliforms are not considered pathogenic. As discussed in Chap. 2, they are important in water examination as indicators of contamination. Coliforms in water, sewage, and decomposing organic matter are exposed to an unfavorable environment. They cannot reproduce and

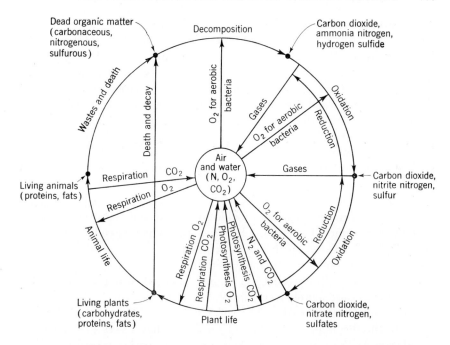

FIGURE 4-2 Carbon, nitrogen, and sulfur cycles in aerobic decomposition. (*From E. W. Steel, "Water Supply and Sewerage," 4th ed., McGraw-Hill Book Company, New York, 1960.*)

will die out at a rate that depends on the environmental factors. The teeming life of a rapidly decomposing sewage is especially unfavorable. Their numbers, therefore, will decrease in sewage as it passes through a sewage treatment plant. Length of life in a relatively unpolluted stream will be longer and will depend upon time and temperature, an average death rate being about 40 per cent in the first 10 hr and 50 per cent of the remainder in each 25 hr thereafter. This assumes no additional pollution.

PATHOGENIC ORGANISMS. Human excreta will at times contain organisms of the diseases mentioned in Chap. 1, but in very small numbers compared with the coliforms. A sewage containing discharges of many persons can be expected to contain some types. They also are exposed to an unfavorable environment outside the body, do not increase in numbers, and tend to die out, generally at about the same rate as the coliforms. Some investigations indicate that the bacilli of typhoid fever and dysentery will die in a septic sewage in 1 to 5 days. Less is known about the longevity of waterborne viruses. A sewage, no matter how well treated by biological means, may contain pathogens unless it is carefully disinfected. Also, water contaminated by sewage cannot be considered safe to drink unless it is adequately treated.

STREAM POLLUTION. When sewage is discharged into a stream, decomposition of its organic matters will start unless the water temperature is below 40°F. Water normally contains some dissolved oxygen, frequently about 7 mg/l.[1] If large amounts of sewage are present, the organic matter soon uses up the free oxygen in solution, and anaerobic decomposition is established. This is characterized by septic conditions. Settlement of suspended solids may occur, and these will also undergo anaerobic decomposition. As the water moves downstream, with some of its oxygen demand satisfied and with oxygen dissolved at the water surface, aerobic conditions will be established, and the stream is recovering. Recovery is complete when the oxygen content of the water again approaches saturation. Recovery is assisted by algae, which release free oxygen from carbon dioxide to supplement the oxygen takeup at the water surface. Fish cannot live in waters which have been denuded of their dissolved oxygen through decomposition. Pathogenic organisms will die in the polluted stream water, but some will survive for long distances of travel. Accordingly, a once-polluted water is never safe to drink unless adequately treated.

4-5. Soil Characteristics. The soil has important characteristics that relate to the disposal of excreta and sewage. It has a very high bacterial population in the upper layers. The population varies according to the nature of the soil, the amount of organic matter present, and the depth below the surface. Bacterial activity decreases with depth, until at 4 to 6 ft there is little or none and at 10 to 12 ft it is completely sterile. Conditions may be different, of course, if there are cracks or fissures in the ground.

Nearly all the soil bacteria are saprophytic, *i.e.*, living on dead organic matter. Pathogens do not find conditions in the soil favorable to existence for any length of time, and they soon die. There are several exceptions to this rule, however. The spores of tetanus, anthrax, and the so-called gas bacillus, which may cause wound infections, will remain viable in soils for long periods.

The soil is a filter. If sewage, with its suspended solids,[2] is applied to it, the solids—including bacteria—will be held on the soil grains or in the voids between them. If there is sufficient free oxygen present, aerobic decomposition of the retained organic solids will take place. The soil grains also become coated with bacteria, and these act upon the dissolved organic solids of the sewage as it passes through. On the other hand,

---

[1] The solubility of oxygen in water varies with its temperature. At 68°F it is about 9 mg/l (or 9 ppm). At 80°F it is 7.8 mg/l. Decomposition of vegetation, etc., tends to keep the oxygen content of natural waters somewhat below saturation.

[2] As will be discussed later, sewage is usually passed through some type of sedimentation tank to remove its larger suspended solids before it is applied to soil or to artificial filters.

if insufficient free oxygen is present, anaerobic conditions will develop, and the soil will become dark-colored and odorous. Aerobic conditions are more likely to be maintained if the sewage is applied intermittently.

Filtration through soil is not effective in removing the synthetic detergents now much used in the home (Art. 2-4). They are in solution in sewage, and they are not biologically degradable; *i.e.*, they are not decomposed to any extent by aerobic or anaerobic bacteria. They have been noted in contaminated ground waters to the extent that foam will appear on the water when drawn from a faucet. Slight tastes have been noted in some cases, but there has been no hazard to health.

The earth is utilized in a number of ways to dispose of feces and sewage. In the open-back privy, excreta are deposited directly on the ground surface. Excreta may be deposited in earth pits, as in the pit privy. Sewage may be discharged into leaching pits or cesspools; discharged as septic-tank effluent to soils from open-jointed subsoil pipes; or discharged as settled sewage to the ground surface for irrigation purposes. It is important, therefore, to know how far contamination will travel underground under the conditions stated.

Excreta deposited on the ground surface will be exposed to rain, which will cause some material to seep into the soil and will wash some into surface water that may enter a stream or possibly into an unprotected well. The excreta are also exposed to flies, rodents, cockroaches, and other vermin. Surface soil pollution also presents a hookworm hazard (Art. 1-9). Anaerobic decomposition will result in bad odors.

When excreta are deposited in a pit, typhoid and dysentery organisms do not move horizontally into the soil to any extent. It should be recognized that contamination, as indicated by bacteria, does not move of itself; it must be carried in some way. Therefore, if a pit privy receives rainwater or surface water, washing of material downward into the soil will occur. It has been observed that in porous soils, typhoid organisms were washed downward for 2 ft. Coliforms, under the same conditions, will be washed downward for 3 to 5 ft. In closer soils, presumably they would not travel so far before being all filtered out and would be retained until they died.

If a pit extends below the ground-water table (Fig. 2-3), which should be avoided if possible, conditions are different, for there will then be a lateral movement of the water into and out of the pit. The investigations of Caldwell and Parr [1] are of interest here.

A bored-hole latrine 15 in. in diameter and 16 ft deep was located in soil of varying characteristics, ranging from fine sand and sandy clay near the surface to coarse sand with little clay at the bottom. The water table varied from 5 to 11.5 ft below the ground surface, and the ground-water velocity varied from 3 to 8 ft/day. Wells were driven at various distances from the boring. Human feces, without water, were placed in the boring daily. The results were as follows: (1) Coliforms were recovered from the wells at a distance of 15 ft downstream from the latrine in 3 days. In the upper strata, where the ground-water velocity was only 3 ft/day, coliforms appeared at a distance of 10 ft after 5 weeks. After 2 months the greatest distance of coliform travel was noted—considerable numbers at 25 ft and occasional organisms at 35 ft. There were none in the upper strata, however, at 15 ft. Thereafter, clogging of the sand caused a recession of the coliforms, and by the end of 7 months they had retreated practically to the latrine. This effect of clogging upon the movement of pollution is known as "defense." (2) Chemical pollution traveled faster and farther than the coliforms, the maximum distance being 80 ft. Defense tended to reduce it also. (3) Pollution of both types moved in a well-defined stream bounded by unpolluted water. The stream tended to rise and fall vertically with the rise and fall of the water table. The coliform stream attained a maximum width of 3 ft at a distance of 15 ft from the latrine and thereafter narrowed, while the figures for chemical pollution were 5 and 25 ft, respectively.

The same investigations also included observations of a pit privy 8 ft 8 in. deep which extended into ground water moving through fine sand. Here coliforms reached only slightly beyond 10 ft in 3 to 4 months. In 9 months they could be found no farther than 5 ft from the pit. The maximum width of the stream was 4 ft at a distance of 5 ft from the pit. Chemical pollution, however, traveled a maximum distance of 310 ft, and at 80 ft, gross chemical pollution was noted. Odors could be noted in the water up to a distance of 195 ft. The maximum width of the stream was 25 ft at 80 ft from the privy, and its depth was a maximum of 7 ft after 6 months. It tended to drop toward the impermeable stratum which underlay the waterbearing material.

Dyer et al. [2] in India also experimented with a bored-hole latrine 16 in. in diameter and 20 ft deep in an alluvial soil which was sandy loam near the surface with decreasing amounts of clay to all fine sand below 14 ft. The water-table level varied from 3 to 13 ft below the ground surface. Wells 12, 15, and 18 ft deep were driven around the latrine and were pumped daily. Human feces without water were placed in the latrine daily. Pollution appeared only down the ground-water stream from the latrine. Observations were made from November, 1941, to April, 1943. Coliforms were recovered 10 ft away from the latrine after 2 months, with large numbers at 5 ft. Thereafter the numbers diminished, and organisms were virtually absent at 5 ft at the end of the period of observation. Chemical pollution was noted to a distance of only 15 ft and was more pronounced in the shallow wells. Investigations of the discharging of sewage into underground waters on a large scale have led the California State Water Pollution Control Board to report [3] that "reclamation of sewage waters by direct recharge into underground aquifers is practical, and that operational considerations rather than public health considerations are the controlling factors."

From the investigations reported, a few conclusions can be drawn:

1. Privy pits, bored-hole latrines, and cesspools should not penetrate the ground water. Preferably pits and latrines should terminate at least 5 ft above the water table, and cesspools, 10 ft. If this requirement can be complied with, the chance of ground-water pollution is practically nonexistent.

2. Occasional rises of ground water, caused by heavy rainfall, into pits or cesspools should be of no significance. Much of such pollution will probably be held in the capillary water as the water level falls again. In any case a continual feeding of bacteria into the water apparently is necessary for pollution to be noted at any great distance.

3. Wells should always be placed upstream in the ground-water flow from privy or cesspool. The upstream distance need not be far, but it should be remembered that heavy pumping of a well and a surcharge of liquid in a pit or cesspool above the water table may result in a temporary flow upstream.

4. Where a well must be placed downstream from a privy or cesspool which penetrates the ground water, the distance should be as great as convenient. There should be no danger of pollution with coliform organisms if the distance is at least 50 ft. If, however, the stream of chemical pollution enters the well, its effects may be noted, although chemical pollution is not a cause of disease.

5. Ground water moving in limestone or other fissured rock must be looked upon with suspicion. Tests will indicate its safety, but a newly constructed cesspool or other new source of pollution may make the water unsafe.

Individual Sewage Disposal Systems

4-6. The problems of excreta disposal with water carriage are generally categorized as either those of individual sewage disposal systems or those of municipal sewage disposal systems. Classed with individual sewage disposal systems are those serving residences, schools, camps, institutions, tourist courts, and other places where municipal sewerage systems are not available. Municipal sewage disposal involves a collection system for an entire community and a central plant for treatment prior to final disposal of the waste.

In the case of individual sewage disposal systems, too often the means of disposal to be used are a mere afterthought, to be solved by the digging of a cesspool or the building, by a local workman who knows nothing of the principles of sewage treatment, of a septic tank that permits the septic effluent to run to any ditch or stream. Consequently, it is not strange that septic tanks are sometimes causes of trouble. Quite frequently in the neighborhood of the finest residences there are ditches receiving tank effluent, or partially treated sewage, that vie with the more primitive toilets in terms of unpleasantness. In view of the difficulties encountered with such systems, individual sewage disposal systems cannot be recommended where a community sewerage system is available or could be organized.

Individual sewage disposal systems are likely to receive only a minimum amount of attention; therefore, the installations should be such that little maintenance is required. The system should create no health hazards through contamination of drinking-water supplies or through exposure of excreta to rodents or insects, and it should create no nuisances in terms of odor or appearance. For individual sewage disposal systems, the septic tank is one of the most acceptable methods of treatment prior to disposal. Cesspools are still used in some favorable areas, although they are not generally recommended.

4-7. The Cesspool. The cesspool is the reverse of a well. The untreated liquid wastes are run into a hole in the ground, from which they seep off into the soil. The sides are usually lined with brick, concrete block, or stone masonry, and the joints are laid without mortar so that the sewage will leach out. In the course of time the pores of the soil surrounding the cesspool may choke up, causing overflow. This results in a very offensive condition, one that is quite often encountered where cesspools are in use. The remedy is to dig a new pool. Clogging is less likely to occur if the masonry lining is spaced 6 in. from the earth sides and this opening is filled with coarse gravel. Cesspools sometimes receive the effluent from a septic tank, in which case they are less likely to clog, although this does not make them more acceptable from the sanitary standpoint. Others are constructed to receive wash water only, the closet wastes being conducted to a septic tank. When poorly covered, they allow odors to escape and are breeding places for mosquitoes. Cesspools are not, in general, recommended by health authorities because of the possibility of their contaminating shallow wells and the other disadvantages cited. A cesspool might be used to advantage at an isolated home where underground formations are suitable and where there is no danger to the water supply. Cesspools are especially dangerous if they are located in limestone because unfiltered sewage may then pass through crevices for long distances or so deeply as to penetrate waterbearing strata.

4-8. The Septic Tank: Principles. The septic tank is simple to construct and requires little care or operation. It should be recognized, however, that it does not "purify" sewage. The tank effluent may contain disease bacteria, and it is septic and putrescible.

Sewage is discharged into the tank, where it is retained, as quiescently as possible, for a period of about 24 hr in residential tanks or for 8 to 12 hr in tanks serving large numbers of people. During the retention period, from 60 to 70 per cent of the suspended solids of the sewage is removed, mostly by sedimentation, to form a semiliquid called sludge, which accumulates at the tank bottom; some of the solids, however, form floating scum. Both sludge and scum are acted upon by anaerobic bacteria to form gases and liquids. This is known as digestion, and during the process, pathogenic organisms are largely or completely destroyed in the sludge (the tank effluent is more likely to contain them); the solid matter is reduced in volume and changed in character. During the digestion process, gas formation at times will disturb the sludge and cause small particles to rise, and they may either become part of the scum or leave with the effluent.

Well-digested sludge is very dark in color and is homogeneous; it has a tarry odor and dries readily on sand beds. Dried sludge that is well digested forms a cake that is dark brown in color and granular in structure, with a slightly musty odor. Hookworm eggs may survive digestion and drying, but dried sludge is considered safe to use as fertilizer.

4-9. Septic-tank Capacity. Sewage is discharged from the house sewer into the tank as it is produced. Tank capacity as stated above should be such that the sewage from a single residence is retained, on an average, about 24 hr. Table 4-1 gives capacities required, based upon number of bedrooms in the house [4]. The bedroom is the basic unit since it indicates the maximum occupancy of the house, at two persons per bedroom. Note that Table 4-1 provides capacities that allow for use of garbage grinders, automatic washers, and other commonly used household appliances. The reason for smaller allowances in capacity for the larger tanks is that the greater the number of persons contributing, the less the fluctuations in flow rates in terms of the average will be. The capacities given also provide space for storage of sludge between cleanings. An additional space, usually 12 in. or about 20 per cent of the liquid depth, is provided between the flow line and the tank cover to provide space for floating scum. Some scum will also encroach upon the space below the flow line. Table 4-2 gives some tank dimensions, which

Table 4-1.   LIQUID CAPACITIES OF SEPTIC TANKS
(Gallons)

Number of bedrooms	Recommended minimum tank capacity	Equivalent capacity per bedroom
2 or less	750	375
3	900	300
4*	1,000	250

NOTE: Capacities allow for use of garbage grinders, automatic washers, and other household appliances.

* For each additional bedroom, add 250 gal to tank capacity.

SOURCE: Manual of Septic Tank Practice, *Public Health Service Pub. 526.*

Table 4-2. CAPACITIES FOR SEPTIC TANKS SERVING INDIVIDUAL DWELLINGS

Number of bedrooms	Maximum number of persons served	Nominal liquid capacity of tanks, gal	Recommended dimensions			
			Width	Length	Liquid depth	Total depth
2 or less	4	750	3'6''	7'6''	4'0''	5'0''
3	6	900	3'6''	8'6''	4'6''	5'6''
4	8	1,100	4'0''	8'6''	4'6''	5'6''
5	10	1,300	4'0''	10'0''	4'6''	5'6''
6	12	1,500	4'6''	10'0''	4'6''	5'6''

approximate the required capacities previously mentioned. Liquid-tank capacities are those below the waterline or flow line, as shown in Fig. 4-3.

4-10. Septic-tank Details. Tanks are frequently built, in place, of reinforced concrete and are rectangular in shape (Fig. 4-3). Liquid depths are 4 to 6 ft, and lengths are usually slightly more than twice the width. The optional sloping bottom shown in Fig. 4-3 makes removal of sludge slightly more convenient.

For the usual rectangular tank, a cover is provided, as shown in Fig. 4-3. This requires a manhole. An alternative is to cast the cover of reinforced-concrete slabs 8 to 12 in. wide and to place these across the short dimension of the tank. The slabs can easily be removed when cleaning or inspection is necessary. For ease of lifting, a loop or handle of reinforcing steel should be cast near each end of each slab.

In order to obtain as good an effluent as possible, direct currents from inlet to outlet should be prevented. This is done by placing tees at the end of the inlet pipe and beginning of the outlet pipe. An alternative is to use small baffle walls extending across the tank as shown in Fig. 4-3. Such walls should be of concrete. If they are made of wood, the material should be creosoted and supported in grooves in the sidewalls.

Precast septic tanks are purchasable. These may be concrete cylinders made of several lengths of large-diameter concrete pipe joined together and laid with axes horizontal. They should be of such size that the depth from flow line to bottom of the pipe is not less than 3 ft and also provides clear space above the flow line of about 15 per cent of the total cross-sectional area. This will be satisfied with liquid depths of 79 per cent of the total diameter. A manhole will be required to allow inspection of the interior and to permit cleaning.

If the tank is to discharge into a tile disposal field greater than about 500 lin ft of tile, a dosing tank and siphon should be used in conjunction with the septic tank [4]. Figure 4-4 shows such a combination. The rush of sewage which occurs when the siphon discharges provides

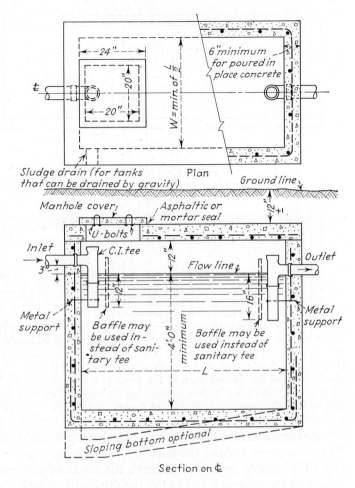

FIGURE 4-3 Single-chamber septic tank. (*From Individual Sewage Disposal Systems, Reprint 2461, Public Health Service.*)

better distribution throughout the system, and the resting periods, while the dosing tank is filling, are favorable to maintaining aerobic conditions in the receiving soil. The dosing tank should have a capacity equal to about 60 to 75 per cent of the interior capacity of the tile to be dosed at one time, and it should be so designed that the automatic dosing siphon will discharge once in 3 or 4 hr.

If the tank is to serve 1,000 ft or more of tile, the dosing tank should be provided with two siphons to discharge alternately, each to serve one-half of the tile field. Siphons require an operating head varying from 1 to 5 ft. They may also require attention if the vents clog.

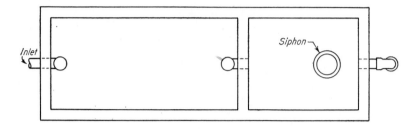

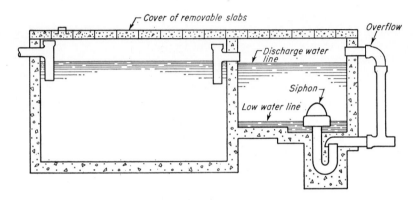

FIGURE 4-4 Septic tank and siphon chamber. Siphon-chamber dimensions should provide the desired dose. If the cover is a solid slab, a manhole will be required for each chamber. Alternating siphons, if required, are placed side by side. Concrete reinforcing is not shown.

Anaerobic action in septic tanks produces gases which must escape. The open upper ends of the inlet and outlet tees shown in Fig. 4-3 will allow the tank to be vented through the stacks of the house plumbing system at the inlet end and to the tile disposal system at the outlet. The gas has some odor, but usually it is not a nuisance. If ells are used instead of tees, ½-in. holes should be drilled into the ells well above the flow line to act as vents.

Two-compartment tanks are occasionally constructed. They are slightly more efficient in removing suspended solids, and this may be important where the tile disposal field is in very dense soil [5]. About 75 per cent of the tank capacity is allotted to the first compartment. In rectangular cast-in-place tanks, a concrete wall is constructed with the opening between baffles or having inlet and outlet tees. Access to each compartment is necessary.

4-11. Large Septic Tanks. Tanks must frequently serve large installations, such as schools, motels, country clubs, etc. This raises the question as to what the sewage flow per day will be. Table 4-3 gives expected flows per person per day at such establishments. Tank capacities [4] to

Table 4-3. QUANTITIES OF SEWAGE FLOW

Type of establishment	Gallons per person per day
Small dwellings and cottages with seasonal occupancy.	50
Single-family dwellings	75
Multiple-family dwellings (apartments)	60
Rooming houses.	40
Boarding houses.	50
Additional kitchen wastes for nonresident boarders	10
Hotels without private baths	50
Hotels with private baths (2 persons per room).	60
Restaurants (toilet and kitchen wastes per patron).	7–10
Restaurants (kitchen wastes per meal served)	2½–3
Additional for bars and cocktail lounges	2
Tourist camps or trailer parks with central bathhouse.	35
Tourist courts or mobile-home parks with individual bath units . . .	50
Resort camps (night and day) with limited plumbing	50
Luxury camps	100–150
Work or construction camps (semipermanent)	50
Day camps (no meals served)	15
Day schools without cafeterias, gymnasiums, or showers	15
Day schools with cafeterias but without gymnasiums or showers . .	20
Day schools with cafeterias, gymnasiums, and showers	25
Boarding schools	75–100
Day workers at schools and offices (per shift)	15
Hospitals.	150–250+
Institutions other than hospitals	75–125
Factories (gal per person per shift, exclusive of industrial wastes) . .	15–35
Picnic parks (toilet wastes only, gal per picnicker)	5
Picnic parks with bathhouses, showers, and flush toilets	10
Swimming pools and bathhouses	10
Luxury residences and estates	100–150
Country clubs (per resident member)	100
Country clubs (per nonresident member present)	25
Motels (per bed space)	40
Motels with bath, toilet, and kitchen wastes	50
Drive-in theaters (per car space)	5
Movie theaters (per auditorium seat)	5
Airports (per passenger)	3–5
Self-service laundries (gal per wash, i.e., per customer)	50
Stores (per toilet room)	400
Service stations (per vehicle served)	10

SOURCE: Manual of Septic Tank Practice, *Public Health Service Pub. 526.*

care for flows greater than 1,500 gal/day can be arrived at by using the following formula:

$$V = 1,125 + 0.75Q$$

where V is the liquid volume of the tank in gallons, and Q is the daily sewage flow in gallons. An example of its use will be given.

Example: A motel providing bath, toilet, and kitchen facilities is to serve a maximum of 80 persons. Determine the capacity and dimensions of the septic tank needed. Table 4-3 indicates 50 gal of sewage per capita per day, or a total of 4,000 gal. This is Q in the formula. Then $V = 1,125 + 0.75 \times 4,000 = 4,125$ gal. There are 7.48 gal in a cubic foot. Then $4,125 \div 7.48 = 552$ cu ft. A tank 5 ft deep (liquid), 7 ft wide, and 16 ft long will provide 560 cu ft.

Where flows exceed 14,500 gal/day, consideration might be given to the Imhoff tank (Art. 4-24), and where they exceed 100,000 gal/day, some other type of sedimentation tank may be desirable (Art. 4-24). Article 11-23 also gives some applicable recommendations for sewage treatment combinations for relatively large installations. See Art. 4-26 for a discussion of "package plants."

4-12. Operation of Septic Tanks. The usual amounts of detergents, drain cleaners, and bleaches used in household operations will have no bad effect upon the operation of a septic tank. Large amounts of disinfectants should not be placed in tanks. Rainwater drains should not be allowed to discharge into them because the large amounts of clear water may wash out sludge.

Septic tanks should be cleaned at intervals, and there is no rule as to the length of the interval. If too much sludge and scum are allowed to accumulate, they will approach too closely to the outlet opening, and solid matters will be swept out with the effluent. The solids will eventually clog the tile of the disposal field. The effects of this may be sewage standing in pools on the ground and/or backing up into the tank and finally up the house sewer and to the plumbing fixtures.

A tank may operate for years without difficulty. The safe rule is to make yearly inspections to determine the volume of sludge and scum. Table 4-4 shows maximum allowable sludge accumulations. Scum should

Table 4-4.   MAXIMUM ALLOWABLE SLUDGE
ACCUMULATIONS

Liquid capacity of tank, gal	Liquid depth		
	3 ft	4 ft	5 ft
	Distance from bottom of outlet device to top of sludge, in.		
500	11	16	21
600	8	13	18
750	6	10	13
900	4	7	10
1,000	4	6	8

SOURCE: Manual of Septic Tank Practice, *Public Health Service Pub.* 526.

not extend downward to less than 3 in. above the bottom of the outlet pipe or baffle. Sludge and scum soundings can be taken with a stick about 6 ft long to which another stick has been attached at the lower end at a right angle but hinged so that it can fold up to the longer stick. A weight is attached to the cross stick. As the stick is pushed through the scum, the hinged cross stick will fold to the upright. As it is raised the cross stick will drop to the horizontal, and resistance can be noted as it strikes the underside of the scum. If it is lowered slowly, resistance will be encountered as the cross stick strikes the sludge.

Cleaning of tanks is done by means of a long-handled dipper or some type of pump. Diaphragm pumps or special types of centrifugal pumps can be used. In areas where there are many septic tanks, there usually are persons with pumps and tank trucks to clean them.

The tank should not be completely cleaned. Some sludge should be left to "seed" the new raw solids that are deposited after operation is resumed.

4-13. Grease Traps. Grease traps or separators are not a necessity in the usual household system. In any case, drain lines conveying ground garbage should not pass through a grease trap. In large installations which include kitchens it may be advisable to install grease traps in the waste lines serving them. Figure 11-10 pictures a simple type. Others constructed of ceramic material are purchasable. A grease trap is of no value unless it is cleaned regularly, and this is seldom the case.

4-14. The Tile Disposal Field. This method of treating and disposing of septic-tank effluents, also known as the soil-absorption field, is frequently used where a sufficient area of suitable soil is available. It makes use of concrete or clay pipe laid with open joints so that the sewage can percolate into and through the soil. Filtration will remove suspended matter, and aerobic bacteria will stabilize organic matter, both suspended and dissolved. A favorable soil is permeable and naturally well drained. Heavy clay soils are unsuitable since they have little permeability. Limestone formations receiving sewage may endanger water supplies since they are frequently fissured and permit unfiltered sewage to enter springs or wells.

The absorption ability of the soil indicates the amount of water and organic matter that the soil can take. This should be determined by test. A test is made as follows: A hole is dug or bored to a depth of the proposed pipe trench. It may be bored with an earth auger anywhere from 4 to 12 in. in diameter. The 4-in. hole is satisfactory and requires less work and water. After the hole is bored, the bottom and sides of the hole are scratched with a sharp instrument to provide a natural soil surface for the water to enter. All loose earth is then removed, and 2 in. of coarse sand or fine gravel is placed in the bottom to protect it from scouring or clogging by sediment.

The hole is then filled with clear water to a depth of 12 in. over the

Table 4-5.   ABSORPTION-AREA REQUIREMENTS FOR PRIVATE RESIDENCES

Percolation rate (time required for water to fall 1 in.), min	Required absorption area per bedroom* for standard trench† and seepage pits,‡ sq ft	Percolation rate (time required for water to fall 1 in.), min	Required absorption area per bedroom* for standard trench† and seepage pits,‡ sq ft
1 or less	70	10	165
2	85	15	190
3	100	30§	250
4	115	45§	300
5	125	60§,¶	330

NOTE: Areas provide for garbage grinder and automatic-sequence washing machines.

* In every case, sufficient area should be provided for at least two bedrooms.

† Absorption area for standard trenches is figured as trench-bottom area.

‡ Absorption area for seepage pits is figured as effective sidewall area beneath the inlet.

§ Unsuitable for seepage pits if over 30.

¶ Unsuitable for tile disposal system if over 60.

SOURCE: Manual of Septic Tank Practice, *Public Health Service Pub.* 526.

gravel. If necessary, it is refilled so that water will remain in it for at least 4 hr and preferably overnight. This is to allow saturation of the soil and also swelling of the soil grains, which is the condition when the absorption field is operating. In very sandy soils swelling does not occur, and only saturation is needed.

If the water remains in the hole after the overnight period, the depth is adjusted to about 6 in. over the gravel, and after 30 min the drop in water level is measured. This drop is used to calculate the percolation rate, which is the time required for the water level to fall 1 in., expressed in minutes. Additional water may have to be added during the test. For example, if the water level drops 10 in. in 30 min, the percolation rate is 3 min/in. If no water remains overnight in the hole, clear water is added to bring the water level to about 6 in. over the gravel. The drop in water level is then measured at 30-min intervals for 4 hr, more water being added as necessary. The drop that occurs in the last 30 min is used to calculate the percolation rate. Table 4-5 shows the absorption area, in square feet, required on the bottom of disposal trenches for different percolation rates. In the absence of percolation tests, percolation areas provided per bedroom may vary from 50 sq ft for most favorable soils to 100 sq ft in average soils and 200 sq ft or more in heavy soils. In any case, a minimum of 150 sq ft should be provided for each individual dwelling unit.

Trenches have been made from 12 to 36 in. wide, and as indicated above, trench-bottom area is considered to be the absorption area. Therefore, a trench 18 in. wide and 50 ft long will provide 75 sq ft. The pipe

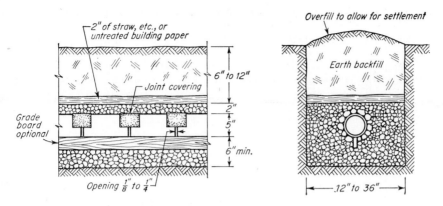

FIGURE 4-5   Absorption trench.

used may be 4-in. plain-ended agricultural drain tile in 12-in. lengths or clay or concrete sewer pipe in 2- or 3-ft lengths. Perforated pipe may be obtainable. Pipe is laid with 2 to 4 in. fall, with a maximum of 6 in. per 100 ft. Use of a grade board, as shown in Fig. 4-5, will facilitate obtaining the desired grade, particularly when plain-ended pipe is used. Pipes are laid with a gap about ¼ in. between joints. The upper half of such a joint should be protected with a piece of tar paper, or a combined spacer and cover made of plastic can be used. Individual laterals or branches should preferably not be more than 60 ft long and never more than 100 ft.

Minimum distances between the center lines of the trenches are related to their widths as follows: 12 to 18 in. wide, 6 ft; 18 to 24 in. wide, 6.5 ft; 24 to 30 in. wide, 7 ft; and 30 to 36 in. wide, 7.5 ft.

The pipe is surrounded with a fill of clean gravel, crushed stone, or broken brick ranging in size from ½ to 2½ in. See Fig. 4-5. A layer of straw, hay, etc., 2 in. thick or untreated building paper should be placed over the fill before backfilling. This prevents the earth backfill from clogging the gravel or crushed stone. An impervious material is considered undesirable as it will prevent evapotranspiration from soil and grass above the trench. This probably adds efficiency to the system. From Fig. 4-5 it will be seen that the minimum depth of the trench will be about 19 in. and that widths are from 12 to 36 in.

4-15. Tile Layouts. Figure 4-6 shows pipe layouts for level and sloping grounds. Care must be taken that distribution to the various branches is as uniform as possible. This is accomplished by using a well-designed distribution box. During construction the outlet openings must be carefully placed on the same level, with their inverts (lowest points of inside pipe surfaces) 4 to 6 in. above the bottom of the box (Fig. 4-7). If it is desired to rest a portion of the bed, provision should be made for

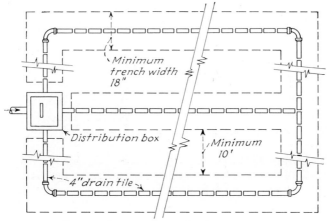

Disposal trench system for level ground

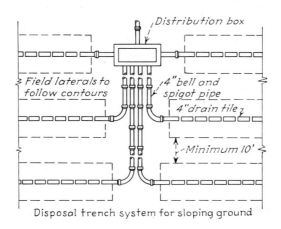

Disposal trench system for sloping ground

FIGURE 4-6 Disposal systems. (*Courtesy of Public Health Service.*)

closing the outlets of the diversion box. Temporary stoppage can be obtained by stuffing a sack of earth into the opening.

Series application of septic-tank effluent to a disposal field has been advocated for steeply sloping ground, where use of the standard trench system might result in overdosing of some parts of the system and pooling of sewage on the ground surface. Consideration should be given to this method wherever the fall of the ground surface exceeds 6 in. in any direction in the area to be utilized [4, 6]. Figure 4-8 shows a plan and section of such a layout. There is no distribution box unless separate systems are considered necessary, and all the sewage passes from one trench to another. Should the first trench become filled with sewage, it will overflow to the next lower trench through a pipe with tight joints.

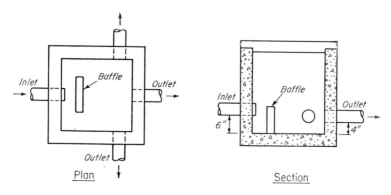

FIGURE 4-7   A distribution box.

As indicated, there should be a minimum of 6 ft of undisturbed earth between trenches. Absorption area required is determined in the same manner as for standard trenches. The bottom of each trench and its distribution line should have a relatively level grade. The invert of the overflow pipe in the first relief line must be at least 4 in. lower than the invert of the septic-tank outlet. There should be a minimum of 12 in. of ground cover, and the usual layer of straw, etc., should be placed between soil and filling medium. On very steeply sloping ground there is a possibility of surface erosion and a breakthrough or seepage from the trench to the ground surface. These troubles may occur if the ground surface has a fall greater than 1 vertical to 2 horizontal.

4-16. Seepage Pits. The seepage pit differs from the cesspool in that the latter usually receives untreated sewage. Seepage pits should not be used where there is a possibility of contaminating underground water supplies. Permission should be obtained from health authorities before they are used. They may be used alone or in combination with standard trench systems when it is feared that they will not function adequately. They are useful where the upper soil strata are impervious and these are underlain by pervious material. Determination of the absorptive capacity of a pit is rather difficult. It is done by digging a pit to the pervious material of sufficient diameter for entrance and then boring a test hole into the pervious material. The testing procedure described in Art. 4-14 is then followed. The absorption area is the vertical-wall area of the pit in the pervious material. In the excavation, care should be taken to avoid "smearing" or sealing of the earth sidewall. This difficulty can be reduced or avoided by keeping the blades of excavating machinery sharp. Pits excavated with bucket augers should be reamed with a cutting point extending from the edge of the bucket [7]. Pits are sometimes filled with rock larger than 2 in. in size, or they may be lined with bricks or concrete blocks laid without mortar. Where a lining is used, the bottom of the pit

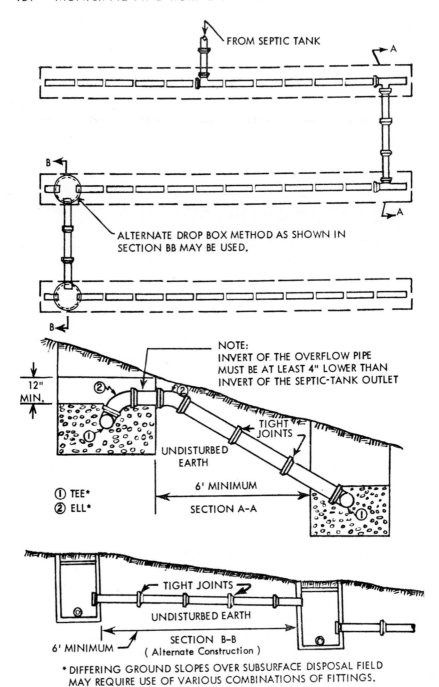

FROM SEPTIC TANK

ALTERNATE DROP BOX METHOD AS SHOWN IN
SECTION BB MAY BE USED.

12"
MIN.

NOTE:
INVERT OF THE OVERFLOW PIPE
MUST BE AT LEAST 4" LOWER THAN
INVERT OF THE SEPTIC-TANK OUTLET

TIGHT
JOINTS

UNDISTURBED
EARTH

6' MINIMUM

① TEE*
② ELL*

SECTION A-A

TIGHT JOINTS

UNDISTURBED EARTH

SECTION B-B
6' MINIMUM (Alternate Construction)

* DIFFERING GROUND SLOPES OVER SUBSURFACE DISPOSAL FIELD
MAY REQUIRE USE OF VARIOUS COMBINATIONS OF FITTINGS.

FIGURE 4-8 Series type of distribution system. (*From Manual of Septic Tank Practice, Public Health Service Pub. 526.*)

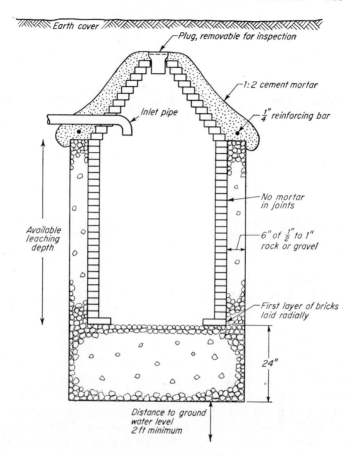

Earth cover

Plug, removable for inspection

1:2 cement mortar

Inlet pipe

$\frac{1}{4}''$ reinforcing bar

No mortar in joints

6" of $\frac{1}{2}''$ to 1" rock or gravel

Available leaching depth

First layer of bricks laid radially

24"

Distance to ground water level 2 ft minimum

FIGURE 4-9 Section of a seepage pit. (*From Manual of Septic Tank Practice, Public Health Service Pub. 526.*)

should first be filled with 24 in. of gravel or crushed rock to provide a foundation. A fill of crushed rock or coarse gravel should be placed between the lining and the sidewall (Fig. 4-9). If more than one seepage pit is required, a distribution box will be needed. Spacing between pits should be at least equal to three times the pit diameter, and if the pits are over 20 ft deep, the spacing should be at least 20 ft.

4-17. Causes of Disposal-field Failures. Failures have occurred in many tile disposal systems. They are usually indicated by appearance of sewage on the ground surface. In some cases they are caused by accumulations in the distribution tile of sludge from a septic tank that requires cleaning, and in other cases the trouble may be ascribed to an unfavorable soil. There have been failures, however, where absorption tests indicated favorable soils and the absorption areas required were provided. Such failures have stimulated investigation of the absorption test and its limitations [14].

The principal weaknesses of the absorption test are that it is made in a short time and with clear water. It should be recognized that two processes take place during the test—infiltration, or entrance of the liquid into the soil, and percolation through the soil. The infiltration rate is largely dependent upon the characteristics of the liquid, while speed of percolation depends upon the soil characteristics.

When clear water is applied continuously to a soil, there is first a drop in the infiltration rate for 1 to several days. As air escapes from the soil, the rate rises to a maximum after a time measured in days, and thereafter it slowly decreases to a small percentage of the original rate. The slow decrease is caused by the following phenomena, which are dependent upon soil characteristics: migration of fine particles with water movement to accumulate and clog pore spaces; ion exchange, which affects the cohesive force between particles and deflocculates materials; and the continued swelling of colloidal materials. Even with water as the liquid, there will be microbial growths that will clog soil pores and interfere with infiltration and percolation. Obviously, substitution of septic sewage for water will increase the number of fine particles and will encourage microbial growth. Ion exchange and colloidal swelling will depend upon the chemical activity of the soil. So far no soil test or examination method has been devised that will indicate the suitability of a soil for absorption of sewage over a long period. It is apparent, however, that a soil composed of sand or gravel, which are inert chemically, would be affected only by the fine particles and microbial accumulations.

In the absence of a more effective procedure than the absorption test, precautions should be applied that will prevent disposal-field failures or at least postpone them for a long period. Important is resting, which permits air penetration, the establishment of aerobic conditions in clogged areas, and digestion of solid accumulations. With food no longer available, the bacteria will also die. This housecleaning requires days, not the hours that will be provided by the usual sewage-flow variations of a residence. Aerobic action cannot be expected if the soil is continuously saturated by capillary action, and this may occur if the soil is within 3 ft of the water table. Of course, anaerobic digestion would continue in the absence of oxygen until bacterial food was used up during a resting period and thus would help to restore some of the absorptive capacity of the soil.

Results of the absorption test have been used to determine areas of trench bottoms. Observations indicate that the infiltration into the sides of the trenches is more important than has been recognized. The trench bottom soon becomes clogged, and its absorptive power is greatly reduced. The greater efficiency of the sidewalls is ascribed to the better filtering effect of the gravel as the sewage moves laterally through it toward the soil and to the varying level of the saturated soil as sewage discharge into the system varies. Clogging can be expected to occur, but it should be greatly delayed. This situation is exemplified by the seepage pit, in which the bottom is neglected in considering the absorption area. There will be fluctuations in sewage level with a gradual permanent rise until overflow occurs. This would require construction of a new pit.

Certain precautions should be taken to promote infiltration into the soil and prevent or postpone failure. These are:

1. Fine gravel, preferably not larger than ¼ in., should be in contact with the soil surface. Larger material not only has less filtering capacity but also seals off more soil surface. An inch or more of coarse sand between the gravel and the soil would be highly desirable but would add to the cost of construction.

2. Construction methods should avoid "smearing" of the trench walls, which would reduce their absorptive capacity.

3. Resting periods should be provided. Siphon chambers will be of some small value. The disposal field could be divided into two sections with a distribution box that will allow diversion of flow at intervals of 1 or 2 weeks.

The conclusion that must be drawn from the contemplation of the potential difficulties of sewage disposal fields is that they are suitable for city lots. An engineer should exert all possible pressure for sewer systems in real estate developments, and if for political or other reasons he is overruled, he should see that the systems are carefully designed and constructed.

4-18. Subsurface Sand Filters. *The underdrained sand-filter trench* may be used where soils are impermeable, where there is head available to permit discharge of effluent from the underdrains, and where there is a suitable watercourse into which the effluent can be discharged. Figure 4-10 shows the arrangement of distributor pipes, sand, and underdrain pipes. Preferably the distributor pipes should be perforated but the underdrain pipes may be of the bell-and-spigot type, laid with open joints. Distributors should be laid on a grade of about 0.5 per cent, and the underdrains at 0.5 to 1.0 per cent. The trenches should not be less than 10 ft apart. Table 4-6 gives dosing rates per bedroom.

Fine sands will soon clog and require replacement. A coarse sand should be used, preferably with an effective size between 0.4 and 0.6 mm and a uniformity coefficient of not over 4.0 (Art. 2-17). Since it is frequently difficult to obtain sand as coarse as that specified, effective sizes as small as 0.25 mm may be used. The sand should be settled by flooding or otherwise before the distributors are placed. The coarse crushed stone or gravel should pass a 2½-in. screen and be retained on a

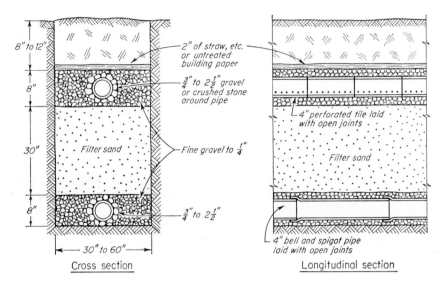

FIGURE 4-10   Underdrained sand-filter trench.

¾-in. screen. It is placed around the pipes. Fine gravel down to ¼ in. in size may be used above and around the coarse material. Table 4-6 shows area requirements.

Sand-filter trenches are not economical for large installations. The *subsurface sand filter* should then be used. A rough guide is that the subsurface sand filters should be used when the total length of the distributors requires the use of a dosing siphon (Art. 4-10), or about 500 ft. The subsurface sand filter is a bed filled with sand. The sand used for filtration and the gravel or crushed rock used for distribution and drainage are as specified for sand-filter trenches. Plan and section of a system are shown in Fig. 4-11. Dosing tanks should be provided when the total area exceeds 800 sq ft and the total length of the distributors exceeds

Table 4-6. LOADING RATES FOR SUBSURFACE SAND FILTERS

Type of service	Area requirements		
	Sq ft per bedroom	Gal per acre per day	Gal per sq ft per day
Without garbage grinder or automatic washer . .	150	50,000	1.15
With garbage grinder	180	41,500	0.95
With automatic washer	200	50,000	1.15
With both garbage grinder and automatic washer . .	240	41,500	0.95

SOURCE: Manual of Septic Tank Practice, *Public Health Service Pub.* 526.

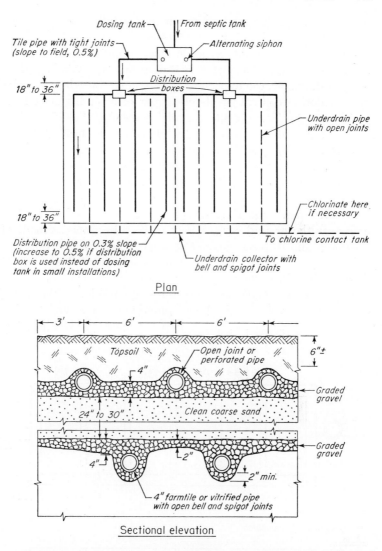

FIGURE 4-11   Subsurface sand filter, plan and section. (*From Manual of Septic Tank Practice, Public Health Service Pub. 526.*)

300 ft. If the distributor system has over 1,000 ft of distributors it is advisable to provide two or more sections of bed, each dosed by a separate siphon. Table 4-6 gives dosing rates per bedroom.

The effluent of subsurface filters that are properly designed and operated will be clear and odorless. Most of the bacteria will have been removed, but some pathogenic organisms may remain. For safety, the effluent should be *chlorinated.* The usual dosage of sand-filter effluents is about 6 mg/l (ppm) to obtain a residual (Arts. 2-18 and 2-19) of 0.5

to 1.0 mg/l. This dosage amounts to about 0.5 lb of available chlorine per 10,000 gal, or less than 1 oz per 1,000 gal.

Chlorine gas is obtainable in steel cylinders and is fed through an apparatus called a chlorinator. It is used principally in large installations. Small installations use hypochlorite of lime (or bleaching powder), which has a chlorine content of about 35 per cent, or high-test hypochlorite, which contains 70 per cent of available chlorine. Solutions of these compounds are made and fed into the effluent to be treated just ahead of a contact tank. The health departments of most states require a contact period of about 15 min to ensure destruction of disease organisms. Figure 4-12 shows a contact tank baffled to ensure mixing of the chlorine and effluent.

4-19. Open Sand Filters. The occurrence of a high water table or rock near the ground surface may make subsurface methods of sewage treatment and disposal difficult or impossible. The solution, particularly for large installations, may be open sand filters. These are the intermittent sand filters described in Art. 4-25.

4-20. Sewage Collection. For the single residence, the sewage-collection system consists of the house plumbing system and the building or house sewer, which discharges into the septic tank. Plumbing systems

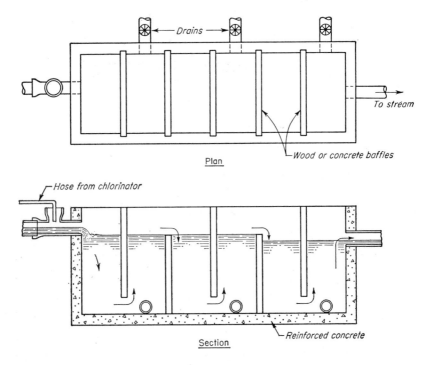

FIGURE 4-12 Contact tank for chlorine disinfection.

are discussed in Chap. 11, and building sewers in Art. 11-10. In large installations, such as institutions or hospitals, there may be separate buildings, each requiring its own building sewer. Sizes of these sewers can be arrived at by determining the fixture units served and providing house sewer size and grade as needed. Table 11-3 gives fixture-unit values of various plumbing fixtures, and Table 11-4 gives the sizes and grades of sewers needed.

Municipal Sewage Treatment and Disposal

4-21. The principles that have been discussed in connection with residential sewage treatment are also applied by municipalities. The differences are due to the larger volumes of sewage treated and the greater size of the plants required. Wastes from industrial establishments create problems in municipal sewage treatment plants. Also, more complicated methods are applicable because of the continuous and more expert attention that may be expected. The information given here is designed to aid operators of small municipal sewage treatment plants. Additional information on design and operation of sewage treatment plants and the significance of sewage tests will be found in books listed in the bibliography.

4-22. Dilution. Sewage disposal by dilution has been used to a considerable extent by cities, particularly by those situated on the seacoast, large rivers, and the Great Lakes. As populations have increased, the volumes of sewage requiring disposal have reached the point that treatment is necessary where dilution alone was formerly sufficient. Large volumes of water are required to dispose of raw sewage without offensive conditions. In general, twenty to forty times as much water as sewage is needed. Even with this volume of water available, however, other conditions in a stream or along a seacoast, such as currents and depth, must be considered in order to prevent nuisances or hazards in some areas.

The dilution available affects the amount of treatment which must be given to the sewage. A city situated near a large river may be required by the state or Federal authorities to provide screening or sedimentation of the sewage, at least. If little dilution can be obtained, very complete treatment may be necessary. Also governing completeness of treatment is the necessity for protecting existing water supplies, bathing beaches, and shellfish beds.

4-23. Preliminary Treatment. Sewage frequently contains sand and other inorganic matter which should be removed before it is given further treatment. This is particularly true if the sewer system also receives storm water. The sewage, therefore, is passed through grit chambers, enlargements of channels in which the velocity is decreased sufficiently so that the heavy inorganic materials will settle, with the

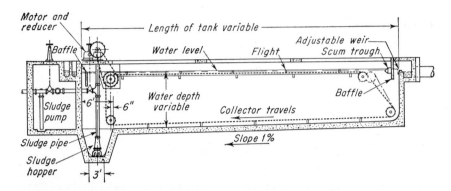

FIGURE 4-13 Link-belt straight-line sludge collector. (*From E. W. Steel, "Water Supply and Sewerage," 4th ed., McGraw-Hill Book Company, New York, 1960.*)

lighter organic matter remaining in suspension. Usually there are at least two grit chambers arranged so that the sewage flow can be diverted from one to the other. This permits removal of the grit when a chamber needs cleaning. In small sewage treatment plants, the grit is shoveled by hand from the chamber to wheelbarrows and is used to fill lowlands around the plant. A well-designed grit chamber should produce grit relatively free from organic matter. Cleaning is likely to be needed immediately after or even during a rainstorm; hence, the operator should be prepared to start cleaning operations promptly to prevent accumulation of grit throughout his plant. Apparatus for cleaning grit chambers mechanically, either intermittently or continuously, is used at some plants.

It is also necessary to remove sticks, rags, and other large floating materials which otherwise would form large amounts of scum on the sedimentation tank or clog the pumps. This is done by means of screens, usually constructed of iron bars with 1-in. or larger clear openings between them. Such screens need frequent cleaning, or they will clog and cause the sewage to overflow. The cleaning is done by means of rakes, and to facilitate this process the screen is placed at an angle of about 30 deg to the bottom of the conduit and in such a manner that the openings allow an upward stroke of the rake. Large plants employ automatically cleaned screens. The screenings contain much water and are very offensive. They are sometimes allowed to drain for a time on a platform over the conduit. A liberal application of lime will prevent odors during this period. At small plants the screenings are usually buried.

4-24. Sedimentation of Sewage. Sedimentation consists in allowing sewage to run through a tank of such size that the velocity is low. This process has been universally used either as a preliminary treatment or as

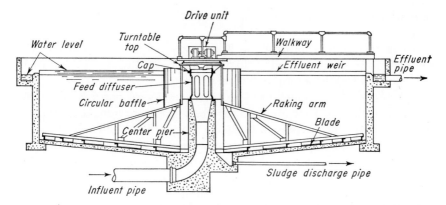

FIGURE 4-14 Dorr-Oliver sludge collector used in circular sedimentation tanks. (*From E. W. Steel, "Water Supply and Sewerage," 4th ed., McGraw-Hill Book Company, New York, 1960.*)

the only treatment if a large body of water is available for final disposal. The tanks operate continuously, and the retention period of the sewage may be from 30 min to 3 hr, depending upon the character of the sewage and the further treatment to be given. The sludge may be removed continuously with the aid of mechanical contrivances or drawn off at intervals from hoppers in the bottom. Septic and Imhoff tanks are special kinds of sedimentation tanks.

Plain sedimentation with separate sludge digestion is much used in present practice. The tanks may be rectangular or circular. They are usually constructed with slowly moving mechanisms having plows or blades which push the settled sludge to a hopper at the center or at one end of the tank. The sludge-moving mechanism may operate continuously or intermittently, as the operator deems necessary. Skimmers to remove the scum and discharge it to the sludge are usually included. The sludge may run by gravity or, more likely, may be pumped to a separate tank for digestion. The duties of the operator of a tank of this type are simple. He should see that the mechanism is operating properly and that he is withdrawing sludge frequently enough. Stale sludge on the tank bottom tends to rise and leave with the tank effluent. On the other hand, care should be taken that sludge pumping is stopped when there is no more sludge in the tank, for it is highly undesirable to pump a large volume of sewage to the sludge-digestion tank. Figures 4-13 and 4-14 illustrate two types of sludge-collection mechanisms.

Chemical precipitation of sewage is also used. In this method certain chemicals are added to the sewage before it enters the sedimentation tank. The chemicals have the property of forming a heavy gelatinous floc which settles rapidly, carrying with it most of the suspended solids of the sewage. Lime, alum, ferrous sulfate, and particularly ferric chloride are used. Lime is used principally to add alkalinity to the sewage. Chemical precipitation has the advantage of greatly increasing the efficiency of sedimentation, but it is costly, requires careful chemical control, and produces a bulky sludge. This method is used for treatment of industrial wastes but rarely by cities.

Septic tanks are much used for single residences but rarely by cities, even of small size. They are used for treating sewage from country clubs, rural schools, and public institutions. For such installations they are usually designed for a sewage-retention period of 8 to 12 hr, and with sludge-retention capacities of 2 to 3 cu ft per capita. Such tanks should be designed with hopper bottoms and pipes leading from them to allow easy withdrawal of sludge, or the sludge may be removed with a diaphragm pump. Partial withdrawal of the sludge, say, at 4- or 6-month intervals, is more desirable than complete emptying. The raw sludge may be "seeded" by leaving some sludge, thus encouraging rapid digestion of the new raw solids.

The Imhoff tank, which gained its name from its inventor, Karl Imhoff, of Germany, has been widely used. This tank is a variation of the septic tank. Two chambers are provided: the upper, or flow, chamber, through which the sewage passes at a very low velocity; and the lower, or sludge, chamber, in which anaerobic decomposition takes place. The solids of the sewage settle to the bottom of the upper chamber, which has sloping bottom walls. At the lowest point of the flow chamber is a slot through which the settled solids fall into the lower chamber. The slot is overlapped or trapped in such a way that gases generated in the sludge chamber cannot enter the flow chamber. A gas vent, also known as a scum chamber, is connected with the sludge chamber. The retention period in the upper chamber is short, usually about 2 hr. The capacity of the lower chamber is such that 2 to more than 3 cu ft is provided for each person contributing sewage. Northern climates require the greater digestion space because of their lower mean annual temperatures.

Nuisance is sometimes caused at the gas vents by a black foam, which may reach such proportions as to spill over into the flow chamber. The foam is sometimes accompanied by very offensive odors. The odors can usually be reduced by placing lime in the gas vents, although this procedure may not stop the foaming. From 5 to 10 lb of hydrated lime per 1,000 persons should be added daily until improvement is noted. This may require several weeks. Permanent improvement may be obtained by drawing off some of the sludge and using a hose to run water into the gas vents. Dumping well-rotted horse manure into the gas vents has resulted in improvement in some cases. This should also be done if the tank is completely emptied.

The sludge from the Imhoff tank is drawn off at intervals of from 1 month to 6 weeks. Only the lower layers which have completely decom-

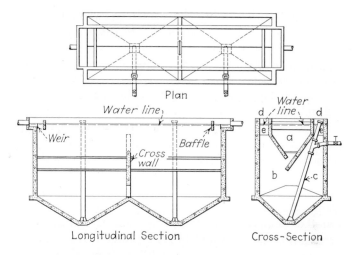

FIGURE 4-15   Plan and sections of an Imhoff tank. (*a*) Sedimentation chamber; (*b*) sludge-digestion chamber; (*c*) sludge-withdrawal pipe, (*d*) gas chamber; (*e*) scum chambers.

posed are drawn, however, some sludge being left to keep the tank seeded with anaerobic bacteria. The tank operator should remove all scum at least once a day from the sedimentation chamber. Disposal of the scum is most conveniently accomplished by placing it into the gas vents. The gas vents should be vigorously agitated daily by means of a wooden T-shaped contrivance to push down partially dried scum and release gas which is keeping it at the gas-vent surface. If this is not done, a heavy and deep plug of scum may form at the gas vents which will be difficult to remove. Careful attention to the operation details given here will increase efficiency of the plant and minimize odors.

4-25. Filtration. The treatment measures heretofore described reduce the oxygen required by the sewage to bring about stability, but the remaining demand must be satisfied to a large extent, or nuisance will result. The sewage filters described here are not true filters and provide little or no straining action. Primarily they serve two functions: to provide oxygen from the air and to provide surfaces where certain types of bacteria, the aerobes, can live and use that oxygen to oxidize the putrescible matter in the sewage to stable and inoffensive compounds, including nitrates and sulfates (see Fig. 4-2). Filters are frequently employed to accomplish this, and the two general types that are in use will be briefly described.

The *intermittent sand filter* consists of a layer of sand, not less than 30 in. deep, with underdrains, surrounded by gravel, to carry off the effluent. The settled sewage is applied by means of a dosing tank and siphon which discharges into troughs on the beds. The troughs have side openings which allow the sewage to flow on the sand, and blocks are placed under each sewage stream to prevent sand disturbance. After being applied to the filter for 24 hr, the sewage is switched to a second bed while the first bed rests. Usually three beds are worked in rotation. Intermittent sand filters must be dosed rather lightly, only 100,000 gal/(acre)(day) (considering the total acreage of the three beds; *i.e.*, beds totaling 3 acres could care for 300,000 gal/day), but the effluent is better in quality than that resulting from any other type of treatment. The operator must be careful to see that dosing is properly done and that the beds are rotated. During the resting period, he should sweep or scrape off the dried sludge which accumulates on the sand surface. It may be advisable to rake the sand surface occasionally. In the Northern states, where beds may freeze, the sand surface is raked into furrows leading from the dosing trough. Ice will form on the sewage surface between the furrows. This remains and forms a protective covering over the channel between the ridges. The principal field of use for this filter is for institutions, large hotels, etc.

Trickling filters are constructed of crushed stone or gravel of varying size placed in beds of varying depth. The sewage is applied to the bed surface, allowed to trickle over the stones, and collected in underdrains in the bed bottom. The oldest method of application is by means of sprays located at the surface of the bed. The sprays are operated intermittently by means of a dosing tank and siphon. A more favored method, now in general use, employs rotary distributors. The rotary distributor consists of two or more arms which are turned in a horizontal plane by the sewage as it escapes from orifices to fall on the bed. During the percolation through the bed, the sewage comes into contact with the bacterial film which has accumulated on the stones. The film is rather complicated biologically. Aerobic bacteria are the most important inhabitants, but there are also protozoa, algae, and, in the thicker portions, worms of various species. Organisms other than bacteria are of less importance than the aerobic bacteria, which reduce putrescibility by their oxidizing action. The film absorbs solids which are worked upon by the organisms, after which they are released as a coagulated suspended material which is rather heavy and settles readily. A settling tank is provided to remove these solids before the effluent is discharged into a stream or otherwise disposed of.

Trickling filters are of two types: conventional, or standard, and high-rate, sometimes known as biofilters or aerofilters. In both types the sewage is first passed through a sedimentation tank, frequently called a primary tank. In the standard filter the bed is usually not less than 5 ft deep, and the filter medium is crushed stone or gravel. A very commonly used size is 2½ to 3½ in., although 1½ to 2½ in. has been used. The dosing rate, or loading, is sometimes expressed as 2 to 4 million

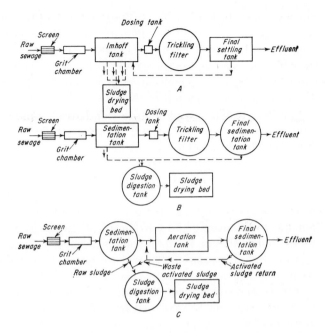

FIGURE 4-16   Flow diagrams of sewage treatment plants.
(A) Imhoff tank and trickling filters; (B) sedimentation,
separate sludge digestion, and trickling filter; (C) activated sludge. Dashed lines show path of sludge.

gal/(acre)(day), with 2 to 2.5 million most common. A more logical
method of expressing loading is in pounds of 5-day biochemical oxygen
demand per acre-foot of filter medium. State health departments specify
limits for this, and they vary from 250 to 600 lb/acre-ft.[1]

The high-rate filters are loaded much more heavily—from 2,000 to
5,000 lb of biochemical oxygen demand per acre-foot, with 3,000 most
commonly used. The sewage loads are from 10 to 30 million gal/(acre)
(day), including any recirculated sewage. Filter media tend to be
larger than for standard filters, at least 2½ to 3½ in. and in some
cases 3 to 4 in. Standard filter depths are usually less than those of the
high-rate type. An important feature of the high-rate filter is the
recirculation of sewage through the filter. Various recirculation schemes
are used. A part of the filter effluent may be pumped back to the primary
sedimentation tank to pass through it and the filter again, or effluent from
the final tank may be pumped back to the entrance to the filter. Recirculation improves results by giving longer contact with the organic film
on the stones, but the passage of a large volume of water through the

---

[1] An acre-foot is a volume equal to an acre of area 1 ft thick, or 43,560 cu ft,
or 1,613 cu yd.

filter washes off film before nitrification has had time to take place. Consequently, high-rate filter effluents may show good oxygen-demand reductions but little or no nitrification. Reduction of oxygen demand is by far the more important as far as quality of the effluent is concerned. Results of single-stage high-rate filtration, as described, are not as good as those of the standard filter.

Where results comparable to standard filters are desired, two high-rate filters are constructed and operated in series, sometimes with an intermediate sedimentation tank between them. Again, various recirculation schemes are used, the most common being to return part of the effluent from each filter to the influent of the same filter. The amount of sewage recirculated varies in different plants, the most widely used being a 1:1 recirculation, which means the recirculated sewage is equal in amount to the average flow to the plant. Loadings, where two filters are used, are based upon the total volume of filter medium.

Multiple high-rate filters, when properly designed and operated, can frequently accomplish results comparable to standard filters, at smaller first cost and with negligible addition to operating cost. In general, trickling filters can be designed to meet the sewage treatment needs for any situation. They are particularly well adapted to small installations because of their ability to take shock loads and their relative freedom from operating difficulty.

Sedimentation tanks generally have sludge-moving mechanisms and present no operating difficulties. Sludge and recirculation pumps will require attention. The devices used to apply the sewage to the filters, fixed sprays or rotating pipes, have nozzles or openings which clog and require cleaning. Should sewage stand on the bed or "pond," breaking the bed surface with a pick will remedy matters, although such a condition on a standard filter may indicate overloading. A small gray fly (*Psychoda*) sometimes breeds in filters in such numbers as to be a nuisance. A method of controlling them is to close the bed underdrain for 24 hr at intervals of a week or two. This floods the bed and drowns the fly larvae. Adults can be controlled by spraying resting places with DDT—a 5 per cent solution, emulsion, or suspension—at the rate of 1 qt per 250 sq ft.

4-26. Activated Sludge. This method is used by both large and small cities but has been favored by the former. Sludge which has been aerated and thereby "activated" with aerobic bacteria is added to the settled sewage that is to be treated. The mixture of activated sludge and sewage is thoroughly agitated by compressed air, which is applied through porous diffusers, jets, or otherwise at the bottom of the tank. At some plants mechanical methods, such as paddle wheels or impellers, are used to agitate the sewage-sludge mixture so that air will be absorbed from the atmosphere. The sludge, in its movement around in the sewage,

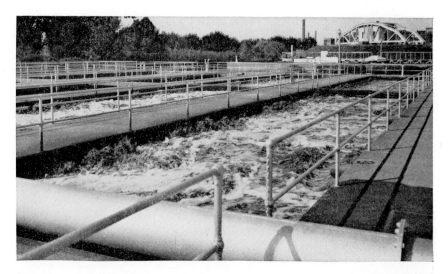

FIGURE 4-17   Activated sludge plant at Peoria, Ill. Diffused air is employed for aeration. (*Courtesy of Pacific Flush Tank Company and Public Works Magazine.*)

together with the air, accomplishes the treatment. The solids in the sewage themselves coagulate into more sludge, leaving the liquid in a fairly well-nitrified condition. The sewage-sludge mixture is then allowed to settle, and the clear liquid is drawn off and discharged. Some of the sludge is retained for aeration and future addition to incoming sewage, while the balance must be disposed of by digestion or some other means. This system has the advantages of having a low first cost, being very flexible in its action, and giving a good effluent. The disadvantages are the skilled attention necessary, the high operating cost, and the large amounts of sludge which are produced and which must be disposed of.

The activated-sludge plant requires considerable attention on the part of the operator. He must ascertain the proportion of sludge which must be retained in the sewage-sludge mixture to obtain best results and so manipulate sludge wastage that this proportion is held. This is most easily done by taking a sample of the mixed liquid at the mid-point of the aeration tank in a liter graduate, allowing it to settle for 30 min, and noting the amount of sludge. About 20 per cent is commonly found to be desirable. An occasional trouble at activated-sludge plants is sludge bulking. This is characterized by a light, fluffy sludge which will not settle normally in the secondary sedimentation tanks. The condition may be due to various causes, such as underaeration; overaeration; the presence of certain industrial wastes, especially those containing sugar or starch; or the presence of a filamentous fungus (*Sphaerotilus*) in the sludge, although this may be an effect rather than a cause. Chlorination of the sewage or the use of lime to obtain a pH of 8 or more will help reduce

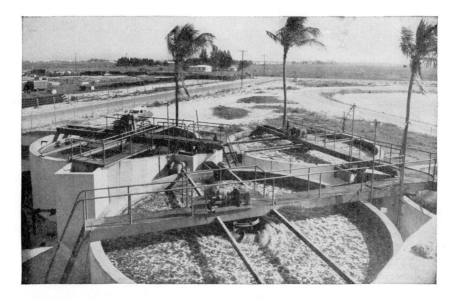

FIGURE 4-18   Activated-sludge plant at Carol City, Fla. Mechanical aeration is used. (*Courtesy of Yeomans Brothers Co. and Public Works Magazine.*)

fungi. Underaeration can be remedied by using more air or, if this is not possible, by reducing the volume of sludge in the sewage-sludge mixture or bypassing the sludge around the aerating tank for a time until the sludge recovers. If injurious, industrial wastes may have to be eliminated from the sewage or perhaps treated at the industrial plant.

Modifications of the activated-sludge process are in use under various names. Usually the variations relate to the length of the aeration period, points of application of the compressed air, etc. Extended aeration [13] is being used to a considerable extent for such small installations as shopping centers, suburban communities, etc. In this type of plant, screened but not settled sewage is given a 24-hr aeration period followed by sedimentation, and all sludge is returned to the aeration tank. Little or no excess sludge is produced.

Another method of treatment which uses compressed air is contact aeration. In this type of plant, settled sewage is applied to a tank in which asbestos-cement sheets are suspended vertically. Compressed air is applied at the bottom of the tank to bubble up between the sheets, on which an active biological film has established itself. Sedimentation of the aeration-tank effluent is needed to remove film which is washed off the plate surfaces.

For small installations, commercial firms fabricate and sell "package plants." They usually operate on the activated-sludge or contact-aeration principle and include tanks for sedimentation, aeration, and sludge digestion and necessary piping, pumps, and air compressors. Tanks are usually of steel. The buyer needs to furnish only the site, including room for a sludge-drying bed. Package plants have given satisfactory service for hotels, motels, schools, and suburban communities. The plants should, of course, be approved by the state health department. The prospective buyer should consult an engineer before choosing a plant.

4-27. Stabilization Ponds. These are sometimes called oxidation ponds. If sewage is retained in a pond or a lagoon for a sufficient time, its biochemical oxygen demand will be satisfied in large part, and it will cease to be putrescible. This change is effected by aerobic bacteria, which use oxygen dissolved in the liquid from the atmosphere, and from the work of algae. They are active in sunlight and break down the carbon dioxide, which is produced during the carbon cycle from the carbohydrates, and they release the oxygen into the water. Settled sewage is generally applied to ponds, and 1 acre of pond area is commonly provided for each 50 lb of oxygen demand that must be satisfied each day. As an example: A sewage flow is 200,000 gal/day, and its biochemical oxygen demand after sedimentation is 110 ppm. The pounds of oxygen demand to be satisfied daily will be $(200,000 \times 8.34 \times 110) \div 1,000,000$, or 183 lb. (*Note:* 1 gal of water weighs 8.34 lb.) This weight of oxygen demand would require 3.66 acres. A rough method of approximation is 1,000 persons to 1 acre of pond area.

Oxidation ponds are constructed by building embankments of earth; more than one, operating in parallel or series, may be used. They must be properly designed. Shallow ponds permit penetration of sunlight to all parts of the sewage and thus encourage algae growth. On the other hand, rooted aquatic plants may then cause trouble and encourage mosquito breeding. A compromise is a depth of 3 ft. It is usual to discharge influent to the middle of a pond so that wind currents will cause some mixing; otherwise a concentration of influent sewage may result in odors. At some plants influent points may be changed to prevent such concentration.

Operation is simple and consists in little more than changing the sewage-entrance point, if this is possible and desirable; the removal of weeds which may grow on the embankments at the water edge; and mosquito control. Mosquitoes should give no trouble if marginal weeds are absent, but if they develop, the methods described in Chap. 9 can be applied. Effluents can be used for irrigation or discharged into streams.

4-28. Disinfection. Since the methods of sewage treatment described cannot be depended upon to eliminate all disease bacteria from sewage, the state health departments require that sewage be disinfected before it is discharged into a body of water which is used for bathing or other recreation or for a water supply. The action and use of the various forms of chlorine in purifying water are described in Art. 2-18, and a similar method is used in disinfecting sewage, except that larger doses are required because the larger amounts of organic matter in sewage tend to neutralize the chlorine. Chlorine residuals are not generally obtained, and dosages may be regulated by reductions in coliform organisms or total count. A 99.9 per cent reduction in coliforms, for example, may be considered to have eliminated the less resistant disease bacteria. Recommended dosages in parts per million by weight are as follows: sewage which has been settled only, including Imhoff-tank effluent, 10 or more; trickling filter effluent, 3 to 7; intermittent-sand-filter effluent, 2; and activated-sludge effluent, 5. A contact period provided by a contact tank (Fig. 4-12) or otherwise is necessary.

4-29. Sludge Disposal. In Art. 4-8, anaerobic sludge decomposition or digestion in septic tanks was briefly described. In Imhoff tanks and separate sludge-digestion tanks, a similar process takes place. Speedy digestion is desirable, and this is obtained when the sludge temperature is fairly high (100°F) and when the acidity and alkalinity of the sludge are in proper balance—in other words, when the sludge is slightly on the alkaline side. Some digestion tanks are heated by means of pipe coils circulating hot water, while the slight alkalinity is retained by a proper relation between the amount of the incoming raw sludge and the amount of the well-digested sludge already in the tank. To ensure adequate capacity, tanks should be designed so that 2 to 6 cu ft is allowed per person served. It is important that engineering studies be made in each case to determine the proper design figure. The operator must not, however, draw off too much well-digested sludge at one time, or the balance will be upset, with resultant odors and foaming. The separate digestion tank presents another problem. As sludge is pumped into it, an equal amount of liquid, known as supernatant liquid, is displaced and overflows. This is much clearer than the sludge, but it is very strong and will make trouble in a stream. It is usually returned to the plant with the raw sewage, but even there it places a heavy burden on the plant. Its volume should be kept as small as possible by careful control of sludge pumping.

The digested sludge is usually placed on beds of sand for drying. It dries into a dark-brown porous material, which is used for fertilizing or filling low places. The sludge which is produced by the activated-sludge treatment, unless it is digested, does not dry well on beds. If land is available, the sludge is sometimes discharged into lagoons or into low areas, where it forms a pond. Through vacuum filtration and chemical treatment, the sludge may be readily dewatered, and advantage may be taken of its fertilizing value, which is much higher than that of the sludge produced by other processes. When dried, it can be sold to commercial fertilizer manufacturers.

The gas produced by digesting sludge is normally composed of about 65 per cent methane, 30 per cent carbon dioxide, and the rest hydrogen and nitrogen. It resembles natural gas and can be used as fuel. Since about 0.6 cu ft is produced per day per person contributing sewage, the amount is considerable, and at some municipal sewage treatment plants the gas is used for operating engines or, more often, for heating the sludge to promote quick digestion.

4-30. Irrigation. One of the earliest methods of disposal of sewage was to apply it to the land in intermittent doses, thereby taking advantage of the capacity of the soil for mineralizing nitrogenous material. This, however, requires a large area of porous, open soil to take care of large amounts of sewage. Crops such as hay or other cattle feed have been raised on land so treated. The growing of vegetables for human consumption in this manner is discouraged by health authorities.

While this means of sewage disposal is no longer a major method of treatment, it is being used to a considerable extent in the western part of the United States, where the rainfall is light and water is comparatively scarce. The sewage is applied in the same manner as irrigation water. The sewage has some nitrogenous elements which are useful as plant food, but they are present in such small amounts that they are of little consequence. The value of sewage in irrigation for cropping lies in its moisture content, not in its organic constituents. Application to the land must be carefully supervised, or nuisances may result. It should be emphasized that irrigation with sewage is primarily a disposal method, and in some cities no soil cultivation or crop raising is practiced.

4-31. What Can Be Expected of Sewage Treatment. Sewage treatment has several purposes: (1) to render the sewage inoffensive as far as nuisances are concerned; (2) to prevent destruction of fish and other wildlife; and (3) to reduce or eliminate the danger of contaminating water supplies, bathing areas, and shellfish. Insofar as these ends are accomplished, stream pollution is prevented. There are several factors which enter into a solution of the problem: (1) bodies of water which receive sewage, raw or treated, have a capacity for self-purification; (2) water which is to be used for public purposes will usually require treatment of some sort if it is derived from surface sources, and such treatment can take care of a considerable degree of pollution; and (3) cost of sewage treatment and water treatment must be kept at a reasonable figure, and degree of treatment directly affects cost.

A decision as to the amount of treatment a sewage will require calls for competent sanitary engineering judgment. State health department requirements must be satisfied, and these are based upon engineering knowledge. Such requirements, however, are subject to modification according to the situation. The preceding articles have indicated that there are many methods of sewage treatment, and various combinations of them will produce results that the engineer can predict with as much accuracy as is needful. He can also predict, after appropriate studies, the self-purifying capacities of a stream and its possible sanitary hazards. He can, therefore, prescribe sewage treatment that will meet the existing situation at a minimum cost. Accordingly, some sewage treatment plants provide screening only to remove large floating matter which might be unsightly in a ship channel or outer harbor. Others, which discharge into large rivers, may provide only sedimentation, with or without disinfection. Still others give full treatment, which includes sedimentation, then one of the oxidizing treatments, such as filtration or activated sludge, and disinfection.

Just as important as good engineering in plant planning and design is adequate operation of the plant. The skill and technical knowledge required will depend upon the size and complexity of the plant, but even the smallest plant deserves an operator who is conscientious and who has some knowledge of the principles of sewage treatment; otherwise the public investment in the plant will be largely wasted.

4-32. Industrial Wastes. Liquid wastes produced by meat-packing plants, creameries, breweries, textile plants, oil refineries, paper mills, and many other industries are known as industrial wastes. They are growing in volume and constitute an increasingly serious problem. In cities they are discharged into the sewers and add to the volume and strength of the sewage. This places a financial burden upon the city for treatment cost, which may be very great in the case of a small city which has a large waste-producing industry. The city which encourages the establishment of such an industry within its limits should also insist upon the industry's paying its share of treatment costs. Industries outside of city limits which pollute streams must be controlled by the state department of health or other governmental agency. Pollution of navigable streams or boundary streams is controlled by the Federal government or by interstate compacts.

Some industries, such as creameries, oil refineries, or manufacturers of chemicals, may produce wastes which are inimical to the bacteriological processes used in sludge digestion, sewage filtration, and activated-sludge treatment. These may have to be eliminated from the sewers and given special treatment at the industrial plants. It is encouraging to note that many industries in cities and elsewhere are assuming responsibility for reducing the strength and volume of their wastes and for treating them to prevent stream pollution.

The logical approach to the industrial-waste problem would be (1) to study the plant processes and reduce the volume of waste, if possible; (2) to control the discharge of the waste so that the wastes reach the plant during periods of low flow or to discharge the wastes at a constant rate over the 24-hr period so that large amounts of waste are not discharged into the sewerage system in a short period of time; (3) to provide pretreatment so that the municipal sewage treatment plant is not overloaded or its operation interfered with; and (4) to provide separate complete treatment for the industrial wastes.

In pretreatment or separate treatment of wastes, screening is an important initial step. Methods employing fine screens are available that in some instances provide sufficient solids removal. Removal of settleable solids by sedimentation, occasionally augmented by coagulation, will provide partial treatment that may be adequate for the larger receiving streams. Where chemicals are used for flocculation, increased efficiency of solids removal is gained at the expense of aggravating the problem of sludge disposal. Biological treatment is the most economical method for treatment of highly diluted organic wastes. Aeration facilities have been developed that are amenable to industrial-waste treatment, and activated sludge is used in this field. Certain wastes ordinarily considered to be toxic, such as kraft-paper-mill and phenolic wastes, have been successfully handled in activated-sludge systems. Biological filters, particularly of the high-rate type, have been used for economical treatment of numerous types of wastes. Anaerobic treatment processes have been successful in removing 95 per cent of the 5-day biochemical oxygen demand and 90 per cent of the suspended solids at loadings up to 0.2 lb of biochemical oxygen demand per cu ft of digester volume per day. Toxic materials, such as cyanides and hexavalent chromium, may be rendered innocuous through chemical treatment. Land disposal methods have found their use in this field as well as in domestic sewage treatment; here spray irrigation, stabilization ponds, and deep injection wells have been used. The disposal of radioactive wastes is discussed in Chap. 17.

4-33. Training of Sewage-works Operators. It has long been recognized that a sewage treatment plant cannot perform efficiently unless it is under the supervision of an operator trained in sewage-works operation. It is generally accepted that certification or licensing of sewage-plant operating personnel is advantageous, not only to the individual concerned but also to the general public, the local officials, and the state and local health departments. Training programs for treatment-plant operators have a history of more than thirty years in the United States. Training programs in most states have been set up by the state or regional waterworks or sewage-works association in cooperation with the state health department and a college or university. Training is provided in the form of annual short schools at colleges or universities, correspondence courses, district or regional short schools, district water and sewage conferences, and state health department in-plant training programs.

Some states have laws requiring licensed or certified operators, but the training programs in most states are operated on a voluntary basis. The sewage-works profession recognizes the need for a certification or licensing program and generally recommends that the program be compulsory, not voluntary. It is further recognized that the agency passing on the qualifications of the sewage-plant operators should be the same agency that has supervision of plant operation. The personnel of the supervising agency may be assisted by a leading educator in the field of sanitary engineering in the state and also by a leader in the sewage-works profession in the state, preferably a superintendent of sewage-plant operation.

Excreta Disposal without Water Carriage

4-34. At the present time excreta are disposed of without water carriage at many farmhouses, at residences in the smaller towns and villages, and in the unsewered sections of the cities; in all probability this situation will continue for many years to come. While disposal with water is desirable, it is not practical under many conditions. It is possible, however, to dispose of the body wastes in a manner that will minimize or eliminate the transmission of disease and the pollution of soil and water.

It should be recognized that many existing outdoor toilets are grossly insanitary—for example, the open-back surface type, which is little better than no toilet at all. At some rural schools the same condition applies, and also in the small villages and unsewered portions of the larger towns. In the small town which boasts of its sewer system it is quite common to find that one-third of its area has no sewers and that the excreta disposal methods used there are as primitive as in a backward rural area. This is one reason why some small towns have an unenviable record of incidence for typhoid fever, dysentery, and "summer complaint" of infants.

4-35. Requirements for Satisfactory Excreta Disposal. An excreta disposal method should satisfy the following requirements:

1. There should be no contamination of ground water that may enter springs or wells.
2. There should be no contamination of surface water.
3. The surface soil should not be contaminated.
4. Excreta should not be accessible to flies or animals.
5. There should be freedom from odors and unsightly conditions.
6. The method used should be simple and inexpensive in terms of construction and operation. This applies particularly to rural areas, where the farmer may construct his own facilities.

Privies which are now approved by health authorities will be discussed, and brief mention will be made of some that are of historical interest.

4-36. The Concrete-slab Pit Privy. The pit privy, with the wood floor of the privy house serving as the pit cover, has long been used. There are obvious objections to wood covers, and health authorities favor the concrete-slab type. Figure 4-19 shows a type developed by the Public Health Service [11], and similar designs are suggested by the state health departments. Usually the slab is 4 ft square, and it rests upon a concrete sill 5¾ in. wide and 4 in. high, usually cast in four pieces. The pit curbing is of wood with ½-in. spaces left between the boards, except between the top two. Note that the earth is mounded and tamped up nearly to the slab level. The concrete riser for the seat is sometimes made oval rather than rectangular and is placed parallel to the sides of the slab rather than diagonally. Vents are sometimes brought through the roof. The long overhang of the rear end of the roof is to prevent rain-

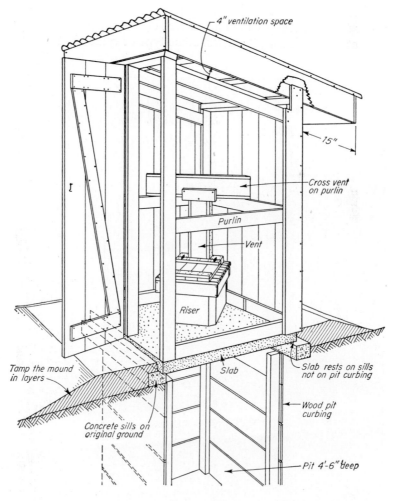

FIGURE 4-19   Concrete-slab pit privy. (*Courtesy of Public Health Service.*)

water from entering the pit. Figure 4-20 shows a completed concrete-slab pit privy.

A pit privy should be located so that contamination of a well or spring will not occur. Ordinarily this means that the pit should be down-slope from the well or spring. This cannot always be done, but there should be no danger if the pit does not penetrate the ground water (Art. 4-5). Pit privies do not function well if water stands in them. They are then odorous; pit contents do not compact; and they probably fill up sooner. If ground water does not enter the pit and the soil is uniformly compact, there should be no danger to a well at very short distances, although prudence dictates a distance of at least 50 ft. Some state health departments prescribe at least 100 ft, and this should be the rule if the ground-water table rises into the pit during a rainy period. If the ground water is permanently within a few feet of the ground surface, conditions are not favorable for pit privies. Some type of vault toilet might be used.

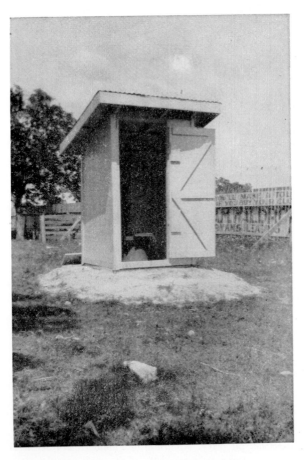

FIGURE 4-20   A sanitary concrete-slab pit privy.

Pit privies need little attention. The ventilation provided helps to keep the contents dry and small in bulk. Consequently a pit should serve for 10 years or more, provided toilet paper is used and no garbage or other refuse is thrown in. Insofar as possible, water should be prevented from entering, but if it does, a cupful of kerosene dropped in at weekly intervals will discourage mosquito breeding; if, however, the seat cover is kept down and the ventilator is screened, there should be no breeding. Odors which occur can, in some cases, be controlled with lime. No disinfectants should be used in the pit.

Privies for rural schools will require more seats. The slabs for such privies are made 2½ by 6 ft, with a riser and seat centered in the 2½-ft dimension, 6 in. from the back. The pit in this case would be 5 ft 4 in. wide, with a length of 2½ ft for each seat. Cross bracing in a long pit would be advisable to prevent caving.

In underdeveloped countries, variations of the concrete-slab pit privy are sometimes used. The riser and seat are dispensed with, and an opening or slot is left in the slab. Slightly elevated areas may be cast on the slab surface for the user's feet.

The bored-hole latrine has been used in some countries. A hole 16 in. in diameter and 20 ft deep is bored with an earth auger. If caving of the soil is feared, the hole can be revetted with a cylinder of woven brush which is lowered into the hole. A small concrete slab with a slot or hole is placed over the boring. This type of toilet should not be used where it would endanger water supplies.

4-37. Other Types of Privies. The *vault toilet* is a tank constructed underground and lined with stone, brick, or concrete, with the seat or seats over the cover. This is the type of toilet that was much used in ancient, medieval, and modern cities until the late nineteenth century, when water-carried sewerage was developed. When the vaults became full they were emptied, or they overflowed. Vault contents tend to become semiliquid and highly odorous. Brick and stone walls frequently leaked, and nearby soil pollution occurred. Vault cleaning was an industry in the larger cities and was more or less regulated by authorities, particularly as to the disposal of the material dipped from the vaults. Cleaning was unpleasant for all concerned, particularly when containers of vault contents had to be carried through the house to a wagon in the street. Cleaning was usually done at night; hence the term "night soil," which even now is sometimes applied to fecal matter in privies.

The *septic privy* is also a tight tank with the seat located over it. Anaerobic action similar to that which occurs in the sludge of a septic tank was encouraged by placing a bucket of water in the tank every day. This required an overflow pipe in a trench, the pipe being surrounded by gravel for leaching. Few septic privies were constructed.

The *chemical toilet* is a tight tank with a toilet seat located over it. It was formerly made by commercial firms and sold under various trade names. The tank was charged per seat with 10 to 15 gal of water in which 25 lb of caustic soda had been dissolved; a charge lasted for 6 to 9 months. A stirring device was needed. The caustic soda caused the tank contents to become a sterile, odorless, thick brown liquid which, when the tank required emptying, was discharged through a valve and pipe to a seepage pit.

The *box-and-can privy* consisted of a box with a seat opening and cover over a metal can. The box had a hinged top or back from which the can was removed, emptied, cleaned, and replaced. In some small cities the cans were city-owned; city employees served the toilets, and a monthly charge was made. Theoretically the toilets were flyproof. Can contents were dumped into a sewer if sewers were available; otherwise they were placed in a surface dump, with unfortunate results, or in a trench and covered with earth.

Bibliography

1. Caldwell, E. L., and L. W. Parr: *J. Infect. Diseases*, vol. 61, pp. 148, 180, 1937; vol. 62, pp. 225, 272, 1938.
2. Dyer, B. R., *et al.*: Investigations of Groundwater Pollution, *Indian J. Med. Res.*, vol. 33, pp. 17, 23, 1945.
3. Gotaas, H. B.: Report on the Investigation of Travel of Pollution, *State Water Pollution Control Board Pub.* 11, p. 8, 1954.
4. Manual of Septic Tank Practice, *Public Health Service Pub.* 526.
5. "Studies on Household Disposal Systems," pt. III, Public Health Service, 1954.
6. Coulter, J. B., and T. W. Bendixen: Serial Distribution of Septic Tank Effluents, *Public Works*, vol. 90, no. 2, February, 1959.
7. Thomas, R. E., and J. B. Coulter: "Notes on the Construction of Seepage Pits," Public Health Service, Robert A. Taft Sanitary Engineering Center, Cincinnati, Ohio, 1959.
8. Steel, Ernest W.: "Water Supply and Sewerage," 4th ed., McGraw-Hill Book Company, New York, 1960.
9. Hardenbergh, W. A., and E. B. Rodie: "Water Supply and Waste Disposal," International Textbook Company, Scranton, Pa., 1961.
10. Fair, G. M., and J. C. Geyer: "Elements of Water Supply and Waste-water Disposal," John Wiley & Sons, Inc., New York, 1958.
11. The Sanitary Privy: Plans and Specifications, Supplement no. 108 to *Public Health Repts.*
12. "Standard Methods for the Examination of Water, Sewage, and Industrial Wastes," 11th ed., American Public Health Association, New York, 1960.
13. Porges, R., *et al.*: Sewage Treatment by Extended Aeration, *J. Water Pollution Control Federation*, vol. 33, no. 12, December, 1961.
14. McGauhey, P. H., and J. H. Winneberger: "Summary Report on Causes and Prevention of Failure of Septic-tank Percolation Systems," Sanitary Research Laboratory, College of Engineering, University of California, Berkeley, Calif., 1963.

5

REFUSE SANITATION

5-1. The dweller in the modern city expects regular collection of household wastes as a city service. He is less concerned with the disposal of those wastes after they are collected, unless the method used causes a nuisance to him. Furnishing of this service is an important item in the city's budget, varying from $1.50 to $8 per year per capita and tending to be larger in the larger cities. From the standpoint of engineering and planning, it presents difficulties. Large amounts of materials must be collected, and those amounts vary throughout the year and, of course, increase as the city grows. Disposal of the large volumes of wastes presents the difficulties of disposal-site location and adoption of methods that will be economical and nuisance-free. Health problems may arise since some of the refuse is attractive to insects and rodents, and always there is the possibility of such nuisances as odors and street litter.

Metropolitan areas are already meeting difficulties in solving the refuse problem. As they increase in size, disposal sites are located farther from the inhabited areas, and hauls become longer and more costly. Planning on an area basis is not easy because of the numerous separate cities, towns, and villages that comprise an area. The most economical solution to the problem may be an area-wide or perhaps a countywide refuse collection and disposal service. In a few areas this has been done, but inertia, distrust of innovations, and, in some cases, legal difficulties are delaying organization that may have to be established sooner or later. The sooner it is done, the more effective the planning can be, particularly in regard to the sites of disposal works with relation to their suitability, proximity to populated areas, and access by roads.

5-2. Quantities. Table 5-1 gives quantities of the various wastes that may be expected. The figures, however, are merely indicative, for wide variations are found. Planning of refuse collection and disposal for a city should be preceded by a study which should include the following: total amount of the refuse and amounts for various areas of the city, such as the commercial and the various residential areas; monthly variations in amount; and characteristics of the refuse, such as proportions of garbage, combustible and noncombustible rubbish, and ashes and the weights, volumes, and amounts of each produced in various areas of the city. Commercial areas will produce refuse high in combustible rubbish. The

Table 5-1.   REPORTED QUANTITY RANGE OF MUNICIPAL REFUSE COLLECTED
(Pounds per capita per day)

Type of refuse	Summer*		Winter†		Yearly average
	Minimum	Maximum	Minimum	Maximum	
Garbage	0.2	2.2	0.1	1.4	0.6
Rubbish	0.5	1.8	0.4	1.4	0.9
Ashes.	0.1	1.5	1.4	3.0	1.1
Garbage and combustible rubbish	0.4	3.7	0.3	2.6	1.2
Ashes and noncombustible rubbish	0.2	3.5	0.4	5.4	1.5
All refuse combined . .	1.4	4.6	1.6	5.1	2.2

* Summer season: May 1–October 31.
† Winter season: November 1–April 30.
SOURCE: "Sanitary Refuse Practices," pt. I, Public Health Service, 1953.

rubbish of some residential areas will be high in grass cuttings and shrub trimmings at certain times of the year.

5-3. Refuse. The materials that are collected and disposed of under the term "refuse" include many different substances from a multitude of sources. The amounts and characteristics of the various types of refuse differ with the time of year, the geographical location, and the habits of the contributing population. Table 5-1 illustrates seasonal fluctuations in quantities of municipal refuse. Terms used in connection with refuse and its various components are not well recognized by the general public; however, most writers and other technical persons associated with refuse programs have recognized the need for uniform terms for maximum understanding by those working together in the same field. These terms have been used in this chapter. Generally accepted components of refuse include all putrescible and nonputrescible solid wastes, with the exception of body wastes. Such wastes include garbage, rubbish, ashes, street sweepings, dead animals, and solid market and industrial wastes.

Some collection and disposal systems allow the collection of all solid wastes from a common receptacle for removal to the same disposal site. The term "mixed refuse" denotes combinations of all components. It weighs 500 to 1,000 lb/cu yd.

From an over-all standpoint, the collection and removal of refuse from the environment of man in a sanitary manner are of importance in effecting vector control, nuisance abatement, aesthetics improvement, and fire protection.

5-4. Garbage. The term "garbage" is used to designate those putrescible wastes resulting from the growing, handling, preparation, cooking, and consumption of food. Quantities of garbage vary throughout the year, being greatest in amount during the summer months, when vegetable wastes are more abundant. The increased use of processed and packaged foods has reduced garbage production and increased the combustible rubbish. Garbage weighs 800 to 1,500 lb/cu yd. It requires careful handling with frequent removal and adequate disposal because it attracts and breeds flies and other insects, supplies food for rats, and rapidly ferments, resulting in the production of unpleasant odors. Garbage is probably the most valuable component of refuse in that it yields fertilizer or soil conditioner through composting processes and is utilized as hog feed.

5-5. Rubbish. The term "rubbish" denotes all nonputrescible wastes except ashes. It consists of both combustible and noncombustible substances, such as cans, paper, brush, glass, cardboard, wood, scrap metals, bedding, yard clippings, crockery, etc. Rubbish weighs 100 to 700 lb/cu yd. Before compaction it will weigh 250 to 350 lb/cu yd. Garbage and rubbish are difficult to separate entirely because those materials classed as rubbish are often used to package food or food products, and various amounts of garbage remain attached to paper, boxes, cans, etc. Rubbish is frequently responsible for the creation of nuisances when it becomes scattered by the wind and careless handling.

5-6. Ashes. Ashes are the waste products of coal and other fuels which have been used for industrial purposes and in homes for cooking and heating. Ashes weigh 1,150 to 1,400 lb/cu yd. Ash production varies greatly with geographical location and, of course, with the time of year. Use of natural gas and oil as fuels has greatly reduced the quantity of ashes that must be collected.

5-7. Dead Animals. The problem of the removal and disposal of large dead animals, *i.e.*, cows, horses, mules, hogs, etc., in many cities is handled by privately owned rendering plants. However, these concerns do not collect small animals in most cities, and their collection is usually left to the municipal collection system. Some municipalities have solved the small-animal disposal problem by providing collection and delivery of these animals to a local rendering plant where disposal is accomplished, often without charge to the city. Other satisfactory small-animal disposal methods include incineration and deep burial in specified locations.

5-8. Street Sweepings. These consist principally of materials worn from street surfaces, dirt and other materials dropped or worn away from vehicles, leaves, sweepings from sidewalks, and bits of wastepaper. Street sweepings are not usually putrescible enough to cause concern as a possible source of fly breeding or odors and may frequently be used for fill, although some dust nuisance may be created. They usually weigh 1,150 to 1,400 lb/cu yd.

5-9. Industrial Wastes. The solid wastes resulting from many manufacturing processes are often a cause for concern to public health authorities. Some wastes, if not properly handled, will produce obnoxious odors, and in the case of putrescible wastes, health hazards will be created. Most municipalities require that industrial concerns maintain their own waste collection and disposal facilities, including those for ashes and cinders, although many producers of industrial wastes arrange for the use of municipal disposal facilities.

Refuse Storage

5-10. The maintenance of adequate sanitary facilities for temporarily storing refuse on the premises is considered a responsibility of the individual householder or businessman. Not only is the proper premises storage of refuse essential from a sanitation viewpoint, but the efficiency of the entire collection and disposal system is partially dependent upon the degree of individual cooperation accorded the storage phase. While many cities have enacted ordinances regulating the refuse-sanitation program which contain specifications for home storage, the most desirable approach in improving home-storage conditions lies in public education. Although a suitable ordinance is necessary, legal enforcement should have a minor role, with dependence placed on the willingness of individuals to cooperate when they are made aware of the hazards and nuisances associated with insanitary practices.

5-11. Separation of Refuse. The separation required depends largely upon the method of disposal to be utilized. Where no separation is required and frequent collection service is provided, a single container may be utilized for storing the mixed refuse. Garbage may be segregated from ashes and rubbish to allow its utilization as hog feed. Some systems using incinerators require the separation of combustible from noncombustible materials, and in a few instances a three-can system is utilized wherein separate receptacles are provided for garbage, rubbish, and ashes. Although separation has the advantages of facilitating the disposal method, it has the disadvantage of increasing the cost of collection, for special equipment and workers are necessary to collect each type of material, and each pickup route must be traveled more than once.

5-12. Storage Containers. Receptacles for the temporary storage of refuse should be designed specifically for the waste to be stored. They should be covered. Since the loaded container must be hoisted to the collection vehicle, often by one man, the size should be given consideration and should be limited in the regulatory ordinance. Containers for mixed refuse should not exceed 30 to 32 gal in capacity and should be equipped with side handles to facilitate handling. Burlap bags furnished by the city have been used for rubbish. Full bags are replaced by empty ones. Those containers utilized for garbage storage, whether separate or in combination with other refuse, should be constructed of 26- to 30-gage galvanized metal and should be equipped with tight-fitting lids. Cans used expressly for garbage storage should not exceed 12 to 20 gal in capacity and should preferably be equipped with a lock-type cover. Plastic cans are light in weight but are easily gnawed through by rats. To avoid odors and the accumulation of fly-supporting materials, garbage containers should be washed at frequent intervals. A few cities remove full cans in double-decked trucks and replace them with clean cans which have been washed at the disposal point. Cans in this case are city-owned and uniform in size.

A household paper-bag container system of collection has been employed, largely on an experimental basis, in this country and is in use on a modest scale in several European communities [18]. The plan necessitates the city's furnishing bags and holders to the individual householders. The bag, of 30 gal capacity or more, is disposable and is constructed of one- or two-ply moisture-resistant kraft paper. Holders vary from enclosed steel cabinets to open stands equipped with hinged flytight lids and animal guards. Among the claimed advantages of the system are that it makes collection faster and easier, keeps garbage dry for incineration, eliminates the garbage-can fly-breeding problem, and reduces injuries to collection forces. The plan has been studied under one of the research programs of the American Public Works Association [19].

Ashes should be placed in strongly constructed fireproof receptacles, and covers should be provided to prevent dust and the possible scattering of embers. Again, the container should not be so large that convenient handling by one person is impossible.

Where disposal methods allow the collection of mixed refuse, rubbish as well as garbage should be stored in a well-covered galvanized container of convenient handling size. Some cities allow the separate storage of tree limbs, lawn clippings, etc.; however, the materials should be stored in such a manner that scattering is limited and ease in handling is provided. Storage will be facilitated by cutting limbs in convenient lengths and bundling them, placing lawn clippings in disposable bags, etc.

5-13. Point of Collection. The location of the refuse containers for collection can have an important bearing on the speed—and therefore the cost—of the collection service. Many cities require that the individual householder transport the container to the curb or, in the case of alleys, to the rear property line. Curb collections require a rigidly scheduled collection service since nuisances are likely to be created if containers are left in the front yards of homes for long periods. Where traffic conditions permit, curb collections probably allow the most rapid pickup service. An additional service is provided in a number of cities where the pickup men enter the yard for back-door collections. Usually refuse is dumped by the collector into a transfer can or large plastic barrel, which is then carried to the collection vehicle. This procedure is considerably more expensive than either alley or street collection and leads to complaints, from the householder, of damage and spillage.

Extensive studies at the University of California [2] reveal significant conclusions with respect to the location of storage containers for collection. The approximate manpower requirements for the pickup operation (time required to load the refuse on the collection vehicle) varied rather consistently from an average of 100 man-min/ton for 100 per cent alley or curb collection to 165 man-min/ton for 100 per cent rear-of-house (back-door) collection. For 100 per cent rear-of-house collection, approximately 28 per cent of the pickup time is spent walking on private property.

If program economy is essential, the individual must assist collection personnel by placing containers in a convenient location.

5-14. Special Treatment. The requirement that garbage be drained and wrapped prior to being placed in containers for mixed-refuse collection is stressed in some cities. Draining and wrapping have a tendency to assist in drying the garbage, thus slowing down its fermentation. This procedure also partially prevents the exposure of garbage to flies and the buildup of organic accumulations within containers, which can support fly breeding. Where garbage is utilized as hog feed, wrapping cannot be allowed.

A few municipalities require that garbage and rubbish containers be placed on racks or other suitable platforms above ground level. Such racks, usually constructed of wood or metal tubing, serve to lengthen the useful life of metal containers (because corrosion is reduced), to permit the cleaning of spilled wastes around the container, and to prevent the spillage of container contents by dogs. Racks are especially well suited where alley or back-door collections are made and for apartment houses or other multifamily residences.

5-15. Public Education. The regulations governing the individual treatment of refuse must be brought to the attention of the householder to ensure his compliance with them. Cards giving instructions as to the degree of separation required, the location of containers for collection, and the collection schedule should be distributed when necessary to each resident, together with information concerning changes in established schedules. Very often, however, it will be found that regulations have been violated for various reasons. In this respect, tags on which various violations may be designated and attached to the container have proved helpful. Householders are usually willing to comply with the recommendations or directions on the tag, but some follow-up activity is necessary to ensure compliance in a few instances.

Refuse Collection

5-16. The refuse collection system furnishes an intimate contact between the taxpayer and the municipal administration. Therefore, deficiencies are very likely to result in criticism. Furthermore, the collection phase is almost always the most expensive portion of the refuse-sanitation program because of equipment and labor requirements. To satisfy the demands of public approval, municipal economy, and public health, careful consideration must be given to organizing the collection system, selecting and training labor, purchasing equipment, and planning collection routes.

5-17. Organization for Collection. Several possibilities for establishing the collection system are available to cities. These include contractual operations, municipally administered programs, and a scavenger system in which private individuals are licensed to collect refuse in certain defined areas.

A number of cities have attempted to operate the refuse collection

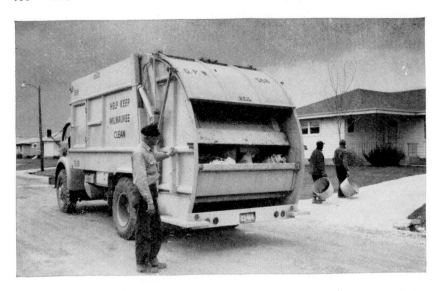

FIGURE 5-1   This 20-yd collection unit enables a Milwaukee crew to collect all day with only a single trip to the incinerator. Collectors are using "carry barrels" for backyard collections. (*Courtesy of Public Works Magazine.*)

system by contract. Some advantages are inherent in this method in that the system can remain free of the influence of local politics and the private contractor is more likely to apply business methods to the operation. In most contracted operations a known and definite sum is fixed in advance of the work, with the contractor usually being paid from general fund revenues or from revenue received from refuse service charges. There are several disadvantages in contractual services, particularly in view of the fact that profit, and not service or the welfare of the public, is often the predominant concern. Sanitary control of the program is not easily obtained, and the response to unforeseen emergencies is often slower than in the case of municipally operated systems.

Those systems operated directly under an agency of the municipal administration are usually in a better position to care for the sanitary needs of the public than a private concern is. Modern trends in municipally administered programs include the designation of a responsible and qualified person as head of a sanitation division which operates within the authority of the public works department or some other comparable organizational unit. The over-all responsibility for the entire refuse program might appropriately be divided into two general areas: (1) the direction of personnel and operation and maintenance of equipment; and (2) the development and enforcement of desirable sanitation standards in the program. Frequently, responsibility in the latter area is delegated to public health agencies.

Scavenger operations are rarely suitable in large cities and must be rigidly controlled by health authorities wherever practiced. Scavengers are often interested in limiting their collections to garbage and, for this reason, must be forced to comply with the necessary sanitary regulations concerning the removal, handling, and disposal of putrescible wastes. In some instances scavengers will be interested in the collection of scrap metals, rags, paper, etc. Sanitary regulations for the handling of these materials should also be rigidly enforced.

5-18. Collection Personnel. The selection and training of the proper type of labor are important factors in the efficient operation of the collection system. With shorter working hours, clothes provided by employers, and generally improved labor-employer relations, the lot of collection personnel has improved during recent years. However, improved labor conditions have also resulted in increased operational costs. Frequent labor turnover is costly, and some cities have found that economies can be effected by rewarding attendance and meritorious work. Uniforming of personnel is reported as improving morale, rendering the service more attractive, adding safety, and providing identification as city employees [3]. Some cities have placed the collection personnel on an incentive basis whereby the working day can be completed when a fairly allotted number of collections are made. This requires careful supervision, or employees may neglect the work. Usually there is the provision that no overtime will be paid at periods, such as Christmastime, when the work load is temporarily heavier.

5-19. Time of Collection. A majority of the refuse collections in most cities are made during the regular working day. However, night collections in business areas are sometimes favored in larger cities to avoid the difficulty of maneuvering the large collection trucks in heavy traffic. Residential collections during night hours are ruled out in most cities because of noise nuisances and difficulty of locating storage containers in the dark.

5-20. Frequency of Collection. For best results, from both the aesthetic and the sanitation viewpoints, garbage should be collected at least two times weekly in residential sections in summer and winter. Most commercial establishments should be accorded daily collection service throughout the year. Rubbish is generally collected weekly in residential areas and daily in business sections. Mixed refuse should be collected twice weekly from residential areas and daily from most commercial concerns. An important consideration in providing frequent collection service is the prevention of fly breeding in garbage. Since the time required for the development of flies from eggs to mature larvae may be less than 1 week, weekly collections do not remove the larvae prior to their migration from the garbage in order to pupate in the surrounding soil. The provision of frequent collection services can also

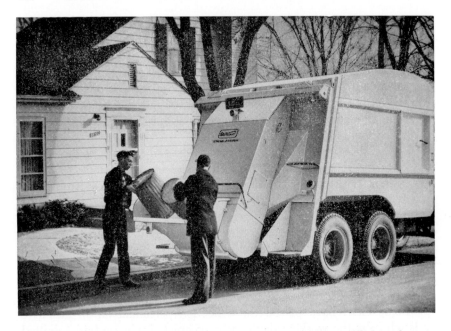

FIGURE 5-2   A packer-type truck in which the hopper loader is filled at the rear of the truck, with the refuse crushed into fragments and then fed into the truck body. (*Photograph courtesy of Gar Wood Industries, Inc., Wayne, Mich.*)

be an important asset in the premises storage of wastes. Householders cannot be expected to provide storage capacity greater than their minimum requirements, and irregular collections can contribute to the nuisances and hazards which result under poor storage conditions.

5-21. Collection Equipment. The equipment used by various cities for the collection of refuse differs considerably in size and character. To achieve sanitation requirements, equipment should include a suitable cover to prevent the exposure of contents, except during loading and unloading. The vehicle should be of watertight construction, preferably metal, to prevent leakage and facilitate thorough cleaning. Other considerations in equipment selection include truck capacity; type of waste collected; loading height; specific problems associated with alley, curb, or carry-out pickup service; and manpower requirements, which are all-important in their relation to the over-all cost of the collection operation.

Some municipalities utilize open-body trucks with capacities of 2 to 20 cu yd or more for collection vehicles, although most cities have replaced open equipment with the more modern enclosed packer-type collection vehicles. Tarpaulin covers and special construction which reduces loading height enable open trucks to perform certain collection jobs adequately, and such equipment is sometimes superior where bulky rubbish is collected separately.

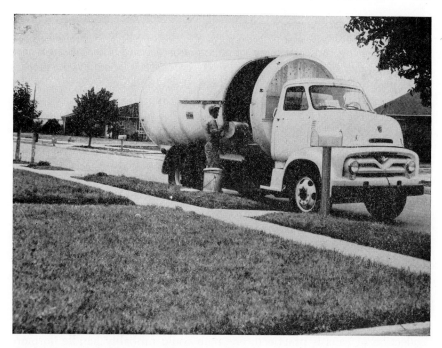

FIGURE 5-3 A packer-type collection vehicle in which refuse is loaded through sliding doors at the front of the truck body and is compacted. (*Photograph courtesy of Pak-Mor Manufacturing Co.*)

Mixed refuse can be satisfactorily handled by the enclosed packer-type vehicles. Several types have been produced, utilizing different mechanical devices for performing the loading, unloading, and packing operations. One type is equipped with a loading bucket at the rear which, when filled, is raised and dumped mechanically into a door in the top of the body, which opens as the bucket moves into position to empty into the garbage compartment of the truck. In another type, the batch or hopper loader is also loaded at the rear of the body, and the refuse is pushed by means of a hydraulic mechanism directly into the body. The truck is unloaded by hydraulically elevating the front of the body. A vehicle of this type is illustrated in Figs. 5-1 and 5-2. A variation of the rear-loading type utilizes an escalator device to transport refuse from the loading port to the interior of the truck. Still another recent variation includes equipment for shredding refuse prior to escalator-type loading into the packing compartment, as shown in Fig. 5-2. Figure 5-3 pictures a refuse collection vehicle which is loaded through sliding doors situated at the front of the body. A plate is utilized to push and compact the refuse against the rear of the bed and to unload the vehicle. Packer-type trucks vary in capacity from 5 to 30 cu yd, sizes between 12 and 16 cu yd being the most popular [3].

Dempster-Dumpster and others have produced portable containers for refuse storage and collection that are applicable to large apartment houses, housing projects, some commercial areas, and other places where large amounts of refuse are produced. Refuse is placed by the householders or other producers in a closed steel container. A specially designed truck hoisting unit makes routine rounds to each container, replaces it with an empty container, hoists the full one to the truck, and hauls it to the disposal area. Only the truck, driver, and containers are required in this collection scheme.

5-22. Factors Affecting Collection. The time required for collection may be divided into productive and nonproductive periods. Productive time is that during which collections are actually being made, and nonproductive time includes the time employed in traveling to and from the disposal point, the unloading period, and the time lost by pickup personnel in waiting during the compaction cycle of packer-type trucks.

The number of workmen used per truck, location of containers, collection frequency, and population density are other factors in the organization of the collection phase. In a densely populated district where cans are placed at the property line or curb by householders, one workman should handle about 500 cans per day. On the other hand, if rear-door collection of cans is practiced, one man could probably handle no more than 200 or 300 cans per day. Collection time required on a ton basis is discussed in Art. 5-13. While twice-weekly collections of refuse are recommended for residential areas, it has been observed that two collections per week result in a considerable increase in refuse produced when compared with once-weekly collection. Economies will likely result if one man in the crew is designated as full-time vehicle operator in densely populated areas. Where stops are less frequent, the driver may assist with the collection procedure.

5-23. Planning a Collection System. The planning of a refuse collection system is essentially a matter of making the most efficient use of equipment and working force. The following factors must be studied and considered to permit adequate planning [3]: (1) types of refuse produced, volume, weight, compressibility, and method of separation and storage at origin; (2) number of service stops, quantity of refuse per stop, and location of refuse for collection; (3) type and capacity of collection equipment available or to be selected; (4) organization of crews; (5) topographic features of the area, street layout, and traffic pattern; (6) disposal method or methods; (7) type of zoning—residential, business, or industry; (8) climate; and (9) extent to which municipal, contract, and private methods are used.

The process of laying out routes is one of trial and error. A course of travel is laid out for a crew. The time of loading and hauling for each load can be obtained by using collection-speed and production data. After a day's work has been laid out, the area served can be indicated on a map, and another route begun in the same way. Such routes will be tentative at first and may require later adjustment. Thereafter permanent routes and areas can be shown on maps and on daily route schedules for each truck. These are carried by the truck driver and are also on file in the office. Costs per ton for collection should be computed for various types of vehicles and crew sizes before routes are established.

In actual practice, some flexibility of operation will be needed to meet emergencies or unexpectedly high loads. Emergency crews may be available, or the crew chief may call a dispatcher to report that he will not finish his route or will finish early. He may then receive help or give help to another collecting crew.

As cities grow larger and as metropolitan areas develop, supplemental transportation, to obtain greater speed of haul to the point of disposal and thus reduce the nonproductive time of the collection crews, becomes economical. Removable bodies may be taken from the collection vehicles and stacked on large trucks or trailers for the long haul, or collection vehicles may be coupled together and hauled by a tractor. Another method requires transfer of the refuse from the collection vehicles to some other kind of transportation equipment. The shifting may be done by dumping directly from one vehicle to another or by dumping into hoppers and then into the transfer vehicles. Transfer has been into railway cars, in some cases, and into barges, where final disposal is into the sea. Transfer stations, if close to populated areas, must be so designated and operated that odor, dust, fly, and rodent troubles will not occur.

5-24. Records. Appropriate records form the basis upon which financial and operational controls may be developed. Fundamental data are the daily refuse collections, expressed in both tonnage and cubic yardage; personnel records; financial data; and operational reports.

While it may be impractical to weigh all loads, it is important to make routine check weighings to keep abreast of any changes in the quantity of refuse produced in any particular district or in the city as a whole. Personnel records should provide data indicating the performance of each employee, including attendance and conduct, and payroll information. Financial reports from the various supervisors, of course, enable the administrator to evaluate his financial status with respect to his budget. Reporting should permit a ready interpretation of the unit-cost status for each of the principal operations in the department.

The daily operational report made by the collecting unit should include the following: vehicle number and capacity and miles traveled; number of loads collected and their volume and, if known, their weight; number of collections made and number of premises from which no collection was made and the reason therefor; complaints and their disposition; and payroll data for workmen. Additional operational reports in the departmental office should include expenses for repairs and maintenance and other equipment costs. The "Manual of Public Works Records and Administration" and the "Manual of Public Works Records and Accounting," prepared by the Committee on Street and Sanitation Records, both published by the Public Administration Service, Chicago, Ill., provide useful information on records.

5-25. Cost of Collection. Because of variations in labor costs, frequency and type of service provided, disposal methods, terrain, and other local factors, it is difficult to arrive at an average unit cost for the collection service. For purposes of comparison, some engineers recommend the ton-mile as a unit. This enables consideration not only of the quantity of wastes collected but also of the number of miles the load must be hauled. Sometimes collection costs are expressed in terms of per capita costs. Cost comparisons between cities mean very little except in the case of cities of comparable size and with similar collection practices. Per capita costs reported in 1958 [3] for collection varied from $8.35 to 82 cents per year, with $3 to $4 the most common.

Refuse Disposal

5-26. The refuse-sanitation program cannot be satisfactorily completed until necessary measures have been taken to ensure the inoffensive disposal of these wastes. In primitive times, solid wastes were merely thrown upon the ground. Unfortunately, some municipalities have refined this procedure only by stipulating that the materials be deposited at a single location. The establishment of a point of disposal is an advantage in itself as it prevents unauthorized and promiscuous dumping, which would probably produce objectionable conditions. Rapidly expanding modern urban areas, however, have surrounded the areas which were originally intended as isolated disposal sites. This expansion necessitates a thorough evaluation of disposal methods suitable for semi-populated areas since isolated sites are now beyond convenient access for most large cities. Methods have been developed wherein the final disposition of refuse can be accomplished without the creation of undue nuisance. It is the purpose of this section to review several disposal methods in some detail and the advantages and disadvantages associated with each method.

5-27. Dumping. Some components of refuse are suitable for open dumping. These include street sweepings, ashes, and incombustible rubbish. However, serious nuisances and hazards will result if garbage or mixed refuse is disposed of in this manner. They include odors, dust, wind-borne paper, fires, flies, rats, and mosquitoes that will breed in rainwater held in cans. Low areas which may be brought up to grade by filling are generally chosen for the dump. Ashes and street sweepings, though dusty, permit the construction of a fairly stable fill. Carefully selected rubbish may also be utilized, although fires often occur, and some settling of the filled areas will result. Dump locations must be carefully chosen so that there will be a minimum chance of complaint from nearby residents.

While some municipal ordinances prohibit the placing of garbage and some rubbish, *i.e.*, paper, food cartons, cans, etc., on open dumps, most dumps invariably receive some of these materials because the difficulties of inspection make rigid enforcement impossible. This, together with lack of adequate supervision of open dumps, has resulted in unsatisfactory conditions in many cities.

5-28. Hog Feeding. The feeding of garbage to hogs has been practiced for many years. Some cities formerly operated hog farms, but municipal piggeries at present are few or nonexistent. It is estimated, however, that about 25 per cent of the total quantity of garbage produced is fed to hogs by private individuals. That garbage feeding is profitable if properly handled is shown by the fact that most hotels and restaurants can dispose of their garbage to farmers who are willing to collect it themselves. Usually they collect daily and furnish clean cans. While garbage is the most potentially valuable element of refuse, it is most difficult to handle in a sanitary manner and is responsible for the majority of the nuisances and health hazards associated with the refuse program. Hog feeding, like other methods of garbage utilization, still involves the necessity of providing for the proper disposal of other refuse.

GARBAGE-FED HOGS AND HEALTH. Health authorities recognize the danger of contracting trichinosis from the consumption of improperly cooked pork products. This disease is caused by trichina worms. The larval worms are encysted in the muscle tissue of the hog, and if the pork is not properly cooked, a dangerous infection may result. See Art. 7-3. Hogs fed with uncooked garbage have been found to harbor up to five times as much trichina infestation as grain-fed hogs, and trichinosis in humans has been reported most frequently where large numbers of hogs so fed are raised.

Prior to 1952, health and agricultural agencies were generally unsuccessful in stimulating hog feeders to cook garbage preliminary to feeding. However, in 1952, a new swine disease, vesicular exanthema, occurred in this country, and its rapid spread brought about a change in the attitude of garbage feeders. It was determined that vesicular exanthema among hogs was chiefly due to the feeding of uncooked garbage. Now all states prohibit the feeding of raw garbage to animals. Public Health Service studies reveal that the subjection of raw garbage to a temperature of 212°F for 30 min is necessary to remove the threat of vesicular exanthema and trichinosis, and equipment has been developed which affords a convenient means for cooking garbage [5]. Cooking the garbage does not reduce its food value. The pork produced compares favorably in quality to that which has been grain-fed.

ORGANIZATION. Disposal of garbage by feeding it to animals may be controlled in various ways. The garbage may be collected by the hog owners under city license or regulation; the city may collect the garbage and give or sell it to hog feeders; or the city may wish to establish a farm and control the entire program under municipal direction, although this is now unusual. In any event, rigid specifications should be adopted and enforced concerning frequency of collection, type of collection vehicle, cooking of garbage, and, where possible, regulation of the animal-feeding area. Some cities realize an appreciable revenue from garbage sold to farmers and at the same time realize a saving in the final disposal of their solid wastes since volume is somewhat reduced.

SANITARY CONSIDERATIONS. Hog farms are frequently the cause of complaints of odors, flies, rats, and other nuisances and sanitation hazards. With proper operation and supervision, many of these conditions can be eliminated or minimized. Flies, however, are always attracted to animals, and hog farms should be located in areas where complaints will not result from flies or other nuisances. Impervious, easily cleaned feeding platforms should be provided to prevent the trampling of garbage into the ground, a condition that is especially favorable for the production of flies and odors. A well-designed feeding platform may be constructed of reinforced concrete poured as dry as possible and cured to assure long service. A "rat wall" (Fig. 9-26) should be placed around each feeding platform. Feeding areas should also be equipped with properly located drains to facilitate cleaning. Manure and uneaten garbage may be collected daily and placed in a compost pit. Each daily accumulation of the material is covered with dry earth, and the compost produced in such pits is an excellent fertilizer. An alternative is to spread the material daily on fields.

ECONOMICS. The presence of extraneous matter and dangerous materials, such as razor blades and glass, in residential and institutional garbage makes it the least desirable garbage for hog feeding. Garbage from hotels and restaurants is much higher in nutritive value, and that from military installations, where there is good separation of refuse, is best of all. Studies made in California [4] indicated a gain of 70 to 75 lb of pork per ton of cooked residential garbage. A gain of 193 lb/ton and a gain of 1.44 lb per hog per day were reported for military garbage. Each hog can, on an average, eat 20 to 24 lb of garbage per day and will gain 1 lb in weight per day.

5-29. Incineration. This is a widely used method of refuse disposal. Whether it should be used will depend upon its applicability to local conditions and consideration of its advantages and disadvantages.

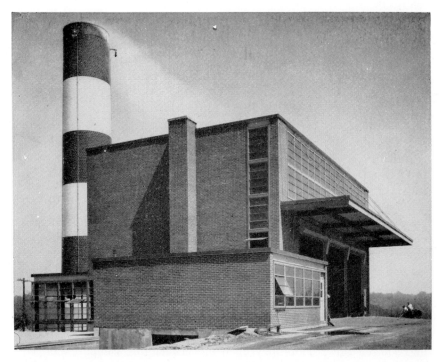

FIGURE 5-4 Municipal incinerator, East Hartford, Conn. (*Courtesy of Public Works Magazine.*)

ADVANTAGES. The important advantages [4] are:

1. Less land is required than for landfills.

2. A central location is possible. A well-designed building, careful operation, and landscaped grounds are acceptable in many neighborhoods, certainly in industrial areas. This may allow short hauls for the collection service.

3. Ash and other residue produced are practically free of organic matter, nuisance-free, and acceptable as fill material.

4. Many kinds of refuse can be burned. Even the noncombustible materials will be reduced in bulk.

5. Climate or unusual weather does not affect it.

6. Flexibility is possible. Incinerators may be operated for 8, 16, or 24 hr/day.

7. It is possible to get some income through the sale of waste heat for steam or power. Some cities charge industries and businesses for incinerator service.

DISADVANTAGES. These should also be considered. They are:

1. Incinerators are high in first cost. This is likely to be from $3,500 to $5,000 per ton of rated 24-hr capacity to build and equip.

2. Operating costs are relatively high, and skilled employees are required for operation and maintenance. The high temperatures, dust, and type of

materials handled have such an effect upon machinery and furnace interior that expensive repairs are frequently needed. Costs are widely varying and will depend in large part on whether operation is in one, two, or three shifts, decreasing with the number of shifts and amount of automation. Not including fixed charges, costs will vary from $3 to $7.50 per ton.

3. There may be difficulty in getting a site. Many property owners will object to refuse disposal in any form near their property. Many will also object that track traffic to and from the plant is a hazard and a nuisance.

PRINCIPAL FEATURES OF AN INCINERATOR. Design of an incinerator requires expert knowledge in this field [6, 7, 8]. There are various types of incinerators, which are usually classified by charging method and type of grates used.

1. *Charging Apparatus.* The simplest method of charging is to dump the collection trucks on the charging floor. The refuse is then pushed into charging doors by hand or bulldozer. This method has the disadvantages of requiring extra handling of the refuse, small storage capacity, and varying loads on the incinerator. Larger incinerators usually have storage bins into which the refuse is dumped by the trucks. A crane and bucket is then used to move the refuse to the charging doors. This permits more uniform loading of the furnace, and the crane operator can mix wet and dry or highly and less combustible materials to provide more even burning. The charging doors may open into a charging compartment, with the upper door closed when the lower door is open to the furnace. This reduces the possibility of great temperature reductions during charging.

2. *The Furnace, or Primary, Chamber.* This chamber includes the grates on which the material is deposited for burning. The grates may be in round or rectangular units, and they may receive batch charges or be continuously charged. Grates will allow fine ash to fall through to the ash pit below, but some types will require rocking to permit larger clinkers to pass. Some hand manipulation will also be necessary to remove the large clinkers and other noncombustible objects. Moving grates are sometimes used. These are fabricated as endless belts to move from the charging point toward the stoking door. They allow ash to drop through and deposit clinkers into the ashpit at the end of the travel. Some furnaces have drying grates or hearths to receive wet material before it is moved to the burning grates. Grates are rated in pounds of refuse burned per square foot per hour. Hand-stoked grates will usually burn 40 lb/hr, while other types will burn up to 70 lb/hr. Traveling grates are often rated at 300,000 Btu/(hr)(sq ft). Refuse fed is likely to average 4000 to 5000 Btu/lb, with 50 to 25 per cent moisture and 12.5 per cent ash or inert material [6].

Separate furnace cells or units, all discharging into the same combustion chamber, are sometimes provided. Since only one cell is charged at a time, higher temperatures can be maintained in the combustion

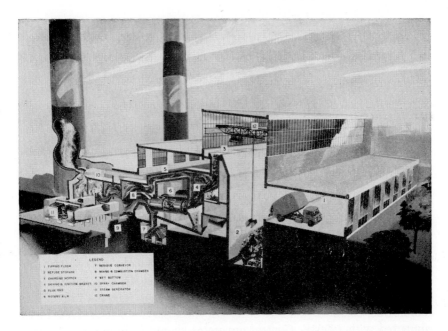

FIGURE 5-5   Section of Southwest incinerator, Chicago. (*Courtesy of Department of Public Works, Chicago.*)

chamber. The furnaces shown in Fig. 5-5 are rotary kilns which discharge the ash to a conveyor.

3. *The Combustion, or Secondary, Chamber.* This is located between the furnace and the stack, and its purpose is to permit mixing of the hot gases and allow time for combustion to take place. Some plants provide for the burning of dead animals in this chamber. It also allows completion of burning of fly ash, which otherwise would be emitted from the chimney to present a fire hazard. A temperature of at least 1250°F is necessary for complete burning of combustible gases, and 1400°F is desirable to ensure against escape of odorous gases. Temperatures in the furnace or combustion chamber should not exceed 2000°F, or the refractory brick lining may be damaged and require replacement. Successive heating and cooling is undesirable as it encourages spalling. Continuous operation of incinerators reduces this effect.

4. *The Chimney, or Stack.* The incinerator stack serves to discharge the gases into the atmosphere and is also a means for providing air movement or "stack draft" through the incinerator system. The wide use of forced-draft systems has had the effect of lowering chimney heights; however, the chimney height should be designed to enable adequate dilution of gases with air and to minimize fly-ash problems.

5. *Miscellaneous Features.* Provision must be made for temporary storage and removal of ashes. Most plants utilize a system of *ashpits,*

which receive the noncombustible wastes and are equipped with a water-spray system or other quenching device. Many ashpits are hopper-shaped and located so that removal trucks may be loaded by gravity. *Air supply* is important. Forced draft is generally used, which requires a fan or blower and the necessary ducts to force air below the grates and up through the bed of burning material, but no farther. The chimney should then supply the remainder of the necessary draft. Not all incinerators employ forced draft, but the practice of including it is increasing. Additional air is usually supplied to the furnace above the grates and to the combustion chamber. The theoretical total requirement is 5 lb of air per lb of combustible refuse, but this is usually doubled in designing air requirements. Preheating of the air supply is also an operational practice that is considered economical in plants of more than 75 tons capacity. The air discharged below the grates is preheated by passing it through ducts where it may absorb heat from the chimney gases. *Steam-generating apparatus* has been installed at some plants. It usually consists of a water-tube boiler placed between the combustion chamber and the chimney. Steam generation requires a higher temperature in the combustion chamber than is otherwise necessary—1600 to 1900°F, as compared with 1250°F. *Control apparatus* should include thermometers for checking temperatures of the burning chambers, the preheated air, and the stack gases. Scales for weighing the refuse are a necessity, and provision for weighing ashes is desirable. Special fly-ash removal apparatus may be necessary, or the incinerator may violate the local air-pollution-control requirements. Filters, baffle devices, centrifugal or cyclonic separators, water-spray chambers, and electrostatic devices have been developed for this purpose.

INCINERATOR OPERATION. The quality of operation and maintenance received by an incinerator will determine its success or failure. Care in charging will prevent reduction of furnace temperature and thereby avoid excessive smoke, odors, and escape of unburned material. It is important that moisture and volatiles be driven off and burned in the combustion chamber while solid materials are being consumed in the primary chamber. To ensure this and to avoid a "flashy" fire, firing should not be infrequent and at long intervals, but rather as continuous as furnace construction permits.

PURCHASE OF INCINERATORS. In contracting for the construction of an incinerator, definite specifications should be formulated, and certain requirements should be established in detail. The kind and condition of the refuse to be destroyed should be specified as definitely as possible, or facilities for prospective bidders to review local operations should be provided. Various operating conditions should also be specified. These include furnace temperature desired; amount of refuse to be destroyed within a certain time; amount of fuel, if any, that is required; and quality and quantity of ashes and clinkers. It should also be recognized that forced draft, preheaters, top-quality refractory materials, and automatic temperature and air-valve controls are all requirements for good incinerator operation and not merely "frills." Contracts should not be awarded on the basis of price if any of the above have been omitted.

Contracts should also guarantee a satisfactory test run of several days' duration under the supervision of the contractor. Some municipalities require the builder to supervise the operation of the incinerator for a month or longer, with the city paying all expenses and furnishing materials but assuming no responsibility and accepting the plant only after a 24- or 48-hr test run at the end of that time. This may necessitate storage of materials in order to ensure that the incinerator can be tested at rated capacity.

5-30. On-site Incineration. This term applies to incineration of refuse at the home, apartment house, commercial building, hospital, or industrial site. Backyard burning by open fires or in simple outdoor incinerators is banned by many cities because of fire hazard and air pollution by particulates and hydrocarbons. Refuse collection and disposal could be much reduced by satisfactory on-site incineration. New York City has an ordinance requiring that all new multifamily dwellings have approved incinerators [4]. A study indicated that by 1970 there would be 13,000 domestic incinerators and that these would burn 2,250 tons of mixed refuse per day, with a residue of 550 tons, which would have to be hauled away. Unfortunately, many on-site incinerators cause local air pollution and complaints. The flue-fed incinerator is often a culprit. This type has openings on each floor to the flue serving the incinerator, and tenants deposit refuse in them. When the furnace is full, the attendant burns the material. There may be difficulties from flame-back and smoke to the floor openings unless all doors are locked during burning. This is prevented in some cases by providing a separate chute to the furnace. Generally, air-pollution troubles can be expected from this and from any type of incinerator unless it has a combustion chamber and adequate air supply. This also applies to incinerators serving hospitals and commercial buildings. The American Gas Association has studied gas-fired hand-charged incinerators suitable for residential use that should present no air-pollution difficulties provided they are properly operated [9].

5-31. Sanitary Landfill. Sanitary landfill differs from ordinary dumping in that the material is placed in a trench or other prepared area, adequately compacted, and covered with earth at the end of the working day. The term "modified sanitary landfill" has been applied to those operations where compaction and covering are accomplished once or twice each week.

GENERAL CONSIDERATIONS. As in other methods of disposal, satisfactory sanitary landfill operation demands careful preliminary evaluation of local conditions. Landfills are designed to care for the complete disposal of all refuse produced, with the possible exception of bulky building wastes and the like. For this reason, sanitary landfill capacities usually are designed for the total refuse produced. Where compacted refuse is placed in the fill to a depth of 6 ft, it is estimated that 1 acre of land per year will be required per 10,000 population.

Prospective landfill sites should be evaluated with respect to type of soil available, drainage, prevailing winds, availability of access roads, and haul distance involved. Possible contamination of ground and surface water should be considered in choosing a site. In some areas of California, limitation of refuse materials is applied to certain sites for this reason [4, 11]. Sandy loam is considered the most suitable landfill soil, although other soils can be utilized. Poor surface drainage may hinder the operation, and care should be exercised to prevent interception of an underground water stratum in constructing the fill. Other considerations governing the planning of sanitary landfill sites are contained in a publication of the Texas State Department of Health [10]. They are as follows:

1. Scavenging materially interferes with the overall efficiency of the operation, and should be discouraged. If it is permitted, strict regulations should be formulated and rigidly enforced.

2. Provision should be made for temporarily fencing the leeward side of the landfill so that the nuisance of blowing papers will be held to a minimum. This is economically accomplished with light chicken wire.

3. Regulations governing the operation and maintenance of the landfill should be predetermined and publicized. Printed instructions should be distributed to all concerned. This is particularly significant if private hauling is permitted.

4. Signs should be erected at the disposal ground which clearly indicate the correct procedure for depositing refuse. The entrance sign should have something similar to "Sanitary Landfill Refuse Disposal Area" clearly indicated.

5. The landfill disposal area should be fenced and have an entrance gate. The gate should be locked during non-operating hours to discourage indiscriminate dumping of refuse.

6. A responsible attendant should be at the disposal site during the operating hours.

OPERATIONAL TECHNIQUES. Methods of landfill operation are largely determined by the information obtained during the preliminary evaluation of prospective sites. Also, the population to be served and the type of equipment available will influence the choice of methods. Three broad classifications of operational methods have been developed: the trench method, the area-ramp method, and the area-fill method. The three

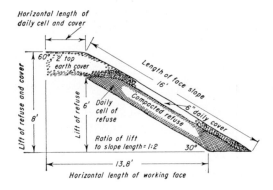

FIGURE 5-6 The working face of a sanitary landfill. (*From "Refuse Collection and Sanitary Landfill Operational Methods," Texas State Department of Health, Division of Sanitary Engineering, Austin, Tex., 1954.*)

methods are similar in many respects, and the principles of each can often be combined to serve specific local conditions. Figure 5-6 is a cross section of the working face, or slope, of a typical landfill. No matter what operational method is chosen, the working face should be maintained at about a 30-deg slope and kept as narrow as practicable. Dumped refuse is spread over the slope, compacted, and covered as a part of the daily operational routine. Six inches of earth is placed over the compacted refuse on the slope, and at least 2 ft of compacted earth should be placed on top of that portion of the fill that is completed each day. Earth cover must be compacted to prevent fly emergence; 6 in. will be sufficient. Uncompacted cover up to 48 in. in depth will not prevent fly emergence. Figure 5-7 shows the trench method, with a side ramp that allows several trucks to dump at a time.

Where level terrain is available, the trench method is usually chosen. The trench may be completely excavated prior to beginning the operation, or it may be excavated progressively as the work proceeds. Trenches are usually 6 to 10 ft in depth and, depending on local conditions, 12 to 36 ft in width.

The area-ramp method is well suited for moderately sloping terrain. Actually, this method can be utilized to bring a sloping area to grade by an operation similar to that depicted in Fig. 5-8. Some excavation is done to secure cover materials and side ramps. Refuse is placed in the excavation to the desired height above the original ground level.

Figure 5-9 depicts a typical area-fill operation where two separate fills are utilized to bring a deep depression to grade. This method often has the disadvantage of requiring supplemental earth from outside sources.

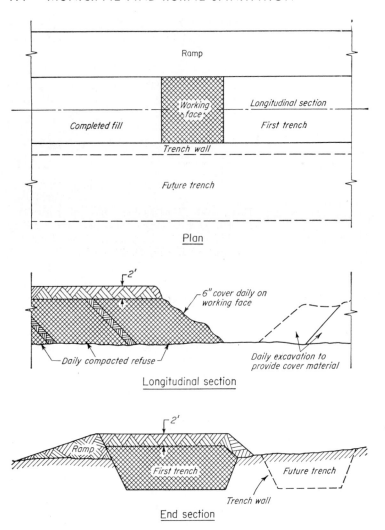

Figure 5-7 Trench method of disposal with side ramp.

Suitable equipment has been developed to perform the complete landfill operation—excavation, spreading and compacting refuse, and moving earth to serve as cover material. Track-type equipment fitted with an appropriate bucket, clamshell, or blade can easily accomplish the landfill operation in smaller cities. Larger cities sometimes prefer to use power shovels or draglines for the excavation of trenches, with tractors being freed for the other operational phases.

CHARACTERISTICS OF THE FILL. Chemical, bacteriological, and physical changes occur in buried refuse. In about 4 days after placement and at

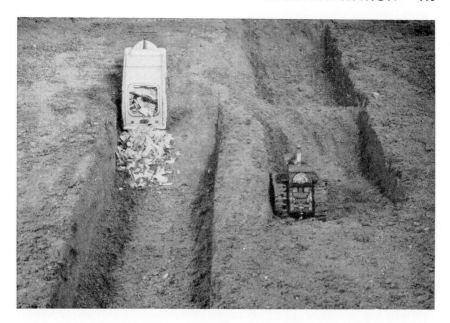

FIGURE 5-8 Trench method of disposal in a prepared trench with earth cover obtained by excavating an adjacent trench. (*Photograph from "Refuse Collection and Sanitary Landfill Operational Methods," Texas State Department of Health, Division of Sanitary Engineering, Austin, Tex., 1954.*)

about 3 ft below the surface, temperatures rise rapidly to 130 to 150°F. They remain at this point for about 60 days and then fall gradually for about 10 months to near air temperatures. It appears from observation of deposited materials that decomposition proceeds very slowly. The composition of landfill materials, which include only about 15 per cent garbage, is probably responsible for this slow decomposition. An important factor in the development of temperatures is the type of material incorporated in the fill. In some cases cells containing "mixed" refuse do not attain temperatures much higher than 100°F.

Some settlement of the fill should be expected, and if the desired elevation of the finished fill is known, allowance for settling can be made during construction. Most of the final settlement will probably occur

FIGURE 5-9 Area-fill operations in deep ravines. (*From "Refuse Collection and Sanitary Landfill Operational Methods," Texas State Department of Health, Division of Sanitary Engineering, Austin, Tex., 1954.*)

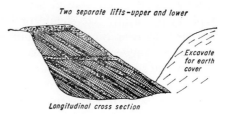

within the first 12 months, and by the end of 2 years most fills have completed settlement. The actual amount will vary with the character of the wastes, the compaction given, and the depth of the fill. Uneven settlement may be caused by improper placement of bulky rubbish and no provision for a well-mixed refuse. An ultimate settlement of between 10 and 30 per cent is to be expected at most fills.

USE OF FILLED LAND. The potential use of filled land should receive careful consideration during the planning stage of landfill construction. Sanitary landfills have been used to improve eroded areas, marshes, and other marginal lands. Following the settling period, such filled areas have been used for parks, golf courses and other recreational areas, airports, parking lots, and small construction. It is usually recommended that construction be limited to single-story buildings, although heavier buildings may be constructed if foundations are carried through the fill to undisturbed earth or if reinforced-concrete mat foundations are utilized. Water pipes and sewers passing through the fill will probably require special precautions against corrosion, contamination, and settlement. Methane gas is produced in the decomposition process. Consequently any construction which might allow seepage into areas that are restricted in air movement, such as a basement, should receive very careful attention with respect to mechanical ventilation facilities.

ADVANTAGES AND DISADVANTAGES OF SANITARY FILL. As compared with the ordinary dump, sanitary fill has the advantages of minimizing odor and fire nuisances and of eliminating such health hazards as insect and rodent breeding. Over such other disposal methods as incineration, reduction, and hog feeding, it has the advantages of cheapness and simplicity, since no separation of refuse is required. Costs per ton in the United States vary from about 50 cents to $1.50. The only manpower requirement at many landfills is a machine operator. Smaller cities find it possible to utilize landfill equipment for other municipal activities, although allowance must be made for the daily use of the equipment at the landfill. Landfill operations are usually elastic enough to care for usual quantities of refuse caused by expanding populations. Properly operated fills can be located in such a way that collection trucks have convenient access. Finally, marginal land can often be reclaimed for profitable resale.

The principal disadvantage is that unless careful and continuous supervision is given, the fill may deteriorate into an ordinary dump. A sanitary fill of any size should preferably be under the supervision of a sanitary engineer. Since land requirements for sanitary landfill operations are large, bigger cities sometimes experience difficulty in obtaining suitable sites at reasonable prices.

5-32. Composting. During recent years, considerable interest has been developed in the composting of municipal refuse as a method of waste disposal [12]. Europeans recognize the process as one of waste recovery, for composted refuse is considered an excellent organic additive for agricultural soils, and composting operations are common in European countries. Because of the availability of cheap inorganic fertilizers in this country, a widespread demand for compost has not yet materialized. Composting should, however, be considered by the engineer in evaluating the various methods of refuse disposal.

THE COMPOST PROCESS. Anaerobic processes have been tried in this country with little success, but trial of aerobic methods indicates that decomposition in the presence of oxygen is much more rapid and affords freedom from odors and other nuisances associated with the older anaerobic method. Operations fundamental to the composting of municipal refuse may be listed as follows:

1. *Removal of Noncompostables.* Several components of mixed municipal refuse are of no value in the compost process. Some of these, such as cans and other metals and glass, can sometimes be recovered for sale. While magnetic devices will remove the ferrous metals, some provision must be made for hand picking the wastes. California studies [13] indicate that after initial segregation, the refuse from a number of California cities is 66 per cent compostable.

2. *Grinding or Shredding.* To speed up bacterial action, the raw refuse is shredded prior to placement in piles, digesters, or bins for decomposition. It is recommended that shredders reduce the refuse to particles having no greater dimension than 2 in. [12].

3. *Blending or Proportioning of Materials.* The optimum carbon-nitrogen ratio in the refuse for speedy bacterial action is 30–35:1, *i.e.*, 30 to 35 parts carbon to 1 part nitrogen [11]. A ratio above 35–40:1 will require a considerable increase in composting time. Blending is considered unnecessary, however, when the carbon-nitrogen ratio is 25–50:1. This may be done at the plant if loads containing much paper, straw, and sawdust, which are deficient in nitrogen, can be combined with other loads high in nitrogen, such as slaughterhouse wastes, fish scrap, blood, night soil, or sewage sludge. The optimum moisture content for aerobic composting is 40 to 60 per cent, depending on the character of the material. Materials which become a soggy mass will soon become anaerobic at a moisture content of 70 per cent. Blending should be done with concern for moisture.

4. *Placement for Composting.* Open piles or windrows are placed on the ground, on a paved area, or in shallow pits. If aerobic conditions are to be maintained by frequent turning, windrows or piles are used, the former being the most convenient. Piles and windrows should not be greater than 5 to 6 ft high and not less than $3\frac{1}{2}$ to 4 ft. Windrows should be about 8 to 12 ft wide at the bottom, and piles about the same diameter. The windrows or piles are turned at such intervals that

aerobic conditions are maintained. This may be every 2 or 3 days if the moisture content is high or a total of three or four times in a 15- to 21-day composting period. Mechanical methods have been developed for turning windrows [11]. Temperature is an important factor, the optimum range being from 122 to 158°F, with about 140°F usually the most satisfactory. Temperatures will be established naturally and will be highest in the middle of the pile or windrow. Excessively high temperatures, over 167°F, will be injurious to bacterial action. Turning has little effect upon temperature, but excessive temperature can be controlled by lowering the windrow height. In order to maintain optimum temperature in cold weather, the height may be increased. A drop in windrow temperature may mean that anaerobic conditions have developed.

5. *Mechanical Methods.* Private companies have successfully used composting methods in European cities, but only a few cities in the United States have entered into contracts for such service. A plant using mechanical methods may be described as follows: The refuse is received on a conveyor and transported to a building where salvable material such as white glass, cardboard, nonferrous metal, rags, and paper are removed and where paper sacks and containers are torn open. Thereafter a magnetic separator removes ferrous metals. The remainder is then ground and conveyed to a digester for a varying period during which moisture, temperature, and aeration are closely controlled. Upon the digester the material is screened to remove large undigested items and is passed through a separator to remove glass. It is then trucked to an adjacent area where, if digestion is incomplete, it is windrowed for further aerobic action. Some companies use a bacterial inoculum to speed digestion, but studies made at the University of California indicated that the necessary bacteria are naturally present in the refuse.

CHARACTER AND VALUE OF THE COMPOST. Composted material is stable, *i.e.*, undergoes little or no further decomposition, and has only a slight musty or earthy odor. Its color will be grayish or brownish black. Its principal value when applied to the soil is as a conditioner. It lightens the soil, promotes aeration, and helps to retain moisture by adding humus. It has some fertilizing value, as revealed by an analysis of compost derived from municipal garbage and refuse containing a large amount of paper [14] which showed average values on the dry basis as follows: nitrogen, about 1.4 per cent; phosphorus (as P_2O_5), about 1.1 per cent; potassium (as K_2O), about 0.8 per cent; carbon, about 28 per cent; and ash, about 37 per cent. The amount of organic matter was not given.

HEALTH PROBLEMS. Compost itself presents no health hazards. The heat developed in the composting process will kill pathogenic bacteria and the eggs of parasites. The killing temperature usually extends only to within 4 to 8 in. of the surface of the pile. Turning, therefore, also plays a part in ensuring destruction of pathogens and parasites.

Fly production can be expected where composting is conducted in the open. The grinding process should kill many fly maggots and eggs already in the refuse, but some will survive, and eggs will be laid on the pile surfaces, particularly if there is much garbage or feces in the material. High temperatures of the pile interior will kill the eggs, but maggots will migrate to the cooler surface layers of the piles, and there pupation will occur. The fly-control measures discussed in Art. 9-32 can then be applied. Completely composted material is not attractive to flies.

FUTURE OF COMPOSTING. The possibility of recovering valuable material from the huge volumes of municipal refuse appeals to the imagination. The hard facts of economics, however, indicate that wide adoption of the process under present conditions is improbable. Compost is in demand by the farmers of some countries [15], but in the United States inexpensive inorganic fertilizers are in common use. Hauling compost at, say, 10 cents per ton-mile makes it more costly, as far as its fertilizing value is concerned, than inorganic fertilizers for most farms [16]. The lack of a market for compost has caused failures of municipal composting ventures in the United States. Composting, however, may become more popular in the future if farmers recognize its considerable soil-conditioning value as an adjunct to its modest fertilizing value. This is a possibility for use for certain soils and for farms and market gardens near cities. There is some evidence [11, p. 142] that operating costs of composting plants are less than the cost of incineration at large plants and that the first costs of the two plants will be about the same. The composting plant will be at a disadvantage because of its greater volume of residue, but if this can be disposed of, free of charge to the city or by sale at some price, composting can compete with incineration.

5-33. Discharge to Sewers. Three methods for the disposal of garbage with sewage are in use in the United States: the installation of individual grinders in homes and commercial establishments; the installation of municipally operated centrally located grinding stations; and the installation of grinders at sewage treatment plants and discharge of the ground materials directly into incoming raw sewage or to the digestion tanks.

HOUSEHOLD GRINDERS. Household grinders contribute no difficulties in sewer collection systems. At the sewage treatment plant, the load of solids is increased by 0.07 to 0.10 lb per person on the dry basis. A few cities have forbidden grinders, and this restriction is justified where existing sewerage facilities are overloaded. Most cities, however, have no restrictions.

Universal adoption of household grinders will be necessary if the process is to have a material effect upon the over-all refuse program.

The total volume of refuse will not be substantially reduced because garbage constitutes only 10 to 15 per cent of the refuse in many cities. Collection of rubbish would remain a necessity. Jasper, Ind., became the first community in this country to attempt city-wide installation of grinders. A report [17] of the system in that city is generally favorable.

MUNICIPAL GRINDING STATIONS. The location of central grinding stations at convenient points along the sewer system or at the sewage treatment plant is favored in some cities. Again, garbage must be separated from other refuse by the householder prior to collection. Ground garbage is introduced directly to the sewer system, or if the grinder is located at the sewage treatment plant, ground materials are sometimes sent to digesters, with other phases of treatment being by-passed. Central grinding stations need not be objectionable, although care should be taken to provide treatment of odors that arise from the accumulated garbage. The solids are ground to $\frac{1}{4}$ in. or smaller.

The discharge of ground garbage into sewer systems has not been reported as causing trouble, although an increase of cockroaches and rats has been noted in some trunk sewers. If garbage of all the population contributing sewage is ground at a central grinding plant and then discharged into the sewers, the suspended solids will be increased 50 per cent or less, and the biochemical oxygen demand will be increased 30 per cent or less. The water consumed with the grinding will amount to 1 gpcpd (gallon per capita per day).

5-34. **Salvaging.** Although objectionable and often economically unsound, salvage operations are sometimes practiced in connection with other disposal methods, particularly composting. Salvaged materials must also be properly stored, pending their utilization, or nuisances will result. If householders are required to segregate and store refuse separately for salvage purposes, the revenue from salvaged goods must be weighed against the additional costs entailed by multiple-collection systems.

Paper, cardboard, glass, metals, rags, garbage, and miscellaneous commercial wastes are the principal elements of refuse having marketable value from time to time, although this market is subject to wide fluctuation. If clean paper can be reclaimed, it can be re-used in the manufacture of paperboard or cardboard. Glass has some value, especially if it can be hand sorted according to size and color. Broken glass is quite limited in value. Cans and other metals are of some value because of their tin coating and solder. Commercial areas are often the source of such salvable refuse as cloth and leather trimmings, some wood materials, and, of course, cardboard cartons. Careful evaluation of potential local markets for salvable goods should precede municipal salvage activities. Salvaging concessions at open dumps and sanitary landfills are sometimes sold.

The Refuse Problem in Small Towns and on the Farm [13]

5-35. In many of the smaller cities and towns there are no organized efforts to collect and dispose of refuse. Business establishments and some householders may make private arrangements for collection, usually at irregular intervals. This results in unsightly and offensive accumulations between collections and is uniformly unsatisfactory as far as disposal is concerned. The piles of cans and other refuse, even dead animals, so frequently found in highway ditches at the outskirts of the town and in vacant lots testify to the irresponsibility of the casual collector. Often the total payments made to private collectors who serve only a fraction of the city amount to nearly enough to give regular service to all the city. Annual cleanups are substituted for regular collection in some small cities. This practice results in some temporary betterment and considerable civic complacency, which is not justified. Cleaning should be a continual process, not just an annual affair.

In general it is recommended that the small city collect refuse itself rather than by contract. In any event, municipal authority should adopt a suitable ordinance regulating the entire program and specifying the storage, collection, and disposal procedures to be observed. Technical assistance in financing, organization, and operational methods should be sought.

Many small cities have found that a complete refuse collection and disposal system can be operated for approximately $1.50 per month per resident and $5 per month per commercial establishment. Some municipalities prefer a fee system by which bills are mailed monthly or quarterly for refuse service, often with the water or other utility bills. Other cities prefer tax-supported systems, with revenue being taken from general funds.

Residents of sparsely populated rural and suburban areas usually find the solution to refuse problems through a combination of incineration and burial. The farmer or suburbanite usually must find a safe, convenient method of disposal within the confines of his own property. Since open burning will not achieve complete combustion of all refuse, the removal and burial of ashes and noncombustibles are necessary for adequate disposal. For the small organized communities, sanitary landfill probably is the best disposal method.

Bibliography

1. "Sanitary Refuse Practices," Public Health Service, 1953.
2. An Analysis of Refuse Collection and Sanitary Landfill Disposal, *Univ. Calif. Sanitary Eng. Research Center Tech. Bull.* 8, 1952.

3. "Refuse Collection Practice," American Public Works Association, Public Administration Service, Chicago, 1958.
4. "Municipal Refuse Disposal," American Public Works Association, Public Administration Service, Chicago, 1961.
5. "Equipment for the Heat Treatment of Garbage to Be Used for Hog Feed," U.S. Agricultural Research Service and Public Health Service.
6. Meissner, H. G.: Municipal Incinerator Selection, *Public Works*, vol. 90, no. 11, November, 1959.
7. Nickelsporn, H. B.: Factors in Incinerator Design, *Public Works*, vol. 93, no. 3, March, 1962.
8. "Incinerator Standards," Incinerator Institute of America, New York, 1963.
9. "A Study of Effluents from Domestic Gas-fired Incinerators," American Gas Association, New York, 1959.
10. "Refuse Collection and Sanitary Landfill Operational Methods," Texas State Department of Health, Austin, Tex.
11. "Sanitary Landfill," American Society of Civil Engineers Manual of Engineering Practice no. 39, New York, 1959.
12. Gotaas, H. B.: "Composting," World Health Organization Monograph Series, no. 31, Columbia University Press, New York, 1956.
13. Reclamation of Municipal Refuse by Composting, *Univ. Calif. Sanitary Eng. Research Center Tech. Bull.* 9.
14. McGauhey, P. H., and H. B. Gotaas: Stabilization of Municipal Wastes by Composting, *Trans. Am. Soc. Civil Engrs.*, vol. 120, p. 897, 1955.
15. Shuval, H. I.: Economics of Composting Municipal Refuse, *Proc. Am. Soc. Civil Engrs.*, vol. 88, no. SA4, pt. 1, July, 1962.
16. Stone, R.: Economics of Composting Municipal Refuse (Discussion), *Proc. Am. Soc. Civil Engrs.*, vol. 88, no. SA6, November, 1962.
17. Community-wide Installation of Household Garbage Grinders, *Public Health Service Pub.* 224.
18. Rogus, C.: Refuse Collection and Disposal in Modern Europe, pt. 1. *Public Works*, vol. 93, no. 4, April, 1962.
19. "Paper Bags for Municipal Refuse Handling," Report of Research Project no. 115, American Public Works Research Foundation, Chicago, 1963.

6

MILK SANITATION

The Dairy

6-1. Milk is not a mere beverage; it is an important food which supplies protein, fat, carbohydrates, mineral matter, and vitamins to the human body. Its chief advantages as a food are that it is a fairly well-balanced ration; it is easily digested; it contains no waste materials, such as bone, peelings, skin, or shell; it requires no cooking; and it is cheaper than many other products having the same food value. A quart of milk furnishes 500 to 600 calories. The protein in milk is the flesh-, muscle-, tissue-, and bone-building constituent; the fat supplies energy and provides fatty tissue; and the carbohydrates, mainly as milk sugar, furnish energy or are converted into fat. Mineral matter, or ash, is necessary for bone and tooth formation. Vitamins A, B, and C are also present in milk, and these promote growth in the young and aid in the prevention of rickets, beriberi, and scurvy. Even under the best conditions, however, normal milk lacks adequate amounts of vitamin C. Also, since this vitamin is not heat-stable, its concentration may be further reduced through pasteurization. For this reason physicians recommend that infants or young children fed on milk from cows be given a small quantity of orange or tomato juice to make up any vitamin C deficiency. Milk is also frequently fortified with vitamin D and is relatively rich in vitamins E and K.

Providing sanitary conditions for the handling of milk and milk products causes many problems for the sanitarian. The conditions under which it must necessarily be produced, the ease with which it may be contaminated, and the rapidity with which it spoils—all these factors contribute to the difficulties confronting the public health official who is responsible for the safety and quality of a city's milk supply.

6-2. Milk as a Vehicle of Infection. The diseases which may be spread by infected milk include tuberculosis, typhoid fever, dysentery, diphtheria, septic sore throat and other streptococcal infections, staphylococcal toxins, salmonellal gastroenteritis, brucellosis, and Q fever. Table 6-1 is a summary of reported milk-borne disease outbreaks. Note the drop in outbreaks from 1950 due to improved milk supplies.

Bovine tuberculosis is transmitted by the ingestion of unpasteurized milk or dairy products from tuberculous cows, by airborne infection in barns, and by handling of contaminated animal products. Transmission of tuberculosis from human origin through milk is usually the result of careless handling of the milk by infected persons or of exposure of milk to flies or dust. The bovine type of tuberculosis is now rare in the United States, Canada, Scandinavia, and the Netherlands. It is rapidly being eliminated in Great Britain, Switzerland, and parts of France and Germany, but it is still a problem in South America, southern Europe, parts of Africa, Asia, and Australia.

Typhoid, dysentery, and *Salmonella* organisms may reach milk from the unclean hands of milkers or other dairy employees who are carriers or are in the early stages of illness. For that reason, dairy workers should wash their hands thoroughly and disinfect them before milking. The importance of clean habits, such as washing the hands after excretion of urine or feces, should be impressed upon all milk handlers. Disinfection of the hands before milking or handling the milk is also necessary. Exposure of the milk to flies, particularly if there are insanitary toilets in the neighborhood, is dangerous. Allowing cows to wade in sewage-polluted water at the dairy may also result in dangerous milk.

Those diseases transmitted by throat and nose discharges, such as diphtheria, septic sore throat, and scarlet fever, usually reach milk from

Table 6-1. SUMMARY OF MILK-BORNE DISEASE OUTBREAKS REPORTED BY STATE AND LOCAL HEALTH AUTHORITIES AS HAVING OCCURRED IN THE UNITED STATES DURING THE YEARS 1923–1960, INCLUSIVE

Year	Typhoid Outbreaks	Typhoid Cases	Typhoid Deaths	Paratyphoid Outbreaks	Paratyphoid Cases	Paratyphoid Deaths	Scarlet fever and septic sore throat Outbreaks	Scarlet fever and septic sore throat Cases	Scarlet fever and septic sore throat Deaths	Diphtheria Outbreaks	Diphtheria Cases	Diphtheria Deaths	Dysentery Outbreaks	Dysentery Cases	Dysentery Deaths	Food infection, food poisoning, and gastroenteritis Outbreaks	Food infection, food poisoning, and gastroenteritis Cases	Food infection, food poisoning, and gastroenteritis Deaths	Undulant fever Outbreaks	Undulant fever Cases	Undulant fever Deaths	Miscellaneous Outbreaks	Miscellaneous Cases	Miscellaneous Deaths	Total, all diseases Outbreaks	Total, all diseases Cases	Total, all diseases Deaths
1923	15	423	31	0	0	0	7	406	6	1	5	0	0	0	0	0	0	0	0	0	0	0	0	0	23	834	37
1924	25	693	48	10	372	16	6	354	0	1	23	0	2	110	1	0	0	0	0	0	0	0	0	0	44	1,552	65
1925	31	580	43	2	37	4	10	1,108	8	1	14	1	0	0	0	0	0	0	0	0	0	0	0	0	44	1,739	56
1926	49	1,189	83	2	19	1	11	1,789	10	2	24	0	0	0	0	1	150	0	0	0	0	3	192	1	68	3,363	95
1927	24	430	35	2	53	0	4	389	5	2	15	1	0	0	0	1	50	0	3	17	0	0	0	0	36	954	41
1928	25	421	48	0	0	1	11	1,449	55	2	48	0	1	126	16	2	104	0	5	21	0	0	0	0	46	2,169	120
1929	29	541	36	1	38	0	19	1,891	14	0	0	0	1	8	1	1	24	0	0	0	0	0	0	0	51	2,502	51
1930	30	575	41	0	0	0	11	1,158	7	0	0	0	1	64	2	6	171	6	0	0	0	0	0	0	48	1,968	56
1931	21	217	16	1	22	0	9	1,059	8	1	22	0	1	65	0	1	13	0	0	0	0	0	0	0	34	1,398	24
1932	23	254	22	0	0	0	9	356	6	0	0	0	0	0	0	1	32	0	0	0	0	0	0	0	33	642	28
1933	25	299	26	1	17	0	10	753	9	2	19	3	0	0	0	0	0	0	0	0	0	4	260	1	42	1,348	39
1934	26	345	27	1	400	0	9	478	8	1	9	0	1	131	0	4	292	0	0	0	0	0	0	0	42	1,524	35
1935	16	172	14	2	50	0	11	1,065	7	0	0	0	0	0	0	13	411	0	1	15	0	0	0	0	43	1,829	21
1936	15	114	5	1	21	0	18	1,553	23	0	0	0	0	0	0	8	188	0	0	0	0	0	0	0	42	1,891	28
1937	15	208	11	0	0	0	14	1,384	3	1	31	0	2	166	0	8	523	0	1	4	0	2	35	0	43	2,150	14
1938	18	187	17	0	0	0	12	674	7	0	0	0	2	324	3	8	627	0	0	0	0	2	33	0	42	1,685	27
1939	6	51	1	2	24	0	9	1,324	6	0	0	0	2	197	0	18	749	0	4	19	0	0	0	0	41	2,509	7
1940	14	120	10	0	0	0	5	482	0	1	5	0	3	126	0	16	855	0	3	96	0	1	5	0	43	1,678	10
1941	12	120	4	0	0	0	3	219	0	1	36	4	1	40	0	15	483	2	5	42	0	0	0	0	37	1,049	10
1942	5	42	0	1	4	0	7	620	0	1	20	2	0	0	0	25	1,341	0	4	22	0	2	68	0	45	2,193	2
1943	6	37	1	0	0	0	3	200	0	0	0	0	0	0	0	26	1,278	6	4	42	0	1	33	0	40	1,590	7
1944	8	359	18	1	6	0	2	171	0	0	0	0	2	34	0	23	816	0	3	20	0	2	43	2	41	1,449	20

185

Table 6-1. SUMMARY OF MILK-BORNE DISEASE OUTBREAKS REPORTED BY STATE AND LOCAL HEALTH AUTHORITIES AS HAVING OCCURRED IN THE UNITED STATES DURING THE YEARS 1923–1960, INCLUSIVE (*Continued*)

Year	Typhoid			Paratyphoid			Scarlet fever and septic sore throat			Diphtheria			Dysentery			Food infection, food poisoning, and gastroenteritis			Undulant fever			Miscellaneous			Total, all diseases		
	Outbreaks	Cases	Deaths	Outbreaks	Cases	Deaths	Outbreaks	Cases	Deaths	Outbreaks	Cases	Deaths	Outbreaks	Cases	Deaths	Outbreaks	Cases	Deaths	Outbreaks	Cases	Deaths	Outbreaks	Cases	Deaths	Outbreaks	Cases	Deaths
1945	3	72	4	0	0	0	3	308	0	1	53	2	1	22	0	18	1,673	11	2	19	0	1	14	0	29	2,161	17
1946	1	7	0	0	0	0	0	0	0	0	0	0	1	15	0	11	696	0	5	66	0	1	11	0	19	795	0
1947	3	57	7	1	28	0	0	0	0	0	0	0	0	0	0	16	162	0	2	6	0	0	0	0	22	253	7
1948	1	11	0	0	0	0	1	67	0	0	0	0	2	126	1	11	350	1	0	0	0	2	59	0	17	613	2
1949	1	7	0	0	0	0	0	0	0	0	0	0	0	0	0	10	218	0	2	4	0	2	17	0	15	246	0
1950	0	0	0	0	0	0	0	0	0	0	0	0	0	0	0	7	54	0	3	8	0	0	0	0	10	62	0
1951	1	2	0	1	10	0	1	20	0	0	0	0	0	0	0	7	46	0	0	0	0	2	12	0	12	90	0
1952	0	0	0	0	0	0	2	143	0	0	0	0	1	639	0	3	51	1	0	0	0	0	0	0	6	833	1
1953	0	0	0	0	0	0	0	0	0	0	0	0	1	59	0	3	38	1	0	0	0	0	0	0	4	97	1
1954	1	6	0	0	0	0	0	0	0	0	0	0	0	0	0	6	182	1	1	4	0	1	8	0	9	200	0
1955	0	0	0	0	0	0	0	0	0	0	0	0	0	0	0	3	302	0	0	0	0	0	0	0	3	302	0
1956	0	0	0	0	0	0	0	0	0	0	0	0	0	0	0	30	869	0	1	4	0	0	0	0	31	873	0
1957	0	0	0	0	0	0	0	0	0	0	0	0	0	0	0	5	48	0	1	2	0	2	17	0	8	67	0
1958	0	0	0	0	0	0	0	0	0	0	0	0	0	0	0	13	441	0	0	0	0	0	0	0	13	441	0
1959	0	0	0	0	0	0	0	0	0	0	0	0	0	0	0	10	44	0	1	5	0	0	0	0	11	49	0
1960	0	0	0	0	0	0	0	0	0	0	0	0	0	0	0	5	48	0	0	0	0	0	0	0	5	48	0
Total	449	7,539	548	29	1,101	22	207	19,420	182	18	324	13	25	2,252	21	336	13,329	23	50	374	3	28	807	4	1,142	45,146	816

SOURCE: Public Health Service. Data for years from 1950 to 1959 from Dauer, Sylvester, and Davids, Summaries of Disease Outbreaks, National Office of Vital Statistics, published annually in *Public Health Repts*. Data for 1960 from C. C. Dauer, "1960 Summary of Disease Outbreaks and a 10-year Résumé," National Center for Health Statistics, Public Health Service.

the dairy workers who are carriers or who are in the early stages of the diseases. Spitting, sneezing, coughing, or even forcible speaking during the process of milking or while in the vicinity of uncovered milk may result in infection. Sneezing into the hands or handling of handkerchiefs during milking is dangerous unless the hands are washed and disinfected before milking is resumed. Streptococci, staphylococci, and other organisms of human origin may gain lodgment in the teats and udder of the cow and grow there. This condition is known as bovine mastitis [1]. It may be responsible for human infections that cause scarlet fever or septic sore throat, and the toxins generated in the milk by the latter may cause severe gastroenteritis (Art. 6-9).

Undulant fever, or brucellosis, is caused by three closely related bacteria: *Brucella melitensis, B. abortus,* and *B. suis.* Cattle, swine, sheep, goats, and horses are reservoirs of infection. One method of transmission to man is by ingestion of unpasteurized infected milk and milk products. Pasteurization of the milk is the best safeguard, although efforts should be made to eliminate contagious abortion from dairy herds [2].

Milk has also been found to be involved in the transmission of Q fever, which is increasing and is now considered endemic in the United States [3]. See Art. 6-24 for special requirements in pasteurization. This disease is caused by a *rickettsia.*

There is no scientific knowledge at the present time concerning the role of milk in the transmission of viral diseases.

6-3. Essentials of Milk Sanitation. The prevention of milk infection is the most important feature of milk sanitation, not only as a means of preventing disease but also as a measure that inspires public confidence, thereby leading to a higher milk consumption, a result that all health workers desire. But disease prevention is only one aspect of the subject. Clean milk is also a necessity, and clean milk is that which has a small number of bacteria in it. Unclean utensils, the entrance of dust and manure, and storage at high temperatures all directly affect the bacterial population. Large numbers of bacteria also cause quick-souring and bad-tasting milk. Odors may be absorbed by milk which is left standing in a cow stable or refrigerator, although odors also appear in milk soon after they are inhaled by the cow. Milk sanitation then has two objects: the production of *safe* milk and the production of *clean* milk. The essentials to attaining these objectives are given below:

1. *Healthy cows.* This implies freedom from tuberculosis, contagious abortion (Bang's disease, or brucellosis), mastitis, and other specific diseases.

2. *Clean and healthy workmen.* The freedom of dairymen from communicable disease is of vital importance. Their personal cleanliness is of little less moment.

3. *A clean environment.* This means a clean, airy, dustless barn with sanitary cow yard and surroundings.

4. *A separate milk room.* This means a room for the handling of milk that is separate from the barn, well constructed, properly screened, and supplied with safe water.

5. *Utensils and equipment of proper design.*

6. *Effective sanitization and scrupulous cleanliness* of pails, cans, coolers, bottles, and other equipment with which milk comes into contact.

7. *Prompt cooling and proper handling of milk,* including milking, storage and transportation if needed, bottling, capping, and delivery.

8. *Pasteurization.* This is essential for the production of *safe* milk, for experience has shown that even though all other possible precautions are taken, infection may still enter. Pasteurization is the most practicable method of overcoming such danger.

In the following articles further details of the above essentials will be set forth.

6-4. Milk and Bacteria. As it is removed from the cow's udder, milk contains some bacteria. Ordinarily these are harmless, but if the animal is diseased some may be pathogens. Inevitably, other bacteria enter the milk from the air and through contact with dust, the milker's hands, and the surfaces of milk pails, cans, coolers, and other utensils. How many enter thus depends upon the skill, cleanliness, and carefulness of the dairyman. Pathogens enter by the methods given in Art. 6-2. Under favorable conditions some of them may increase. However, the rapid increase of bacteria as shown in Fig. 6-1 is caused by the growth of nonpathogens, including those which cause souring.

The bacteriological tests of milk include obtaining the "total count," which means determining the number of organisms which will grow on agar plates under the standard laboratory conditions [4]. The total count is also obtained by counting with the microscope the clumps of bacteria seen in the field and by counting individual organisms. The clump count and the plate count are comparable, but the individual organism count is normally four times the others. They are all expressed as the count per milliliter.

Reduction tests with methylene blue or resazurin have been utilized as a quick method of estimating the quality of raw milk [4]. Because

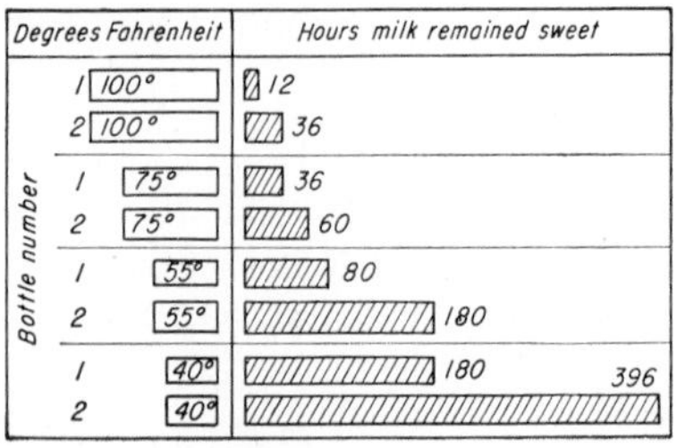

FIGURE 6-1 Effect of high count and temperature of storage. Milk from bottle 1 contained 280,000 bacteria per milliliter; that from bottle 2 contained 16,400 per milliliter. (*Courtesy of U.S. Department of Agriculture.*)

of many limitations, however, decreasing emphasis is placed on them as control tests. In fact, the "Milk Ordinance and Code: 1953 Recommendations of the Public Health Service" [5] omits mention of them in the definition of average bacterial plate count and direct microscopic count; however, communities that find it necessary to permit use of the reduction tests may do so by making suitable modifications in the Ordinance.

Pasteurized milk should be tested for coliform organisms. These bacteria are killed by pasteurization, and their presence in pasteurized milk is an indication of dangerous aftercontamination.

Thermophilic bacteria are nonpathogenic organisms which flourish and increase at high temperatures. They are believed to enter milk with dust, and therefore they can be generally related to conditions at the dairy. They give trouble by causing high counts in pasteurized milk. Thermoduric bacteria are also nonpathogenic and are frequently found in the raw milk. They are able to withstand the pasteurizing temperature and thus are also responsible for high counts. They are especially likely to occur in milk from dairies where milking machines are used and where the methods of cleaning, sanitizing, and storing the machines are poor. The milk stone which accumulates on poorly cleaned equipment is likely to be high in such bacteria. Psychrophilic bacteria are nonpathogenic and will multiply at low temperatures. Their presence in milk is established by incubating samples before plating at 44.6°F [6].

6-5. Foreign Substances in Milk and Milk Products. The term "foreign substances" as used here does not apply to bacteria, dust, hairs, insects or insect debris, manure, or other dirt which may appear in milk products. The other foreign substances that constitute a potential health hazard are pesticides and antibiotics which may appear in milk or milk products. Pesticides may enter milk through the careless or uninformed use of insecticides in the barn or milk room. They may also enter milk when applied to the cows or put in the forage fed to them. Antibiotics are used in the treatment of diseases of diary cattle. Penicillin, for example, is used in the treatment of mastitis, an udder infection. Regulations require that milk be wasted for 3 days after treatment, but this is hard to enforce. If it is not done, penicillin will be in the marketed milk. The Food and Drug Administration has established no tolerances for any foreign substances in milk or milk products [6]. The use of certain insecticides in dairy animals as well as in the dairy and milk room is approved by the Public Health Service. Approval is based on reports of the Entomological Research Division of the U.S. Department of Agriculture, which revises its publications periodically and gives acceptable uses and strengths of these insecticides [7]. Table 9-4 gives names and methods of use in dairies of some approved fly-control chemicals.

Other foreign substances in milk may be derived from plastics, which are now replacing metals in certain processing equipment and which have components that may migrate to the milk. Chemical sanitizing agents may enter from treated surfaces. Radionuclides appear in milk after weapons testing, principally from fallout upon grasses or forage consumed by cows. Methods are being developed to remove certain radionuclides from milk [8, 9]. The Public Health Service (Art. 17-12) conducts a program monitoring radioactivity of milk.

6-6. Legal Responsibility for Quality Control of Milk and Milk Products. The Food and Drug Administration of the U.S. Department of Health, Education, and Welfare enforces the Federal Food, Drug, and Cosmetic Law. Under it the FDA controls the safety of milk and other foods which enter into interstate commerce. With regard to milk quality, it sets up the requirements for, and makes tests regarding the use of, insecticides on forage for dairy cattle or in barns.

The Public Health Service of the same department exerts no legal control but has done much to aid in the production of safe and clean milk by the development of procedures for the production and handling of milk. These are incorporated in the Standard Milk Ordinance and Code [5]. It is currently the basis of milk regulation in 37 states, and its provisions have been voluntarily adopted by 1,435 cities and 512 counties.

State health departments exert the police powers of the state as they apply to health protection. The local health departments, city and county, exert as much control as they are permitted by the state and also, practically speaking, as much as they are willing to pay for. The cities are more important than counties in this activity since most market milk, though produced in rural areas, is sold in the cities, which can control the quality of milk brought in for sale. Adoption of the Standard Milk Ordinance by a state generally means that it has authorized its cities to adopt the Ordinance through their own legal action. Some may adopt it with variations, particularly as to bacterial content and requirement of pasteurization.

6-7. Physical and Chemical Tests of Milk. While bacteriological tests, as indicated in the above article, are important, certain other tests are routinely made in milk-control laboratories [4]. The test for butterfat content determines whether the cream content is up to standard. The specific-gravity test and the cryoscope, or water-freezing-point, test are used to determine the content of solids-not-fat and to indicate whether milk has been watered. Chemical tests are made when it is suspected that preservatives have been added. Some laboratories also check all samples of raw milk for the presence of bacterial inhibitors, such as penicillin. The sediment test consists in forcing a sample of milk through a disk of filtering material; the visible dirt on the disk gives an indication of the amount of dirt in the milk.

The phosphatase test shows that this enzyme has been destroyed by heat and indicates whether milk has been properly pasteurized or not. If it is suspected that the temperature has not been high enough or that the holding time has been too short, the test should be applied. The Milk Ordinance and Code states that this test should be routinely performed by every pasteurization plant. This test is also reliable in the detection of underpasteurization of cream, ice cream, sherbet, chocolate milk drinks, butter, sweet buttermilk, cultured buttermilk, most of the principal kinds of cheese, and cheese whey. Care should be taken when making this test that the milk is not rewarmed after collection, or the phosphatase may become reactive and give a false indication of improper pasteurization [6, 10].

Surveillance of milk for radionuclides is discussed in Art. 17-12.

6-8. The 3A Sanitary Standards for Dairy Equipment. Three groups that are interested in milk sanitation on a national basis—the public health authorities, dairy-equipment manufacturers, and the users of dairy equipment—collaborate in developing a set of standards recommending the observance of certain sanitary principles in the design of various items of dairy equipment. These three groups are represented by the Committee on Sanitary Procedures of the International Association of Milk and Food Sanitarians, Inc., the Milk and Food Program of the Public Health Service, and the Sanitary Standards Subcommittee of the Dairy Industry Committee. The latter subcommittee is composed of members from the American Butter Institute, American Dry Milk Institute, Dairy Industries Supply Association, Evaporated Milk Association, International Association of Ice Cream Manufacturers, Milk Industry Foundation, National Cheese Institute, and National Creameries Association.

The development of standards is a continuing program, with revisions being made as deemed necessary. As the standards are established, they are published in the *Journal of Milk and Food Technology*. Among the items covered by the standards are fittings used on milk-products equipment, thermometer fittings and connections, storage tanks, milk pumps, weigh cans and receiving tanks, homogenizers, automotive transportation tanks, electric motors and motor attachments, can-type milk strainers, filters using disposable filter media, determination of holding time of high-temperature short-time pasteurizers, plate-type heat exchangers, milk pumps, internal tubular heat exchangers, installation and cleaning of cleaned-in-place pipelines, holding and/or cooling tanks, thermometer fittings and connections, and automotive milk-transportation tanks for bulk delivery and/or farm pickup service.

6-9. Healthy Cows. All cows from which milk is obtained and sold in towns under the Milk Ordinance are required to be tested at least once every 6 years if located in an area accredited by the Animal Disease

Eradication Division, U.S. Department of Agriculture, as having a bovine tuberculosis incidence of 0.2 per cent or less. Where this standard is not maintained, the herds should be subjected to annual tuberculin tests until that incidence is reduced to 0.2 per cent. All cows discovered to be reactors must be immediately removed from the herd, branded with the letters TB, and slaughtered under the direction of the livestock sanitary officials in the presence of an accredited veterinarian.

Milk yielded during a period of 15 days before calving and usually 4 or 5 days (occasionally several weeks) afterward is not normal and should not be sold. Slimy, ropy, or bloody milk may indicate udder infections. The cow should be separated from the herd, and the milk should not be sold.

The slightest suspicion that a cow is not in good health should result in the rejection of its milk, pending thorough examination of the animal by a veterinarian. The dairy inspector should look for abnormal conditions of teats and udders, particularly inflammation and lumps, and should recommend the services of a veterinarian. If the lumpiness or induration is extensive, affecting one or more quarters of the udder, the cow should be excluded from the milking herd, even though its milk seems normal. Such conditions in cows are known as bovine mastitis, and they are caused by a number of organisms including streptococci, staphylococci, *Salmonella,* and others which are transmissible and pathogenic to man. In addition, the enterotoxin produced by staphylococci, which are not destroyed by pasteurization, will cause poisoning (Art. 7-4). Preventive measures applied to the cows are periodic examinations by veterinarians, segregation of infected animals, sanitation and good milking practices, and good herd management [1].

The Milk Ordinance and Code requires that a certain number of years after its adoption—usually 3—all milk and milk products to be sold be from herds following one of the brucellosis-eradication plans recommended by the Meat Inspection Division of the U.S. Department of Agriculture and administered by the state livestock sanitary authorities. These plans involve brucellosis-free testing routines aimed at making the dairy herds in the United States free of brucellosis [2]. Q fever has been mentioned in Art. 6-2.

6-10. Health and Habits of Dairy Workmen. Dairy workers should be given physical examinations, and their histories should be taken. If the health officer considers it necessary, laboratory examinations are made to determine whether they are carriers of disease. Should any illness occur upon a dairy farm, the producer or distributor should immediately notify the health authorities.

Personal cleanliness of the milk handler is, of course, necessary, particularly during milking and other periods of contact with the milk. This applies to the clothing as well as to the hands. Hands should be washed, rinsed with an effective bactericidal solution, and dried immediately before milking, and should there be any interruption whereby the hands may have become contaminated, such as handling a handkerchief or touching the floor or any unclean object, the disinfectant should again be used. The worker should never indulge in sneezing, coughing, spitting, or the use of tobacco while handling milk. Since colds and other respiratory irritations are sometimes the first symptoms of serious diseases, it is advisable to exclude persons so affected from milking or other close proximity to the milk.

The bactericidal solution used for hands can also be used for other purposes. Compounds of chlorine are most suitable and can be purchased in solution, with directions and instructions for the making of dilutions. Bactericides other than those mentioned should not be used unless approved by the health authorities.

6-11. The Dairy Barn and Surroundings. The dairy barn must be kept clean lest dust and dirt from its atmosphere enter the milk during the milking and affect its quality. Barns should be well ventilated, and there should be no crowding. Efficient artificial illumination must be provided for milking during the hours of darkness. To allow easy cleaning, the floor and gutters must be constructed of concrete or some other impervious material and must be graded to drain properly. The walls and ceilings should be painted once every 2 years or whitewashed every year. This allows easy inspection and encourages the dairyman to keep walls and ceilings clear of cobwebs and other dirt and dust. Tight ceilings are necessary if cattle feed is stored above the barn.

Weather conditions in certain areas of the country are such that "loafing" pens, called pen-type stables, may be provided for cows waiting to be milked. They can be located adjacent to, but not actually in, the

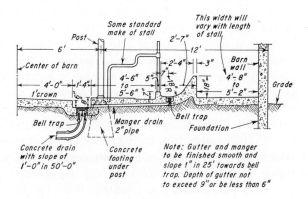

FIGURE 6-2   Half cross section of a well-designed dairy barn, showing dimensions based on best practice. (*Courtesy of Portland Cement Association.*)

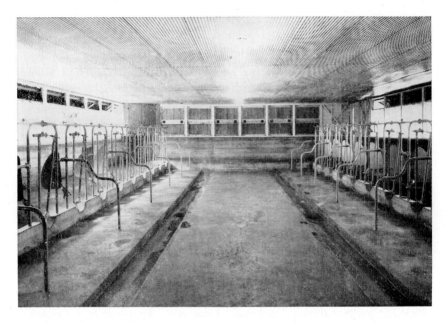

FIGURE 6-3   Interior of a dairy barn.

milking area. However, they are not permitted in the southern section of the United States, where indoor pens create a tremendous fly-control problem.

The water used at a dairy farm to cleanse surfaces that come in contact with milk should be obtained from a supply which meets all public health standards with regard to location, protection, and operation (see Arts. 2-36 to 2-40). Generally, well water should be used except when other sources, such as a cistern or surface-water supply, have been given sufficient treatment in the judgment of the public health authority to render them safe for this use. The well, of course, should be located so that it is not subject to contamination from privies, cesspools, barnyard areas, and similar sources. Cross-connections should be avoided; these include submerged inlets in cattle drinking cups, wash vats, etc. The water supply should preferably be piped into, or otherwise made easily accessible to, both the milkhouse and the dairy barn. The method of sewage disposal employed for the farmhouse as well as any other toilets in the establishment is important from several standpoints, including effective fly control, protection of the source of water supply, and maintenance of a generally clean area.

6-12. The Toilet. Too often the toilet on the dairy farm is far from sanitary. The open-back surface toilet is especially undesirable here because of the danger of infected flies reaching the milk. Most dairies have, or should have, an abundant water supply, so that there is no

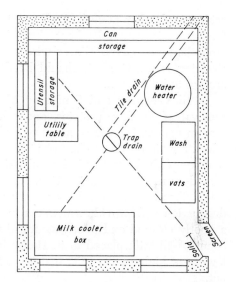

FIGURE 6-4 Recommended design for a milk room.

reason why flush toilets with a septic tank and disposal field should not be used. If there is not sufficient water, pit toilets of the improved type with self-closing seats, properly located with respect to the water supply, may be used. See Art. 4-36. The method for disposal of dairy wastes should meet all state standards.

6-13. The Milkhouse. All handling of milk, with the exception of the actual milking, should take place in a separate structure designated as the milkhouse or milk room. In order that no odors will be absorbed by the milk, and as a protection against flies and dust, the milkhouse should not open directly into the barn or into a room used for sleeping or domestic purposes, and it should be used for no purpose other than the handling or processing of milk. The practice of handling milk previous to sale in the farm kitchen, where it is likely to be tampered with by children, perhaps suffering with one of the children's diseases, is not to be tolerated. A completely satisfactory milkhouse is well lighted and ventilated, having a window area equal to 10 per cent of the floor area, with walls and ceilings that can be easily cleaned and painted or otherwise finished in a satisfactory manner, and with a tight floor of concrete, or other impervious material, graded to drain. All openings are screened to exclude flies. The screen doors must open outward and be provided with springs to ensure prompt and automatic closing. Water should be piped into the milkhouse.

6-14. Design of Utensils. Milk pails and cans should have as few seams as possible, and the necessary ones should be soldered flush so that there will be no cracks to prevent efficient cleaning; better still, the improved seamless pails and cans may be used. The same applies to coolers and other utensils. Badly rusted and dented tinware is unsatisfactory as it cannot be kept clean. Milk cans should preferably have umbrella-type covers. Woven-wire milk strainers are not permitted. If straining is practiced, it should be done with single-service pads that are not to be re-used.

6-15. Cleaning and Sanitizing of Equipment. *Cleaning* means the removal of all fats, proteins, and salts of the milk, as well as other foreign matter, from the surface of milk utensils. Destruction of bacteria which remain on the surface of utensils after cleaning, when such action is accomplished by physical or chemical agents, is termed "sanitizing." This does not imply sterilization. Efficient cleaning aids sanitization because films of grease, salts, or other matters protect the bacteria from destruction and provide a medium in which they will grow. Therefore, a poorly cleaned and poorly sanitized utensil will increase the bacterial count of all milk placed in it. Hence it is essential to the production of low-count high-quality milk that these two processes be properly carried out.

6-16. The Cleaning Process. Various cleaners are available for the purpose, but regardless of the type of cleaner used, the final results depend upon the conscientiousness of the worker. Clean equipment is bright and shining and sheds water evenly. If drops of water adhere to surfaces, there is some grease film present, and further cleaning is necessary. Good cleaning also eliminates bacteria from surfaces, for most of them are removed mechanically by the washing process and rinsing.

All equipment which is not designed so that it can be cleaned in place should be disassembled for cleaning. This applies to such dairy-farm and milk-plant apparatus as milking machines, valves, coolers, pasteurizers, and pipelines, and the cleaning should be done daily. A thorough brushing aids the cleaning agent in removing all soil, and disassembling makes brushing easier. Warm water should always be used, preferably at a temperature of 115 to 120°F, for cold water will not remove grease. Warm water also aids the action of cleaning agents.

Properly designed pipelines may be cleaned in place by circulating appropriate cleaning solutions through them at relatively high velocities. First, usually, a rinse water at 100 to 120°F is circulated for a short period of time, the rinse water being continuously discarded. After this initial rinse, an alkaline nondepositing cleaning solution, heated to 120°F or above, is circulated for 15 min and then discharged. Sometimes an alternate acid cleaning solution heated to 120°F or above is circulated for 15 min. After the acid or alkaline solution is used, a thorough rinsing of the lines is required, and a bactericidal solution is run through the lines immediately prior to their next usage period.

A good cleaning agent will dissolve in the wash water to make a clear mixture free from floc, and it should remove the fats, proteins, and salts without forming combination curds. Strongly alkaline cleaners act as saponifiers of the fats; if a wetting agent is also included in the cleaner, an emulsifying effect is obtained which speeds up the flowing of the film from the surfaces. Such alkaline cleaners as trisodium phosphate and sodium metasilicate, working at pH 10.5, are good protein-dissolving agents [5, 11]. At other pH values they are less effective.

Hard waters affect the action of cleaners. A detergent such as trisodium phosphate will unite with calcium and magnesium salts, which are the causes of hardness in water, to form an insoluble precipitate. Until all the calcium and magnesium are so combined with the phosphate, i.e., until the water approaches zero hardness, the detergent does little or no good. This explains why more cleaner must be used with some waters than with others. Unfortunately, too, the precipitated salts unite with the milk solids to form a film which sticks to the utensil surfaces. The film is known as "milk stone" or "water stone," and bacteria trapped on its rough surface will increase the bacterial count of milk that comes in contact with it.

There are three compounds in general use that operate in hard waters without forming stone: pyrophosphates, tetraphosphates, and hexaphosphates. The first is the least effective, and the last the most effective. They will also remove milk stone, but only gradually. A number of compounds that dissolve calcium and magnesium salts are on the market as stone removers. As Mallmann points out, where milk-stone removers are used intermittently in conjunction with an inefficient cleaner, intermittently good and bad cleaning and intermittently good- and poor-quality milk result.

6-17. Sanitizing with Chemical Agents. Sanitizing or disinfecting by chemical agents is not a shortcut to obtaining clean utensils. They must first be cleaned, and then the sanitizing agent will destroy any bacteria remaining on the surfaces. The best time for sanitizing is just before the utensil is used; however, if cleaning and sanitizing are properly done and if the utensils are properly stored, there should be no great danger of high bacterial counts.

The principal sanitizing agents used in dairy practice are the oxidizing compounds, the sodium and calcium hypochlorites, the former being sold in liquid form and the latter as a powder. They are sold under various trade names, and the containers give the percentage of chlorine and the methods of use for various purposes (see Arts. 2-18 and 2-20). Use involves making solutions or dilutions of a required strength of available chlorine. The chloramines are another group of chlorine oxidizers. They are more stable than the hypochlorites and give good results when used in hot-water rinses. The chlorine here is liberated more slowly than from the hypochlorites, and accordingly more contact time must be allowed.

Several precautions are necessary in the use of chemical disinfection: (1) The surfaces should be clean because films will protect the bacteria. (2) Sufficient time should be provided. Most bacteria are killed within 10 sec of contact, but those which are surrounded and protected by other organisms require a longer time. Hence the contact period should be at least 2 min, and longer if possible. (3) The strength of the bactericidal solution should be so much in excess of the killing dose that, as its strength is dissipated by use, there is still sufficient residual strength to kill all the organisms on the surface. At least 100 ppm should be in the applied solution, and the solution must be discarded when the concentration drops below 50 ppm available chlorine. (4) The water in which the chlorine disinfectants are diluted should not be too alkaline. It will take four to five times as much chlorine in solution to kill at a pH of 9 as it will at a pH of 7, and the time of exposure should be lengthened. This is another reason for using the high concentrations recommended under (3) if the pH of water is variable or unknown. At a milk plant, however, this important information should be available. (5) Temperature is important. An increase of 10°C or 18°F doubles the activity of the chemical. It would be inadvisable, however, to use chlorine solutions in water having a temperature of more than 160°F because the chlorine may be driven off.

The strength of the chlorine solution can be checked in several ways. The orthotolidine solution (Art. 2-19) or the starch-iodide method may be used to determine the available chlorine in solutions. Test sets with instructions are available. Starch-iodide papers are also used; these are strips of sensitized paper immersed in the solution, and a change of color is noted. The results given are only roughly quantitative. Bacterial tests can also be made. A sterile cotton swab is rubbed over the surface, or sterile water is flushed over it, and the swab or rinse water is examined for the number of bacteria (see Art. 7-14). The plate count should not be more than 100 from 8 sq in. of swabbed surface.

6-18. Heat as a Sanitizing Agent. Heating, as a method of sanitization, penetrates the film on the surface of utensils and provides disinfection even though the utensils have not been properly cleaned. The high temperatures required, however, generally discourage the use of this method, and it is therefore not recommended for dairy farms.

If dry heat is used, the temperature must be at least 180°F with an exposure of at least 20 min in a properly designed oven or cabinet equipped with a thermometer.

Moist heat, however, is widely used at milk plants by one or more of the following methods:

1. Exposure to steam for at least 15 min at a temperature of at least 170°F, or at least 5 min at 200°F, in a steam cabinet equipped with an indicating thermometer located in the coldest zone

2. Exposure to an enclosed steam jet for not less than 1 min

3. Immersion in hot water at a temperature of at least 170°F for at least 2 min, or exposure to a flow of hot water at a temperature of at least 170°F (at the outlet) for at least 5 min, as determined by a thermometer

6-19. Milking. Bacterial contamination of the milk during the milking process will provide the maximum opportunity for the bacteria to multiply, resulting in an increased count and a lowering of the quality of the milk by the time it reaches the consumer. It is necessary, therefore, for dairy workmen to be extremely careful in observing all standards of cleanliness during the milking process (see Art. 6-10). Dust in the air is likewise a source of contamination and should be kept to a minimum by maintaining cleanliness in the barn. One good practice to observe is that of placing the feed and allowing the dust to settle before the cows are milked. The cleanliness of the cow is equally important. The cow's flanks should be carefully brushed to remove all visible dirt, and the teats and udders should be washed and sponged with water containing a bactericidal solution similar to that used by the milkers in disinfecting their hands, as mentioned in Art. 6-10. The excess solution is removed with a cloth, which has also been subjected to the disinfecting treatment. It is recommended that the hair on the tail and under the flanks of the cow be clipped at periodic intervals.

Wet-hand milking is not permissible. As each cow is finished, the

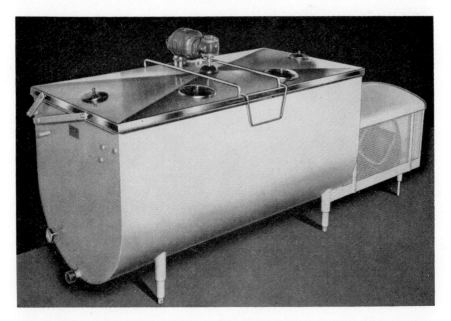

FIGURE 6-5   A farm bulk milk tank. (*Photograph courtesy of Creamery Package Manufacturing Company, Chicago.*)

milk is carried directly to the milk room to be strained and cooled. In lieu of using the milkhouse for the straining operation, an effectively screened straining room may be provided in or near the barn or stable but not opening into it. This procedure, however, is not recommended because it delays the cooling of the milk. An alternative is pouring and/or straining from the milk pails or milking-machine pails into a 5- or 10-gal clean milk can provided with a well-fitting cover. In this case, the cans are placed at a distance from the cows or raised above the floor so that they are protected from manure or splash, with the cover closed when milk is not being poured. Self-closing covers are recommended.

The milking stool must be kept clean. A dirty, manure-encrusted stool will contaminate the hands of the milker and increase the bacterial count of the milk. Aluminum stools or other kinds which can be scrubbed and cleansed with hot or boiling water may be used. In any case, they should be handled as little as possible by the milker.

6-20. Milking Machines. The use of milking machines has some advantages and some drawbacks. Danger of infection from the hands of the milkers is lessened, and there is less opportunity for dust, manure, and other bacteria-containing material to fall into the milk. In many cases, however, the use of milking machines has resulted in high-count milk. Upon investigation, this was found to be due to the difficulty of sanitizing the materials used, particularly the rubber hose. Very high temperatures are injurious to the hose, and yet the minute cracks which appear in it after use make necessary the most careful and thorough treatment. Milking machines also tend to accumulate milk stone, which furthers the production of thermoduric bacteria and results in unduly high bacterial counts in pasteurized milk. It is important, therefore, that cleaning and sanitization of milking machines be very carefully done. In poorly designed machines, it has been found that milk sometimes gains entry into the air line. If such air lines are not properly cleaned, this milk drips back into the container and results in contamination. In any event, whether machines are well or poorly designed, airline hoses should be maintained in a sanitary condition.

Mallmann and coworkers [12] conducted a series of experiments in the cleaning and sanitizing of milking machines. Groups of milk producers were chosen, each of whom followed a different but generally acceptable method of cleaning and sanitizing the milking machines. All groups disassembled and washed the apparatus daily. Group 1, the control group, followed its usual procedures. Group 2 used an alkaline cleaner (Solvay 600) and BK powder as a hypochlorite. After the cups and tubes had been cleaned, they were stored in the hypochlorite, and a hypochlorite rinse was given just before using. Group 3 also used Solvay 600 as a cleaner, BK powder, and an alkali (Rubberkleen). After being cleaned, the cups and tubes were stored in the alkali, and the hypochlorite was used as a rinse just before milking. Group 4 used Solvay 600 for cleaning. Storage was in a 1:6,400 dilution of a quaternary ammonium compound (Art. 8-10) for sanitizing, and there was a rinse before use in the same compound at the same dilution. Group 5 used a combined cleaner-sanitizer compound. This was a mixture of alkaline cleaners, a wetting agent, and a quaternary ammonium compound. It was used as recommended, in such concentration that the quaternary compound would be 1:4,000. The producers of this group used the compound, followed by a clear-water rinse. All equipment was stored dry, and there was no rinse before using. The milk samples obtained from all the producers were pasteurized in the laboratory and then tested for total count.

The conclusions that can be drawn from the investigation are interesting. The quaternary compounds were most effective in sanitizing the equipment. This was the method used by Group 4. Group 3 also showed uniformly good results. No method was noticeably inadequate. The rinse with a sanitizing agent just before milking is apparently important. The effect of careful operation was well brought out. The good producers were able to obtain better results with any of the methods described than the poor producers attained by the best methods. This emphasizes what milk sanitarians have long known, that care and intelligence must be combined with proper agents and equipment in order to produce good milk and that the former requirements are the more important.

6-21. Straining. The milk-straining process should take place immediately after the cow is milked. This is preferably done in the milkhouse, but if it is done in the barn, the conditions explained in Art. 6-19 should be observed. There is a tendency for the uninformed dairyman to place too much reliance upon straining. It removes hair and the larger particles of dust and manure, but some of the manure goes into solution, and the bacteria, of course, tend to remain in the milk. Straining, no matter how efficiently done, is never a substitute for cleanliness and care in milking. The best strainer is composed of two pieces of perforated metal holding a thin layer of sterilized absorbent cotton between them. After use, the cotton is thrown away. The metal apparatus with supplies of cotton can be obtained from manufacturers of dairy equipment. Since wire strainers cannot be properly cleaned, they are not permissible. Straining will indicate unclean milking methods.

6-22. Cooling. Milk is an ideal medium for the multiplication of most disease-producing organisms. Their activity ceases, however, at temperatures of 45°F and below, and therefore prompt cooling of the milk to that point is an important factor in the production of low-count milk. Milk that is to be delivered raw to the consumer should be cooled immediately after the milking process to 45°F or less. This is desirable under all conditions, but if the milk is to be delivered to a milk plant for pasteurization or separation within 2 hr after milking, it need not be cooled. The Standard Milk Ordinance (1953) states that the cooling temperature should be 50°F or less, but it has been discovered that 45°F or below is essential in order to prevent growth of *Brucella* organisms. More than cooling is necessary; the low temperature must be maintained until the milk is delivered to the consumer. Milk should not be allowed to freeze.

Cooling is accomplished in various ways. The crudest method consists in submerging the cans of milk in troughs or tanks of ice water. This is frequently the only method of cooling at many farms which sell or ship milk in bulk. In this case, the troughs should be of concrete, preferably insulated by layers of cork, with insulated covers. A removable wooden rack should be placed on the bottom of the tank. It should be borne in mind that a 30-gal tank of water at 37°F will cool a 10-gal can of milk from 85 to 50°F in half an hour and will keep it at that temperature as long as the can remains in the tank. A mechanical stirrer should be used to keep the cold water circulating around the cans. Ice, of course, should never be placed in the cans themselves.

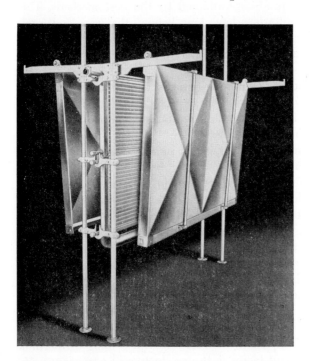

FIGURE 6-6   A surface cooler, with covers partially removed. (*Courtesy of Cherry-Burrell Corp., Chicago.*)

Another method of cooling uses coils or pipes over which the milk trickles in a thin film and through which ice water or cold brine is circulated (see Fig. 6-6). This, of course, implies a refrigerating system and in general is used only at the larger dairies and at pasteurizing plants. Surface coolers in milk plants are covered to protect the milk from dust and flies. Coolers require careful cleaning and sanitizing. The latter should be done preferably just before using, or a rinse with a sanitizing agent should be used.

6-23. Bottling, Capping, and Delivery. Bottling in small dairies is usually done by small machines which fill only one bottle at a time. At large dairies or creameries, more elaborate bottling and packaging machines, capable of filling many bottles or cartons at a time, are used.

Hand capping of milk bottles has the defect of permitting contamination of the milk or the cap by the hand of the worker. Approved types of caps for milk bottles may be constructed of paperboard; metal foil, such as aluminum foil, is also approved and commonly used. Cartons of plastic or paper of approved design have largely replaced glass bottles.

As the bacterial count of milk immediately starts to climb when the temperature rises above 50°F, it is necessary in warm weather that milk be kept iced during delivery. This is done by packing fist-sized lumps of ice around the necks of the bottles.

Pasteurization

6-24. Pasteurization is the application of heat to milk for the purpose of destroying disease-producing organisms. It is the one practical method of ensuring safe milk. On the other hand, it is not to be considered a palliative measure to apply to unclean milk or milk that is far advanced in decomposition. In fact, undesirable tastes or odors of milk, if already present, are likely to be intensified by the heating.

Opponents of pasteurized milk frequently harp on the fact that its vitamin C content is destroyed in the process and that children consuming it are therefore deprived. As mentioned in Art. 6-1, however, the vitamin C content of raw milk is an uncertain factor, and the diet of babies requires reinforcing with orange or tomato juice. Opposition to pasteurized milk, although it still exists among some of the "natural food" faddists, is unimportant at this time.

The destruction of bacteria by heat is dependent upon the temperature and also upon the length of exposure to that temperature. While pathogenic organisms are more susceptible than most of the harmless bacteria, the susceptibility varies with the species. Diphtheria organisms are most easily killed, a temperature of 130°F with an exposure time of 30 min being effective. With a like exposure, streptococci succumb at 133°F; typhoid bacilli, at 136°F; and tubercle bacilli, the most resistant to heat, at 139°F. Shorter exposures—for instance, a 20-min period—require higher temperatures. A 10-min exposure requires about 3° still higher. Still higher temperatures kill the pathogens in very short times. At 160°F, for example, the desired result is obtained in 15 sec.

Too high temperatures are undesirable because of their destructive effects upon the normal cream line of the milk and the enzymes. They cause coagulation of the albumin, produce a "cooked" taste, and bring about chemical changes in the salts, fats, casein, and sugar. The cream-line effect is the earliest noted if the temperature is increased or the period prolonged over and above that necessary for destruction of the pathogens. The temperature of change of the cream line varies from 3° above the killing temperature of tuberculosis organisms with a 40-min exposure, to 7° above with a 10-min exposure; it is 5° above with a 30-min exposure. The wide use of homogenized milk, in which no cream line appears, has lessened the importance of this objection. A 30-min period for milk pasteurization has been established as being convenient in the operation of many commercial pasteurizers. Since the tuberculosis organisms with this exposure are killed at 139°F and since the cream line is affected at 5° higher, or 144°F, it will be seen that there is a range between the two values that permits pasteurization with safety and without damage to the other qualities of the milk. This led to the usual requirement by state and city health authorities that milk pasteurization be accomplished by heating to at least 142°F and holding that temperature for 30 min. However, to allow for fluctuations, it is recommended that in the low-temperature pasteurizers the minimum temperature be placed at 143°F, which is the temperature required by the Milk Ordinance and Code: 1953 Recommendations of the Public Health Service. The Ordinance also permits use of 161°F for at least 15 sec. This is known as the high-temperature short-time (HTST) method. Investigations indicate that the organism responsible for Q fever—the rickettsia *Coxiella burnetii*—requires a temperature of 145°F for 30 min. Accordingly, this temperature is necessary for such protection [13]. This is even more important when dairy products containing sugars and high fats, such as cream, chocolate milk, and ice cream mixes, are pasteurized. It is also recommended that when high-temperature short-time pasteurization is employed, a temperature of 166°F or higher be used instead of 161°F [14]. A modern trend is to use ultrahigh temperatures, a method described in Art. 6-25.

Pasteurization is fatal to pathogens and to nearly all other bacteria; the total reduction in bacterial count is usually close to 99 per cent, varying with the number of thermophilic and thermoduric bacteria present. It will be seen, therefore, that pasteurization is not sterilization. High-count raw milk, which is likely to contain high concentrations of thermophilic and thermoduric bacteria, after pasteurization will show considerable numbers of bacteria. Souring of milk is delayed by the process but is not prevented. It should also be recognized that pasteurized milk may become contaminated with pathogenic organisms through careless handling after pasteurization.

6-25. Pasteurization Methods. Those types of pasteurization equipment that are used, and the sanitary problems connected with them, are briefly described in this article.

VAT TYPE. This consists of a vat into which the cold or partially heated raw milk is run until it is filled, after which heat is applied to bring the milk to the pasteurization temperature; that temperature is then maintained until the required 30 min has elapsed. The milk may be heated by steam or hot water which circulates through a pipe coil in the vat or through a hollow vat wall. In order to ensure uniform temperature throughout the milk, some method of agitation is used. After the pasteurization period is over, an outlet valve is opened, and the milk runs through piping to the cooler and bottler. This pasteurizer is manually operated.

HIGH-TEMPERATURE SHORT-TIME TYPE. The high-temperature short-time type (HTST) pasteurizer is a continuous flow pasteurizer. After the milk has been preheated in the regenerator, its temperature is rapidly brought up to that of pasteurization, at least to 161°F, and is held there by passage of the milk through a holding tube for a period of 15 sec, after which the milk is returned to the regenerator, cooled, and bottled. Where the milk is high in fat or sugar, and particularly where Q fever is endemic, the temperature should be increased to 166°F or higher [6, 13]. It has also been found that a temperature of 170 to 175°F will not cause a cooked taste and will provide a longer shelf time.

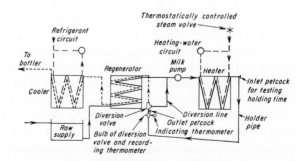

FIGURE 6-7 Diagrammatic elevation of automatic high-temperature short-time pasteurizer. (*From A. W. Fuchs, Automatic Control of Pasteurization: Advantages and Safeguards, Am. J. Public Health, vol. 30, no. 5, May, 1940.*)

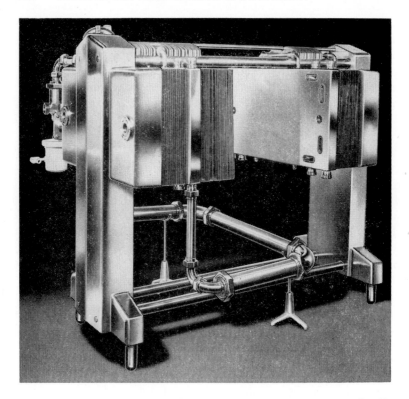

FIGURE 6-8 High-temperature short-time pasteurizer. Hot water and milk or coolant pass between alternate metal plates. Large pipe below is the holder. The three sections (shown separated) permit regeneration, heating to pasteurizing temperature, and cooling. (*Courtesy of Creamery Package Manufacturing Company, Chicago.*)

Figure 6-7 is a diagram of the HTST pasteurizer. Since they require far less space, HTST pasteurizers have mostly replaced the holder types at the larger milk-processing plants.

ULTRAHIGH-TEMPERATURE PASTEURIZATION. A late development is the use of 194°F as the pasteurization temperature. The action is practically instantaneous, although in apparatus using it the holding time is about 0.75 sec. It appears [6] that this method provides a greater margin of safety than other methods and that the surviving bacteria are somewhat impaired in their subsequent growth after such a heat treatment. The Public Health Service has approved this method, but not all states and local authorities have approved installations, and it is little used. A difficulty is the extreme sensitivity of control needed. Pasteurization at 194°F is effected by such units as the Vacreator, Mallory, Roswell, and others.

Pasteurization at 220 to 250°F for a 1-sec or instantaneous hold is being investigated and may be widely adopted in the course of time.

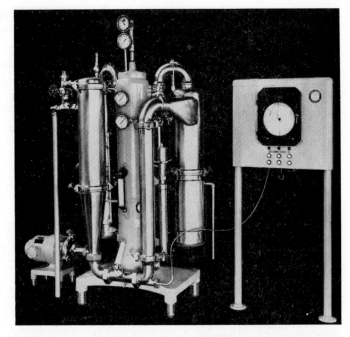

FIGURE 6-9   Vacreator (ultrahigh-temperature) pasteurizer with control panel. (*Photograph courtesy of Cherry-Burrell Corp., Chicago.*)

Pasteurization of this type, it is claimed, allows survival of only the sporeforming bacteria and permits effective refrigeration at 50°F instead of at much lower temperatures, with a shelf life of 3 to 4 weeks [6]. This will have the important economic effects of allowing longer bulk storage in wholesale and retail outlets and bulk delivery to homes instead of the expensive daily delivery.

6-26. Sanitary Control of Pasteurization. If pasteurization is to render milk safe and free from cooked taste, all practical precautions should be taken to ensure the attainment of the proper temperature throughout all the milk and the maintenance of that temperature for the required length of time. This is accomplished through properly designed apparatus, the use of thermometers, and the use of safeguards to prevent raw or partially pasteurized milk from leaking into completely pasteurized milk.

VAT TYPE. The temperature of the vat pasteurizer is controlled by means of a recording thermometer which records on a chart the temperature obtained and the elapsed time. The charts become a permanent record. Recording thermometers, however, may not be sufficiently accurate for the purpose, and accordingly an accurate indicating thermometer is also placed on each vat as a check upon the recording thermometer.

Foam will not be properly heated, and the same applies to milk splashed on the vat surfaces above the milk. Accordingly, a small amount of live steam or hot air is allowed to enter the vat above the milk. An indicating thermometer to show air temperature above the milk is used, and a temperature at least 5°F higher than the milk temperature is maintained. The steam line is provided with a trap to prevent discharge of water into the milk.

A defect noted in the earlier vat pasteurizers was a pocket of cool milk between the outlet valve and the wall of the vat. A close-coupled outlet valve should be used with a flaring passage from the inner wall of the vat to the valve. The diameter of the flare at the inner wall must be equal to the distance from the inner wall to the inlet side of the valve. The valve should be of the "leak-protector" type; i.e., if any leakage occurs, the leaking milk is wasted and does not pass down the discharge pipe, or the discharge pipe may be disconnected during the holding period. The inlet valve should also be of the leak-protector type and so arranged that wasted milk does not enter the vat.

AUTOMATIC CONTINUOUS-FLOW TYPES. It was formerly supposed that the manual control of the batch-type vat pasteurizer would be more likely to produce safe milk than the automatically controlled continuous-flow types. Checks made by the phosphatase test have indicated, however, that the human equation involved in manual control is less reliable than automatic control, although the latter is by no means perfect.

Temperature control is important. Thermostats are installed to maintain proper temperature, but since they occasionally get out of order or the heat source fails, an automatic milk-flow stop is necessary to stop the forward flow of subtemperature milk. There are two types of automatic milk-flow stops. One automatically shuts off the milk-pump motor whenever the milk temperature falls below the pasteurization tempera-

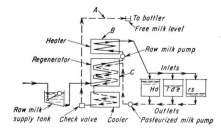

FIGURE 6-10 Diagrammatic elevation of an automatic pasteurizer illustrating how proper pressure is maintained in the regenerator. →→, Raw milk; ←←, pasteurized milk. Raw-milk supply-tank overflow is lower than lowest raw-milk point in regenerator and hence ensures negative raw-milk pressures. Raw-milk pump sucks raw milk through regenerator heater and holders. Pasteurized-milk pump forces pasteurized milk through regenerator, cooler, and check valve to point A in pasteurized-milk line, which is above the highest raw-milk point B by at least 3 per cent of difference in elevation between B and lowest raw-milk regenerator point C, thus maintaining proper relative pressures during shutdowns. Check valve prevents reduction of pasteurized-milk pressures during shutdowns.

ture and automatically starts the pump when the milk again reaches the proper temperature. The other type is a flow-diversion valve, which automatically diverts the milk back to the heater whenever the temperature is too low and reestablishes forward flow when the temperature has risen.

Milk-flow stops should be sealed so that they cannot be changed without the knowledge of the responsible persons. There should be no chance of bypassing milk around them, and they should be set to operate at a temperature sufficiently below the routine temperature to avoid unnecessarily frequent operation. This is undesirable as, with each cut-out, there is a surge forward of subtemperature milk for a few seconds. The bulbs of indicating and recording thermometers should be located as near as practicable to the bulb of the milk-flow stop so that all may react to the same temperature. These requirements apply to both types of milk-flow stops.

In the case of milk-pump stops, some special precautions are advisable. These are as follows: (1) The stop should be located within the influence of a heating unit, or the pump will not restart; (2) manual electric switches on the pump motor should be prohibited, or an operator may reestablish forward flow without regard to temperature; and (3) all forward gravity flow of milk during the pump shutdown should be prevented. In the case of flow-diversion valves, the following must be guarded against: (1) failure of the electric power that operates the valve, (2) omission or jarring loose of the clip that connects the valve seat and the actuating mechanism, (3) tightening of the valve stem packing so that the valve cannot move properly, (4) absence of a leak escape that will prevent leakage forward during diversion, and (5) incomplete closing of the forward-flow seat so that leakage past it exceeds the capacity of the leak-escape device.

The proper holding time must also be safeguarded. No milk should be added to a tank or pocket after the beginning of a holding period, and overflow from one pocket to another should be impossible. Unless tubular heaters have an air vent, they should be sloped so that air or other gases cannot accumulate and thereby reduce the cross section, increase the velocity, and reduce the holding time. Tests of holding times should be made when pasteurizers are installed and after alterations.

A 3A standard method has been developed [15] for determining the holding time of high-temperature short-time pasteurizers by injecting a salt solution and measuring conductivity. An electrode equipment with a syringe connection is installed in a sanitary tee at the upstream end of the holder, and another electrode is installed on the indicating thermometer fitting at the downstream end of the holder. Fifty milliliters of saturated salt solution is injected by means of the syringe in the upstream electrode. The time interval occurring between the first change in conductivity noted in the upstream and downstream electrodes is measured by a stopwatch. The procedure is repeated until the variation between minimum and maximum readings is not more than 0.5 sec in six successive tests. Since this test has to be conducted with water in the pasteurizer, correction should be made to compute the actual holding time for milk. On a volume basis, this correction is applied by means of a simple proportion relating holding times in volumes. If the correction is on the basis of weights, the specific gravity of milk must be taken into consideration. (For definition of 3A standards, see Art. 6-8.)

In tubular holders the holding time is sometimes checked by injecting a dye solution through a petcock at the inlet to the holder and observing the time required for the color to appear at the outlet. Air and foam heaters are required in the holding tanks or pockets. Where regenerators are employed, the raw milk must be automatically kept at a lower pressure than that of the pasteurized milk, and this condition must be maintained during both operation and shutdowns. This is required so that any leakage which may occur will be from the pasteurized milk into the raw milk. Accomplishing this requires a knowledge of hydraulics, and solution of the problem depends upon the layout of the pasteurizing system and the necessary piping. In general the raw-milk pump is placed on the upstream side of the regenerator so that the pipe to the pump is, during normal operation, a suction pipe and under very low or negative pressure. The outlet of the pasteurized milk is placed so that the free level of the milk is above the highest point to which the raw milk rises in the system. This difference in levels should be at least 3 per cent of the difference in elevation between the highest point of the raw milk and the lowest point the raw milk reaches in the regenerator. In Fig. 6-10, which also shows an enclosed cooler, point A must be higher than point B by at least 3 per cent of the difference between B and C.

6-27. The Pasteurization Plant. The plant should be so constructed that the pasteurizing, processing, cooling, and bottling operations shall be carried on in a room separate from that where containers are washed and given bactericidal treatment. Cans of raw milk should not be unloaded directly into the pasteurizing room, and a separate receiving room is desirable. Rooms in which milk, milk products, or cleaned containers are handled or stored should not open directly into stables or living quarters, nor should pasteurization plants be used for any purposes other than the processing of milk and operations pertaining thereto. Pasteurized milk and milk products should not be permitted to come in contact with equipment that has been in contact with raw milk, unless such equipment has been cleaned and given bactericidal treatment.

The floors of pasteurizing plants should be constructed of concrete or some equally impervious material, be graded to drain, be provided with trapped drains, and be kept clean. Walls and ceilings should have a smooth, washable, light-colored surface and be kept clean. Flies must be excluded by screens or fans at entrances. Openings through which cans or crates are loaded may be protected by flaps or fans. Good ventilation and lighting are necessary. The latter requirement will usually be satisfied by providing window space equal to 10 per cent of the floor space. For artificial lighting, the intensity should be a minimum of 10 ft-c on all working surfaces. Toilets and hand-washing facilities must be provided, but the toilet rooms should not open directly into a room in which milk, milk products, containers, or equipment are handled or stored. The toilet room should have self-closing doors, be kept clean, and have a sign directing employees to wash their hands before returning to work. Warm running water, soap, and individual towels should be provided. The water supply should be safe, easily accessible, and adequate in quantity.

The piping and fittings used to convey milk or milk products are of the so-called sanitary type. These are standardized equipment made of noncorrosive metal so constructed that all interior surfaces, including valves and connections, are of such size and shape that they are easily accessible to sight and touch and are so designed as to permit easy cleaning. This requires dismantling of the piping system for cleaning and bactericidal treatment. All necessary joints and seams are soldered flush, and the same requirements hold for cans and other utensils. With special types of piping and fittings, including plastic pipe in some places, it is feasible to clean the piping system without dismantling.

The milk and milk products should be bottled and capped mechanically. Hand bottling and capping, with the accompanying danger of contaminating the pasteurized milk, obviously should be discouraged.

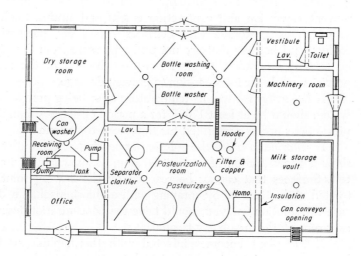

FIGURE 6-11   Plan of a pasteurization plant.

6-28. Operation of the Plant. The operating personnel of the plant should be free from disease, wear clean clothing, and keep their hands clean at all times while handling milk, containers, or equipment. They should also be conversant with the principles of sanitation as they apply to the milk plant. It is especially important that they be instructed in the importance of preventing contamination of the milk after pasteurization. Outbreaks of typhoid fever, for example, have been caused by an unsuspected typhoid carrier adjusting by hand the caps of bottles which had been capped in a faulty manner by the mechanical capper. Such an occurrence would indicate violation of the requirements that a worker thoroughly wash his hands before resuming work after a visit to the toilet and that milk in bottles improperly capped be returned to the raw milk.

The plant and all its equipment should be kept scrupulously clean. The equipment requires washing with a solution of alkaline washing powder followed by a bactericidal treatment, immediately after the day's run of milk is completed, as described in Arts. 6-15 to 6-17. But this is not sufficient. Just before the next run is started, and after the piping, etc., has been reassembled, another bactericidal rinse is given.

If *steam* is used for this purpose, each group of assembled piping is treated separately by inserting the steam hose into the inlet and maintaining steam flow from the outlet for 5 min after the temperature of the steam at the outlet has reached 200°F. A 5-min period is required here rather than the 1 min required for cans, etc., because of the loss of heat resulting from the relatively large surface exposed to the air. All closed equipment connected with the pipe system can be considered adequately treated by means of the above procedure. Covers, unions, etc., should be cracked to allow steam to enter the joints and also to prevent expansion and contraction cracks and strains. Such equipment as weigh cans, storage vats, clarifiers, separators, pasteurization vats, coolers, and bottlers that are not under pressure from the pipeline must be treated separately. Coolers must be drained of the refrigerant or provision made for its expansion to prevent damage.

If *hot water* is used, its temperature after being pumped through the system should be at least 170°F for a period of not less than 5 min. Other precautions are as prescribed for the steam treatment.

If *chlorine* is used, the solution appearing at the outlet end should show a concentration of at least 50 ppm as shown by the orthotolidine test. Surfaces that cannot be reached by the flowing solution may be treated with steam or by spraying with a chlorine solution. In the latter case the solution sprayed should have the concentration indicated above as it runs off the area being treated.

If the plant becomes infected with thermophilic or thermoduric bacteria, more intensive bactericidal treatment will be required, or a change in methods is advisable. If the steam or hot-water method has been used, a temperature of 200°F for over 10 min or 200 ppm of chlorine for 2 min or more may be needed.

Bottles and cans may be washed as indicated for dairies. In large plants, however, it is recommended that automatic bottle washers be used. These machines soak the bottle in an alkaline solution having a strength of at least 2.4 per cent, including at least 1.6 per cent of caustic soda [5].

After bactericidal treatment, all multiuse milk containers and equipment must be so stored that they are protected from dust, flies, and splash. They should be handled so that the hands and clothing of workers do not touch the cleaned surfaces that come in contact with the milk. Bottle caps, cap-paper stock, parchment paper, and single-service containers must be stored where they will remain clean and dry. At the beginning of each run, the first cap from each tube, the first few caps from each roll of cap stock, and the first parchment paper should be discarded as they have been exposed to contamination.

Municipal Regulation of Milk Supplies

6-29. Most cities which are making any pretense of carrying on public health work exercise some sort of supervision over the milk supplies. In some cases it consists only of ordinances, with little or no attempt at enforcement. In other cases good control is obtained through wise ordinances and an efficient inspecting force and laboratory. Many of the larger cities require that all milk be pasteurized. It is estimated that more than 90 per cent of the market milk consumed in the United States is being pasteurized. In general, the use of pasteurized milk is growing.

While inspection alone can do much toward controlling the quality and production of milk, it is handicapped without frequent laboratory tests of the milk. The counts, therefore, supplement the reports of the inspector; persistently high counts of milk from an apparently good dairy may lead to the inspector's finding an unsuspected trouble, such as infected udders, inefficient sanitization of utensils, or poor cooling.

6-30. **The Milk Ordinance and Code.** There are three general types of milk ordinance now in use in the United States. One requires all milk to be pasteurized; another classifies milk as raw or pasteurized but does not grade either; and a third classifies milk as raw or pasteurized and provides for a number of grades in each class. All these ordinances set up minimum standards concerning milk handling and bacterial counts. The Public Health Service [5] of the U.S. Department of Health, Education, and Welfare has promulgated a milk ordinance and code which is a modification of the third type. The states have been encouraged to assume leadership in the obtaining of better milk by approving the Milk Ordinance and Code and by stimulating the cities to pass it. After passage, in many instances, state personnel aid in the building of the city's enforcement organization. Alabama adopted the program in 1924, and its example has been followed by many other states with satisfactory results. The Ordinance not only has improved the quality of the milk in those cities which passed it but also has increased the consumption of milk.

A further advantage of the Milk Ordinance and Code is that it allows rating or scoring of a city's milk supply by the state health department upon the basis of the percentage of the total milk which is of high grade or pasteurized. Competition between cities in this respect effects a gradual improvement in the quality of the city's milk supply and increases the interest of public and city councils, thereby assisting the health officer in his work.

The Ordinance requires that the grade of milk appear on the bottle cap or carton, thereby tending to place the buying of milk upon the same basis as for most commodities, its quality. Grading also has a tendency to drive poor milk out of the retail market, particularly as people become educated to the meanings of the different grades. It also tends to reward the dairyman who is careful and clean and protects him from the unfair competition of the unclean, careless, and unscrupulous dairyman.

The Ordinance may require that all the milk be pasteurized if the state of public health education is such that this requirement does not cause too much opposition. In any event it states the grades to which sale is restricted, as decided by the city itself. In most cities applying the Ordinance, only Grade A raw and Grade A pasteurized milk or milk products may be sold to the final consumer or to restaurants, soda fountains, grocery stores, or similar establishments. This requirement does not, however, exclude milk that cannot qualify as to the above grades, for it may, after pasteurization, be used in the manufacture of such products as butter and cheese.

Enforcement of the Ordinance is usually effected through a permit, which is granted if the dairyman conforms to the requirements of the Ordinance and revoked if he violates the Ordinance. If he persists in selling milk in the city without a permit, he is subject to a fine, although he may also be fined for selling milk with false or misleading labels. The health officer may also degrade the milk if he finds violations of the provisions of the Ordinance. If violations of any of the items of sanitation are found upon any inspection of a dairy or milk plant, a notice is given, and a reasonable time is allowed, never less than 3 days, to make the required improvement. If improvement has not been made by the second inspection, the grade of the milk is determined by conditions then existing.

The outstanding features of the Ordinance are as follows:

1. REQUIREMENT OF STATED CONDITIONS FOR PRODUCTION AND HANDLING. The Ordinance requires testing of cows; healthy cows; proper construction and cleanliness of the dairy barn, milkhouse, and equipment; health and cleanliness of the workmen; cleanliness and sanitization of equipment; a safe water supply; and adequate sewage or excreta disposal. Cooling-temperature requirements are based upon an average of three out of four samples taken. These requirements have been discussed in detail earlier in this chapter. As an aid to the inspector, an inspection blank is used that lists all the requirements. Should he find the dairy or milk handling deficient in one or more items, he so designates upon the blank by a check against the item. Standard inspection blanks for dairies and milk plants are illustrated in the public health bulletin previously referred to [5]. Violation of dairy requirements on two successive inspections results in the revocation of the dairy's Grade A permit.

Grade A pasteurized milk must be processed in a plant which has all the safeguards previously discussed. All bottles in which Grade A milk is sold are required to have a lip-protecting cap which extends to cover the largest diameter of the pouring lip. Milk which is not processed in accordance with Grade A requirements is not permitted to be sold under Grade A labels but may be used for manufacturing purposes.

2. BACTERIOLOGICAL STANDARDS. In addition to satisfying the standards governing handling and production, the milk must conform to bacteriological requirements. Since poor production and handling methods are usually indicated by high bacterial counts, the two requirements constitute a useful correlation.

The bacterial plate count of Grade A raw milk, if permitted for retail sale by the Ordinance, or the direct microscopic clump count cannot exceed 50,000 per milliliter. That for Grade A raw milk for pasteurization should not exceed 200,000 per milliliter, as delivered from the farm; however, the raw milk should at no time between dumping and pasteurization have a plate count or clump count exceeding 400,000 per milliliter, although some sanitarians advocate a clump count not exceeding 200,000 per milliliter. Grade A pasteurized milk is Grade A raw milk which has been subjected to pasteurization, the effectiveness of which is determined by a phosphatase test. The bacterial plate count of pasteurized Grade A milk prior to delivery must not exceed 30,000 per milliliter, or the coliform count of the milk should not be greater than 10 per milliliter. Grade B raw milk for pasteurization should have a plate count or direct microscopic clump count not exceeding 1,000,000 per milliliter. Grade B pasteurized milk, made from raw milk for pasteurization of a quality of not less than Grade B, must not have a bacterial count exceeding 50,000 per milliliter. Grade C pasteurized milk is milk that does not conform to the requirements for Grade B pasteurized milk.

The bacterial standards used in grading milk are doubled for cream and omitted in the case of sour cream and buttermilk.

3. THE GRADING FEATURE. It should be recognized that the grade of the milk depends upon all the requirements mentioned above. Once it is determined, the grade of the milk is emphasized. The caps of all milk bottles must be plainly marked with the grade determined at the previous grading period. Milk must be served in restaurants in the original containers only or from an approved bulk dispenser. The grading period is not more than 6 months, and at least once in that period the dairies and milk plants must be inspected.

In addition to the more important features given above, there are the usual definitions and the prohibition of adulteration and use of preservatives. There is also the requirement that milk contain not less than $3\frac{1}{4}$ per cent milk fat and not less than $8\frac{1}{4}$ per cent solids-not-fat.

In many states it is legal for the cities to adopt a short form of the Ordinance [5]. It makes the Code, and further revisions of it, a part of the Ordinance without the necessity of passing it in detail or printing it in the local newspapers. A state law recognizing the Ordinance is useful as it may forbid dairymen to use Grade A bottle caps unless their milk has actually been subjected to regulation under the Ordinance.

6-31. Inspection and Sampling. An efficient dairy inspector must have a great deal of specialized knowledge in addition to keen powers of observation, tact, and firmness. The best inspectors are not necessarily former dairymen. Veterinarians and agricultural school graduates who have specialized in dairy science have been successful, while sanitarians and sanitary engineers are entering the field to a large degree, the last-named particularly in connection with pasteurization plants.

Inspections should be made at least monthly, with follow-up visits if necessary. Under the Milk Ordinance and Code, the grading visits are usually made every 6 months, although inspections should also be made at shorter intervals. Inspections should, as far as possible, be made at milking time.

The collection of samples is also a part of the inspector's duties. Since knowledge of the condition of the milk when it reaches the consumer is desired, the samples are collected from the delivery wagons in the case of retail dealers and from the cans at the milk plants if the milk is delivered to a creamery or pasteurization plant. Samples of the pasteurized milk are also collected before it is delivered to the consumer.

If bottles are collected, they should be selected at random, and the tops should be covered with paraffin paper or parchment to avoid contamination en route to the laboratory. They should be kept at temperatures below 45°F; however, when the sample is plated for the plate count within 4 hr from the time of collection, the temperature may be as high as 50°F. When samples are collected at milk plants or receiving stations, they may be taken from well-stirred cans, storage tanks, or the weigh vat. The importance of stirring is emphasized because the cream usually has a higher bacterial count than the balance of the milk. After each usage, stirrers, thermometers, sampling tubes, and dippers should be rinsed in clean water of not more than 80°F and placed in a hot-water solution maintained at 180°F or in a hypochlorite solution with a concentration of at least 100 ppm available chlorine. The utensils are allowed to remain in the sterilizing solution for a minimum of 1 min. The samples should consist of at least 10 ml of milk.

The samples have tags attached to them, showing date and time of collection and an identifying number. The name of the dairyman or milk plant is not shown, so that the laboratory personnel do not know the source of the milk.

When insufficient funds are available for complete inspection service, the Milk Ordinance permits the local health officer to accept the inspection reports covering producer dairies which are made by inspectors of the receiving milk plants. This is permissible, however, only if such reports are officially checked periodically and found satisfactory.

6-32. The Laboratory and Testing. The laboratory is important in the control of the quality of milk. It should be ample in size for the amount of work that it has to do and should be staffed with persons who are acquainted with the technique of milk testing. In cities which have a public health laboratory as a part of the city health department, the milk work is taken care of there. In small cities it is possible to use a well-trained inspector who can do his own testing, and in this case the testing may be confined to butterfat and solids-not-fat. In either case, testing methods should follow those given in the book "Standard Methods for the Examination of Dairy Products" [4]. The Milk Ordinance permits recognition of the reports of commercial laboratories covering raw milk to be pasteurized if they are officially checked periodically and found satisfactory.

The laboratory makes routine tests of the butterfat content of milk and cream and milk solids-not-fat to determine whether the requirements of the Ordinance are satisfied. Other tests sometimes made are the tests for determination of the presence of preservatives, bacterial inhibitors, and pesticides and the sediment test, which shows the presence of dirt as caught on a filtering disk.

Most important of the tests is the bacterial plate count, which gives the count per milliliter as determined by incubation on a nutritive medium, and the counting of colonies, or the microscopic clump count. The plate count and the clump count are comparable and are generally used unless otherwise indicated. In enforcement of the Ordinance and determination of the milk grade, logarithmic averages are used. The use and value of the logarithmic average can be shown by an example. Common logarithms are used. For grading purposes it is usual to take the last four counts as determined by the laboratory. It is assumed that the figures are as follows:

Counts	Logarithms
33,000	4.52
21,000	4.32
12,000	4.08
220,000	5.34

$$4)\overline{18.26}$$

4.56 = average logarithm

The count corresponding to the average logarithm is 36,000, whereas the arithmetical average of the counts is 71,000, which is too high for A grade. The logarithmic average is used because it does not penalize the dairyman so heavily for high counts that are in the nature of accidents. It is obvious, in the example given, that the milk produced is, in general, satisfactory as to count, and it would be unfair to degrade the milk because of the effect of the one unsatisfactory count. Tables of logarithms can be furnished to the record clerk, who can use them without having a knowledge of mathematics.

In the grading of milk supplies, coliform counts are also required to be taken on Grade A products. These counts are allowed a maximum of 10 per milliliter. Whenever more than one of the last four consecutive coliform counts of samples taken on separate days is beyond the prescribed limit, the health officer notifies the plant of its excessive count and then takes an additional sample after 3 days. If this additional sample exceeds a prescribed limit, an immediate degrading is called for.

6-33. Collection and Delivery of Milk. Vehicles used for collecting milk from dairies or milk stations and for retail delivery should be constructed with permanent tops and with permanent or roll-down sides and backs. They must be kept clean, and no materials capable of contaminating the milk should be transported at the same time as the milk. Vehicles should display the name of the milk dealer.

Delivery of milk from farms to plants has been expedited in certain areas by the development of the farm-tank pickup system. This system utilizes a refrigerated bulk-holding tank on the dairy farm for the collection and storage of milk until the time of delivery to the plant. There are a number of designs of bulk farm tanks, but they usually have the common features of being constructed of stainless steel throughout and being provided with a removable measuring-stick device which positively measures the milk level in the tank. Farm tanks are provided with mechanical agitators and with an indicating thermometer to show the

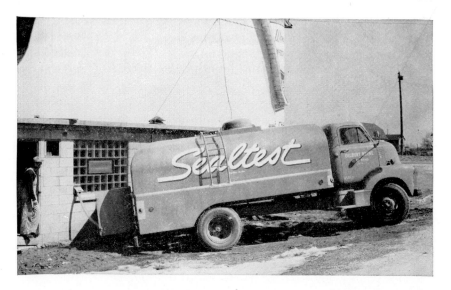

FIGURE 6-12   Farm-tank pickup truck. (*Photograph courtesy of Heil Co., Milwaukee, Wis.*)

temperature of the contained milk. See Fig. 6-5. Several different types of emptying valves are provided, but all such valves are required to be designed so that they are easily inspected and cleaned. The farm-tank pickup trucks are similar in design to other milk transports. They are usually provided with a pump and a refrigerated compartment for carrying the milk hose and butterfat samples.

In the operation of the tank-truck pickup system, the tanker driver arrives at the diary farm and connects the hose from the pickup tank to the dairy farmer's bulk-holding tank. Before the connection is made, however, both the valve on the holding tank and the fittings on the end of the tanker hose are uncapped and given bactericidal treatment. A measure of the gallonage contained in the holding tank is also taken by the tanker driver. The holding-tank agitator is started, and after 5 min of agitation a butterfat sample is taken. After the tank is completely loaded, the truck returns to the milk plant, where the milk is then drawn off into the plant holding tank.

Raw milk which is delivered must be placed in its container at the farm where it is produced, and pasteurized milk must be placed in the delivery container at the plant. No transfer of milk from one container to another is permissible in the vehicle or in a store or anywhere except at a bottling or milk room especially equipped for the purpose. This requirement prevents the dangerous practice of filling returned milk bottles with milk or milk products while on the milk route.

Hotels, soda fountains, etc., should serve milk only in the original

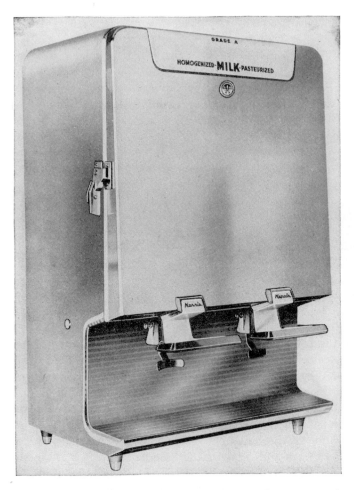

FIGURE 6-13 Bulk milk dispenser. (*Photograph courtesy of Dispenser, Inc., Meim, Minn.*)

containers or from approved milk dispensers. Until served, the milk must be kept below 50°F.

Outstanding among a number of modern developments in the retail handling of milk is the use of bulk milk dispensers in eating establishments.

Bulk milk dispensers are designed so that the milk container cans may be filled in the milk plant and can then be delivered to the eating establishments, where they are placed in a bulk milk dispenser cabinet. This cabinet is designed to meet sanitary standards and has doors of sufficient size to receive the dispenser cans. In the bottom of these cans are fittings where a plastic or rubber tube is attached. After the can is placed in the dispenser cabinet, this tube is threaded through the dispenser valve, which controls the flow of milk through a pinchcock arrangement. When a can is emptied, it may be removed from the dispenser cabinet to be replaced by another full can. There are also other arrangements for controlling the flow of the milk from the dispenser can.

Since bulk milk dispensers are not generally designed to agitate the milk after cans are placed in the cabinet, they may be used only for homogenized milk. Advantages claimed for bulk milk dispensers are the abilities to maintain lower temperatures in the milk and to provide certain economies in handling the product. They also eliminate accumulations of dirty bottles around eating establishments.

Dispenser cans are usually required by enforcement agencies to be sealed at the plant. These seals are not broken until the cans are again returned to the plant for cleaning, bactericidal treatment, and refilling.

The delivery of milk or milk products to, and the collection of milk or milk-product containers from, residences in which there are cases of communicable disease transmissible through milk are subject to special requirements to be prescribed by the health officer.

6-34. Rating of Cities. In states where the Milk Ordinance and Code is in use, the Public Health Service has listed semiannually those cities which have a market milk rating of at least 90 per cent. Listings are made in two classes: cities in which all milk is pasteurized and those in which both raw and pasteurized milk are sold. A market milk rating in cities of either class means that the weighted average of the percentages of compliance with the various items of sanitation required by the Ordinance for Grade A raw milk or Grade A pasteurized milk is 90 per cent or more. The weighting is done according to the amount of milk produced by each dairy. It is possible, of course, to compare scores between cities as a means of encouraging competition.

The ratings must be determined by the state milk-sanitation authority in accordance with the method prescribed by the Public Health Service [16]. A listing is good for not more than 2 years. When a city falls below the 90 per cent mark, it will not be resurveyed for at least 6 months, so that it will be penalized by being dropped from one listing. The Public Health Service makes occasional check surveys of the cities listed by the states. If a check rating shows less than 90 per cent but not less than 85 per cent, the city is removed from the list after 6 months unless a resurvey in the probationary interim shows a rating of 90 per cent or more. If the check rating is less than 85 per cent, the city is removed from the list immediately.

6-35. Interstate Milk Shipments. Formerly the problem of interstate milk shipments was not serious for any metropolitan area other than the extremely large ones such as New York. Now, however, interstate shipment of milk and cream is widespread not only to metropolitan areas but also from areas of high milk production to those where a shortage exists. Among the factors influencing this trend were the development of refrigerated transport, industrialization, accelerated urbanization, and increase in population. The practice regarding sanitary control of milksheds originally consisted in each community's being responsible for inspections and the institution of control measures wherever the milk was produced, regardless of the distance from the community. The economic problem this practice produced soon became evident with increased interstate shipment. In fact, trade barriers were consciously or unconsciously established to the extent that interstate and intrastate commerce was being seriously interfered with.

In October, 1950, the Supreme Court ruled that a city could not adopt discriminatory health regulations which act as trade barriers against interstate commerce and pointed out two alternatives for remedial action, namely, having the city rely upon its own officials for inspection of distant milk sources or upon the inspections made by health authorities at the source, as provided in the Milk Ordinance and Code of the Public Health Service. The Ordinance establishes reciprocity as a basis of acceptance of outside milk, defining the criteria to be met. In the following year the Senate Committee on Agriculture and Forestry held public hearings concerning the cause and effect of restrictive regulations and endorsed a plan for the Public Health Service to increase its efforts to develop a cooperative program with the states for the certification of interstate milk shippers.

At national conferences on interstate milk shipments, representatives of various state health departments have met periodically to study this problem. They have recommended that states receiving interstate milk shipments recognize the inspection and supervision by full-time health and agricultural department personnel, either local or state. They selected the 1953 recommendations of the Public Health Service embodied in the Milk Ordinance and Code as the basic standard. Also, they recognized a certified rating plan whereby receiving states would accept ratings made by certified rating officials of either the Public Health Service or the health departments having sole jurisdiction of milk sanitation in a particular area. Certification includes survey ratings on producing farms, receiving stations, or plants and enforcement ratings of the supervisory agency. It was agreed that the Public Health Service would standardize the rating procedure of its own personnel and state rating officials, spot-check laboratories of the state agency participating in the shipment of milk, and publish lists of interstate shippers for semiannual distribution [17].

6-36. Certified Milk. In 1912, the American Association of Medical Milk Commissions formulated certain rules for the production of certified milk. These are complete and somewhat stringent regulations governing the conditions of the dairy and its surroundings, utensils, methods of milk handling, and health of workmen, with prescribed chemical and bacteriological standards. The total count must never exceed 10,000 bacteria per milliliter. The milk is certified by a local or county commission of physicians who give their services gratis to enforce the rules of the parent organization. It may be certified raw or certified pasteurized milk.

6-37. Milk Products. Under the Public Health Service Milk Ordinance, milk products include cream, sour cream, half and half, reconstituted half and half, whipped cream, concentrated milk, concentrated-milk products, nonfat milk, flavored milk, flavored reconstituted milk, cultured buttermilk, cultured milk, cottage cheese, creamed cottage cheese, homogenized milk, goat milk, vitamin D milk, buttermilk, skim milk, reconstituted or recombined milk, milk beverages, and any other product designated as a milk product by the health officer. Some of the above terms may require definition. Homogenized milk is milk which has had its fat globules broken up to such an extent that no visible cream separation occurs on the milk within 48 hr of storage and in which the top 100 ml of a quart bottle (or proportionate amount in another container) differs no more than 10 per cent of itself in fat percentage from that of the remaining milk, as determined after thorough mixing of each portion. The Milk Ordinance and Code prohibits the mixing of homogenized milk or cream with unhomogenized milk or cream. This "partial homogenization" has been practiced by some milk plants to increase the apparent butterfat content when the milk is viewed in a bottle, for the homogenized material would come to the top. Vitamin D milk is that which has had its natural vitamin D content increased by an approved method to at least 400 USP units per quart. Reconstituted or recombined milk results from recombining milk constituents with water so that it will comply with the requirements as to butterfat and solids-not-fat. Reconstituted or recombined cream results from the combination of dried cream, butter, or butterfat with cream, skim milk, or water.

Milk products, as defined above, should be controlled and graded in the same manner as milk. As mentioned previously, however, bacterial standards differ in the case of cream, where designated counts are doubled, and in the case of sour cream, buttermilk, and cottage cheese, where they are omitted entirely.

6-38. Dry Milk and Dry-milk Products. Dry milk and dry-milk products are widely used, and the Public Health Service has prepared a sanitation ordinance and code to control their sanitary quality [18]. This ordinance requires that the milk used for drying comply with requirements for Grade A raw milk for pasteurization as defined in the Milk Ordinance and that the milk be pasteurized at the drying plant. After pasteurization such milk and milk products shall at no time have a bacterial plate count or direct microscopic clump count exceeding

30,000 per milliliter, although these counts may be increased in case of concentrated products in proportion to the degree of concentration. Grade A dry-milk products must have a bacterial plate count not exceeding 30,000 per gram and a coliform count not exceeding 90 per gram. They shall be free of unwholesome and deleterious materials and shall comply with the U.S. Extra Grade spray-process products as promulgated by the U.S. Department of Agriculture. Plants must be inspected every 6 months, and products sampled and examined each month. Sanitary requirements concerning plant, etc., approximate those of the Milk Ordinance, as they are applicable. The final product must be so packaged that it will be protected against contamination. In cities where this ordinance is in force, no dry-milk products may be sold unless they are produced under the same conditions as required by the Milk Ordinance.

6-39. Butter. Butter, while not herein defined as a milk product, should be controlled as to sanitary quality. The butter-making process cannot be depended upon to kill disease bacteria. Therefore, the milk and cream used should be produced under sanitary conditions and should always be pasteurized before using. A problem arising in connection with butter is that sour cream is sometimes purchased by milk or cream depots from farms where there is no control over sanitary conditions. Much of this cream is filthy and should not be considered suitable for human consumption, even though it is pasteurized by the milk plant. Responsibility should be placed upon the milk plants for the cleanliness of the milk and cream that they process. State laws or city ordinances may prescribe the minimum allowable butterfat content of butter and may also prohibit the sale of reworked or "renovated" butter.

6-40. Cheese. Cheese should be subjected to sanitary control, for investigations indicate that staphylococci may be found in cheese either as a result of using unpasteurized milk or as a result of poor handling [19]. Some investigators believe that a concentration of 500,000 coagulase-positive staphylococci per gram of food is required to cause food poisoning. Probably there are many unrecognized outbreaks. The rule should always be that cheese be made from pasteurized milk and cream. Aging of cheese at not too low a temperature will destroy disease bacteria even if the cheese is made from raw milk. Some states are not requiring the pasteurization of all milk or cream for cheese and allow, as an alternative, aging for at least 60 days before sale. This appears to be too short a time for cheddar-type cheese. A recently reported outbreak of 200 cases of food poisoning [20] was due to staphylococci in cheddar cheese that was 4 to 8 months old and made from unpasteurized milk.

6-41. Frozen Desserts. Sanitary control of frozen desserts has been very unsatisfactory. The Public Health Service has studied the problem and proposed standards that have been embodied in an ordinance and code which is recommended for adoption by cities and promulgation by the state health departments [21]. It is offered in two forms: one allowing enforcement by grading, degrading, and permit revocation, and the other enforceable by permit revocation only and not having the grading feature. The grading type is probably more desirable, and its provisions are discussed here.

This ordinance governs primarily handling and quality of the frozen desserts, but, wherever possible, sanitary control should also be applied to the milk and milk products from which they are made. A frozen dessert is defined as any frozen or partially frozen combination of two or more of the following: milk or milk products, eggs or egg products, sugars, water, fruit or fruit juices, candy, nutmeats, other wholesome food products, flavors, color, and harmless stabilizer. A frozen dessert is considered to include ice cream, ice milk, milk sherbet, frozen custard, ices, and similar products. Standard compositions for the various frozen desserts are determined by the Food and Drug Administration of the U.S. Department of Health, Education, and Welfare. The "mix" in preparation of frozen desserts is the unfrozen combination of all the ingredients with or without fruits, fruit juices, candy, nutmeats, flavor, or harmless color.

The grading ordinance defines three grades—A, B, and C—and it is suggested that in those cities which already enjoy good sanitary control of frozen desserts, only Grade A be sold. In other cities it may be advisable to permit sale of both A and B grades. For qualification as Grade A, the dessert must be prepared in a plant that conforms in construction, cleanliness, use of sanitary piping, washing and bactericidal treatment of equipment, and cleanliness of personnel to the standards required in a pasteurization plant by the Public Health Service Milk Ordinance. Milk and fluid-milk products as they arrive at the plant must be immediately cooled to 50°F or below unless they are to be pasteurized within 2 hr, and the pasteurized mix must be immediately cooled to 50°F or less. The mix must be pasteurized at a temperature of at least 155°F with a holding time of at least 30 min, although the state health authority may approve some other method which has been demonstrated to be equally efficient. One acceptable alternative is the use of a pasteurization time of 25 sec and a temperature of 175°F. The average bacterial count of the pasteurized mix or the frozen dessert shall at no time before delivery exceed 50,000 per gram for Grade A. Average counts are obtained from the last four consecutive samples, and they may be obtained from the plate count or direct microscopic count of clumps, in which cases the logarithmic average is determined, or the reductase test may be used. The raw milk and milk products used as ingredients must have bacterial counts not exceeding

200,000 per milliliter or gram, if the count or direct microscopic clump count is used, or 800,000 if individual organisms are counted, or have an average reduction time of not less than 6 hr. Milk and milk products that are used in the pasteurized, condensed, evaporated, or dried state must have an average bacterial plate count not exceeding 50,000 per milliliter or gram. These limits on the ingredients should be doubled in the case of cream.

Grade B frozen desserts comply with Grade A standards with the following exceptions: Floors of the manufacturing plants may be of tight wood or linoleum instead of concrete, tile, etc., and flood drains are not required. Walls and ceilings need not have light-colored surfaces, provided that they are kept clean. The lighting requirement is not so stringent as to even distribution. The average bacterial count of the pasteurized mix or frozen dessert must at no time prior to delivery exceed 100,000 per gram. Milk and milk products used as ingredients must have average counts not exceeding 1,000,000 per milliliter or gram by the plate count or direct microscopic clump count; 4,000,000 by the count of individual organisms; or an average reduction time not exceeding 3½ hr. Milk and milk products used as ingredients in the pasteurized, condensed, evaporated, or dried state must have a bacterial plate count not exceeding 250,000 per milliliter or gram. This limit on the ingredients is doubled in the case of cream. Grade C frozen desserts are those which violate any of the requirements for Grade B.

The grading period is 6 months; that is, the health officer announces the grades of all frozen-dessert plants at least once every 6 months, and the plants are inspected at least once during that period. All containers enclosing mix or frozen desserts except those filled from bulk containers in retail dispensing must be plainly labeled with the name and grade of the contents, whether raw or pasteurized, and the name and street address, or permit number, of the manufacturing plant. A descriptive word or phrase indicating composition or flavor may be added.

Bibliography

1. Bovine Mastitis, *Public Health Rept.*, vol. 75, no. 10, October, 1960.
2. "Uniform Methods and Rules for the Establishment and Maintenance of Certified Brucellosis-free Herds of Cattle in Modified Certified Areas," Animal Disease Eradication Division, U.S. Department of Agriculture, 1955.
3. Luoto, L.: Report on the Nationwide Occurrence of Q Fever Infections in Cattle, *Public Health Rept.*, vol. 75, no. 2, February, 1960.
4. "Standard Methods for the Examination of Dairy Products," 11th ed. American Public Health Association, New York, 1960.
5. Milk Ordinance and Code: 1953 Recommendations of the Public Health Service, *Public Health Service Pub.* 229, 1953.

6. Milk Sanitation Administration, *Public Health Service Pub.* 728, 1959.
7. Insecticide Recommendations, *U.S. Dept. Agr., Agr. Handbook* 120, 1962.
8. Murthy, G. K., *et al.*: Method of Removing Cationic Radionuclides from Milk, *J. Dairy Sci.*, vol. 44, no. 12, December, 1961.
9. Murthy, G. K., *et al.*: Method of Removing Iodine 131 from Milk, *J. Dairy Sci.*, vol. 45, no. 9, September, 1962.
10. Lyster, R. L. J.: The Reactivation of Milk Alkaline Phosphatase after Heat Treatment, *J. Dairy Res.*, vol. 29, no. 1, February, 1962.
11. Mallmann, W. L.: Notes on Dairy Cleaners and Cleaning Dairy Equipment and Notes on Sanitization of Dairy Equipment, *Mich. State Univ. Agr. Exp. Sta. Quar. Bull.*, vol. 27, no. 1, August, 1944.
12. Mallmann, W. L., *et al.*: "The Influence of the Method of Sanitizing Milking Machines on the Bacterial Counts of Milk," Twentieth Annual Report of the New York Association of Milk Sanitarians, reprint 1946.
13. Enright, J. R., *et al.*: Thermal Inactivation of *Coxiella burnetii* and Its Relation to Pasteurized Milk, *Public Health Monogr.* 47, 1960.
14. Enright, J B.: The Pasteurization of Cream, Chocolate Milk and Ice Cream Mixes Containing the Organisms of Q Fever, *J. Milk Food Technol.*, vol. 24, no. 11, November, 1961.
15. 3A Standard Method for Determining the Holding Time of High-temperature Short-time Pasteurizers by Means of the Salt Conductivity Test, formulated by the International Association of Milk and Food Sanitarians, Public Health Service, Dairy Industry Committee, reprinted from *J. Milk Food Technol.*, vol. 13, no. 5, September–October, 1950.
16. *Public Health Rept.*, vol. 53, p. 1386, reprint 1970, 1938.
17. Procedures Governing the Cooperative State–Public Health Service Program for Certification of Interstate Milk Shippers, *J. Milk Food Technol.*, vol. 25, no. 8, August, 1962.
18. "Grade A Dry Milk Products: Recommended Sanitation Ordinance and Code," Public Health Service, 1959.
19. Mickelsen, R., *et al.*: The Incidence of Potentially Pathogenic *Staphylococci* in Dairy Products at the Consumer Level, *J. Milk Food Technol.*, vol. 24, no. 11, November, 1961.
20. Hendricks, S. L., *et al.*: *Staphylococci* Food Intoxication due to Cheddar Cheese, *J. Milk Food Technol.*, vol. 22, no. 10, October, 1959.
21. "Frozen Desserts: Ordinance and Code," Public Health Service.

7

FOOD SANITATION

7-1. Food affects health in many ways, and scientific knowledge of the subject is increasing continually. The vitamins, unbalanced diets, the effects of diet deficiencies, allergies to certain foods, and overeating are all matters of importance to the physician, dietitian, and nurse. The person interested in sanitation, however, is primarily concerned with five agencies through which food may cause suffering or death. These are:

1. Animal parasites, such as tapeworms and trichina worms. These gain entrance to the human body through the eating of infected meat or fish which has not been cooked sufficiently to kill the immature worm.

2. Microorganisms which enter food in various ways and then infect the consumer, such as the bacteria which cause typhoid fever, dysentery, and

salmonellosis; the rickettsia which causes Q fever; and the virus which causes infectious hepatitis.

3. Toxins given off by certain bacteria growing in the food. Botulinus organisms and some of the staphylococci are important in this respect.

4. Harmful substances illegally or ignorantly used in foods for preserving purposes, coloring, or adulteration or those entering by accident, such as insect poison mistakenly used for flour or sugar, poisonous spray residues left on fruits or vegetables, or poisons from containers, although this is rare.

5. Use of poisonous plants or other materials as foods. Instances are eating of poisonous toadstools mistaken for edible mushrooms and out-of-season consumption of the mussel of the Pacific Coast, which is poisonous during the months of June to September.

It will be noted that ptomaine poisoning has not been included in the list. What is popularly called ptomaine poisoning may be either or both of the second and third classifications given above.

7-2. Food and Drug Laws. The Federal Food and Drug Act of 1906, as amended in 1938 (the Federal Food, Drug, and Cosmetic Act), prohibits the adulteration of foods for interstate shipment [1]. To protect their citizens from injurious and fraudulent foods prepared within the same state, many states have also passed food and drug acts. They usually follow closely the Federal law. The provisions concerning foods, which include drinks, flavorings, and condiments, are considered to be violated in the following cases:

1. If the food bears or contains any poisonous or deleterious substance which may render it injurious to health.

2. If it bears or contains any added poisonous or added deleterious substance which is unsafe. This section has resulted in much controversy and investigation. It is aimed at the practice of adding chemical preservatives to foods. These include formaldehyde, boric acid, borax, salicylic acid, and others. There is difference of opinion as to whether, in the small amounts generally used, such preservatives are injurious or not.

3. If it consists in whole or in part of any filthy, putrid, or decomposed substance, or if it is otherwise unfit for food. Examples are dried fruits which are wormy or spoiled, chocolate or candy which has been nibbled by mice or rats, and oysters polluted with sewage.

4. If it has been prepared, packed, or held under insanitary conditions whereby it may have been contaminated with filth or otherwise rendered injurious to health.

5. If it is, in whole or in part, the product of a diseased animal or of an animal which has died otherwise than by slaughter.

6. If its container is composed, in whole or in part, of any poisonous or deleterious substance which may render the contents injurious to health.

7. If any valuable constituent has been in whole or in part omitted or abstracted therefrom, if it is damaged, or if inferiority has been concealed in any manner. An example of this is skimming of milk and selling it as

regular milk. There is no objection, however, if the milk is afterward sold a
skim milk.

8. If it bears or contains a coal-tar color other than one that has bee
certified in accordance with regulations.

9. If it is a confectionery and it bears or contains any alcohol or nor
nutritive article or substance except harmless coloring; harmless flavorin;
harmless resinous glaze, not in excess of 4 per cent; natural gum; and pecti
This paragraph does not apply, however, to any confectionery by reason c
its containing less than 0.5 per cent by volume of alcohol derived sole
from the use of flavoring extracts or to any chewing gum by reason of i
containing harmless nonnutritive masticatory substances.

It will be seen that the food section of the Federal Food, Drug, an
Cosmetic Law mentioned above is concerned not only with the safety c
food products that move in interstate commerce but also with fraudulei
practices. The law and the fair enforcement by the Food and Dru
Administration have had a stabilizing effect on industry, promoted fa
practice, and made a great contribution to public health.

Misbranding is also made unlawful. This calls for honest labeling c
the product as to its character, origin, and constituents and as to th
amount in the container.

7-3. Parasites. This subject is also discussed in Art. 1-15. The bee
tapeworm is common in the United States, residing in its human ho
without injurious effect except as a possible cause of anemia and nervou
symptoms. The adult worm lives in the intestines of man and perpe
uates the transmission cycle by depositing eggs which leave with th
feces. Cattle may ingest the eggs with egg-infected food or water. Larva
worms issue from the eggs into the intestines of the animal. From th
intestines they enter the muscles and there encyst themselves to wa
until the animal is slaughtered and the beef eaten. The cysts, also know
as measles, are visible to the naked eye. Effective cooking of beef wi
kill tapeworm larvae.

The pork tapeworm is less common in this country than the bee
tapeworm. It is somewhat similar to the latter except that hogs instea
of cattle are involved. There is one important difference. The perso
harboring an adult worm may infect himself with eggs from his ow
excreta, larval worms hatched in his own intestines encysting themselve
in his muscles. Should they choose the eye or the brain for this purpos
there may be serious results. This parasite is therefore considered mor
dangerous than the beef tapeworm. The practice of allowing hogs acce:
to human excreta in open toilets or elsewhere is responsible for muc
infection, although the hogs also infect each other. Effective cooking c
pork will kill the larvae in the measle form.

The fish tapeworm causes anemia. It is very likely to occur amon
people who eat much freshwater fish, particularly if it is eaten rav

The life cycle of this parasite is somewhat more complicated than that of the other tapeworms mentioned. The adult lives in the human intestines; the eggs are in the feces and infect the water of rivers or lakes. In the water the eggs hatch into small motile embryos, which at the first opportunity enter the body of a small crustacean (*Cyclops*). If the crustacean is eaten by a fish, the larva makes its way somewhere into the muscular tissue of the fish, there to wait until it is eaten by man. Preventive measures are thorough cooking of fish or freezing at minus 10°C and proper disposal of sewage.

Trichinosis, which is due to the worm *Trichinella spiralis*, is quite common abroad and occurs in the United States, more often, no doubt, than is reported or recognized. This is indicated by the fact that investigations made by the New York State Trichinosis Commission, based on numerous autopsies, indicated that 17 per cent of the people of the United States had had trichinosis at some time during their lives.

Its greater prevalence in Europe, especially in Germany, is due to the custom of eating raw pork in sausage. The larvae are embedded in the muscles in an oval cyst about $\frac{1}{25}$ in. long. When the flesh containing them is eaten, they are set free in the stomach, move into the intestines, and there reach maturity. The adults are not long-lived, but the larvae will survive for many years in their cysts before dying or being absorbed. The females are $\frac{1}{12}$ to $\frac{1}{6}$ in. long, and the males are about $\frac{1}{17}$ in. long. The females are viviparous and in about a week produce young totaling 1,000 to 2,000 over a period of 6 weeks, although most will be born in the first 2 weeks. The young migrate over a period of 3 days to encyst in muscular tissue. Trichinosis, the disease, occurs only if the infection is severe, and then signs of the disease occur in 1 to 2 weeks after the trichinous meat has been eaten. The movement of the worms into the muscles is accompanied by intense pain, fever, and other symptoms. Autopsies indicate that in fatal cases millions of larvae have become encysted. Infection is not obtained through feces but only through infected meat. Therefore, hogs which have been fed on garbage containing pork scraps and slaughterhouse offal are very likely to be infected. Rats living around slaughterhouses are usually heavily infested, and it is possible that the hogs may eat dead rats. It is estimated that about 0.15 per cent of all hogs in the country are infested. The cooking of garbage before it is fed to hogs on hog farms, as now required by most of the states, has reduced *Trichinella* in the animals to somewhat over 2 per cent in areas where it was formerly 11 per cent. It is still too high and indicates that possibly the garbage cooking is sometimes carelessly done [29]. Meat inspection is of little avail against this disease. Thorough cooking is necessary, although the trichina worm is easily killed, only 137°F being required. The pork should be cooked until it is white all through. Refrigeration at 5°F for a period of 20 days will also kill larvae [2, 29]. Pickling, salting, and smoking also kill when done thoroughly. Some hams and other pork products are commercially processed in such a manner that all trichinae are destroyed and no further cooking by the housewife is necessary. These products are generally labeled accordingly.

7-4. Food Poisoning. This term is loosely used to cover both infections and intoxications caused by eating contaminated food. Food poisoning is often characterized by vomiting, abdominal pain, diarrhea, chills, prostration, and gastroenteritis. These signs usually occur 4 to 12 hr after ingesting the food, although the extreme limits may be 2 to 72 hr even in the same outbreak. It is quite common, but the fatality rate is low. Reporting is far from complete [3, 4]. Outbreaks are said to be increasing, not only because of population increase, but because of the greater use of public eating places.

The distinction between food poisoning or intoxication and food-borne infection should be understood. In an official report of the American Public Health Association [5] food poisoning is distinguished from food-borne infection:

> The effects of food poisoning are promptly evident, and the amount of particular food ingested has a relation to severity, suggesting the importance of preformed elements [see p. 80 of the report]. Food-borne infection with a number of intestinal pathogens, with streptococci, and with agents of diphtheria, tuberculosis, and undulant fever follows a usual incubation for the particular disease, and clinical course and manifestations are not as a rule materially altered by the circumstances of the food serving as a vehicle of infection.

1. *Staphylococcus intoxication* is a poisoning (not an infection) of abrupt and often violent onset with nausea, vomiting, and sometimes severe diarrhea. This is the commonest of the food-borne illnesses, but fortunately deaths are very rare. Certain strains of *Staphylococci* will multiply in foods under favorable temperature conditions and will there form an enterotoxin that is stable at boiling temperature. The symptoms will appear in $\frac{1}{2}$ to 4 hr after taking the food, usually 2 to 4 hr. See Art. 6-40 for numbers in food required to form sufficient poison to be troublesome. Staphylococci are supposed ordinarily to be of human origin. They obtain entry to food from the hands of food handlers with skin infections, such as boils or pimples, or from nasal carriers. The foods involved are usually types that are handled and stored at temperatures too high to prevent bacterial multiplication before consumption. Reheating the stored food before consumption does not, of course, provide protection. The poisoned foods reported include custards; cream-filled cakes, including eclairs; processed meats [6] such as hashes and ham; poultry and poultry products; salads; and milk from cows with

infected udders. Dried milk has also been incriminated. Investigation of outbreaks should include bacterial examination of suspected foods. Preventive measures include:

a. Prompt refrigeration of chopped and sliced meats and of custards and cream fillings to avoid multiplication of staphylococci introduced; filling of pastries with custard immediately before sale or subjection of the finished product to adequate heat treatment to kill the organisms; and prompt disposal or refrigeration of leftover foods.

b. Education of food handlers in the role of staphylococci in food poisoning, the importance of hand washing, the danger of working with hand infections, and the necessity of refrigeration of foods. Management should require temporary exclusion from food handling of persons with skin or respiratory infections.

2. *Botulinus intoxication* is caused by the sporeforming organism *Clostridium botulinum,* of which there are several types. Most outbreaks are due to type A or B, and in a few instances type E is involved, mainly in relation to fish. The disease is an afebrile poisoning (not an infection) characterized by headache, weakness, constipation, oculomotor or other paralysis, and absence of diarrhea. Symptoms usually occur within 18 hr after the food has been eaten. Death by heart or respiratory paralysis occurs in about two-thirds of the cases, usually within 3 to 7 days. Biological and toxicological tests may confirm presence of the bacterium or its toxin in suspected foods or stomach contents. The toxin is produced in improperly processed foods, particularly nonacid foods, and only under anaerobic conditions. The toxin is easily destroyed by boiling, but the spores require higher temperatures. The reservoirs of the botulinus bacillus are the soil and the intestinal tracts of animals. Vehicles of infection are usually home-canned vegetables or meats, eaten uncooked. In Europe, cases have been ascribed to eating sausages or other preserved or smoked meats. Involvement of commercially canned foods is very rare. Signs of spoilage in the food may or may not be obvious. The toxin is so virulent that even the tasting of inspected foods has caused deaths. Preventive measures include:

a. Destruction of the spores of the organism during home canning. The home-canned foods should be heated to the boiling point before consumption.

b. Disposal of all preserved foods that show signs of spoilage.

3. *Clostridium perfringens (welchii) intoxications* are occasionally reported, particularly in Great Britain, although lately this organism has been attracting the attention of health authorities in the United States. Outbreaks reported have been caused by meat which has been cooked, allowed to cool slowly, insufficiently refrigerated, and served the next day or later, either reheated or cold. Apparently spores are not killed by the cooking, and during storage the toxin is formed. Signs and symptoms

appear after 8 to 22 hr and are acute abdominal pain and diarrhea, rarely nausea and vomiting. Prevention consists in excluding food handlers known or suspected to be infected and in cooking meat immediately before consumption or cooking it rapidly and following with rapid cooling and refrigeration.

4. *Salmonellosis infection* (not a poisoning) may be indicated by a variety of signs and symptoms. The most common is an acute gastro-enteritis with diarrhea and abdominal cramps. Fever, nausea, and vomiting are frequently present. Deaths are uncommon but are somewhat more frequent than in the case of staphylococcal food poisoning. *Salmonella* organisms may be recovered from feces or from the site of a localized infection during the acute illness. There are numerous species of *Salmonella*. Of the group pathogenic for animals and occasionally for man, the source and reservoir of infection are feces of patients or convalescent carriers; feces of domestic fowl, household pets, rodents, and domestic animals; and eggs of ducks and less commonly of chickens. Outbreaks are frequently traced to:

a. Improperly prepared food, especially meat pies and roast fowl. This means insufficient cooking, either at too low a temperature or for an insufficient period.

b. Insufficiently cooked foods containing dried hen eggs or duck eggs.

c. Unpasteurized milk or dairy products.

d. Pastries or other foods contaminated by rodent feces, or possibly through the medium of cockroaches, and served with no further cooking.

e. Food prepared by an infected food handler.

Sporadic cases probably originate through direct contact with an infected person or animal. The incubation period in an epidemic is from 6 to 48 hr, usually about 12 hr. The principal preventive measures are:

a. Thorough cooking of all foodstuffs derived from animal sources, with particular attention to preparation of fowl, egg products, and meat dishes.

b. Protection of prepared food against rodent and insect contamination.

c. Refrigeration of all prepared foods during storage. This will prevent *Salmonella* organisms from increasing in number.

5. *Other food infections.* Organisms other than those already mentioned use foods as vehicles of infection. Some, such as typhoid fever, paratyphoid fever (which is caused by certain *Salmonella* organisms), bacillary dysentery, and amoebic dysentery, may also be spread by water and involve human excreta.

Streptococcus faecalis is occasionally identified in food-borne disease. A wide variety of foods has been involved, including custards, dried eggs, sausage, and meats [7]. *Escherichia coli* apparently includes some strains which are pathogenic in very heavy doses. *Bacillus cereus*, which has been found in potato products and cornstarch, has caused outbreaks. Infectious hepatitis has been traced to the consumption of raw clams and oysters [8, 9].

"Gastroenteritis" is a term sometimes used for food-borne disease which has not been investigated as to the causative organism or for which the causative organism could not be identified. The unsuccessful examinations of foods and stomach contents indicate that more research of food poisonings and infections is needed [3].

6. *Summary of preventive measures.* Briefly, these include (*a*) protection of foods at all times from insects and vermin; (*b*) employment of food handlers who are free from infections of all kinds and who are clean in their habits; and (*c*) storage of foods subject to infection at temperatures of 45°F or below or 140°F or above, the latter applying particularly to foods kept on steam tables during serving. See Appendix A.

7-5. Sources of Outbreaks and Investigation. Public eating establishments are responsible for about 35 per cent of food-borne outbreaks. This is not surprising since the public of the United States spends about 1 billion dollars a month in restaurants [3]. High on the list of sources is the social occasion, which includes picnics and church suppers. At these, foods are usually eaten which have been prepared in advance in various homes and perhaps stored at temperatures above 50°F and which are finally served with little or no heating. Thus *Salmonella* or *Staphylococcus* organisms may be present to cause infection or poisoning. Also, appearing prominently in the statistics are hospitals, schools, and other institutions and foods consumed during travel in boats, railway trains, buses, etc.

Procedures for investigating outbreaks include (1) questioning affected persons as to foods consumed and comparing results, (2) collecting samples of food, and perhaps of stomach contents of victims, for examination, and (3) investigating the food handlers and the manner of food handling and storage [30].

7-6. Chemicals in Foods. Food poisoning has resulted from the accidental use of the rat poisons, sodium fluoride for milk powder or barium carbonate for flour. Such poisons should not be stored on the same shelves and preferably not in the same room as foods. Cadmium poisoning has resulted from contact of acid foods with cadmium-plated utensils, and antimony poisoning from foods cooked in cheap gray-enameled utensils. An outbreak of zinc poisoning resulted from storage of lemonade in a galvanized steel can.

Popular fears are sometimes aroused against insecticide residues on fruits and vegetables. The Food and Drug Administration controls this by permitting the use of insecticides on food crops only after it has established tolerances in food that are based upon animal experiments. These are related to the dosages used or recommended by the insecticide manufacturers, and agricultural users are informed. There exists a danger that the insecticides may be misused. This is met by inspection and testing by the Food and Drug Administration of such foods that are shipped interstate. With these safeguards, spray residues are not considered an important health hazard at the present time.

7-7. Legal Control of Food Safety. Legal control of foods is exerted in practically the same manner as outlined in Art. 6-6. The activity of the Food and Drug Administration in connection with insecticides is mentioned in the preceding article. In addition, the FDA controls all other chemical food additives, whether for preservation, for coloring, or to improve food characteristics. Chemicals which produce cancer in test animals are not permitted to be added to foods [10, p. 90]. Investigation of this characteristic of chemical additives to food presents difficulties. Sampling of foods for radioactivity is carried on regularly. Adulterations are investigated and prosecuted. The FDA also inspects food-processing plants whose products enter interstate commerce. The Communicable Disease Center, also a part of the Department of Health, Education, and Welfare, investigates food-borne disease outbreaks. The Public Health Service is engaged in food, shellfish, and milk programs designed to assist the state and local health authorities in the development, operation, and maintenance of programs for the prevention and control of food-borne diseases. It has prepared the Food Service Sanitation Manual, which includes a model food service sanitation ordinance and code for adoption by cities [11]. Meat inspection is carried on by the Meat Inspection Division of the U.S. Department of Agriculture on meats that are shipped interstate. Food-processing plants which include meats in their products are also inspected by this organization. State and local health departments are responsible for the local food-processing plants, cafes, restaurants, meat inspection, etc.

7-8. Canned Foods. While, from the epidemiological standpoint, canned foods are the safest foods we have, some control is exercised over them by health authorities. Many states inspect canneries and do not allow the product to be sold unless it conforms to their sanitary requirements. Sanitarians are required to eliminate from the shelves of wholesale and retail groceries and restaurants any canned goods showing signs of spoilage.

Grading of canned goods is attempted by canners on the basis of texture, firmness, and flavor. But it is difficult to keep packs of uniform quality, and in general the labeling by the canners as to whether the product is a fancy grade or otherwise has meant very little. Grading is purely voluntary on the part of the processor; he engages the services of the U.S. Department of Agriculture if he wishes to grade his food and label it accordingly. Some progress has been made in this direction, and some canned foods are graded by Federal inspectors as A, B, or C, corresponding to fancy, extra-standard, or standard. Substandard goods may be sold, if suitable for food, but must be so labeled. The National Canners' Association has established a policy concerning the growers' use of pesticides on products to be canned [12].

The cans used are made of steel coated with tin. The tin coating is not perfect and may contain some small holes. Protective enamels, which are usually synthetic resins baked on the metal sheets at high temperatures, are used on the interiors of many cans. They prevent a harmless but discoloring reaction between certain foods and the metal of the can. The can seams are made by crimping the edges of the metal and sealing with a thin gasket. The cans should be clean before filling.

The following steps are taken in the processing of fruits or vegetables that are to be canned [13]: (1) Sorting, which eliminates rotten or undesirable material. (2) Washing by soaking and spraying. (3) Peeling and trimming. (4) Blanching, which is the application of hot water or steam. It wilts some bulky vegetables, prevents discoloring of others, cleans peas of mucilaginous material, and removes some of the air from the tissues. (5) Placing in the cans. (6) Exhausting, which consists in heating to such a temperature that air and other gases are driven out. Air removal prevents oxidation of the can contents later, while the partial vacuum resulting after the cans are sealed prevents excessive pressures during the processing. It results in concave ends for the cans after the process is complete. A mechanical vacuum may also be applied and cans sealed in it. (7) Covering and sealing of the cans while the contents are at the exhausting temperature. (8) Processing, or the heating or cooking of the contents to prevent spoilage. This does not necessarily ensure complete sterilization because a few resistant thermophilic spores would necessitate such a high temperature that the food would be unsalable. These spores are of no consequence. The processing time and temperature depend upon the nature of the food and have been established by research, much of which has been done in the Research Laboratory of the National Canners' Association. (9) Immersion of cans in cool water to relieve pressure and prevent overcooking and germination of thermophiles, which would occur during slow cooling.

Inspection of cans for spoilage presents no difficulties. The normal can has no leaks around the rims or seams, and the ends are slightly concave. A "swell" has bulging ends. A "flipper" has one end which bulges when the can is tapped sharply against a hard surface and which does not return unless pressed in. A "springer" has a bulging end which, when pressed in, causes the other end to bulge. Swells must pass through the flipper and springer stages.

Swells, flippers, and springers may be caused by overfilling the can, insufficient exhaustion of air, or transportation of cans to high altitudes. The vast majority, however, are caused by fruit attacking the metal of the can and evolving hydrogen gas. Practically all such swelling occurs a year or more after canning. It does not make the food dangerous. It is true that small amounts of tin compounds are formed by reaction with certain foods, but research has shown that these are harmless. There is no basis for the popular belief that some poison is formed if food is left in the can after it is opened, but opened cans that still contain food should, of course, be placed in the refrigerator to prevent contamination of the contents by flies or other agents of disease transmission.

Decomposition caused by the action of microorganisms occurs practically only in nonacid vegetables. It is generally not dangerous, but the possibility of botulism must be borne in mind. Since the public cannot be expected to distinguish between the decomposition of fruits and vegetables, the rule should be that all swells, flippers, and springers be condemned. The sanitarian should also make certain that the contents are destroyed, for swells may be punctured to release the gas, the holes soldered up, and the contents reprocessed and sold.

Inspections of canning plants should be made while the plants are in operation. The following requirements should be enforced: Washers, blanchers, etc., should be emptied and cleaned at least once a day. Overflow brine, syrup, or juice should not be re-used. Protection of cans and covers from dirt and insects should be required; no cans or other containers should be filled by dipping, and no pails or vessels used for food packing should be used in cleaning operations. There should be daily removal of refuse; a tight roof; and watertight and smooth table tops and floors, graded to drain and kept clean. Toilet rooms should be screened and have self-closing doors, and there should be one toilet for each 15 employees. Adequate washing facilities with soap and towels should be available. Personnel should be free from disease and have clean hands and clothing; female employees should wear clean, washable caps. Spitting should not be permitted in rooms where food is processed. There should be a safe water supply, and liquid wastes should be disposed of without danger or nuisance.

7-9. Dried Foods. Dried fruits, vegetables, and meats have not been reported as causing outbreaks of food poisoning. *Salmonella* organisms have been isolated frequently from dried whole egg, and some *Salmonella* outbreaks in man in Great Britain have been suspected on good evidence of having been caused by spray-dried eggs. Reconstituted eggs should be cooked immediately because if they are incubated for some hours so that bacterial multiplication results, only thorough cooking (in terms of time and temperature) will destroy all the *Salmonella* organisms present. Staphylococcus poisoning has been attributed to dried milk. For dry-milk sanitation control, see Art. 6-38.

Insanitary handling of food prior to or during dehydration results in high bacterial content, possibly including organisms of the coliform group, and the presence of yeasts and molds. This condition may lead to poor flavor of the product and early spoilage while the food is being stored. Bacterial standards for dried foods have been advocated as a means of controlling the sanitation of handling, processing, and storing. In the absence of such standards, plant sanitation should be emphasized, since the consumer of dehydrated foods is entitled to an assurance that they have not been prepared under filthy conditions.

7-10. Paper Containers. Containers made of paper, paperboard, and molded pulp are widely used for foods, including milk. Sanitation standards to guide manufacturers of these products have been established through the cooperation of Federal, state, and local authorities; members of the Syracuse University Research Corporation; and representatives of the manufacturers concerned [31].

The standards include the following requirements: (1) The products must be made from clean, sanitary virgin chemical or mechanical pulp or from waste or cuttings of such paper as paperboard, provided they have been handled in a clean, sanitary manner. Stock must be free from slime spots. (2) The use of deleterious or poisonous substances is forbidden, as is the use of any material that will impair the flavor, odor, or bacteriological quality of the contents. This applies to adhesives, lubricants, and moisture-resistant substances used. Products used for packaging milk or milk products shall comply with the Milk Ordinance and Code of the Public Health Service. (3) Products, while in possession of the manufacturer, must be so handled, wrapped, stored, and transported that they will be protected from contamination. (4) Materials used in manufacture must be free from coliform bacteria, and, as determined by disintegration test, the stock used must contain not over 250 bacterial colonies per gram. (5) The sanitation of the plant in which the containers are manufactured requires cleanliness, freedom from insects and from rodents and other vermin, a safe and adequate water supply, freedom from food residues and refuse, and adequate toilet and hand-washing facilities for employees.

7-11. Sanitation of Refrigerated Locker Plants. Refrigerated locker plants are designed and constructed to store food at low temperatures in lockers of about 25 cu ft capacity. The processing requires (1) a chill room, where the food is reduced in temperature; (2) a quick- or sharp-freeze room, in which the food is quickly frozen; and (3) the locker room. In some plants an aging room is also included that is used for a period of storage at moderate temperature after chilling. The plant may also include facilities for butchering cattle, hogs, and poultry for storage in the lockers. Such service may also include curing, smoking, or barbecuing the meat.

In addition to the usual sanitary requirements for food-handling establishments discussed in this chapter, the locker plant presents a few special problems. The temperatures of the various rooms should be as follows: in the chilling room, 34 to 36°F, with a tolerance of 10° for a reasonable time after food has been placed in the room; in the aging room, 38°F, with a tolerance of 4°; and in the quick-freeze room, 10°F or lower when still-air cooling is employed and 0°F or lower when forced-air circulation is used, with a tolerance of 10° for either type of installation for a reasonable time after food has been placed in the room. Accurate thermometers must be kept in each room, and the one in the locker room must be of the recording type with a weekly chart.

At least one gas mask of a type approved by the U.S. Bureau of Mines must be on hand in case of leaks of the refrigerant.

Foods not for human consumption must be so marked. All foods must be quick-frozen before being stored in lockers, and they must be wrapped in nonabsorbent paper so as to exclude air. Each package must be marked with its contents, the locker number, and the date of quick freezing.

7-12. Frozen Foods. This term applies to the more than five hundred frozen fruits; vegetables; fruit-juice concentrates; precooked foods and dinners; and cooked or uncooked fish, meats, and poultry that are displayed in the frozen-food cases of food stores [14, 15]. Frozen foods, according to the records, are not a health hazard. Contamination is of course possible in the processing, and mishandling may occur during packaging, transportation, and storing or in the home. The ubiquitous *Staphylococcus* organisms and *Salmonella* have been found in frozen foods but in such small numbers that they have caused no food-borne outbreaks. Figure 7-1 shows the relationship between food temperatures and food-poisoning and psychrophilic organisms. Psychrophiles are defined as organisms capable of relatively rapid growth at 32°F. The manufacturer, wholesaler, and distributor are concerned with food spoilage, and since storage times are long, slow spoilage must be prevented. Hence the optimum storage temperature is considered to be 0°F. This cannot always be maintained during transportation and handling, and precautions should be taken to prevent higher temperatures and particularly defrosting. In so-called frozen foods, not all the water is frozen except at very low temperatures, and it is in the unfrozen water that bacterial action is presumed to take place. Below 14°F, concentration of various substances is so high in the water that bacterial action is stopped. Storage times can be quite long before detectable taste or odor changes occur. Well-packaged raw chicken may be stored for over 2 years at 0°F but for only 6 months at 20°F; fried chicken, for 2 months at 0°F and for 2 weeks at 20°F (turkey pies and dinners are between these periods); and peas and green beans, for 10 months at

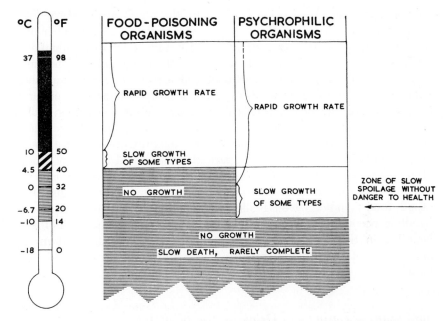

FIGURE 7-1   The temperature range of food-poisoning and psychrophilic organisms. (*From "Conference on Frozen Food Quality," Western Regional Research Laboratory, U.S. Department of Agriculture, Albany, Calif., 1960.*)

0°F and for 1 month at 20°F. Spoilage, it should be pointed out, occurs at low temperatures through the action of oxygen; hence the importance of packaging.

Any increases in temperature above the optimum, even though only temporary, are cumulative in the reduction of shelf time. Retailers, therefore, should keep display cases at proper temperatures, except when defrosting, and should check temperatures there and in storage rooms. Cases should not be filled above the indicated food line, and the newer products should be placed in display cases under the older ones.

7-13. Health Certificates. Laws of some states require that all food handlers employed to serve the public have certificates indicating that they have been examined by competent physicians and have been found free from communicable disease. The certificates have to be renewed at intervals of 6 months or a year, and the employer is required to keep them on file for checking by the inspectors of the food-handling establishments.

Experience with health certificates has been far from satisfactory. Before a physician can be sure that a food handler is free from tuberculosis or venereal disease or is not a carrier of typhoid fever or diphtheria, special examinations and tests are required that would cost too much for either the employer or the employee to pay. Consequently, only a superficial examination is given by the physician in return for a small fee. This procedure also ignores the fact that a food handler may develop disease shortly after he has been examined. Both the employer and the employee realize the small value of the examinations. They may lose respect for the health department which enforces the requirement, while the public may have a false sense of security. The present tendency is to disregard the health certificate and concentrate on listing known carriers of disease and having sick workers report to the health officer. It is useful for the city or county health department to keep a file of known typhoid fever carriers. In part, this file would consist of names of persons known to have developed into carriers, as determined by tests given during convalescence. Such a file, together with registration of all food handlers, would allow elimination of carriers from food-handling occupations. Of assistance, too, would be the education of food handlers in the recognition of the early signs of disease and in the importance of immediately reporting to a physician for diagnosis and treatment.

Sanitation of Eating and Drinking Establishments

7-14. Cleaning and Bactericidal Treatment of Utensils and Equipment. Figure 7-2 is a diagram showing the importance of the multiuse utensils of a public food-handling establishment in transmitting diseases. Respiratory and intestinal infections may be transmitted through unclean eating utensils.

Reference to the diagram will indicate the importance of the dishwater. Unless the water is hot enough or a bactericidal treatment is used, it may serve to transmit disease and may also endanger the workers whose hands are frequently immersed in it; and, of course, if the washing and sanitizing process is not properly done, the danger of the utensils to the patrons is apparent. All washing operations done by hand should be carried on in a three-compartment vat. The complete washing process should include the following: (1) rinsing or thorough scraping to eliminate large food particles—this will keep the wash water in better

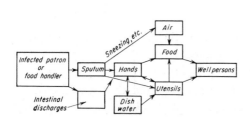

FIGURE 7-2 Principal methods of transmission of respiratory and intestinal diseases at food-handling establishments. The double arrows indicate possible travel of infectious material in each direction. Flies and contaminated water are also possibilities but have not been indicated. (*Courtesy of Public Health Service.*)

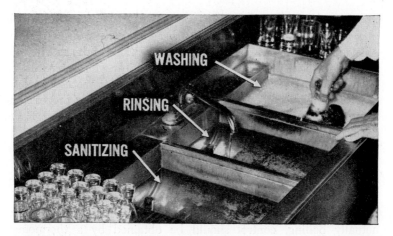

FIGURE 7-3 Three-compartment sink. (*Photograph courtesy of Wyandotte Chemicals Corporation.*)

condition; (2) washing in water at a temperature of 110 to 120°F with a soap or other detergent; (3) rinsing combined with an effective germicidal process.

THE DETERGENT. The detergent is the cleaning agent (see Art. 8-18). It works by dissolving and emulsifying the grease or other soil on the utensils so that it flows off into the water. Bacteria are also carried off in the process, although some remain on the surfaces. The ideal detergent would not be injurious to the hands of the dishwasher and would be efficient in both hard and soft water. In hard waters the calcium and magnesium salts present unite with the detergent to form a sticky curd which causes a film on the surfaces after washing. The film protects bacteria in the sanitizing process. Some detergents include sequestering agents to prevent the formation of the curd or to reduce its stickiness. Choice of the detergent, and particularly the amount used, depends upon whether hand washing or machine washing is used and upon the hardness of the water.

Soap and the foaming commercial detergents as well are good detergents in waters having a hardness of not over 300 ppm. Sodium carbonate is an alkaline detergent which has been much used, although its efficiency is low in all ranges of soft to hard waters. Other alkaline detergents containing the polyphosphates, particularly the hexaphosphates, have the sequestering action mentioned above and are therefore sufficiently effective in hard waters. Some observers also claim that they increase rinsability, *i.e.*, permit quick rinsing without leaving a film. They have high pH values, are hard on hands, and are suitable for mechanical washing. Foaming detergents should not be used in mechanical dishwashing processes.

Sanitization. This term is applied to the treatment of dishes and utensils so that there is no health hazard involved in their re-use. The efficiency of sanitization is based on observations of the survival of various test bacteria on the presumption that the less resistant pathogens have been killed by the process. Actually sanitization is another word for disinfection, usually applied in connection with a cleaning process. Sanitizing agents, however, are not usually called disinfectants since Federal law requires that disinfectants have a phenol coefficient (Art. 8-7) on the container, and the efficiency of some sanitizers cannot be tested by obtaining a phenol coefficient.

Heat is an effective sanitizer if it is properly used. Immersion of the utensils for at least 2 min in clean hot water at a temperature of at least 170°F or for ½ min in boiling water is effective. Unless the water is actually boiling, control should be obtained by a thermometer and preferably by a thermostat placed on the water heater or immersion vat. Pouring hot water over the dishes is not effective, nor is the use of water in which the worker can place his hands. If hand washing is used, metal baskets, lined with wood strips to prevent marking the china, are required to immerse and remove the dishes from the hot water. After removal from the hot water, the dishes should remain in the baskets until dry and should then be stored in such a manner that they will not be contaminated before they are used again. Where heat is used, a three-compartment washing vat will be needed, one for washing, the second for heat treatment, and the third for rinsing. Care should be taken that the wash water does not become excessively dirty before it is changed.

A chlorine solution may also be used for bactericidal purposes. Immersion should be for at least 2 min in a lukewarm solution containing at least 50 ppm of available chlorine if hypochlorites are used, or a concentration of 100 ppm if chloramines are used. The rinse should be made up at a strength of 100 ppm or more of hypochlorites, and it should not be used after an orthotolidine test shows that the chlorine residual has been reduced to less than 50 ppm. Some organic chlorine compounds are sold for this purpose. They produce less chlorine odor but must be used with caution, for they are apparently less efficient than hypochlorite. Their efficiency should be checked by the tests given below. If chlorine is used, a three-compartment washing vat is needed, one for washing, the second for a plain rinse, and the third for the chlorine rinse. If desired, the dishes or glasses may be rinsed again in clean running water, to remove the chlorine odor, and then permitted to dry either in the basket or on a drain shelf or tray. The odor, however, soon leaves in any case. In this or the heat method of disinfection, care should be taken that no air is entrapped in the dishes or glasses to prevent actual contact with the hot water or solution. Chlorine should not be used to disinfect silver or silver-plated articles, for it will turn them black.

Quaternary ammonium compounds are being used as sanitizers to a considerable extent. Compounds containing iodine and bromine have also been found effective for bactericidal treatment.

Combination detergent-sanitizers have been available and may be used to an increasing extent in the future. Since the quaternary ammonium compounds are less affected by organic matter than chlorine is, they are showing promise when combined with alkaline detergents. Mallmann believes that they should be used in the hand washing of utensils and all washing of bottles and glasses. They have proved successful in washing dairy utensils, although it is advocated that just before use the utensils receive an additional rinse with a bactericide.

MECHANICAL DISHWASHING. Mechanical methods of dishwashing are more satisfactory than hand washing if the dishwasher is properly designed and operated. The efficiency of mechanical machines depends upon temperature, spray pattern, time of spraying, nozzle size, and pressure. Mechanical dishwashers used in large kitchens are of the single-

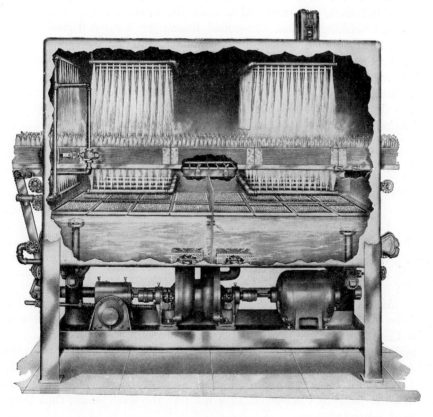

FIGURE 7-4 Cutaway view of a multiple-tank dishwasher. (*Courtesy of Universal Washing Machine Co., Nutley, N.J.*)

or multiple-tank types. The single-tank washer has one tank which contains heated wash water with a detergent. The wash water is pumped from the tank through sprays which direct it against the utensils to be washed, and the water drains back to the tank and is recirculated. Before returning to the tank it passes through a strainer tray which has openings smaller than those of the sprays. After the wash the utensils are exposed to a hot rinsing spray which comes directly from the hot-water heater and which after use is generally discharged into the wash water, after passing through a strainer. The multiple-tank washer has a rinse-water tank and pump in addition to the wash-water tank. Since the rinse water is also recirculated, a curtain rinse of hot water directly from the hot-water source is applied to the utensils as they leave the machine. Thus no recirculated water remains on the washed dish or utensil.

The dishes and silver, after rinsing or scraping, are placed in baskets or trays. The baskets then are placed on an endless belt which automatically moves them through the machine. Push-through types are also made, but these are undesirable since the attendant may reduce the required washing period. Controlled timing for wash and rinse is desirable. The temperature of the wash water should be from 140 to 160°F. Higher temperatures bake some foods, such as eggs, on the utensils. The water pressure and amount should be high enough to get good mechanical action from the jets. The optimum amounts of these have been determined by the National Sanitation Foundation and vary with the size of machine [16]:

> The minimum number of gallons of wash water at 140° to 160°F required to be sprayed uniformly over each rack of dishes in not less than 40 seconds shall be determined by multiplying the total area of the rack by 0.23. The pump delivery capacity shall be determined by multiplying such rack area by 0.35. For racks of all sizes, the pressure at the jet during the washing operations shall be sufficient to deliver the wash water to all portions of the racked dishes with a cutting velocity. Such velocity shall be just under that which will dislodge standard restaurant coffee cups from racks.

After the washing, the dishes are rinsed in water not less than 180°F at the dish for at least 10 sec. It is recommended that the water pressure be 15 to 25 psi, with a flow rate of 9 gpm per 20- by 20-in. dish rack in single-tank, stationary-rack, hood-curtain, and door types. If the racks are of a different size, the flow rate should be varied proportionately [17]. A recirculating pump applies the wash water. In many machines the rinse water is discharged after use into the wash water, thus keeping it relatively clean.

The detergent, which must be kept at proper strength, is added mechanically or by hand, although the latter has not been found to be very satisfactory. Detergents in blocks have been used. They are placed in the wash water and dissolved as the water is used. No rule can be given as to the amount of detergent to be used since it depends upon the character of the water, particularly its hardness. Results should be checked by tests.

The sanitarian, when checking dishwashing machines, should especially note a number of possible deficiencies. The machine may be of the push-through type, which means that the baskets or trays remain in the sprays only as long as the operator permits. The total time should never be under 1 min, preferably more, and as much as possible of this period should be used for the rinse, provided proper washing is obtained. Temperatures of the wash and rinse waters should be checked, as should the amount of detergent in the wash water, which may be highly variable because of the entrance of rinse water. Stacking of the dishes, particularly the cups and the spoons in the trays, should be noted, for they may not be properly exposed to the water. Dishes should be inspected and testing swabs used. The machine should be checked to make certain there are no cross-connections to the public water supply.

Glasses are frequently washed in warm water containing an alkaline detergent having a formula similar to that given above, the cleaning being done by rotating brushes which vigorously scrub the interior and exterior. The glasses are then rinsed in a chlorine solution. This procedure results in fewer broken glasses and a better appearance.

Dishes should preferably dry by drainage, but if towels are used they should be clean. High-temperature rinses promote rapid drying.

The National Sanitation Foundation, in its laboratory, has conducted a series of studies and has developed standards for soda-fountain, luncheonette, and food-service equipment, including standards for spray-type dishwashing machines. Manufacturers meeting these standards may use the National Sanitation Foundation seal of approval. These standards have been most helpful to food regulatory officials.

TESTS. The efficiency of dishwashing and bactericidal treatments can be determined bacteriologically. The swab test is used on cleansed and disinfected utensils.

The laboratory first prepares a dilute phosphate buffer solution that is nontoxic to bacteria. If the utensils to be swabbed are likely to have chlorine and/or quaternary ammonium compound on them, the solution must contain a neutralizing agent. Utensils to be examined should include at least glasses, cups, and spoons, if used. Select at least four of each at random, using one swab and swab container for each group of four or more utensils. When collecting samples, take a swab from the container and press it against the inside of the container to remove excess water, leaving the swab moist, but not wet. Then swab slowly and firmly three times over significant surfaces of four or more similar utensils, reversing the direction each time. Significant surfaces of glasses and cups are the upper ½ in. of inner and outer rim. The entire inner and outer surfaces of the bowls of spoons and tines of forks are significant. Swab completely across plates, each of two diameters at right angles, and around inner surface of bowls halfway between bottom and rim. After swabbing each utensil, return the swab to the container of dilution water, rotate the swab in the dilution water, and press out excess water before swabbing the next utensil. Replace swab in container of dilution water after completing the swabbing of all utensils in a group. Keep the dilution water samples iced while in transit to the laboratory and until samples are plated. Plate the samples preferably within 4 hr of swabbing; but where this cannot be done, samples must be properly refrigerated and analyzed within 24 hr. From the bacterial count of the solutions, the average plate count per cup, glass, or spoon surface can be obtained. The average should be not over 100. Higher counts are presumed to be caused by inadequate cleaning and bactericidal treatment.

Rough tests are available that will demonstrate the presence of grease or film on utensil surfaces. If water will not run completely off a china or glass surface, the presence of some soiling material is indicated. If sugar is dusted over a dry surface and there is adherence, there is evidence of grease.

7-15. Storage and Protection of Food in Restaurants. From a preceding article it has been seen that infection of foods, followed by storage at room temperatures, results in food poisoning or infection. Therefore, protection of foods against infection and proper storage after handling are important. Common practice in the past has been to require the storage of foods at temperatures less than 50°F. This may have been a reasonable requirement when ice was depended upon for refrigeration, but mechanical refrigeration permits storage at lower temperatures with the accompanying additional protection. The National Sanitation Clinic [18] recommends that the maximum air temperature be 40°F for storage of raw meat, raw poultry, eggs, milk, cheese, and butter when the storage period is to be less than 7 days. Foods which have been cooked should be cooled as quickly as possible through the danger zone of quick bacterial multiplication (98 to 50°F) and stored at 40°F or lower until served. The cooling can be done in the refrigerator, preferably in open shallow pans. This procedure applies to cuts of meat, sliced meats, poultry, seafoods, minced foods, sandwich fillings, egg-salad mixtures, and similar foods that are not kept hot while being served.

Custards and custard-filled pastries are frequently involved in disease outbreaks and should be cooled to 40°F within 1 hr after preparation. They should not be taken from the refrigerator for display or sale for periods of more than 1 hr. All such products exceeding 24 hr in age should be destroyed. An exception is made with hot custards, which must be maintained and served at temperatures exceeding 150°F.

Regarding the temperature for hot-food service units, the National Sanitation Clinic [18] recommends a minimum holding temperature of 150°F. If the hot foods cannot be kept at this temperature for any reason, they should be cooled rapidly to 40°F or less and then brought up to 150°F before re-serving. This applies particularly to foods of animal origin and those containing protein. Leafy vegetables and foods of very low protein content may be held for periods not exceeding 2 hr at room temperatures (60 to 90°F). Some of the temperatures specified above differ slightly from those required in the Model Ordinance [11], which gives 45°F as the maximum temperature for foods served cold and 140°F as a minimum temperature for foods served hot. Local health authorities may adopt the stricter requirements if they wish. Other requirements are discussed in Art. 7-16.

Highly important is the exclusion until cured of food handlers who have colds or lung infections or who have pimples or other pus-containing lesions on their hands or arms. Handling of all foods that have been cooked or that are served raw should be kept to a minimum. Butter and ice should not be touched by the bare hands. The tasting of samples of food in the kitchen should be safeguarded by requiring that it be done from special dishes, one for each person, with spoons or other articles that are cleaned and sanitized after use.

7-16. Model Ordinance for Restaurant Sanitation. Satisfactory sanitary conditions in establishments where food is processed, prepared, and served are obtained only if there is an efficient inspecting force, or other legal authority operating under an adequate city ordinance which can, when necessary, be successfully enforced through the courts. Court action is uncertain as to outcome and should be avoided by using more constructive measures, such as seeking the assistance and advice of inspectors who are thoroughly acquainted with the principles of sanitation and their applications to food handling. A well-organized laboratory is important to the sanitarian or sanitary inspector to help in solving food problems and in epidemiological investigations.

The Public Health Service has prepared a model ordinance and code [11] as an aid to cities in obtaining sanitation at restaurants, the term being defined to include cafeterias, taverns, sandwich stands, soda fountains, etc., and also kitchens in which food and drink are prepared for sale elsewhere to the public. The more important features of the Model Ordinance will be given briefly according to its lettered sections:

A. This section defines terms used.

B. *Food.* This requires that food served be from approved supplies, *i.e.*, the milk and milk products from approved sources and complying with local and state laws, meats and meat products federally inspected or inspected by other approved authority, and shellfish obtained from certified dealers. Food considered unsafe or unsuitable for human consumption can be condemned. Potentially hazardous food must be stored at safe temperatures, below 45°F or above 140°F.[1] Pork and pork products not especially treated to destroy *Trichinella* must be cooked to heat all parts to 150°F. Stuffed meats and poultry must be heated throughout to a minimum temperature of 165°F, with no interruption of the initial cooking process. All nonacid hermetically sealed foods must have been processed in commercial food-processing establishments as a precaution against butolithic poisoning. Unwrapped foods on display— for example, at cafeterias, smorgasbords and buffets—must be protected against handling, sneezing, and coughing and against contamination by flies, rodents, or other vermin.

C. *Personnel.* Employees are to keep hands clean, wear clean outer garments, and use hair restraints. Persons with boils, infected wounds, sore throats or other respiratory infections, or any communicable disease are not permitted to work where there is likelihood of transmission of the disease to patrons or fellow employees.

D. *Food equipment and utensils.* This requires that food-contact surfaces of equipment be in good repair with no cracks and no pits or open seams and that they be made of approved material, which excludes cadmium, antimony, zinc, and lead, except that lead may be used in the solder of seams. There shall be no corrosion of surfaces, and construction shall be such that all equipment is accessible for cleaning and inspection. Multiuse utensils must be cleaned and sanitized by methods described in Art. 7-14.

E. *Sanitary facilities and controls.* This requires an adequate, safe hot and cold water supply. Ice is to be from an approved source and handled and stored properly; ice blocks must be rinsed, and all contact surfaces clean. The sewage disposal method must be approved. Plumbing must be properly sized, installed, and maintained. No cross-connections are permitted, and no back siphonage possible. Toilet facilities must be provided for employees. The toilet rooms must be easily accessible but must not open into rooms where food is prepared, and they must be kept clean. Lavatories must be provided, kept in good repair, and furnished with hot and cold running water and with towels or other hand-drying facilities. Garbage and rubbish storage and disposal methods must be sanitary. Rodents, flies, and other vermin must be kept to a minimum. Harborage and feeding of vermin are to be prevented. Outer

---

[1] Other authorities (see Art. 7-15) prefer 40°F as a maximum temperature and 150°F as a minimum temperature.

openings must be protected against flying insects, and the building must be rodentproof.

F. *Other facilities.* This section covers construction and cleanliness of walks, ceilings, and floors and proper lighting of working surface (20 ft-c); rooms, toilets, and hand-washing areas (10 ft-c); and all other areas (5 ft-c). Ventilation is required to remove odors, steam, and smoke. Dressing rooms or areas for employees are required, together with lockers or other suitable facilities. No food-handling operations are permitted in sleeping quarters. The establishment is to be kept clean, with soiled linen and clothing kept in proper containers and laundered clothes and napkins stored in a clean place.

H. *Enforcement provisions.*[1] This covers the issuance, suspension, reinstatement, and revocation of permits. Holders of suspended or revoked permits may request a hearing before the health authority, who thereafter makes a finding that will sustain, modify, or rescind the official notice given to the permit holder. Inspections are to be made at least once every 6 months or as often as deemed necessary. An inspection form is used on which violations of the requirements are checked, and a copy is left at the establishment at the time of the inspection. The violations have different weights, and demerits are given according to those weights. If the demerit score is over 40, the permit is immediately suspended. Time limits are specified for the correction of certain violations which are related closely to health hazards where permit suspension is not required. If the grading system is used, the grades are as follows: a grade of A for a demerit score of not more than 10; a grade of B for a demerit score of more than 10 but not more than 20; and a grade of C for a demerit score of more than 20 but not more than 40.

The ordinance also requires that when a food-service establishment is constructed or extensively remodeled or when an existing structure is converted for use as a food-service establishment, the plans and specifications be submitted to the health authority for approval before work is begun.

Temporary food-service establishments such as those at fairs and carnivals are covered by the Ordinance. For an unrestricted food-service operation, all the requirements of secs. B to F which are applicable to its operation must be met. If, in the opinion of the health authority, no imminent health hazards will result, temporary establishments which do not meet the requirements of secs. B to F may be permitted with certain restrictions, such as prohibition of potentially hazardous foods. These include cream-filled pastries, custards and similar products, and meat, poultry, and fish in the form of salads or sandwiches. This restriction does not, however, apply to hamburgers, frankfurters, and other food which prior to service requires only limited preparation, such as seasoning and cooking. The restriction also does not apply to potentially

[1] There is no subsection G.

hazardous food which is served in individual containers and which was packaged in a commercial food establishment and stored at a safe temperature.

7-17. Restaurant Sanitation in Rural Areas. The above discussion concerns city health departments operating under city ordinances. In rural areas and unincorporated villages, the problem is a smaller one since there are fewer public food-handling establishments, although this statement does not apply to counties having one or more large cities and highways that have become lined with food establishments. Inspectors of the state health departments are usually not able to make regular inspections. Some control should be applied, and a county health department may have this as its responsibility. It may operate to enforce state food laws, although these are rather general in nature, or it may adopt a voluntary grading system patterned upon the items of the Model Ordinance. All restaurants that comply with the requirements are permitted to display a Grade A placard which is granted by the health department. Publicity may be used to make the public cognizant of the significance of the placard.

7-18. Automatic Food Vending. The coin-operated machine for vending of various types of foods and beverages is a familiar sight. It is estimated that about 1.7 million workers, students, and others get at least one meal per day from automatic vending machines and that 80 per cent of industrial plants use vending machines, 20 per cent using them exclusively for employee food services [19]. The magnitude of these food operations justifies health department control.

LEGAL CONTROL. Foods dispensed by the machines are prepared and packaged in factories or commissaries which can be inspected and where food quality can be controlled by the usual methods. Automatic food vending presents the additional problems of prevention of contamination of foods during delivery to, and storage in, the machines and during the dispensing. The design, operation, and maintenance of the dispensing machine are important. The National Automatic Merchandising Association (NAMA), whose membership is made up of manufacturers of dispensing machines and containers, was instrumental in forming a council of representatives from the vending-machine industry, schools of public health, and health regulatory agencies; this is known as the American Merchandising Health-Industry Council (AMHIC). The Council, various health authorities, and the Public Health Service developed a Sanitation Ordinance and Code [20], which is recommended for adoption by local health departments. The Ordinance requires issuance of permits to persons operating one or more vending machines, prohibits sale of adulterated or misbranded foods, and requires the inspection by the health authority of commissaries and of the servicing, maintenance, and operation of vending machines dispensing readily perishable foods at least once every 6 months. Vending machines dispensing other than readily perishable foods may be inspected as often as deemed necessary.

The NAMA conducts research and publishes manuals, evaluation forms, etc., relating to vending machines, with the AMHIC acting in an advisory role. Research has been carried on at Michigan State University (Department of Microbiology and Public Health) and at the Indiana Research Foundation (School of Public Health) with regard to automatic vending. Machines proposed for use are examined and tested according to the "Vending Machine Evaluation Manual" [21]. If approved, the manufacturer is given a letter of compliance. A list of vending-machine manufacturers and their machines which comply can be obtained by health authorities from the NAMA.

VENDING-MACHINE SANITATION. The principles of sanitation for milk and other foods already outlined apply to automatic dispensing machines. It is important, of course, that operators and attendants of the machines also understand them and that the machines be so designed that contamination, spoilage, and food poisoning of consumers will not occur. The Ordinance is particularly concerned with the readily perishable foods. These are defined [21] as any food, beverage, or ingredients consisting in whole or in part of milk, milk products, eggs, meat, fish, poultry, or other food capable of supporting the rapid and progressive growth of microorganisms which cause food infections or food intoxications. The temperature of these foods, in transportation or in storage, should not be permitted to rise above 50°F or fall below 150°F. Temperature controls are required in the machines. All multiuse parts of any bulk milk vending machine which come into direct contact with the milk or milk product shall be effectively cleaned and sanitized at the milk plant. All multiuse containers or parts of vending machines which come into direct contact with readily perishable foods shall be thoroughly cleaned and sanitized at the commissary or other approved place. This does not apply to surfaces kept at temperatures below 50°F and above 150°F. These are to be cleaned and sanitized and then protected from contamination.

Foods other than the readily perishable include candy; nuts; gum; cookies, crackers, and other bakery products; bottled, canned, and bulk soft drinks; powdered or dry coffee and tea; soup; sugar; chocolate, cocoa, and similar products; black coffee; plain tea; fruit juices; water; beverage juices; canned and other foods in hermetically sealed containers; and dry or powdered products so low in moisture that microorganisms will not develop. Some of these will present storage problems, although health hazards are not involved [22].

Other requirements of the Ordinance include the following: insects, mice, and rats are to be prevented from entering the machines by proper safeguards; machines are to be located where they will be easily clean-able, and they must be kept clean; all interior surfaces are to be kept clean, and if in contact with the product, they must be of approved non-toxic materials; pipes, valves, chutes, and faucets which come into contact with foods are to be removable for cleaning, or if not removable, they must be of such design that a bactericidal solution can be passed through them; water used in the machines is to be of a safe and sanitary quality; and there is to be proper disposal of all wastes.

7-19. Aids to Inspection of Food Establishments. From the fore-going articles it is apparent that the sanitary inspector or sanitarian should have a thorough knowledge of food sanitation, including epidemiological procedures used in investigating food-borne disease outbreaks. He should also be an educator in his field as well as an enforcer. He will require access to a laboratory for the bacteriological and chemical examination of suspected foods. He should have, when making inspections, thermometers, a light meter, a flashlight, a water-pressure gage, a metal measuring tape, a stopwatch, and a clipboard. He may at times need a pyrometer and thermocouples to measure high temperatures, a black-light (ultraviolet) generator to demonstrate spoilage, a camera, and an epidemiological kit that includes instructions, forms, sterile sample equipment, and an insulated sample case [11].

The health departments of some cities encourage weekly sanitary inspections by members of the food-establishment staff. The staff members do this in rotation, and they are furnished with inspection forms to assist them. Their reports should be scrutinized by the management.

7-20. Instruction of Food Handlers. Food-service personnel are necessarily recruited from a group that has little or no knowledge of sanitation or of methods of disease transmission. At present, food-handler schools are conducted in cities by personnel of some state health departments or by extension services of universities. The courses include lectures, motion pictures, slides, and exhibits. They have been popular and successful. Restaurant owners are requested to allow their employees the necessary time off for attendance, but their cooperation is entirely voluntary.

The National Sanitation Clinic [18] recommends a course of five lessons, each lasting 2 hr, to be held two or three times a week. The course should cover the following main topics: (1) objectives of the course, responsibility of the food handler, and how the food handler may help himself; (2) how to stay well; (3) flies, cockroaches, and rats, and how they spread disease, and garbage and refuse control; (4) foods—their sources, handling, and protection—and food poisoning; (5) cleaning and sanitization, handling and storage of equipment, paper service, and general housekeeping; and (6) employee cleanliness and good working habits.

It has been suggested that additional specialized courses be given to waitresses, dishwashing-machine operators, pasteurization-plant operators, and bakers and other specialized food-handling workers. The Instructor's Guide: Sanitary Food Service, *Public Health Service Publication* 90, presents a comprehensive outline for instructors conducting training classes for food-service personnel. The Baking Industry Standards Committee has also developed some helpful guides.

Where food-handler training programs have been given, the benefits have been striking in terms of improved sanitation, better health of workers, decreased labor turnover, improved morale among workers, increased efficiency in operation and maintenance of establishments, reduced wastage and spoilage of foods, and reduced likelihood of damage claims. It has been suggested that food handlers be given an examination on the subjects mentioned in this article and that they be awarded a certificate if successful.

Meat Inspection

7-21. Meat requires inspection by competent technologists; usually they are veterinarians. Inspections are necessary for several reasons: the rapidity with which meat decomposes; the possibility of the animal's being diseased, particularly with some disorder transmissible to man; and the ease with which the meat may become infected. Meat inspection is performed by the Meat Inspection Division (formerly called the Bureau of Animal Industry) of the U.S. Department of Agriculture and also by inspectors of many of the cities. That this inspection is necessary is indicated by figures that were published by the Bureau of Animal Industry [23]. In nearly 2 per cent of the carcasses inspected, some disease or condition was found which necessitated condemnation of all or part of the meat. The Meat Inspection Division has jurisdiction only over meat that is shipped from state to state and meat that is for export. Animals slaughtered under other conditions receive either no inspection or only that of local health officials.

When it is considered that most of the inspections mentioned above were made at stock centers where range cattle, comparatively free from disease, were handled, it is apparent that the greatest need for meat inspection is in the smaller cities, where killing of local stock is carried on. The poorer grade of animals or those which may be suspected of disease are not taken to slaughterhouses where there is inspection. Furthermore, the uninspected slaughter pen in the country or small town is usually in a most deplorable sanitary condition. It is a place of foul odors and millions of flies, a happy hunting ground for rats and buzzards. The offal is rarely handled properly but is left to decompose in heaps or is sometimes thrown into neighboring streams.

7-22. Inspections. Meat inspection requires the services of a competent veterinarian capable of recognizing pathological conditions. The ante-mortem examination is made whenever possible and is for the purpose of detecting symptoms of disease. Suspicious animals are slaughtered separately. The post-mortem examination is more important and is applied first to certain glands, the heart, and the tongue, and if these are found suspicious the abdominal viscera, the lymph glands, and the sex glands are examined. There are many diseases and conditions for which meat is rejected, of which the following are most common: tuberculosis, anthrax, hog cholera, tapeworm cysts, septic conditions, pneumonia, bruises, and injuries. In many cases only parts of the carcasses are condemned. Tuberculosis of cattle and hogs in the earlier stages is usually confined to certain glands. If there is no evidence that the tubercle bacilli have invaded the bloodstream, only the infected portions are rejected. Only the tissues containing the tapeworm cysts are condemned unless they are very widely distributed and numerous. Knives which have been used to cut animals found to be infected must be disinfected in hot water at 170 to 200°F before being used again. Meat which is passed is stamped at all primal wholesale cuts, 13 places on each half of beef.

It is frequently necessary for one inspector to cover several abattoirs, and it is impossible for him to make ante-mortem inspections. Under these circumstances the viscera are removed from the carcasses, tagged, and held until his arrival. This is not recommended because of the possibility of switching organs and carcasses.

7-23. Abattoirs. The problem of getting good meat other than that which is federally inspected is greatly simplified by having a municipal abattoir at which all killing must be done. This may be required through the passage of an ordinance which provides that all animals be slaughtered and dressed at the abattoir or under equally good conditions. The city meat inspector may be placed in charge of the abattoir. This allows ante-mortem and post-mortem examinations of all animals and, with proper supervision of the abattoir, ensures sanitary handling of the meat, by-products, and offal.

In a few cities the abattoir is municipally owned and operated. If this arrangement cannot be made, it is sometimes possible to organize a stock company of the local butchers for the purpose of building and operating the plant. In either case all animals to be slaughtered are brought to the abattoir, and a fee is charged per animal handled. In large cities there will be one or more privately owned abattoirs at which the city can arrange for inspections to be made. Cold-storage space should be required. In addition to the possibility of effective meat inspection and better sanitation, the large abattoir allows the use of various products which are commonly wasted at the small slaughterhouse. These include the intestines, which are cleaned and used as sausage casings, and the blood and scraps, which are treated to extract grease and tallow, the remainder being dried and pulverized for fertilizer or animal feed. A city of 8,000 population or more can support a municipal abattoir.

7-24. Markets. The inspection of meat markets has much in common with the inspection of other food establishments. The meats should not be kept unwrapped on open counters exposed to flies, dust, and handling by customers. Special attention must be given to the cleanliness of the counters, refrigerators, meat blocks, iron hooks, meat- and sausage-grinding machines, and knives and their handles. If an ordinance requires that all meat be inspected, search should be made for the official marks of approval on all the meat cuts in stock and also on the meat products.

Poultry Inspection and Sanitation

7-25. With the introduction of new methods of processing and merchandising, the consumption of poultry and poultry products has greatly increased in recent years. Poultry and poultry products are responsible for a number of food-borne illnesses including the virus disease known as psittacosis when it occurs among parrots and parakeets and as ornithosis when it occurs in domestic fowls. A number of outbreaks of this disease among poultry-plant workers have been ascribed to turkeys. The increasing interest in poultry sanitation recently exhibited by states and municipalities, and their requests, prompted the Public Health Service, in cooperation with the Public Health Poultry Liaison Committee, to develop a poultry ordinance [24]. It follows the pattern set by the Milk Ordinance and Code, and if it is adopted as readily by cities, it will bring about uniformity of programs and create greater confidence in the safety of the product among the consuming public.

In addition to requiring that all operations, from the live-bird pens to the retail establishments, including processing, packaging, storage, and transportation, be in accordance with good sanitation practice, the ordinance provides for ante-mortem and post-mortem inspection. Some items covered by the ordinance are:

1. A post-mortem inspection of each carcass shall be performed by an inspector at the time of evisceration. . . .

2. No viscera or any part [of it] shall be removed from any dressed poultry except at the time of evisceration and post-mortem inspection.

3. Each carcass shall be opened so as to expose the organs and the body cavity for proper examination by the inspector and, if passed, shall be prepared immediately after inspection as eviscerated poultry.

4. Poultry and poultry products in which there is no evidence of disease or other condition rendering such poultry or poultry products unfit for use as human food, and which comply with all applicable provisions of this Ordinance, shall be passed [and labeled]. . . .

The Poultry Products Inspection Act, passed by Congress, went into effect in 1959. It requires that all poultry and poultry products in interstate commerce be inspected by a qualified inspector of the Poultry Division, Agricultural Marketing Service, U.S. Department of Agriculture. The Act also provides minimum standards for sanitation, operating procedures, and facilities in the processing plants. It also establishes broad requirements for the building and the design and placing of equipment.

7-26. Operating Procedures. Dead birds must be removed from coops and batteries. Feed must be withheld from live poultry for the time necessary to prevent material from the crops from contaminating poultry carcasses during evisceration. If dressed carcasses are vented (*i.e.*, if fecal contents are expelled from the cloaca by pressure on the posterior portion of the abdomen), the venting must be performed under a flow or spray of water in such a manner that the fecal material is washed away without contaminating the carcass. Cropping, if conducted, must be accomplished by forcing the crop contents out through the esophagus and mouth.

Poultry and poultry products must be chilled or frozen immediately after processing and must be maintained in a completely frozen state. The defrosting and refreezing of poultry and poultry products are prohibited.

In order to prevent ornithosis among workers, poultry buyers should inspect flocks and accept no birds from those which have diseased birds, although some diseased birds may appear healthy. When an outbreak occurs, attempts should be made to discover the source of the birds. This is usually possible since the disease outbreaks are generally explosive. Most cases appear among the poultry-plant workers who pluck or eviscerate the birds, especially the former. Preventive measures include wearing of rubber gloves and use of masks, although these give only partial protection. The most effective plant measure is provision of downdraft ventilation, particularly where cyclomatic pluckers are used. Natural draft upward, horizontal and toward doors and windows, conveys infection to the breathing level. The daily cleanups of the plant and equipment must be carefully planned and carried out [25].

Shellfish Sanitation

7-27. Shellfish produced or handled under insanitary conditions may cause typhoid fever, dysentery, gastrointestinal disturbances, and infectious hepatitis. Oysters, clams, and mussels become infected from the water in which they are grown or during the process of handling, shucking, packing, or shipping. The menace of contaminated oysters is increasing with increased pollution of coastal waters, particularly of the bays and estuaries in which the oyster beds are located. As the oyster requires only a moderately saline water, the oyster-producing areas are necessarily near the mouths of rivers. Since many cities are located near river mouths and discharge their sewage untreated, the danger is apparent.

The discussion given here also applies to clams and mussels, which are as dangerous as oysters. Mussels and clams of the entire West Coast and of eastern Canada are dangerous in another way, as indicated in Arts. 7-1 and 7-36.

7-28. Oysters and Water Pollution. A healthy oyster, under optimum conditions, pumps as much as 4 l of water an hour. From the water it extracts its food, and from the water coliforms and possibly typhoid, dysentery, and other pathogenic organisms may also be accumulated, either in its alimentary canal or in the shell liquor. If polluted oysters are placed in clean water, they are cleaned by the passage of the water through them.

The most important factor in the production of oysters is the control of sanitary conditions in the growing and bedding areas. This, aside from reducing the actual pollution by remedial measures, requires location of beds where the pollution hazard is least. To establish safe areas requires exhaustive studies of the sources and amounts of pollution entering rivers above tidewater and of the approximate dilution (Art. 7-30).

7-29. Certification. The certification of oysters, mussels, and all varieties of clams is a cooperative arrangement. Responsibility for formulating and enforcing control measures and for issuing certificates to the shellfish shippers rests upon the health, agricultural, or conservation departments of the states in which the oysters are produced and from which they are shipped to other states. The Public Health Service specifies the minimum requirements for its approval of state certification [26]. It also inspects and rates a representative number of shucking and packing plants annually in the state and cooperates with the states in making sanitary and bacteriological surveys or makes such surveys independently but in agreement with the states. The entire state procedure and machinery for sanitary control of shellfish are examined and rated annually by the Public Health Service. It also publishes and keeps current a list of interstate shippers of shellfish certified by the producing states for the information of health officers and other interested persons in the consuming states.

Shipments of shucked shellfish and shell stock must be properly tagged, with the tags showing the name and address of the consignee and of the shipper, the state of origin, and the certificate number of the shipper.

The health authorities of the states, cities, and countries where the shellfish are consumed should check the sources of all shellfish consumed in areas under their jurisdiction. Sanitarians should be furnished with the lists of approved shippers and, on their visits to restaurants, should make certain that shellfish served have been received from certified shippers. Dealers are required to keep complete records of shipments so that information will be available in case of epidemics.

7-30. Classification of Waters. A sanitary survey must be made of each shellfish-growing area prior to its approval by the state as a source of market shellfish or of shellfish to be used in a controlled purification or relaying operation. The sanitary quality of the area must be reappraised at least biennially, and if necessary, a resurvey is made. The sanitary survey includes an evaluation of the actual or potential sources of pollution; tests for the presence of industrial wastes or radionuclides that would cause a public health hazard; a study of the effects of winds, stream flow, and tidal currents on the distribution of pollution; and bacteriological examination of the growing waters.

There are three classifications of areas in which shellfish are grown: *Approved areas* are those from which shellfish may be taken without serious question as to their safety because of distance from sources of pollution, dilution, and the time factor. The median most probable number (MPN) of coliforms of these waters, as indicated by samples taken at points most likely to be exposed to fecal contamination, should be less than 70 per 100 ml. Also, the waters must not be contaminated with industrial wastes or radionuclides to a hazardous extent. Bacterial reexaminations of the area must be made whenever sanitary surveys (made not less than every 2 years) indicate a change in conditions.

Conditionally approved areas are those in which permission to harvest shellfish is conditional upon the satisfactory operation of sewerage systems, particularly the sewage treatment plants. This requires the establishment of quality standards for treatment-plant effluents and a relationship to operating personnel that will result in the shellfish-control authorities being informed when it is necessary to bypass sewage around the plant, when the plant is inadequate or operational difficulties occur, and when sewage lift stations fail. Other sources of pollution, which may be seasonal or temporary, are increased population such as at a shore resort, sewage discharges from a recreational area, and sewage from merchant or naval vessels. A closed safety area should be interposed between the source of pollution and the conditionally approved area. It is so chosen that the time of travel of pollution through it will be twice the time required for the notification process to become effective. The time the conditionally approved area should be closed following a temporary closure will depend upon the species of shellfish and the condition of the area.

Restricted areas are established where a sanitary survey indicates a limited degree of pollution which would make it unsafe to harvest shellfish for direct marketing. As an alternative, the states may classify such areas as prohibited. A restricted area is one so polluted that direct consumption of shellfish might be hazardous, although it may not be so contaminated by radionuclides or industrial wastes that a hazard would occur. The median MPN of the coliforms must not exceed 700 per 100 ml, and not more than 10 per cent of the samples may exceed 2,300 per 100 ml in those portions of the area most probably exposed to fecal contamination during the most unfavorable hydrographic and pollution conditions. Shellfish from restricted areas are not marketed without controlled purification or relaying.

Prohibited areas are those which a sanitary survey indicates that dangerous numbers of pathogenic microorganisms might reach, or they may be areas dangerously contaminated with radionuclides or industrial wastes. The median MPN of coliforms exceeds 700 per 100 ml, and 10 per cent of the samples have a coliform MPN in excess of 2,300 per 100 ml. Coastal areas which have not been subjected to sanitary surveys are automatically classified as prohibited. The taking of shellfish from prohibited areas for direct marketing is forbidden, and relaying or other salvage operations must be carefully supervised.

Closure of areas where paralytic shellfish poisoning may occur is a responsibility of the state agency. It should regularly collect and assay representative samples of shellfish collected in those areas. If the poison content reaches 80 micrograms per 100 g of the edible raw meat, the area must be closed until the state agency is convinced that the poison content is below the dangerous level. See Art. 7-36.

7-31. Harvesting. Boats used in the taking of shellfish and "buy" boats must be kept in such a state of cleanliness and repair that shellfish are not subject to contamination from bilge water, leakage, or other sources. Decks, holds, bins, etc., used for the storage of shellfish must not be washed with polluted water. If necessary, the oysters must be cleaned of mud and sediment with water equal in quality to that of the growing water. Reasonable precautions must be taken while the boats are over the shellfish grounds to prevent pollution through the discharge of human wastes. Tight containers for human wastes are required for harvesting and "buy" boats, and the wastes must be disposed of in such a manner that they do not endanger the shellfish.

7-32. Preparation of Shellfish for Marketing. This is necessary when shellfish are taken from restricted or prohibited areas. It is done by relaying or controlled purification.

RELAYING. Shellfish from restricted or prohibited areas are relaid only after written permission has been received from the state authority and only when the relaying operations are under direct supervision of the authority. Direct supervision will not be necessary, however, if the relaying is done when shellfish may not be marketed. Relaying is done in *approved* areas, and the shellfish are held there for a time sufficient to allow them to cleanse themselves. This will depend upon the water temperature and salinity, the initial bacteriological quality, and the species of shellfish. The relaid shellfish are not harvested without written permission from the state control agency. The relaying area is located and marked so that relayers will not place contaminated oysters in nearby approved areas. The area must be patrolled during the period when the shellfish are undergoing the cleansing process.

CONTROLLED PURIFICATION. Shellfish from restricted or prohibited areas may be marketed after effective controlled purification, which is permitted only under the immediate supervision of the control agency. Controlled purification may be accomplished in tanks or in natural bodies of water, but in either case the water used must meet the physical and bacteriological requirements of an *approved* growing area, or if it is a treated water, it must comply with the bacteriological limits of the Public Health Service Drinking Water Standards. The shellfish must be freed from contamination and foreign material adhering to shells before purification. The plant operator must possess a satisfactory knowledge of the principles of water treatment and bacteriology. Laboratory control must be exercised over the purification operation, including water quality, and bacteriological quality of each lot of shellfish purified. Shellfish from prohibited areas are not subjected to purification unless the state control agency can show that relaying or depletion is not biologically feasible and that no public health hazard will result from the use of such shellfish. The use of chlorinated or chlorinated-dechlorinated waters for purification of shellfish is not recommended as the chlorine interferes with the water-pumping processes of the shellfish.

Depletion is the removal of all market-sized and as many of the smaller-sized shellfish as may be gathered by reasonable methods from closed areas to clean areas. This is a precaution against the harvesting and sale of contaminated shellfish by unscrupulous or ignorant persons.

7-33. Bacteriological Criteria for Shellfish. Shellfish will generally reflect the bacteriological quality of the water in which they are grown, but this relationship is not sufficiently constant to permit development of a uniform bacteriological standard applicable to all species of shellfish. Oysters *as harvested* from approved areas of the North and Middle Atlantic regions should not ordinarily exceed a coliform MPN of 230 per 100 g of shellfish meats, although a few samples may approach or exceed 2,400 per 100 g. If the latter value is exceeded in two consecutive samples, the state control agency should investigate to determine the probable cause. Oysters harvested from Chesapeake Bay, South Atlantic, or Gulf states, even though these are approved areas, cannot be expected to meet routinely the standard of 230 per 100 g. They should, however, ordinarily have a coliform MPN of less than 2,400 per 100 g, and if this value is exceeded in two consecutive samples the state control agency should investigate. The bacteriological quality of hard clams will be about the same as that of oysters from the New England and Middle Atlantic coasts. There is no information available about clams from other areas. Soft clams, even from approved areas, cannot always meet the limit of the 230 MPN, but if the 2,400 MPN is exceeded the same procedure should be followed as with oysters. The bacteriological quality of mussels in relation to the growing water is similar to that of soft clams. Examination of shellfish follows procedures described by the American Public Health Association [27].

The bacteriological criteria given above apply to shellfish as harvested. They do not apply to shell stock in storage for any length of time or to shucked shellfish. Bacterial contents generally increase during storage and processing.

7-34. Processing of Shellfish. The shellfish are first washed to remove mud or sediment. This is done as soon after harvesting as possible,

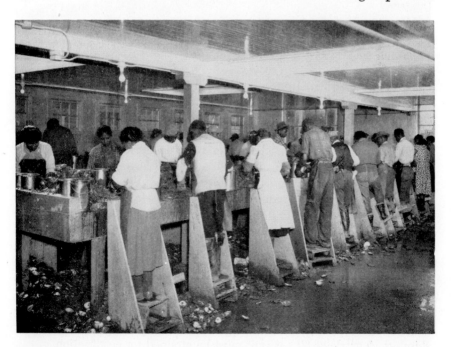

FIGURE 7-5   Shucking oysters. (*Photograph courtesy of Oyster Institute of North America.*)

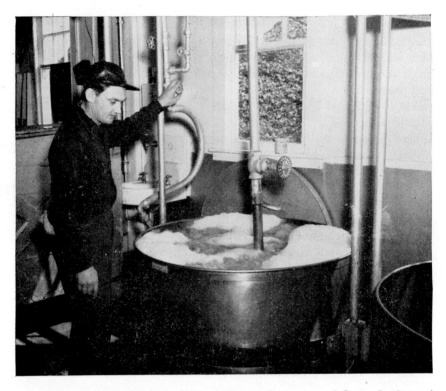

FIGURE 7-6 Washing shucked oysters. (*Photograph courtesy of Oyster Institute of North America.*)

using water obtained from an approved growing area or from another approved source. Wet storage prior to further treatment or shipping is permitted after written approval by the authority. Approval is based upon protection of the storage water from sewage contamination. Dry storage of shell stock must be under conditions that will prevent contamination and allow drainage and cleaning of floors, hoppers, etc.

Requirements concerning building interiors, plumbing, provision of lavatories with hot and cold water and of toilets for workers, cleanliness of workers, and precautions against flies, rodents, and other vermin are the same as for other food-handling operations. Shucking of the shellfish must be done in a room separate from that in which they are packed for shipment. Construction of shucking benches is specified, and also the construction of utensils and equipment must be approved [28]. Utensils must be washed and sanitized within 2 hr after the day's operations have ceased. The Public Health Service has prepared inspection-grading forms for the sanitation of shipping-packing plants and shell-stock shippers. A grade of 80 per cent must be attained for certification.

Shell stock of shellfish species having poor keeping qualities, such as

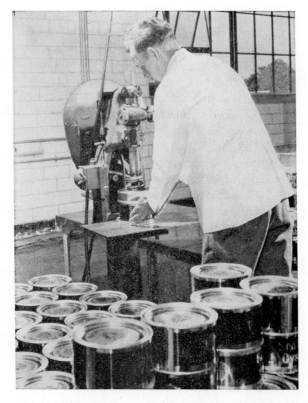

FIGURE 7-7 Oyster meats being packed and sealed.
(*Photograph courtesy of Oyster Institute of North America.*)

mussels and soft-shell clams, must be stored at 50°F or less but not frozen. The shucking of shellfish must be done in such a manner that they will not become contaminated. Water used for washing the shell stock must be from an approved source. The shucked shellfish must not remain on the shucking bench more than 2 hr unless they have an internal temperature of not more than 50°F. Only live shellfish are shucked. If they are not packed for shipment within 1 hr after delivery to the packing room, they must be cooled to 50°F or less within 2 hr. Shucked shellfish must be cooled to 50°F or less within 2 hr after packing. Further cooling to 40°F is recommended. In frozen-storage rooms, a temperature of 0°F or less must be maintained.

Shell stock must be packed and shipped in clean containers bearing a tag or label giving the name and address of the consignee and of the shipper and the kind and quantity of the shell stock. Shucked shellfish must be packed in clean single-service containers made of impervious materials or in clean, properly designed sealed returnable containers.

Each package of fresh or frozen shellfish must have on the package a label giving the packer's, repacker's, or distributor's name and address and the packer's or repacker's certificate number, preceded by the abbreviated name of the state. Frozen shellfish must be kept at temperatures that will prevent thawing during shipment. Unfrozen shucked shellfish must be kept at 50°F or below during shipment.

Shellfish dealers must keep adequate records of persons or firms from whom shellfish were purchased; dates of purchases; areas from which the shellfish were harvested; and names and addresses of persons to whom shellfish were sold Such information will be of value in epidemiological investigations.

7-35. Effect of Cooking. While consumption of raw shellfish is far more dangerous from the standpoint of disease incidence, cooking the shellfish does not always ensure safety. Oyster stews, for example, are sometimes made by bringing the milk to a boil, pouring in the cold oysters, and serving immediately. This is not effective in killing disease organisms. The most satisfactory method is to boil the oysters in their own juice separately, heat the milk separately, and then combine. Frying for 2 min kills most pathogenic organisms, but some may survive for 8 min. Subjecting shucked oysters to live steam for 5 to 10 min, or shell oysters for 10 to 15 min, destroys typhoid organisms. The principal safeguard against contracting disease from shellfish, it will be noted, is control at the source by competent sanitary authorities.

7-36. Poisoning Caused by Shellfish. On the West Coast and in Alaska mussels and clams may be toxic at certain times and cause a paralytic poisoning which has resulted in fatalities. Also, clams and mussels in some areas of the Canadian east coast may be toxic during the colder months. In both the Pacific and the Atlantic, the trouble is caused by a dinoflagellate, a plankton organism on which the shellfish feed. They are likely to be abundant in dangerous numbers at times in certain areas, and they are more likely to be abundant in areas near the open sea. Canadian control measures include the restriction of collection in certain areas at certain times. No commercial fishing is permitted at all in some areas. All commercial fishing is under control, and the output of shucking and canning plants is sampled before it may be sold. Cooking cannot be depended upon to destroy the poison, although commercial canning usually reduces it below dangerous levels.

Bibliography

1. "Federal Food, Drug and Cosmetic Act and General Regulations for Its Enforcement," U.S. Food, Drug and Cosmetic Series, no. 1, rev. 4, June, 1953.
2. Kagan, I. G.: Trichinosis in the United States, *Public Health Rept.*, vol. 74, p. 159, 1959.

3. Report of Committee on Environmental Health Problems—Milk and Foods, *Public Health Service Pub.* 908, 1962.

4. Dauer, C. C., and J. J. Davids: Summary of Disease Outbreaks, 1958, *Public Health Rept.*, vol. 74, p. 715, 1959.

5. "Control of Communicable Disease in Man," 9th ed., Report of the American Public Health Association, New York, 1960.

6. Jay, J. M.: Further Studies on Staphylococci in Meats, *Appl. Microbiol.*, vol. 10, no. 3, May, 1962.

7. Dack, G. M.: "Food Poisoning," The University of Chicago Press, Chicago, 1956.

8. Mason, J. O., and W. R. McLean: Infectious Hepatitis Traced to the Consumption of Bay Oysters, *Am. J. Hyg.*, vol. 75, January, 1962.

9. Rindge, M. E.: Infectious Hepatitis in Connecticut, *Conn. Health Bull.*, vol. 76, May, 1962.

10. Man and His Environment, *Proc. Second National Congress on Environmental Health*, School of Public Health, University of Michigan, Ann Arbor, Mich., 1961.

11. Food Service Sanitation Manual, Including a Model Ordinance and Code, *Public Health Service Pub.* 934, 1962.

12. Bell, J. W.: The Protective Screening Program for Canned Foods, *J. Milk Food Technol.*, vol. 25, no. 6, June, 1962.

13. "Canned Food Reference Manual," American Can Company, New York.

14. "Conference on Frozen Food Quality," Western Regional Research Laboratory, U.S. Department of Agriculture, Albany, Calif., 1960.

15. Sawyer, F. M., *et al.*: "Handling and Merchandising of Frozen Food," Cooperative Extension Service, University of Massachusetts, Amherst, Mass., 1960.

16. "Spray-type Dishwashing Machines," University of Michigan, School of Public Health, National Sanitation Foundation, Ann Arbor, Mich.

17. Mallmann, W. L., *et al.*: "A Study of Mechanical Dishwashing," University of Michigan, School of Public Health, National Sanitation Foundation, Ann Arbor, Mich.

18. "The First National Sanitation Clinic," University of Michigan, School of Public Health, National Sanitation Foundation, Ann Arbor, Mich.

19. Hartley, D. E.: Vending Sanitation, *Sanitation and Building Maintenance*, July, 1960.

20. Sanitation Ordinance and Code: Vending of Foods and Beverages, *Public Health Service Pub.* 546, 1957.

21. "Vending Machine Evaluation Manual," National Automatic Merchandising Association, Chicago.

22. Mallmann, W. L.: Sanitation in Bulk Food Vending, *J. Milk Food Technol.*, vol. 16, no. 6, November–December, 1953.

23. Melvin, A. D.: State and Municipal Inspection and Municipal Slaughter Houses, *U.S. Bur. Animal Ind. Circ.* 185.

24. Poultry Ordinance, *Public Health Service Pub.* 444, 1955, and Supplement 1, 1960.

25. Schulz, R.: "Planned Sanitation in the Poultry Industry," The Sanitarian's Desk Reference, The National Association of Sanitarians, University of Denver, Denver, Colo.

26. Cooperative Program for the Certification of Interstate Shellfish Shippers. Pt. I, Sanitation of Shellfish Growing Areas. Pt. II, Sanitation of the Harvesting and Processing of Shellfish, *Public Health Service Pub.* 33, rev. 1962.

27. "Recommended Procedures for Bacteriological Examination of Sea Water and Shellfish," 3d ed. American Public Health Association, New York, 1962.

28. Shellfish Industry Equipment Construction Guides, *Public Health Service Pub.* 943, 1962.

29. Schwartz, B.: "Trichinosis in the United States," First International Conference on Trichinellosis, Warsaw, 1960.

30. "Procedure for the Investigation of Foodborne Disease Outbreaks," International Association of Milk and Food Sanitarians, Shelbyville, Ind., 1957.

31. "Manual of Sanitation Standards for Certain Products of Paper, Paper Board, or Molded Pulp," Microbiological and Biochemical Center, Syracuse University, Syracuse, N.Y., 1963.

8

DISINFECTANTS AND INSECTICIDES

8-1. There is considerable popular confusion about the meaning of the terms used in connection with disinfectants and allied agents. *Disinfection* is the killing or removal of those agents which cause infection. For instance, *pasteurization* is a certain means of killing typhoid and other disease bacteria; it is therefore a means of disinfection, but it does not destroy all the spores of other bacteria. *Sanitizing* is the cleaning and disinfecting of surfaces of food utensils, etc., so that they do not present a health hazard. *Sterilization* is the destruction of absolutely all life. A *germicide* is an agent which kills bacteria. A *bacteriostat* retards or inhibits the growth of bacteria. A *disinfectant* is therefore a germicide. *Antiseptics* are not germicides but are merely agents that retard the growth or multiplication of bacteria. An antiseptic, therefore, will prevent or delay decay. Many disinfectants are deodorants also, but many deodorants have no effect upon germ life and merely mask one odor with another more powerful one. The distinction between disinfectants and antiseptics is sometimes one of degree. A highly concentrated solution, for instance, will have disinfectant properties, while weaker concentrations are merely antiseptic. Insecticides are not, in general, good germicides.

8-2. Disinfection. The disinfection of water and foods has been discussed elsewhere. Here disinfection will be treated mainly as it is used in the control and prevention of communicable disease. A disinfectant should be used as a bar between the patient and the people about him. Disinfection should be applied, therefore, as closely as possible to the patient. It is frequently used to treat the excretions and discharges of the patient and also fomites, the various objects with which the sick person comes in contact, such as clothing, bedding, handkerchiefs, and eating utensils. It is by means of the discharges and the fomites, particularly the former, that diseases are frequently communicated, although direct contact may also be involved. Concurrent disinfection is the practice of treating all excreta as they are produced and fomites as they leave or sever contact with the patient during the course of the illness. Terminal disinfection is the final treatment given, after the patient is cured or removed, to bedding, fomites, and perhaps to the room which the patient has occupied. Terminal disinfection may also include fumigation.

8-3. Fumigation. Fumigation is the application of disinfectants in gaseous form, although the meaning of the term has been extended to include use of gas as an insecticide. While many cities as a routine measure formerly practiced fumigation at the termination of certain communicable diseases, such as measles, scarlet fever, and smallpox, this practice has been abandoned by health authorities. Observations made as to the number of new cases, in the same house, following a communicable disease indicate that fumigation has but little effect. Also, the greatest danger of communication to others is generally during the early stages of the disease, long before fumigation is applied. Concurrent disinfection, terminal disinfection of fomites, and a thorough cleaning of the room appear to be more effective. In any event, fumigation affects surfaces only and will not exercise any germicidal effect within fabrics. Fumigation has a recognized field, however, in the killing of insects, rats, and mice in buildings, ships, and railroad cars. The agents used in fumigation for this purpose, however, are of little or no value as germicides.

Physical Agents of Disinfection

8-4. Heat. *Fire* is the best sterilizing agent. In the control of communicable disease it can be applied only to those articles which may be destroyed, such as bandages and dressings of various sorts and old bedding. Sputum should be collected in paper cups and burned.

Steam is widely used as a disinfectant. For surface disinfection it can be applied as streaming steam, in which case the steam is not under pressure, and a contact period of 30 to 40 min is required. If the steam is generated in a closed tank or vessel and the articles placed therein are to be disinfected under pressure, a 20-min contact period will be required at 16 psi, and a 15-min contact period at 20 psi. The latter method allows better penetration of the steam, particularly if a partial vacuum is obtained before the steam is generated. Large steam sterilizers are used in hospitals, bacteriological laboratories, and dairies.

Boiling will kill pathogenic organisms in a few seconds, but for sterilization, which includes destruction of spores, 20 min may be required. Boiling can be used to disinfect clothing and excreta. Temperatures lower than boiling are also destructive to bacteria, particularly pathogenic bacteria, if continued long enough. This principle is illustrated by the pasteurization of milk.

Dry heat is also used to disinfect but does not penetrate so well as steam and may injure fabrics. It is much less effective than wet heat. For instance, dry heat at 300°F requires three to four times as long as boiling to destroy bacteria. Disinfection with dry heat may be carried out in an ordinary oven. As a rough test, the oven should be hot enough to brown ordinary absorbent cotton.

Cold is not a disinfectant, or at best it acts too slowly to be so considered. It does, however, prevent the multiplication of bacteria. On the other hand, some types of pathogenic bacteria, particularly typhoid, may be preserved for 3 months or more by freezing.

Dryness is injurious to bacteria. The desiccation of substances containing bacteria will in time cause their death. Clean dry surfaces contain very few live bacteria. Dryness is even more effective in preventing the multiplication of bacteria.

8-5. Light. Sunlight is a disinfectant. The rays toward the violet end of the spectrum have the greatest germicidal power, the ultraviolet rays being particularly destructive. For disinfecting purposes, floors, carpets, etc., may be exposed to sunlight. As the ultraviolet rays cannot pass through ordinary glass, it is preferable that objects to be disinfected be exposed to the direct sunlight.

The Chemical Agents of Disinfection

8-6. General Characteristics. Disinfectants vary in qualities which must be considered when choosing the proper agent for some particular purpose. The faculty of penetration is important as bacteria, particularly in sputum and feces, are embedded in organic matter. The disinfectant, to do its work, must be able to penetrate this material. For this purpose chemical agents in the form of solutions are better than emulsions, although steam, dry heat, and boiling may also be used. Gases have a surface action only, although they will, of course, penetrate porous materials, such as fabrics. The presence of organic matter with the bacteria affects disinfection, particularly of sputum and feces, since those disinfectants which are oxidizing agents react chemically with the organic matter and speedily become ineffective as disinfectants. Formaldehyde is well suited for conditions of this type, although it does have objectionable properties from the standpoints of odor, irritability, and corrosiveness. Phenol, although widely used in the past, has largely been supplanted by more potent disinfectants, such as the chlorophenols and quaternary ammonium compounds, which are less corrosive and irritating. It is necessary that sufficient time be allowed for the disinfectant to make contact. In general, the weaker solutions or dilutions of disinfectants require longer periods to do their work. Raising the temperature of the dilutions materially speeds up the action.

8-7. Phenol Coefficient. As a means of standardizing the killing power of disinfectants, the phenol coefficient has been devised. This is the killing power of the disinfectant in question standardized against the killing power of phenol, typhoid bacilli being used as the organisms to be killed. Although the Rideal-Walker and the Hygienic Laboratory methods were formerly used, the method advocated by the Association of Official Agricultural Chemists is now generally accepted for determining the strength of disinfectant solutions. Disinfectants should be purchased only from reputable manufacturers under a guarantee as to the phenol coefficient. If large quantities are used, a test of the coefficient should be made by a qualified laboratory.

8-8. Lime. This is the cheapest of all disinfectants. It also has the advantages of being odorless and safe to use. Hydrated lime, which may be purchased in sacks, is the most convenient. When mixed with eight to ten times its weight or four times its volume of water, milk of lime is obtained. This is very useful in the disinfection of feces. At least the same bulk of milk of lime as feces should be used. Milk of lime is also used as whitewash in dairy barns, where it is said to kill spores and sporeformers lodged in cracks. Lime is also a deodorant. When air-slaked, it is of no value. The indiscriminate scattering about of dry lime in open toilets, barns, etc., is of little or no use.

8-9. Chlorine. Chlorine is one of the most important bactericides in the field of sanitation. Its principal uses in its various forms in the sanitary field are for disinfecting drinking water, swimming-pool water, sewage, hands of milkers, udders of cows, and glasses, dishes, and other utensils used in handling, preparing, and serving milk and other foods. Its application and the forms in which it is used are given in Art. 2-18.

8-10. Quaternary Ammonium Compounds. These compounds are on sale as sanitizing agents for dishes, glassware, and other food utensils.

Research and field studies have indicated that some of these compounds are effective bactericides for the treatment of various utensils and food-processing equipment. The bactericidal effectiveness of specific quaternary ammonium compounds varies and is influenced by the concentration of active agent, temperature, pH, and exposure time, as well as by interfering substances present in natural waters. The interference of natural waters with quaternary ammonium compounds is due principally to bicarbonates, sulfates, and chlorides of calcium and magnesium. Any treatment which tends to precipitate, remove, or inactivate calcium or magnesium reduces the interference, as do increased pH and temperature.

Not all quaternary ammonium compounds remain bactericidally effective through a wide range of water hardness. The value of sequestering agents in reducing the interference of hard waters has been demonstrated. Products containing alkyl (C_8–C_{18}) dimethylbenzyl ammonium chlorides, paradiisobutylphenoxyethoxyethyldimethylbenzyl ammonium chloride, alkyl (C_9–C_{15}) tolylmethyltrimethyl ammonium chlorides, or didodecenyldimethyl ammonium chloride have been found to be bactericidally effective in waters containing up to 500 ppm of hardness when compounded with sufficient tetrasodium pyrophosphate to provide 0.2 per cent concentration in the solution used and when used (1) at concentrations of 200 ppm or more, (2) at pH levels of 6.0 or higher, (3) at temperatures of 75°F or higher, and (4) for a 2-min exposure period.

The above-named compounds without sequestering agents are also effective within certain limits of water hardness under the conditions of use enumerated above; however, the level of hardness at which bactericidal activity is reduced below that necessary for effective treatment varies among the four named compounds and may be influenced by other ingredients in a proprietary formulation. Accordingly, the limiting hardness should be established for the use of each quaternary ammonium product. Unless it is stated on the label, the health officer should request such information from the manufacturer.

Until such time as a reliable chemical test is developed which will indicate the bactericidal efficiency of quaternary ammonium compounds, bacteriological data should be used to establish the usefulness of quaternary ammonium compounds and sequestering agents other than those named above or to establish the use of the above-named compounds (1) at temperatures less than 75°F, (2) at a pH below 6.0, (3) when combined with a compatible sequestering agent in waters above 500 ppm of hardness, or (4) without, or with less than, the specified amount of sequestering agent [1].

8-11. Carbolic Acid. This is a term applied to a crude mixture of phenols and cresols which is obtained from coal tar. It has a higher phenol coefficient than phenol alone—usually about 2.75. It is used in solutions of 2 to 5 per cent. It cannot be depended upon to destroy spores. With the exceptions of anthrax and tetanus, however, the germs of most communicable diseases are not sporeformers. Carbolic acid is more effective if the solution is warm or hot. This disinfectant and the closely allied substances phenol and cresol are poisonous and cannot be used in relation to foods or eating utensils.

8-12. Phenol. This is a crystalline substance which is soluble in water and is the chief constituent of carbolic acid. It is affected very little by organic matter and is, therefore, useful in disinfecting sputum and feces. It has little effect upon spores.

8-13. Cresol. This term includes a large group of disinfectants which are sold under various trade names. They are mixtures of phenols and cresols with inert tar oils and an emulsifying agent such as soap, tar, or rosin. They have a characteristic carbolic-acid odor. They can be obtained with phenol coefficients up to 6 without organic matter and between 3 and 4 with organic matter. The emulsifying appears to lower their penetrating abilities, and this results in a loss of efficiency in the presence of the organic matter in which bacteria are frequently buried. The soapy emulsion, however, makes this type of disinfectant especially effective on greasy surfaces.

8-14. Formaldehyde. This gas has very little insecticidal value but is very toxic to bacteria. It also acts as a deodorant. Although irritating to the eyes and nasal passages, it is not poisonous. As it is not very efficient in penetrating fabrics, it cannot be depended upon to accomplish more than a surface disinfection. Though fairly effective in the destruction of spores, it should not be relied upon to kill the spores of anthrax or tetanus.

Formalin is a watery solution of formaldehyde containing about 40 per cent of the gas. Formalin is widely used as a disinfectant and is especially valuable for the treatment of body discharges. For fumigation with formaldehyde, the gas is generated from formalin. The usual method of generation is by the aid of potassium permanganate. For every 1,000 cu ft of air space in the room to be fumigated, 50 ml of formalin is required. To this is added 250 g of permanganate. The permanganate is first placed in a deep pan or bucket, and the formalin is poured over it. The chemical reaction which takes place results in the release of formaldehyde gas. Since there is heating and bubbling in the container, it must be deep enough to prevent boiling over, and the floor should be protected by setting the container on a board or bricks. A 6- to 12-hr contact period is required. Fumigating chemicals can be obtained commercially, conveniently arranged for use. Fumigation with formaldehyde is not very efficient at temperatures lower than 60°F.

Disinfection may also be carried out by spraying the formalin on such articles as books or into closets, drawers, etc. Fumigation of small rooms may be accomplished by spraying bed sheets and hanging them up to give off the gas. The ordinary bed sheet will hold 8 oz of formalin without dripping, and this will be sufficient for 1,000 cu ft of air space. The room should be kept closed for 8 hr.

8-15. Ethylene Oxide. This gas is coming into use as a sterilizing agent in hospitals [1]. It is highly effective against all types of organisms, is penetrative, and can be used on objects that would be damaged by heat or moisture. Its disadvantages are that it is toxic by inhalation and skin contact, it requires expensive equipment and a long exposure time, and sterilized objects require time for absorbed gas to dissipate. The gas itself is highly flammable, and it is made safe by the addition of an inactive gas, such as carbon dioxide, Freon, or nitrogen.

8-16. Bichloride of Mercury. This chemical, known as corrosive sublimate, is a powerful bacteriostat, but it has the disadvantage of corroding metals. Also, it is very poisonous. If solutions are made up for use, they should be colored so that there will be no danger of mistaking their identity. The tinting may be done with a few crystals of potassium permanganate or with ordinary household bluing. Bichloride of mercury loses some of its disinfecting power if in contact with albuminous matter, and it is not particularly suitable for feces. It is generally used in 1:500 and 1:1,000 solutions. In the former strength it will kill spores after an exposure of 1 hr. The effectiveness and speed of action of this disinfectant are greatly increased by the use of warm solutions.

8-17. Other Disinfectants. *Alcohol* is both an antiseptic and a germicide. It is effective as a germicide in solutions of 50 to 70 per cent. It has the peculiar faculty of being ineffective if the alcohol is absolute, that is, if no water is present. The reason for this is that the alcohol has no effect upon dry bacteria. The water in the solution, therefore, is needed to moisten the bacteria so that the alcohol can destroy them.

Pine oil is a clear, dark, reddish-brown liquid obtained as a by-product in the turpentine industry. Most pine-odor disinfectants are compositions containing 60 to 80 per cent pine oil and about 10 per cent soap, with the balance water. Pine-type disinfectants are also on the market. Unless they contain some other germicidal ingredient, pine-oil disinfectants are not effective against gram-positive organisms.

Many other acids in addition to carbolic may be used as disinfectants if in sufficient concentration. *Sulfuric acid* in a 1:1,000 solution kills typhoid bacilli in 1 hr. *Hydrochloric acid* is weaker, although a 4 per cent solution of normal acid is antiseptic and will kill many bacteria. *Acetic, citric, formic,* and *salicylic acids* are considerably weaker. *Boric acid* in a 2 per cent solution is a germicide to the less resistant bacteria and antiseptic to others. Salicylic and boric acids are used illegally as food preservatives.

Iodine is generally used in a 2½ per cent solution in 70 per cent alcohol. It is used as a skin disinfectant and in surgery. It may also be used to disinfect water (Art. 2-40).

Potassium permanganate is an effective germicide but is an extremely active oxidizing agent and, therefore, quickly loses its value against bacteria when in the presence of organic matter. This chemical has also been used to disinfect water.

8-18. Detergents. Detergents, including soap, are not disinfectants except as they may act mechanically to remove bacteria along with dirt. A detergent is a *surface-active agent,* that is, a compound that affects the face layer of one surface in contact with another. The surfaces affected may be air and water, oil and water, glass or metal and water, or any surface between two substances. If a surface-active agent combines wetting, dispersing, and emulsifying, it is a cleanser and is called a detergent. A good detergent [3] should (1) be soluble to some extent; (2) permit penetration of the water solution into capillaries by lowering interfacial tension, *i.e.,* permit wetting; (3) disperse or break up particles which have gathered together; and (4) link, by emulsifying, the dirt or grease particles with the water rather than with each other or with the substance to be cleaned.

Soap, which is a chemical combination of a fatty acid and an alkali, is a wetting, dispersing, and emulsifying agent and therefore a surface-active agent and a detergent. Soap acts well only in waters of over pH 10. This means that extra soap must be used to raise the wash water to this high alkalinity. Soap is also a softening agent; *i.e.,* it will combine with the hardness-producing compounds in the water—the carbonates, bicarbonates, and sulfates of calcium and magnesium—to form insoluble compounds. The softening is accomplished before the detergent action takes place. This means a wastage of soap and also the presence of undesirable insoluble compounds in the wash water. Therefore soap is limited in its desirability for household use and for some industrial purposes where wetting and emulsifying action are required.

Other surface-acting agents are synthetic, consisting of manufactured compounds not readily found in nature. A synthetic may accomplish any one of the three actions mentioned above, or it may accomplish all, in which case it is a synthetic detergent.

Synthetic detergents were devised (1) to be effective in neutral or acid solutions, (2) to be effective in hard waters without softening, and (3) to be effective without forming insoluble magnesium or calcium compounds in hard water. Several groups of synthetic detergents are available, including the quaternary ammonium compounds when combined with an alkali. This, as indicated in Art. 8-10, is a combined detergent and disinfectant.

In general the detergent ability of the various groups of agents, including soap, varies not only between groups but also among the individuals of a group according to the dirt to be removed—soil, rust, oil, fat, or soot—and also with the surface to be cleaned—crockery, metal, paint, enamel, skin, cotton, wool, or nylon. The effect of the water characteristics has already been mentioned. Commercial brands of synthetic detergents are built up by the addition of such neutral salts as sodium or calcium chloride to increase detergency properties. Others are mixtures of compounds of the same general type to broaden the range of applicability. Still others contain sequestering agents that will prevent formation of sticky curd in hard water. These are pyrophosphates, tetraphosphates, and hexaphosphates. The buyer must either depend upon the statement of the manufacturer as to the applicability of a particular detergent or learn by trial whether it is the kind best suited to his purposes and the water he uses.

8-19. Methods of Disinfection. In addition to the disinfection of water, milk, and food utensils, which is discussed elsewhere, the usual fields for disinfection in public health work involve urine, feces, sputum, body and bed linen, and bedrooms. At least 2 hr of contact should be provided for all disinfectants. The disinfection of feces is of great importance, particularly in the case of diseases of the intestinal tract. The discharges should be caught in an impervious vessel and immediately treated with the disinfectant. If the feces are in masses, a small stick should be used to break them up and to mix in and incorporate the disinfectant thoroughly. During the period of contact the vessel must be covered to prevent access of flies. Lime is an excellent agent for this purpose. A cupful of hydrated lime is sufficient for one bowel movement. Lime and excreta should then be covered with hot water. The small stick used for mixing may be left in the vessel. If milk of lime is used, at least enough should be added to equal in volume the matter to be disinfected. A 10 per cent solution of formalin is frequently used and is also excellent as a deodorant. A 5 per cent solution of carbolic acid will be effective. Emulsified disinfectant should not be used for feces or sputum.

Sputum is a medium for spreading many of the common communicable diseases, including tuberculosis, the common cold, chicken pox, pneumonia, whooping cough, diphtheria, etc. This matter, therefore, must be carefully disinfected. So far as possible it should be caught in paper cups or gauze cloths and burned. Handkerchiefs so soiled should be soaked for 1 hr in 5 per cent bichloride of mercury before laundering. If the sputum is caught in cups which cannot be destroyed, the cups may first be partially filled with a solution of carbolic acid or phenol. The practice of partially filling cuspidors in public places with disinfectants is a good one. A 5 per cent solution of carbolic acid is the usual disinfectant for this purpose, although pine oil of equal strength has a pleasanter odor.

Sickroom attendants should disinfect their hands after handling patients and soiled clothing. This can be accomplished by wetting the hands with a 70 per cent solution of alcohol.

Bed and body linen, including napkins, towels, sheets, pillow covers, and underwear, may be steamed, boiled, or soaked for 1 hr in a 5 per cent carbolic solution, 10 per cent formalin, or 1:1,000 bichloride of mercury before laundering.

Dead bodies are not likely to disseminate disease. The possibility of spreading of infection may be prevented, however, by wrapping the bodies in a sheet soaked in 1:500 bichloride of mercury solution or 5 per cent carbolic acid until disposed of, or the skin surface may be washed with 10 per cent formalin. With modern methods of burial it is not likely that bodies will be sources of danger.

8-20. Disinfection of Rooms. At the beginning of the sickness all unnecessary objects should be removed from the sickroom. During the period of illness, cleaning should be accomplished by scrubbing and other dustless methods as far as possible. Dusting should be done with a dampened cloth. If the walls have been soiled, painting or repapering may be advisable. This procedure, together with complete airing and as much sunlight as possible, may be applied to replace the old-fashioned fumigation.

Insecticides

8-21. The effectiveness of insecticides for public health usage depends upon a variety of factors which should be considered as they apply to local conditions. It has been demonstrated that such related factors as the adequacy of application procedures, the formulations used, the types of surfaces treated, the local atmospheric conditions, the extent of the insect infestation and breeding potential, and the level of resistance to chemicals in the insect population can affect the results obtained by an insecticide.

Cost is often an important consideration in the choice of an insecticide for a particular usage. The high cost of the trial-and-error method of selecting an effective economic poison may be reduced by critical analysis of the history of insecticides previously used in the area and by simplified field tests for resistance in the insect population coupled with careful field observations.

8-22. Insecticide Formulations. New pesticides for the control of insects and rodents of public health importance continue to be introduced quite frequently. Insecticides are usually commercially available in one or more of the forms in which they are used in public health activities— technical-grade material, dusts, wettable powders, emulsifiable concentrates, solutions, and aerosol preparations.

Technical-grade insecticide is the raw product used in preparing such formulations as emulsions, dusts, solutions, etc., and is not ordinarily chemically pure. Technical-grade DDT, for example, contains approximately only 70 per cent of the isomer effective against insects of public health significance. The material, however, is considered 100 per cent DDT when making up solutions, emulsions, or dusts.

Insecticidal dusts are prepared by grinding toxic ingredients, such as DDT or benzene hexachloride, in inert carriers like talc or pyrophyllite. Dusts are marketed in the concentrations required for field use since the inert and toxic materials must be blended together during the grinding process.

Wettable powders consist of a blend of inert dust and a toxic ingredient, such as DDT or chlordane, to which a suitable wetting agent, such as sodium lauryl sulfate, has been added. Wettable powders are added to water to form suspensions, which require continuous agitation to prevent settling of the considerable amount of inert material present. Suspensions are most often used in spraying such places as stables and other outbuildings when the residue is not objectionable.

Insecticidal solutions are marketed both as concentrates and as finished sprays. Concentrated solutions usually contain the toxic ingredients and a solvent. Concentrated solutions must be diluted for field use with kerosene or similar mineral oils; for example, 40 per cent chlordane concentrate is diluted to 2.5 to 5 per cent, a finished spray, before use. Finished-spray solutions are concentrations suitable for immediate use. Solutions are not emulsifiable or soluble in water.

Emulsifiable concentrates are concentrated solutions to which an emulsifier has been added. When the concentrate is mixed with water, the emulsifying agent forms a very thin coating on each individual droplet of the solvent containing the insecticide, thus preventing separation from the water carrier. A finished *emulsion* is made by diluting a concentrate with sufficient water to form a concentration suitable for immediate use—for example, 5 per cent DDT emulsion.

Aerosol formulations are commercially available in convenient containers (the so-called "aerosol bomb") for producing a fine fog to control flying insects in an enclosed space, such as the home. Typical formulations contain 0.1 to 0.6 per cent pyrethrins, allethrin, or lethane; a synergist such as piperonyl butoxide; 1.0 to 2.0 per cent DDT or methoxychlor; 10 to 12 per cent petroleum distillates; and 85 per cent propellants such as Freon 11 and Freon 12. For control of insects in large buildings or outdoor areas such as picnic grounds or drive-in theatres, there have been developed several types of equipment which disperse insecticides in the particle-size range of 1 to 50 μ and which are generally classified as aerosols.

Synergists are agents added to insecticides to increase their efficiency. Piperonyl butoxide is much used for this purpose.

8-23. Types of Insecticides. Some insecticides are fumigants, such as hydrogen cyanide, methyl bromide, sulfur dioxide, and chloropicrin.

Some are stomach poisons, such as arsenic compounds, which include paris green. Others are contact poisons and are applied directly to the bodies of the insects, to the surfaces with which they will come in contact, or to the air as fogs or mists, which will also provide body contact. Some insecticides combine stomach, contact, and fumigant action.

Insecticides include natural organics, and some of these have been synthesized, such as the chlorinated hydrocarbons, the organic phosphates, the organic thiocyanates, and the organic sulfur group. The development of resistance in insects to certain insecticides may require change from one type to another. Only poisons commonly used in public health work will be discussed here.

Choice of insecticides will depend upon their cost, efficiency, and toxicity to man and warm-blooded animals. Some should not be used around human foods or where animal foods will be contaminated. Some are unsuitable for use in homes or in confined spaces.

Federal regulations require that insecticides be labeled as to their contents and precautions necessary in their use. Manufacturers are prepared to give the concentrations of their products that will be efficient as dusts, emulsions, suspensions, or solutions. Chapter 9 gives formulations and concentrations used for specific purposes.

8-24. Natural Organic Insecticides. Pyrethrum is a powder made from the flower heads of certain daisies, principally types of chrysanthemums. Extracts known as pyrethrins are made for use in the insecticides, although the ground-up flower heads can be used as an insecticidal dust. Pyrethrum is so low in toxicity to humans that it can safely be used in milk rooms and pasteurization plants. It is often mixed with other insecticides in contact or space sprays since it results in a quick knockdown; the other insecticides then complete the killing.

Allethrin is a synthesized compound similar to the pyrethrins. It is also a very safe insecticide. Flies and mosquitoes have not developed resistance to allethrin or pyrethrum in the field.

8-25. Chlorinated Hydrocarbons. The *DDT series* includes a number of insecticides, of which those most used in public health work are DDT, DDD (or TDE), methoxychlor, DMC, and Dilan. Of these, DDT is the most widely used and is the insecticide of choice for the control of flies, mosquitoes, bedbugs, lice, and fleas because of its low cost, lasting power, and safety in use.

DDT is stored in the fat of animals and may appear in milk. It is therefore not used around dairies. Methoxychlor does not have this characteristic and, if permitted by health authorities, may be used, as a dry dust only, to control barn flies, ticks, and lice on cattle. It should not be used less than 5 hr before milking. In its various formulations it is frequently used in a 5 per cent concentration.

The *benzene hexachloride series* includes two important insecticides, benzene hexachloride (BHC) and lindane. BHC has a number of known isomers, of which only one, the gamma isomer, is effectively insecticidal. The technical grade contains 10 to 90 per cent of the gamma isomer. It is more volatile than DDT and thus has a shorter residual life, 2 to 6 weeks. It has been much used in mosquito control. As a larvicide it is less toxic to fish than DDT. It has an objectionable odor. It is frequently used in 5 per cent concentration.

Lindane contains 99.5 per cent of the gamma isomer of BHC. In large doses it is toxic to mammals, but it is rapidly excreted by the kidneys. Lindane is rather expensive. It is more toxic than DDT to most insects and is effective against a wide variety of pests, including cockroaches, bedbugs, fleas, and ticks in homes. It acts as a contact poison, stomach poison, and fumigant. Its residual action is short, and some insects, notably the housefly, have become resistant. A 2 per cent concentration of lindane is as effective as a 5 per cent concentration of DDT. Use of lindane vaporizers to control household pests is not recommended by any agency of the Federal government.

The *chlordane series* includes chlordane, heptachlor, aldrin, dieldrin, endrin, isodrin, toxaphene, and others. Some of these insecticides have killed fish, birds, mammals, and even human beings, through accidents in handling the emulsifiable concentrates. Manufacturers' directions, therefore, should be carefully followed in their use.

Chlordane was formerly much used for controlling cockroaches, ants, and termites, but the German cockroach has developed resistance, and other insecticides, particularly the organophosphorus types, are now preferred. It is used as a 5 per cent emulsion or solution for residual spraying and as a 2.5 per cent emulsion in exterior space sprays. Heptachlor is four to five times as toxic to many insects as chlordane. Since it is also more toxic to humans, it is mostly used outdoors. It is an effective, inexpensive agent as a mosquito larvicide. Dieldrin is more toxic than DDT. It is readily absorbed through the skin, and spray men using it should be especially careful. It has been much used in malaria-control work and for outdoor control of houseflies resistant to DDT. However, they soon develop resistance to dieldrin also. It is used in 1.25 per cent concentrations as a residual spray. It has been used as a residual spray to kill the *Triatoma* bugs, which carry Chagas' disease. Aldrin has been used in termite control, but it and the other insecticides in this group are used mostly for agricultural pests.

8-26. The Organic Phosphorus Insecticides. These are also called organophosphorus compounds. Their toxicity to man differs widely. TEPP, phosdrin, and parathion are highly toxic and should only be used by skilled personnel. DDVP, Bayer 29493, Baytex, and Diazinon are moderately toxic. Dipterex, malathion, and ronnel are only slightly toxic. Some are approved for use in dairy barns (Table 9-4). They are useful where insects have developed resistance to the chlorinated hydrocarbons.

Malathion is widely used as mists, fogs, and residual sprays for mosquitoes, flies, and fleas. As a mosquito larvicide it is recommended for crop areas or where cattle pasture. It has a disagreeable odor, which is masked in formulations used in houses. It is used in spot treatments in buildings against German cockroaches resistant to the chlorinated hydrocarbons. Some mosquitoes are reported as having developed resistance to malathion. It is used in 5 per cent sprays for residual treatments and in concentrations up to 6.5 per cent for fogs and mists.

Ronnel is considered one of the safest insecticides, and it does not have the disagreeable odor of malathion. One and two per cent sprays of ronnel are used for control of flies, cockroaches, and bedbugs. Dipterex is used against cockroaches and flies combined with sugar baits, dry or liquid.

DDVP has a short residual life but quickly produces vapors toxic to insects. It also adds a quick knockdown effect to other insecticides. It is considered promising as a residual fumigant for malaria control in occupied buildings.

Diazinon is used for fly control in food-processing plants in a 1 per cent concentration and, with sugar, as residual bait sprays in a 2.5 per cent concentration. These will give effective control for a month or more. Diazinon is considered valuable for control of German cockroaches that are resistant to chlorinated hydrocarbons and malathion.

8-27. Organic Thiocyanates. These compounds provide a rapid knockdown and are much used in combination with other insecticides. Some, however, are used alone in airplane applications, and they are also used in fog and mist machines and in fuel-oil solutions combined with DDT or malathion. Some have unpleasant odors. Mention will be made of some of these compounds that are used by public health workers.

Loro was used during World War II for louse control. Lethane is used in petroleum house sprays alone or in a combination with DDT and other materials. Fogging with a fuel-oil solution of lethane and malathion is effective against adult mosquitoes. Thanite is also used as a knockdown for flies, and it has been used as a cattle spray and in houses, mills, and warehouses. Its toxicity to mammals is very low.

8-28. The Organic Sulfur Group. This includes the carbamate compounds, sevin, isolane, dimetilan, pyrolan, and phenothiazine. Isolan has a rapid pyrethrum-like action against flies, and it is useful against bedbugs. Phenothiazine has been used as a mosquito larvicide. This group of insecticides may assume greater importance if resistance to other groups of poisons continues to develop.

8-29. Other Insecticides. Paris green is a stomach poison used as a mosquito larvicide. The development of resistance to other poisons has renewed interest in this poison.

Sodium fluoride was long used as a dust for cockroach control. As German cockroaches are becoming resistant to other poisons, its use is increasing, usually as a mixture with pyrethrum and an inert carrier. It is toxic to humans and may cause death if taken internally. It should not be stored with food and should be colored green or blue for identification.

Borax has been used for cockroach control for many years. Roach tablets of borax are useful for controlling cockroaches in bookcases. Borax will kill fly larvae in manure and other feces. If the manure is to be used as a fertilizer, not more than 1 lb of borax should be used to 16 cu ft of manure, and not more than 15 tons of the manure should be applied to an acre of land. The borax can be applied to the manure as a solution, or it may be applied as powder, in which case the manure is wetted with water.

8-30. Resistance. Where insects are exposed to certain insecticides a large percentage may be killed, but a small proportion may survive through their ability to withstand the poison after contact or after it has entered their bodies. If this quality is inherited, a resistant population of the insect will be established. A number of arthropods have developed resistance to some of the generally used insecticides [5]. It has been noticed in mosquitoes, flies, cockroaches, and fleas. DDT is usually the insecticide of choice. If a resistant population develops, a change may be made to another chlorinated hydrocarbon, preferably of a different series. Resistance may again appear, and it will then be advisable to change to an organophosphate, usually malathion. Some mosquitoes, however, have also developed resistance to malathion [6].

Directors of antimosquito or antifly campaigns should be certain that resistance really exists and that the difficulty is not caused by inefficient methods of using insecticides. Methods of testing arthropods for resistance have been developed [5].

8-31. Precautions in the Use of Insecticides. All poisons should be plainly labeled and should be stored away from foods and where irresponsible persons do not have access to them [5]. Toxicity to man and other mammals may be dermal, oral, or by inhalation. Precautions needed will vary according to the insecticide and its concentration [7], but some general rules can be given.

DUSTS AND POWDERS. During the handling, mixing, or application of dusts or powders excessive inhalation or skin contact should be avoided. Clothing should be changed after each day's work, and a bath should be taken.

EMULSIFIABLE CONCENTRATES AND CONCENTRATED SOLUTIONS. Persons handling concentrates should wear protective clothing, such as neoprene-dipped gloves, aprons, goggles, and approved types of respirators. The skin should be protected, and it should be washed immediately if it becomes contaminated. Contaminated clothing should be removed immediately, the skin washed, and clean clothing put on. Clean clothing should be worn every day. Work should be carried on in a well-ventilated area to avoid inhalation of fumes.

DILUTE SPRAYS AND MISTS. The skin should be protected from wetting with the insecticide. Spraying should not be done into the wind. Neoprene-dipped gloves should be worn to protect the hands, and goggles should be used when spraying organic phosphorus compounds.

Bibliography

1. "Cleaning, Disinfection and Sterilization," Bureau of Hospitals, California State Department of Health, Berkeley, Calif., 1962.
2. Milk Ordinance and Code: 1953 Recommendations of the Public Health Service, *Public Health Service Pub.* 229.
3. Larson, T. E.: Synthetic Detergents, *J. Am. Water Works Assoc.*, vol. 41, no. 4, April, 1949.
4. Pratt, H. D., and K. S. Littig: "Insecticides for the Control of Insects of Public Health Importance," Public Health Service, Communicable Disease Center, 1962.
5. Schoof, H. F.: Resistance in Arthropods of Medical and Veterinary Importance, 1956–1958, *Misc. Publ. Entomol. Soc. Am.*, vol. 1, no. 1, pp. 3–11, 1954
6. Pratt, H. D., *et al.*: "Survey and Control of Mosquitoes of Public Health Importance," Public Health Service, Communicable Disease Center, 1962.
7. Insecticide Recommendations of the Entomology Research Division of the Control of Insects Attacking Crops and Livestock for 1963, *U.S. Dept. Agr. Agr. Handbook* 120.
8. Rollins, R. Z.: Federal and State Regulation of Pesticides, *Am. J. Public Health*, vol. 53, no. 9, September, 1963.

9

INSECT VECTOR AND RODENT CONTROL

9-1. By definition, *vectors*, in communicable disease terminology, are "arthropods or other invertebrates which transmit infection by inoculation into or through the skin or mucous membrane by biting, or by deposit of infective materials on the skin or on food or other objects."[1] The vector may be infected itself or may act only as a passive or mechanical carrier of the agent. The *vector* is distinguished from the *vehicle* in disease transmission by the fact that the intermediary is animate and is generally an insect. At various times in history, insect vectors have been the scourge of humanity, being responsible for the great pestilences

[1] F. R. Moulton (ed.), "Human Malaria," American Association for the Advancement of Science, Washington, D.C.

Table 9-1. SOME HUMAN DISEASES TRANSMITTED BY ARTHROPODS IN NORTH AND CENTRAL AMERICA

Disease	Causative agent	Vector	Method of infection	Reservoir
Chagas' disease	*Trypanosoma cruzi*	Kissing bugs: *Triatoma* and related species	Fecal contamination of bite	Rodents, dogs, cats, etc.
Cholera*	*Vibrio cholerae*	Housefly: *Musca domestica*	Contamination of foods	Man
Conjunctivitis . . .	*Haemophilus aegyptius* and others	Eye gnat: *Hippelates pusio* and related species	Contamination of eye tissues	Man
Dengue*	Virus	Yellow fever mosquito: *Aedes aegypti*	Bite	Man
Dysentery, amoebic† . .	*Endamoeba histolytica*	Housefly: *M. domestica*	Contamination of foods	Man
Dysentery, bacillary† . .	*Shigella dysenteriae* and other species	Housefly: *M. domestica*	Contamination of foods	Man
Encephalitis (St. Louis, Western, and Eastern)	Virus	Mosquitoes: *Culex, tarsalis,* and others	Bite	Birds and mammals
Filariasis*	*Wuchereria bancrofti* and possibly *malayi*	Mosquitoes: *Culex, Aedes, Anopheles,* and *Mansonia*	Invasion of bite; also through skin	Man
Leishmaniasis . . .	*Leishmania* spp.	Sandflies: *Phlebotomus*	Bite (?)	Man
Malaria. . . .	*Plasmodium vivax, P. falciparum,* and *P. malariae*	Mosquitoes: *Anopheles*	Bite	Man
Onchocerciasis . . .	*Onchocerca volvulus*	Blackflies: *Simulium*	Invasion of bite	Man
Plague	*Pasteurella pestis*	Oriental rat flea: *Xenopsylla cheopis.* Other fleas	Bite; also by contact with infected rodents	Rats and wild rodents
Relapsing fever . . .	*Borrelia* spp.	Soft ticks: *Ornithodoros*	Bite or contamination of bite	Ticks, rodents, and other mammals
Rickettsialpox . . .	*Rickettsia akari*	House-mouse mite: *Allodermanyssus sanguineus*	Bite	House mice
Rocky Mountain spotted fever .	*Rickettsia rickettsii*	Hard ticks: *Dermacentor* and *Amblyomma*	Bite	Ticks and rodents (?)

Table 9-1. SOME HUMAN DISEASES TRANSMITTED BY ARTHROPODS IN NORTH AND CENTRAL AMERICA *(Continued)*

Disease	Causative agent	Vector	Method of infection	Reservoir
Tularemia	*Pasteurella tularensis*	Deerfly: *Chrysops.* Hard ticks: *Dermacentor*	Bite and contact with infected animal	Rabbits and other wild animals
Typhoid fever† . . .	*Salmonella typhosa*	Housefly: *M. domestica*	Contamination of food and water	Man
Typhus, epidemic* . .	*Rickettsia prowazeki*	Human-body louse: *Pediculus humanus*	Contamination of bite and abrasions	Man
Typhus, murine . . .	*Rickettsia typhi*	Oriental rat flea: *Xenopsylla cheopis*	Contamination of bite and abrasions	Rats
Yellow fever‡	Virus	Yellow fever mosquito: *Aedes aegypti*	Bite	Man and monkeys

* Not known in the United States at present time.
† Disease also spread by other more important carriers.
‡ Not found in the United States. Prevalent in Central America and Mexico.
SOURCE: H. D. Pratt *et al.,* "Mosquitoes of Public Health Importance," Public Health Service, Communicable Disease Center, 1960.

in the Old World and the New—the "Black Death," "yellow jack," and "chills and fever." Fortunately for our modern era, techniques have been developed which have eliminated or minimized the disease potential of the insect vector. In some cases wholesale attack has been unleashed on the insect itself—mosquitoes, in the case of yellow fever and malaria, and fleas, in the case of endemic typhus. In the latter situation, the animal host, the rat, has also been subjected to control efforts.

With the passing of the importance of insect and rodent vectors in disease transmission, in the United States at least, and with the development of techniques for destroying more insects and rats, we have become aware of one phase of a new concept of public health—comfort, physical efficiency, and a sense of well-being. Mosquitoes of the harmless varieties are being destroyed because they interfere with human comfort. While flies remain significant to some extent in disease transmission, fly-control measures are employed largely because flies annoy people. The same may be said of rats. Thus, while their place in disease transmission in the United States is a minor one, insect and rodent vectors may be said to remain of importance in the public health picture.

Table 9-1 lists the important diseases transmitted by arthropods in North and Central America. Arthropods are characterized by articulated bodies and legs, or what may be called an outside skeleton. Arthropods comprise the true insects, of which there are many orders, families, and genera; the arachnids, which include the spiders, scorpions, mites, and ticks; the crustacea, which include crabs, lobsters, crayfish, cyclops, and pillbugs; and the millipedes and centipedes. Of these, the insects are the most important in disease transmission and as a cause of discomfort; also ticks and mites are to be found in Table 9-1. Of course many arthropods are responsible for discomfort by biting, for example, the black widow spider, scorpions, centipedes, bedbugs, bees, wasps, ants, mites, various biting flies, and midges.

9-2. Mosquitoes and Disease. Mosquitoes are of worldwide distribution, and 100 or more species occur in the United States. Most are harmless, some are important as nuisances, and a few are vectors, or links in the chain of disease transmission. The mosquito-borne diseases which occur in North and Central America and their important vectors are listed in Table 9-2. The diseases there listed will be discussed [3].

MALARIA. On a worldwide basis, malaria is considered the most important communicable disease. It is endemic and takes a heavy toll in extensive areas of Latin America, Africa, and Asia. Until late in the nineteenth century, malaria was prevalent in the eastern two-thirds of the United States, with the exception of the highlands of the Appalachians. There was also an endemic area in central California. Since then the incidence has regularly declined, with limited sporadic outbreaks occurring at irregular intervals. The virtual disappearance of malaria in the

Table 9-2. SOME IMPORTANT MOSQUITO-BORNE DISEASES

Disease	Causative organism	Important vectors
Malaria	Protozoa	*Anopheles* mosquitoes:
Benign tertian . .	*Plasmodium vivax*	A. *quadrimaculatus* east of the Rockies
Malignant tertian. .	*P. falciparum*	A. *quadrimaculatus* east of the Rockies
Quartan	*P. malariae*	A. *freeborni* west of the Rockies
Ovale	*P. ovale*	A. *freeborni* west of the Rockies
Yellow fever	Virus	Many mosquitoes, especially:
Urban type . . .	Virus	Yellow fever mosquito (*Aedes aegypti*)
Jungle type . . .	Virus	Jungle mosquitoes, such as *Haemagogus* or *Sabethea* in tropical America and *Aedes* spp. in Africa
Dengue	Virus	Primarily *Aedes aegypti* and A. *albopictus*
Encephalitis	Viruses	Many mosquitoes, including:
Eastern	EEE virus	*Culiseta melanura*
Western	WEE virus	*Culex tarsalis*
St. Louis	SLE virus	*Culex pipiens* complex and *C. tarsalis*
Filariasis	Worm (Nemathelminthes)	Many mosquitoes, especially:
Bancroftian type . .	*Wuchereria bancrofti*	*C. quinquefasciatus*
Malayan type. . .	*W. malayi*	*Mansonia* sp.

NOTE: People may contract a case of malaria, yellow fever, dengue, or encephalitis after being bitten by one infected mosquito. It requires the bites of many infected mosquitoes and the injections of many filarial worms to cause a clinical case of filariasis.

SOURCE: H. D. Pratt *et al.*, "Mosquitoes of Public Health Importance," Public Health Service, Communicable Disease Center, 1960.

United States has been ascribed to the increased prosperity of the country, particularly among the rural population. This has resulted in better medical treatment and in homes which are better protected from mosquitoes. This is important because the vector mosquitoes in the United States are night biters. The balanced farm program has resulted in an increase in cattle raising, and this may also have contributed to malaria reduction since *Anopheles quadrimaculatus*, a very important vector, readily attacks domestic animals as a source of blood. The decrease of the rural population, through migration of farm workers from the marginal or poorer farms to industrial areas, has probably had an effect. The decline has not been due, however, to reduction of the mosquito's efficiency as a vector nor to any change in the characteristics of the malaria parasite.

The causative agents are protozoa or animal organisms called *plas modia*. Four species are involved in human malaria, each type producing differences in the signs of the disease. The organisms have an elaborate life cycle [4] which requires both the mosquito and man for completion.[1] After obtaining a meal of infected blood, the mosquito will be ready to infect another person in a minimum of 7 to 8 days at a temperature of 85 to 90°F or up to 17 days at 65 to 75°F. A person infected by a mosquito will show signs of the disease in 12 to 14 days, except for infections of *P. malariae*, which will require 20 days.

The malaria vectors in the United States are *Anopheles quadrimaculatus*, east of the Rocky Mountains, and *A. freeborni*, west of the Rockies. A few other *Anopheles* of the United States including *A. punctipennis*, *A. crucians*, and *A. walkeri* may be infected in the laboratory but are not believed to transmit malaria in the field. *A. pseudopunctipennis* is not of any importance in the United States, but in some South American countries it is an important vector. *A. albimanus* is an important vector in Latin America. It occurs in southern Texas and the Florida Keys but appears to be of no importance there.

YELLOW FEVER. This disease probably originated in Africa, where it still occurs in the jungle form. It was formerly a very important disease in Latin America, and there were occasional outbreaks in the United States, particularly in port cities where the vector mosquito, *Aedes aegypti*, was prevalent. Discovery of the part played by the mosquito about 1900 resulted in the successful application of control measures at the Panama Canal and in the cities. Yellow fever practically disappeared from America until cases began to appear which were found to be derived from the previously unknown jungle yellow fever. Jungle, or sylvatic, yellow fever is endemic among monkeys and probably other wild animals of the jungles of America from Paraguay to southern Mexico and in central Africa. In the jungles it is spread by various species of *Aedes*, *Haemagogus*, and *Sabethes* mosquitoes, which live in treetops and breed in tree holes. Humans are occasionally bitten by these mosquitoes, and they may then infect the *A. aegypti* in a town, there to produce an outbreak of the classical or urban yellow fever. There have been, however, no *aegypti*-spread outbreaks reported in the Americas since 1942.

The causative agent is a virus. After a mosquito has obtained the virus, it requires from 1 to 3 weeks before it can transmit it to another host. The virus is injected into man with the mosquito's saliva. After a 3- to 6-day incubation period, signs and symptoms of the disease appear. Man is infective to mosquitoes only during the first 3 to 5 days of ill-

---

[1] There are over one hundred known species of plasmodia. The intermediate hosts include frogs, snakes, lizards, many birds, and many mammals other than man. Animal malaria is not transmissible to man, and vice versa.

ness. Fatalities are frequent. Lifelong immunity follows an attack. Vaccination against the disease is effective.

According to Soper [5], yellow fever virus is always present, with variable year-to-year distribution, throughout the tropical and subtropical forests of the Americas from Argentina to Mexico. Jungle yellow fever is a serious threat to rural populations and is a permanent source of virus for such cities as may be infested with A. aegypti. Prevention would include widespread vaccination of rural populations and eradication of A. aegypti from the Americas. Much has been accomplished against this vector. It has been eradicated in many of the countries of Latin America where jungle yellow fever is reported, and it is under heavy attack in others. In the spring of 1964 the United States began concentrated efforts to eradicate this mosquito.

DENGUE. This disease, also known as breakbone fever, is a rarely fatal disease caused by a virus. It is spread by A. aegypti in the Americas and by A. albopictus in Hawaii, the Philippines, and southeast Asia. It may occur in epidemic form in any tropical country when the vectors are present. Four important outbreaks have been noted since 1922 in the southern United States and Hawaii. Mosquitoes become infective 8 to 14 days after biting an infected person. Persons may infect mosquitoes from 1 day before the fever appears until the third or fourth day of the disease. There is no immunity.

ENCEPHALITIS. Three types of this frequently fatal disease occur in the United States: Eastern equine, Western equine, and the St. Louis type. Birds are considered to be the reservoir of the disease, with transmission by mosquitoes from bird to man. Horses, mules, and other animals may also be infected by mosquitoes, but these appear to be dead-end hosts, and infection proceeds no further. There is doubt as to whether mosquitoes can transmit the infection from man to man. Important human epidemics of all these types of encephalitis have been reported in the United States. The incubation period in man is usually from 5 to 15 days.

The Eastern equine type is recognized in the eastern United States, particularly in the Atlantic and Gulf Coast areas; in Canada; and in scattered areas of Latin America, the Philippines, and Slovakia. This disease also commonly occurs among horses and pheasants. Suspect vectors in the United States are Culiseta melanura, Aedes sollicitans, A. vexans, and Mansonia perturbans.

Western equine encephalitis is found in all the states west of the Mississippi, in Minnesota and Wisconsin, in South America, and in Slovakia. Noteworthy outbreaks in horses have also occurred. In the United States, Culex tarsalis is the most important vector.

St. Louis encephalitis has been found in all states west of the Mississippi, the Ohio River Valley, Trinidad, and Panama. Horses do not appear to contract the disease. Mosquitoes of the *C. pipiens-quinque-fasciatus* complex are the principal urban vectors. *C. tarsalis* is the chief vector in some Western states, particularly on the Pacific Coast.

Two other strains of encephalitis virus cause disease in areas outside the United States. Japanese B occurs in the western Pacific islands from Guam to Japan and in many eastern areas of Asia from Korea to Singapore and India. Its most important vectors are *C. tritaeniorhynchus* and *C. gelidus*. The Murray Valley type occurs in parts of Australia and New Guinea. The probable vector is *C. annulirostris.*

FILARIASIS. The causative agents of this disease are two nematode worms (see Table 9-2). They live in the lymphatic systems of humans, where they may cause inflammation and other complications. After long and repeated infections, certain parts of the body may become extremely enlarged, often with thickened and rough skin, a condition known as elephantiasis. The disease is widespread in many tropical and subtropical areas: in the Americas in Colombia, Panama, Venezuela, the West Indies, and the coastal portions of Brazil and the Guianas. Many American servicemen became infected in the South Pacific during World War II, but no cases of elephantiasis developed. An endemic area formerly existed near Charleston, S.C., but it has disappeared.

9-3. Life Cycle of the Mosquito. The life cycle of the mosquito is characterized by complete metamorphosis, with four stages—the egg, the larva, the pupa, and the adult winged insect. See Fig. 9-1. The adult female lays eggs in batches ranging in number from less than fifty to more than two hundred, and one female may deposit several batches in her lifetime. The eggs of some species are glued together in a mass or raft about ⅛ in. long which floats on the water; others are deposited on the soil at the edge of the water or in depressions where water will collect; and still others are deposited singly to float on the water. They are too small to be easily visible. See Table 9-3. The incubation period is usually 2 to 3 days in warm weather; however, the eggs of many species can withstand long periods of drying or cold. The eggs of some of the salt-marsh mosquitoes may remain dormant for years.

The eggs hatch into the larvae, which are aquatic; however, they are air breathers and must renew their air supply occasionally through a breathing tube situated at the tail. During this period of development, usually 4 to 10 days, the larvae pass through four successive stages of growth known as instars, in which the skin is shed four times. Most mosquito larvae are free-swimming and feed by straining minute plants, animals, or particles of debris from the water through action of the mouth parts.

The pupae, commonly called "tumblers," appear with the fourth molt or instar. They are still aquatic and air-breathing but do not feed. The adult winged insect is formed during this period of development

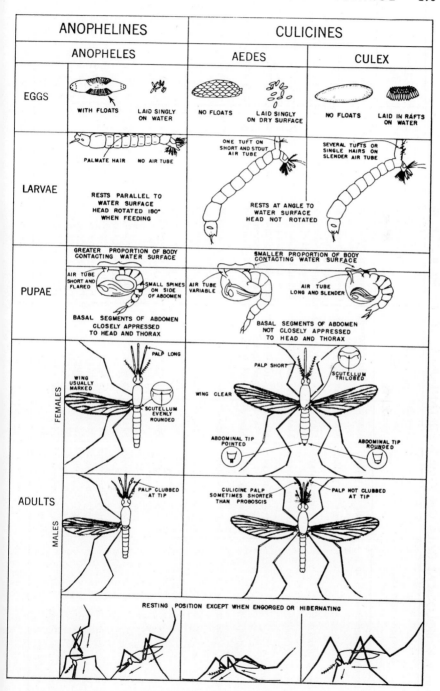

FIGURE 9-1   Life cycles of *Anopheles*, *Aedes*, and *Culex* mosquitoes. (*From H. D. Pratt et al., "Mosquitoes of Public Health Importance," Public Health Service, Communicable Disease Center, 1960*).

Table 9-3. BIOLOGICAL DATA ON SOME IMPORTANT UNITED STATES SPECIES OF MOSQUITOES

Mosquito species	Eggs	Broods per year	Overwintering habits	Preferred larval habitat	Effective flight range
Anopheles quadrimaculatus	Singly on water	Many	As adult females	Clean, partially shaded water; some vegetation	1 mile
A. freeborni	Singly on water	Many	As adult females	Clean, partially shaded water; some vegetation	1–2 miles or more
Culex pipiens	Rafts on water	Many	As adult females	Permanent water with organic matter or pollution	1 mile or more
C. quinquefasciatus	Rafts on water	Many	As adult females	Permanent water with organic matter or pollution	1 mile or more
C. tarsalis	Rafts on water	Many	As adult females and larvae	Almost any collection of water, usually waste water	2–5 miles
Culiseta melanura	Rafts on water	Many	As adult females and larvae	Permanent shaded pools in swamps	100–1,000 yd
Mansonia perturbans	Rafts on water	One	As larvae	Permanent water with some aquatic vegetation	1–5 miles or more
Aedes aegypti	Singly on sides of containers or tree holes	Many	As eggs	Artificial containers	1 block; usually less than ½–1 mile
A. triseriatus	Singly on sides of containers or tree holes	Many	As eggs	Tree holes, artificial containers	1 block; usually less than ½–1 mile
A. sollicitans	Singly on ground	Many	As eggs	Temporary pools, usually brackish or with sulfates	5–20 miles
A. taeniorhynchus	Singly on ground	Many	As eggs	Temporary pools, usually brackish	5–20 miles
A. dorsalis	Singly on ground	Many	As eggs	Temporary pools, pastures, etc.	10–20 miles or more
A. nigromaculis	Singly on ground	Many	As eggs	Temporary pools, pastures, etc.	2–5 miles
A. vexans	Singly on ground	Many	As eggs	Temporary pools	5–20 miles
Psorophora ciliata	Singly on ground	Many	As eggs	Temporary pools	5 miles or more
P. confinnis	Singly on ground	Many	As eggs	Temporary pools, rice fields	5 miles or more

SOURCE: H. D. Pratt et al., "Mosquitoes of Public Health Importance," Public Health Service, Communicable Disease Center, 1960.

and usually emerges in about 2 days. Upon emerging, the adult rests on the surface of the water until its wings dry and harden; it is then capable of flight.

It will be noted that the first three stages of the life cycle require about 7 days. This, for most species, is the minimum period under the most favorable conditions; colder weather lengthens the time. The life-span of the adult mosquito in nature is difficult to determine but probably is only a few weeks during the summer months. A large reduction in broods of certain species of *Anopheles* and *Aedes* has been noted within 2 weeks, while the yellow fever mosquito, *Aedes aegypti,* may live, on an average, a month or more with a maximum of several months. Overwintering habits are shown in Table 9-3.

9-4. Habits of Adult Mosquitoes. Only the female mosquito is able to bite humans or animals, the mouth parts of the male not being adapted to piercing human or animal skin. The male lives upon plant juices, which also support the female in the absence of a blood supply. The female usually must obtain a blood meal prior to the development of viable eggs. Many species of mosquitoes never bite humans and are therefore inconspicuous, while others, mainly swamp and sylvan types, never leave their native haunts but will attack any humans or other animals that come their way. Certain mosquitoes are night biters and spend the daylight hours in dark corners of structures and in high grass, weeds, vines, and shrubbery, where they are sheltered from the sun, wind, and rain. The discomfort that results from mosquito bites is caused by the small amount of liquid which is injected by the mosquito as soon as she has penetrated the skin.

As a rule mosquitoes do not travel long distances. Flight ranges are given in Table 9-3. These are extreme. From a breeding place of small productivity, few or no mosquitoes may travel the extreme distances given.

Anopheles quadrimaculatus is a medium-sized blackish mosquito with four well-defined spots on its wings. It frequents houses more than the other *Anopheles* and is the most dangerous of the malaria carriers. It breeds in fresh water, particularly permanent pools, lakes, or swamps, and is distributed east of the Rocky Mountains from Mexico to New England.

A. freeborni is medium-sized and blackish, with wings resembling those of *A. quadrimaculatus*. It is the most dangerous malaria carrier of the West Coast, besides being something of a pest. It breeds in puddles, preferring permanent water with some protective vegetation. Its habitat is the western United States and Canada.

Aedes aegypti, the carrier of yellow fever and dengue, is a medium-sized mosquito and gives the impression of being gray. When closely examined, the gray color is found to be due to silvery markings on the legs, abdomen, and thorax. Those on the thorax have some resemblance to a lyre. It breeds only in artificial containers of relatively clean water. It bites only in daytime or in artificial light and prefers the ankles as points of attack. Its flight range is not over a block. It is a warm-climate mosquito and in the United States is usually not found farther north than the latitude of Kentucky.

Culex pipiens is a small, brown, night-biting mosquito. The abdomen is blackish with whitish bands connected to the spots on the sides. It breeds principally in artificial containers but will also breed in ground pools and sewage. This is the common house mosquito of Europe, introduced into the United States through commerce and now one of the most important pestiferous mosquitoes in the country from Virginia to Canada on the Atlantic Coast and from California to British Columbia on the Pacific Coast.

C. quinquefasciatus resembles *C. pipiens* in habits, breeding places, and appearance, except that the bands of the abdomen are not connected to the spots at the sides. It is the common house mosquito of the tropics and in the United States ranges as far north as Kentucky.

C. tarsalis is a medium-sized mosquito with a bronze-brown thorax, frequently adorned with a few narrow silver-white lines. The proboscis is dark, with a white ring near the middle; the legs are bronze—the femora are white beneath, and the tarsi have white rings at both sides of the joints. The larvae are commonly found in grassy ponds or marshes, in escaping irrigation water, and in well-treated sewage effluent. They do not breed in artificial containers. This mosquito may enter houses and become a nuisance in the western part of the country and is the generally accepted vector of Western equine encephalitis. It is distributed over the Mississippi Valley and western prairies to the Pacific Ocean.

Aedes sollicitans is a medium-sized to large mosquito with conspicuously ringed legs. The thorax is bronze-yellow, dark bronze at the sides. The abdomen is black with crossbands of pale yellow and a longitudinal band down the middle. The proboscis has a white ring. The larvae occur in salt tidal pools on the coast but sometimes develop inland in association with saltwater wastes from industrial processes. The adult is a strong flier and in many instances travels long distances inland. It is distributed over the Gulf states and over the Atlantic Coast to New England. It and the small salt-marsh mosquito are of importance because of their nuisance effects and because they reduce property values. In the Gulf states they sometimes cause death in cattle.

A. taeniorhynchus is the small salt-marsh mosquito. It is rather blackish in color; the thorax is dark brown, and the abdomen is black with narrow white bands and white spots at the sides. The legs are black, but the femora are white beneath, and the tarsi have narrow white rings which are wider on the hind legs. The proboscis has a narrow white

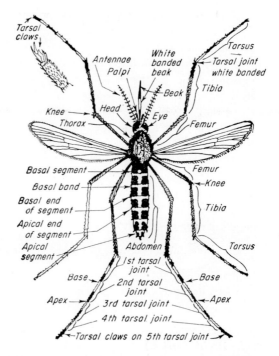

Figure 9-2 Adult mosquito (*Aedes sollicitans*
Wlk.) with parts named. (*After John B. Smith,
New Jersey Agricultural Experiment Station.*)

ring. It breeds in saline or slightly saline pools near the seacoast. It is
very abundant in the Gulf states and Florida but also occurs in the
North Atlantic states and along the Pacific Coast.

9-5. Identification of Mosquitoes. Identification of mosquitoes is
important. The worker in mosquito control soon becomes acquainted
with the common adult mosquitoes in his own area. He may be guided
in part by the very brief descriptions given in Art. 9-4. Some simple
rules are also applicable. All anophelines, except two unimportant
species, have spotted wings. All other mosquito genera have clear wings.
The spot patterns vary somewhat in different anopheline species; these
are shown in Fig. 9-3. Anopheline adults also assume a standing-on-head
position when resting or biting, as shown in Fig. 9-1. All other mosquitoes appear humpbacked when resting or biting.

Mosquito identification in many cases will require the use of a key
[6]. A key gives descriptions of the various parts of a mosquito, and by
following it the identity will be established. Figure 9-2 shows anatomical
parts of the adult mosquito. A hand lens will be necessary in the use of
a key.

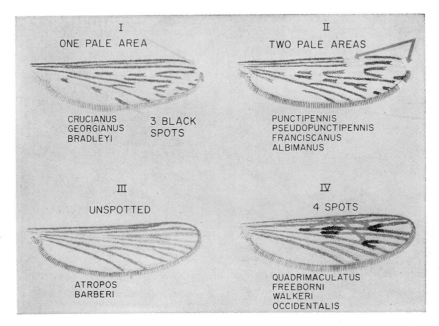

I

ONE PALE AREA

CRUCIANUS
GEORGIANUS   3 BLACK
BRADLEYI   SPOTS

II

TWO PALE AREAS

PUNCTIPENNIS
PSEUDOPUNCTIPENNIS
FRANCISCANUS
ALBIMANUS

III

UNSPOTTED

ATROPOS
BARBERI

IV

4 SPOTS

QUADRIMACULATUS
FREEBORNI
WALKERI
OCCIDENTALIS

FIGURE 9-3 Wing markings of the more common *Anopheles*. (*Photographs by Public Health Service.*)

Anopheles larvae normally remain just below the water surface and parallel to it. They have no breathing tube, only an opening. When alarmed they usually dart along the water surface, but they can and sometimes do dive. Larvae of other mosquitoes have visible breathing tubes, hang at an angle to the water surface when breathing, and dive when alarmed. *Aedes aegypti* have shorter, thicker breathing tubes than *Culex*, but this requires close observation for recognition. Keys [6] are also available to determine the identity of larvae. A microscope will be required.

When identification of larvae or pupae is necessary, it is possible to capture some with the water in which they are living and allow them to hatch. Pupae will usually hatch out, and larvae near pupation will frequently do so. The adults may then be identified.

Pupal differences of culicines and anophelines are shown in Fig. 9-1.

9-6. Mosquito Surveys. A program for controlling mosquitoes, whether for public health purposes or for public comfort, should be preceded by a basic survey and accompanied by an operational survey [7].

A map will be needed for the basic survey. Preferably it should have contours and should also show populated areas, streams, ponds, swamps, and other mosquito-producing areas. On it can be placed locations of adult and larvae collection points and traps and limits of the

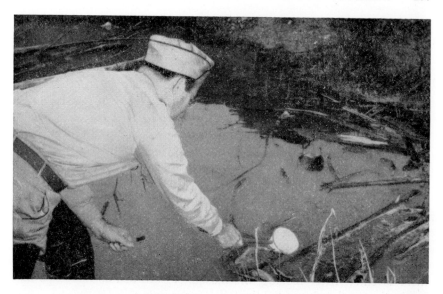

FIGURE 9-4   Dipping for *Anopheles* larvae. Note that collection is made in floating debris. (*Courtesy of Public Health Service.*)

control area. Control-area limits will be set by the flight ranges of the mosquitoes that are to be controlled.

All water in which breeding may take place must be examined. A container of water near a house or a tree hole may be a source, or the mosquitoes may be flying in from a more distant area. In general, the edges of bodies of water where there is vegetation or floating debris are the points where larvae or pupae will be found. In most cases the water in which mosquitoes breed is easy to reach, and the larvae can be picked up in a long-handled dipper. For the collection of anopheline larvae, the lip of the dipper is quickly swept along the surface of the water in such a manner that water is skimmed into the dipper, or if vegetation is dense, the dipper may be submerged so that water flows into it. The aquatic stages of some culicine mosquitoes require a quicker, deeper dip. Mosquito larvae and pupae are wary and will dive when alarmed; therefore, it may require many dips before any are captured, particularly if the breeding is not very heavy.

The quickest indication of the mosquito species present and the type of control that may be required can be secured by capturing adult specimens in traps or by hand. Hand collection of adults from their resting places in dark corners of dwellings, barns, privies, and chicken houses and under bridges and culverts can be accomplished with a flashlight and a "killing tube." A satisfactory killing tube can be made from a test tube or similar container fitted with a cork stopper. Rubber bands or wads of cotton saturated in chloroform and placed in the bottom of the tube under wadding cut from blotting paper kill the mosquitoes. The unstoppered tube is placed under or over the resting mosquito, and the chloroform causes it to fall into the tube. Specimens are removed to pill-boxes and protected with cotton for submission to the laboratory for identification.

The most commonly used light trap is the New Jersey type [7]. This trap consists of a vertical metal cylinder covered by a metal roof. An electric light under the roof attracts the mosquito to the cylinder, and a small electric fan draws it into the cylinder and blows it downward to a jar containing poison, usually calcium cyanide. Light traps are not particularly appropriate for the collection of anophelines.

Another type of trap has been used with success in the tropics but has not been found of value in the United States. A donkey or other animal is placed in a small shed with large screened windows on the sides so arranged that mosquitoes are diverted to slits in the screened wire or louvered areas situated just below the screened area which allow them to enter. After feeding, the mosquitoes are unable to escape and can be captured and counted the following morning.

Because of differences in their habits, the proportions of the different species of mosquitoes present in an area cannot be determined exactly by hand or trap collection, but collection by one or both methods should give a fairly reliable indication of changes in the mosquito populations.

The operational survey is a continual evaluation of the effectiveness of the mosquito-control work and is made by capturing adults, noting species and numbers, dipping for larvae, and recording results. Record forms should be made to ensure easy recording and filing of information.

9-7. Disease Control. Control methods applicable to mosquito-borne diseases will depend upon the habits of the mosquitoes involved. The methods used will only be mentioned here. Discussions of them are given later in the chapter.

MALARIA. Drainage has been employed, but its cost must be justified by comparison with the cost of other methods that will attain the same results.

Larvicidal methods are applicable to malaria control, but they are also expensive and are justified only when a considerable population is protected and when other methods are less economical or cannot be applied.

Protection of rural populations long presented a problem. Mass medication has been employed. Where it was effectively carried out, it reduced malaria death rates but did not prevent transmission of the disease. Screening and other methods of mosquitoproofing homes to give protection against the night-biting anophelines are applicable in relatively prosperous populations, where homes are usually screened in any case as a nuisance preventive. Such methods are not applicable in regions where the economic level is low and where the types of homes used may be impossible to make mosquitoproof.

Residual spraying of rural and village homes with insecticides has been highly successful in giving malaria protection where the malaria-carrying anophelines come into homes to feed and, before or after feeding, rest on surfaces that have been sprayed.

YELLOW FEVER AND DENGUE. Jungle yellow fever does not appear to be amenable to control by antimosquito measures. Urban yellow fever, since it is carried by *Aedes aegypti,* a breeder in artificial containers near and in homes, can be rather easily controlled. *A. aegypti* can be eradicated by the elimination of all water standing in containers or, if they cannot be eliminated, by covering them so that mosquitoes cannot get to the water to lay their eggs on the surface or near the edges. An outbreak of the disease should be followed by systematic, careful inspections of all premises, indoors and out, for the presence of actual or potential breeding places and by the immediate elimination of these breeding places. In a town of any size, this may require a corps of inspectors assigned to districts. Inspection cards containing a list of possible water containers that can be checked for presence of mosquito breeding will be helpful. The inspector makes out a card for each property and gives directions, if necessary, for eliminating or covering the containers; a follow-up visit is then made. Routine inspections should be made weekly. In the early stages of an outbreak, when it is feared that infected mosquitoes are numerous, residual spraying in homes may be applied. Dengue outbreaks should be combated in the same way. Infected persons should be protected from mosquitoes.

Since *A. aegypti* flies only a block or less from its breeding place and breeds only around human habitations, eradication of the species is possible. Concerted action of all the towns and cities of a large area would be necessary since individual female mosquitoes might travel in airplanes, ships, buses, or other public transportation for some distance. The mosquito may, of course, find breeding places on a ship. Eradication of the species in the United States is practicable and has already been accomplished in some Latin-American countries [5].

ENCEPHALITIS. Routine elimination of nuisance mosquitoes is, of course, a protective measure. Infected persons should be protected against mosquitoes. Residual spraying may be applied in the homes of infected persons and in neighboring houses. Outhouses, garages, etc., should also be sprayed. Mosquito breeding places around homes should be eliminated. Ponds and streams, particularly those that are sewage-polluted and within the flight range of the mosquitoes (see Tables 9-2 and 9-3), should be given larvicidal treatment, and possibly measures should be taken for permanent elimination.

9-8. Control of Nuisance Mosquitoes. Drainage is usually employed to control the salt-marsh mosquitoes. Larvicidal methods are sometimes employed near populated areas.

Control of *Culex quinquefasciatus, C. pipiens, C. tarsalis,* and *A. aegypti* requires elimination of water containers around homes and other premises. Larvicidal treatment will be needed for catch basins of storm sewers, water held in culverts, streams, and ponds which cannot be drained and which are within flight range of the mosquitoes.

Adults are controlled by "fogging" areas with insecticidal aerosols at such intervals as may be necessary (Art. 9-27). This procedure will also reduce houseflies and other flying insects, but it has little or no residual effect.

Larvicidal Methods

9-9. Drainage. Drainage improvement includes installing open ditches, subsurface drains, and vertical drains; filling low areas; cleaning and draining natural streams; and controlling impounding reservoirs. In tidal areas it may also include construction of dykes and tide gates. Drainage frequently makes it possible to eliminate permanently not only small pools but also such large breeding areas as swamps. It has some disadvantages, however. The ditches, if not carefully constructed and properly maintained, may themselves breed mosquitoes. This applies particularly to unlined earth ditches. Usually it is not possible to eliminate all natural waters. The streams which drain the area will provide mosquito breeding places unless they are carefully observed and cleared. Heavy rains will cause overflows and temporary pools, which may be very expensive or impossible to drain. The same applies to ponds and lakes.

Drainage for mosquito control differs in some of its details from ordinary drainage. Storm-water drainage, for instance, requires immediate carrying away of large volumes of water, while drainage of water for mosquito control requires only that the water be carried off in less time than the period necessary to produce mosquitoes. Ordinary drainage of agricultural land is concerned only with keeping the land sufficiently dry to produce crops, and little or no consideration is given to small amounts of water retained in the ditches. On the other hand, such small accumulations are more favorable for mosquito breeding than larger bodies of water. Hence, antimosquito drainage must be so arranged that no water is allowed to stand for appreciable lengths of time in the drainage ditches or elsewhere.

9-10. Ditching. The first step in drainage is to make a tentative layout of the system of ditches. If the problem is to drain a swampy area formed by seepage at the bottom of a hill, the main ditch should parallel the bottom or the hill and be deep enough to intersect all the ground-water flow before it appears on the ground surface. Flat, swampy areas and ponds will require a main ditch leading from the deepest point of the area. The main ditch should always be dug first and drainage allowed to occur. After a few days the lateral ditches may be dug, and it may be discovered that not so many will be required as was first supposed. Frequently there will be smaller ditches connecting low areas with the main ditch.

Ditches should have clean sides sloped as steeply as the earth, or other material, will permit. The bottoms should be as narrow as possible in order to confine the stream to a small area. Wide ditches are undesirable since they permit pools of water to stand and breed mosquitoes. Where a very wide ditch is essential, this problem may be eliminated by constructing a small ditch in the bottom of the large one so that small flows will be concentrated and kept moving. Sharp bends should be avoided when making changes of direction, and branch ditches should join the main ditch at acute angles or with a curve. The grade of an unlined ditch should be great enough to give a cleaning velocity, but not so great that erosion will occur. A grade or fall of 0.05 ft per 100 ft is the minimum for an unlined ditch, and 0.6 to 0.8 ft per 100 ft is the maximum. When steeper grades are necessary, spillways or check dams of concrete, rock, brush, or poles are used to reduce the velocity.

Side slopes of earth ditches are usually 1 horizontal to 1 vertical in firm loam or sandy clay. In soft, loose soil it should be 1.5 horizontal to 1 vertical. In hard, rocky material, it may be steeper than 1 to 1.

Where sharp curves are necessary and the grade is near the upper limit suggested above, it may be necessary to place some type of lining at the outer side of the curve to avoid excessive erosion. This can be done by laying stone or concrete blocks on the ditch side or by driving small logs into the ditch bottom at the same angle as the ditch side. This may also be necessary where a lateral ditch enters a main ditch, both in the lateral where it is curved and in the main ditch opposite to the junction. The lateral should have an increased grade just before it enters the main ditch, and its bottom at the point of junction should be slightly higher than that of the main ditch.

Figure 9-5 shows the ditch lining originated at Panama [8]. It consists of a curved section, or invert, which ensures that small flows will be concentrated and that good hydraulic conditions will prevail. Side slabs are placed so that the lined portion extends as far up the ditch sides as the flows may require. For small ditches, the inverts alone may be sufficient. Frequently, however, the inverts are merely half-sections of concrete pipe, or third-sections, if the ditch is to be very wide and the diameter of the invert section is over 24 in. The concrete is usually 1:3:5 mix. The lining here illustrated is precast, but monolithic linings,

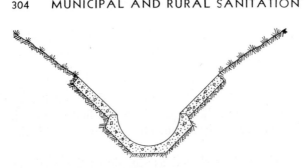

FIGURE 9-5   Cross section of a lined ditch.

i.e., those laid continuously in place, have also been used. Sidewalls, and sometimes the inverts also, have been constructed of rough stones, or riprap, laid to grade and carefully grouted.

If a ditch has a small flow with occasional large flows, the invert may be a half-round channel with the rest of the bottom sloped slightly to obtain proper width and with more steeply sloping sides rising higher. For very infrequent heavy flows, a ditch may be widened still more on a slope of 1½ horizontal to 1 vertical, which is sodded. Bermuda-grass sod 1 in. in thickness is satisfactory. Sod bonds more rapidly to the earth if it is thinner than 2 in. The sod should be carefully tamped with shovels for quick bonding. The lower edge of the sod must rest upon the upper edge of the ditch lining.

Junctions of branch ditches coming into main ditches should be designed so that no injury will be done to the lining of either ditch. If lined ditches are to pass through muck, it may be necessary to remove the soft material and replace it with sand, gravel, or other available satisfactory material. If the ditch is to traverse a seepy area, it may be advisable to lay open-jointed tile drains that will intercept or collect the water and discharge it into the ditch through openings that pierce the ditch lining. If the grade of the ditch is steep, there is a tendency for water to run beneath the lining. This can be prevented by placing cutoff or key walls at intervals of 200 ft. If the velocity in the ditch will be more than 4 fps (feet per second), some authorities recommend that the grade be flattened and that spillways or drops from one elevation to another be constructed. Precautions should be taken at the point of abrupt elevation change so that the falling water will do no damage. Velocities should be more than 2 fps to ensure cleaning, and grades should be increased slightly on curves to prevent deposition of silt.

Ditching in swamps where the earth is saturated with water and perhaps filled with roots is a difficult and expensive undertaking. Under these conditions, ditching with dynamite has been very effectively carried out. This method should not be attempted without an experienced blaster on the job. It is usually cheaper than ditching by hand and is

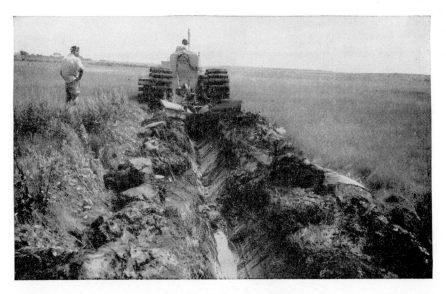

FIGURE 9-6 Widening ditches which checkerboard the salt marshes at Baldwin Harbor in Nassau County, N.Y. (*Courtesy of H. O. Penn Machinery Co. and Public Works Magazine.*)

much faster, since ditching at the rate of 100 to 200 ft/hr is possible. Dynamite manufacturers furnish instruction booklets giving the details of this method of swamp drainage.

9-11. Ditch Maintenance. Ditches should be carefully maintained, or they may themselves become breeders of mosquitoes. This is particularly true where cattle have access to unlined ditches. It is usually necessary to give the ditches a thorough working-over each spring. They may or may not require further cleaning in the middle of the summer.

Extensive improvements are sometimes necessary. Regrading will be needed when ditches have become eroded in some sections and silted in others. Vegetation must be removed. Excessive erosion may be prevented by placing in the ditch key walls of concrete 3 in. wide, 18 in. deep, and 12 to 24 in. longer than the ditch width. The upper edge is set at the permanent grade elevation desired. Eroded banks are protected by log stakes. If the ditch has widened, it may be necessary to dig a small ditch in the bottom to confine small flows.

9-12. Vertical Drainage. Pools and swamps are sometimes due not only to insufficient surface drainage but also to the fact that there is an impervious stratum immediately below the ground surface. Beneath the impervious stratum there may be one that is open and porous, such as sand or gravel, or fissured, such as limestone. If surface drainage in such a case is too costly, vertical drainage may be employed. This requires the sinking of one or more shafts or wells through the impervious

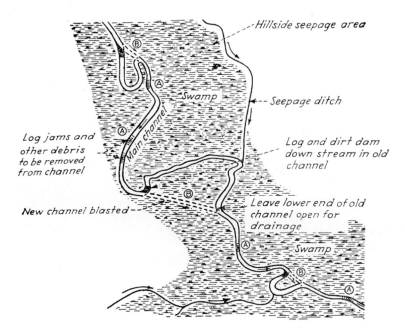

FIGURE 9-7 Stream rechanneling to eliminate a swamp. *A,* points where stream clearing may be needed; *B,* points where new channels may be dug or blasted. Upper ends of old channels are blocked with earth and log dams. Note intercepting ditch for hillside seepage area. (*Courtesy of Public Health Service.*)

stratum to the porous or fissured one. In the case of fissured rock, a hole may be drilled in it at the bottom of the shaft and one or more sticks of dynamite exploded to open up the seams. Inlet ditches may be required to carry the water to the shafts. Such shafts or wells may be lined with tile pipe or sheeted with timber to prevent caving. If of large diameter, they are sometimes filled with large stones.

9-13. **Improvement and Maintenance of Streams.** Mosquitoes do not breed in swiftly running water. This, however, does not eliminate the running stream as a mosquito producer, as there will frequently be found deep pools, obstructions, or vegetation which will retard the flow of the stream sufficiently to allow breeding in favorable places. Conditions in the stream may be improved by clearing it of vegetation and other obstructions. It will sometimes be possible to eliminate deep holes by rechanneling or filling. Swampy areas can often be eliminated by straightening the channel of a slow winding stream. Before this is done, levels should be run to make sure that enough slope is available. Many streams cease flowing in dry periods, leaving water in isolated pools. These should be connected by ditches. Clearing and maintaining

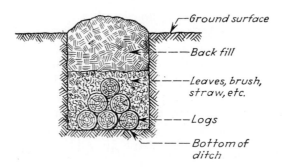

FIGURE 9-8 Log drain. Backfill is mounded to allow for settlement.

of streams will aid minnows and other predators to keep down mosquito production.

9-14. Street Drainage. Mosquito control in towns will be facilitated by giving proper attention to street drainage. All side ditches of unpaved streets should be brought to grade, cleaned, and freed of weeds. Culverts are frequently silted up at the lower end and consequently hold water for weeks if not cleared. Storm-water catch basins may be mosquito breeders. Work that is done on streets should be carried out with mosquito control in view. This calls for cooperation between the street department and the health authorities.

9-15. Subsurface Drainage. Underground tile drainage has been used to advantage in swampy areas, where open ditches quickly become choked with vegetation or trampled by cattle. Tiling of marshy property may also be profitable as a land-reclamation measure.

The tile used varies from 3 in. in diameter upward. Under average soil conditions the laterals may be appropriately spaced and the pipe laid at a depth of 2 to 4 ft. The tile, which is of the plain-ended porous variety, is laid with close joints, which may be covered with straw or sacks to prevent entrance of sand. The usual slope given is not less than 2 in. per 100 ft, and care must be taken that the tile is laid carefully to grade.

A less expensive drain can be made by using logs, as shown in Fig. 9-8. Such drains should slope from 0.2 to 1.0 ft per 100 ft of ditch length.

9-16. Impounded Waters. Marshy areas in stream beds have been controlled by erecting a dam and flooding the area. Under such conditions, particularly if the edges can be kept clear, some degree of control may be anticipated because the natural predators will have access to the mosquito larvae.

Waters impounded in reservoirs for flood control, power, irrigation, or water supply frequently become producers of large numbers of mosquitoes. Mosquito-control principles should be incorporated into reservoir design, construction, and operation.

Mosquito breeding does not occur in the open water of reservoirs, where the larvae would be exposed to injury by wave action and destruction by fish, but usually in the shallow water along the edges, where there is vegetation and floating matter to give protection and concealment to the larvae. Reservoir design for mosquito control should place emphasis on obtaining a maximum of vegetation-free water surface by "building out" the most favorable mosquito-producing areas through shoreline alterations—by deepening and filling or by dyking and dewatering.

Shoreline improvement may not always be practicable, in which case water-level management may be carried on to reduce mosquito production. Effective supplements to water-level management include drift removal, marginal-drainage maintenance, and plant-growth control. Reservoir construction should, therefore, include clearing of the land which will be the margin of the reservoir to prevent protrusion of stumps, branches, etc., which, in turn, would give protection to larvae. Clearing should also be extended a sufficient distance above the high water level so that falling trees will not extend into the water. Wherever erosion may be expected to extend the reservoir margin, such potential extensions should also be cleared. Depressions in the marginal area between high and low water levels should be drained or filled.

It is advisable to fill the reservoir for the first time when vegetation is not in the growing season so that floating leaves and other organic materials which encourage and conceal heavy mosquito breeding will be at a minimum. If possible, the reservoir should first be filled above the normal level so that much of the floating material will be stranded. Thereafter, mosquito control will be greatly aided or perhaps obtained by systematically varying the water level. Whether this can be done will depend upon the continuity of the supply of water to the reservoir and the demand for water. The Tennessee Valley Authority at the Wilson Reservoir obtained good results by lowering the water level a distance of 1 ft in $\frac{1}{2}$ week and refilling 0.9 ft in the rest of the week. This resulted in a gradual net drawdown during the 6 months of the breeding season [9].

Water-level variations are beneficial in several ways. They strand mosquito eggs and protective floating matter. They discourage both land and aquatic marginal vegetation, making the reservoir edge an unsuitable environment for larvae by giving no protection against wave action or fish. Some types of vegetation, however, are resistant to water fluctuations, and clearing or larvicidal measures may be required.

9-17. Other Man-made Mosquito Breeding Places. Careless construction work has been responsible for a large amount of mosquito breeding. Culverts beneath highways and railroads are frequently placed so that a pool is formed on the upstream side which cannot be drained. Or the culvert is placed too low, so that it is continually filled with water. Borrow pits, left without any means of drainage, become filled with water and contribute mosquitoes to the countryside.

Carelessness in the design and operation of irrigation systems has resulted in heavy mosquito populations. Waterlogged soil, with excess water standing in low areas; standing pools formed by overflows from irrigated lands; and leaky ditches are the common faults seen in irrigated sections. Good operating methods and proper drainage are essential if mosquito control is to be obtained.

Rice fields are frequently flooded soon after planting and may be more or less continuously flooded. Control by larvicides is not always practicable, and fish have not proved effective. The most promising method of preventing breeding of anophelines in the rice fields is to drain periodically at such intervals that the life cycle of the mosquito cannot be completed.

9-18. Salt-marsh Drainage. Control of salt-marsh mosquitoes requires knowledge of the breeding habits of the mosquitoes involved, the tidal fluctuations, and the nature of the soil in the marsh [10]. As previously indicated, the eggs are laid on the mud in depressions at the edges of the marsh which will be filled by rainwater or flooded by exceptionally high tides. Hatching occurs rapidly, and adults may emerge, under favorable conditions, within 7 days. Not all eggs will hatch at the first, second, or even later wettings. This helps the mosquito to survive in an area even though the pools may dry up before the first-hatched larvae have had time to emerge. To determine the area to be controlled, it is necessary to determine the highest tidal elevation. The so-called spring tides, which occur several times a month, are the highest. Their heights may be obtained from government records. To this height, an addition must be made for onshore winds, which may force the water even higher. Under some conditions it may also be necessary to make a further addition for waves, although this is of more importance in connection with the design of dykes. Soil conditions are important for several reasons. If the soil is principally peat, it is advisable to draw the water level only below the grass roots. Too great a drawdown will permit shrinkage to such an extent that drainage is interfered with, or fires may occur. Either of these difficulties may require flooding of the area by pumping or otherwise. Some marshy regions are of claylike silt. This may crack when it dries, and the cracks may hold water and breed mosquitoes. The remedial measures are larviciding or plowing of the ground, followed by disking to fill the cracks.

Open-marsh drainage is used in narrow marshes where the longest length of drain to outlet is not in excess of 2,000 ft or where settling may be a problem. Two methods of open-marsh drainage are used. In one, parallel ditches are run at regular intervals, either to a main ditch or directly to the main body of water. A more economical approach is to construct a ditch leading from all low spots holding water to the main body of water or to the natural sloughs or waterways in the marsh. These ditches may be curved somewhat to take in a number of the low spots or pools. Areas that are merely wet are not drained at first, as construction of the first drains frequently lowers the ground-water table sufficiently to dry up many of them. Free circulation of water through the drainage ditches permits the various predators to consume mosquito larvae. The top-water minnow (*Gambusia affinis*), which is discussed in Art. 9-26, is efficient for this purpose, but the stocking of salt water or brackish marshes should be done with specimens that have been accustomed to salt water as this species is primarily a freshwater fish. There are species of small saltwater fish that are common to many sections of the country, and these may be depended upon as an aid in keeping ditches clear of larvae.

The closed-drainage system is also known as the "reclamation method." It is used for large marshes and has the advantage of making the land usable for agricultural or other purposes. It has the disadvantage of allowing cracks and shrinkage, which require expensive remedies. In this method the tide is prevented from entering the area by means of a dyke or levee, and the surface water is allowed to escape in one or more outlets through the dyke. The outlets must, of course, be provided with flap gates of some type that will prevent water from entering the area during high tide. It may be necessary or advisable to pump the water into the sea or bay rather than to depend upon free drainage.

The dyke is usually constructed with a slope of 3 horizontal to 1 vertical if the height is not more than 6 ft, and the construction of a berm may be advisable. Frequently the top is made wide enough to provide a roadway for vehicles. The borrow pit, which provides earth for the dyke, is inside but far enough away so that there is no danger of a slide. The ground surface on which the dyke is to be placed should be scarified, or, better still, a cutoff trench should be dug to prevent leakage. The height must be great enough to protect against the highest tides—wave height and some freeboard. If the dyke fronts on the open sea, local inquiries must be made to determine wave heights to be expected. If the dyke is on a bay or harbor front, the following formula will give the wave height to be expected:

$$H = 1.5 \sqrt{R} + (2.5 - \sqrt[4]{R})$$

where H is the wave height in feet, and R is the reach in miles of the longest straight line that can be drawn from the dyke across the water surface of the bay or harbor.

If excessive wave action is expected, the front of the dyke may be protected with riprap or other facing materials.

The drainage gates, if 8 ft in width or less, are usually of the metal type. If they must be larger, wooden flap gates may be used. They should preferably be creosoted and suspended by 1½- or 2-in. galvanized pipe threaded through galvanized iron or bronze U-bolts. A channel of wood or concrete through the dyke will be necessary. This will require wing walls and an apron on the outlet side and may have to be supported on piling. The capacity must be great enough to carry off the runoff expected during the time the gates are discharging. The "rational" method of computing runoff of rainfall may be followed, as outlined in works dealing with hydrology or storm-sewer design. Runoff need only be rapid enough, however, to prevent the development of a crop of mosquitoes. If the outlets discharge into the open sea, protective works may be necessary to prevent damage by waves. These may take the form of timber structures supported by piles extending beyond the outlets to break the force of the waves.

The ditches used in salt-marsh drainage are often deep and narrow. Sometimes vertical sides are possible, particularly if there is a heavy mat of grass roots. In some cases the top foot is sloped 1:1, and the rest of the ditch has vertical sides. Ditches are excavated with machinery as far as possible. In recent years excavating machinery has been developed which has its weight distributed over a large bearing so that it can operate on soft ground. Ditches must be maintained so that fish can circulate and the water can move out freely.

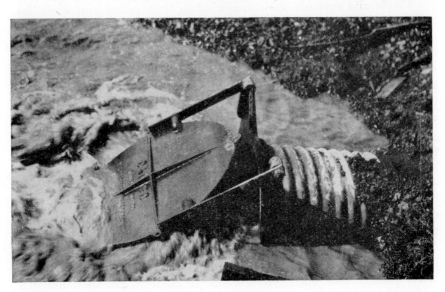

Figure 9-9   Armco flap gate discharging at low tide.

9-19. Filling. Areas that cannot be drained can sometimes be economically and adequately kept from breeding mosquitoes by filling. Large fills along waterfronts may be accomplished with hydraulic dredges. In some cases it is possible to fill low areas on the outskirts of towns with rubbish. The sanitary fill described in Chap. 5 should be used in this type of situation. Street sweepings are also of value for filling purposes.

9-20. Larviciding. The larvae and pupae of the common varieties of mosquitoes are air breathers and must come to the water surface to renew their air supply. Oil, when applied to the water, forms a film over the water surface, and when larvae return to the surface, some of it will enter the breathing tubes. The oils used have a poisoning rather than a mere clogging effect. If mosquito larvae are exposed to kerosene and then removed to clear water, they will die in about 15 min, practically the same length of time required to kill those remaining beneath a kerosene film. With the heavier crude oils, 3 hr may be required before the larvae die. Pupae are somewhat more resistant than larvae.

Other larvicides have superseded oil to a great extent. The choice depends upon economy, ease of handling, and applicability to a situation.

9-21. Oils Used. Petroleum oils are used. Kerosene is a rapid destroyer of mosquito larvae, and it also has the advantage of good spreading ability. Its disadvantages are its cost, compared with some other oils; quick evaporation from the surface of the water, particularly in hot weather; and a lack of color, which makes it difficult for the oiler to be certain that he has adequately covered the water surface.

Crude and fuel oils vary somewhat in toxic power and spreading ability. The latter quality is usually the governing factor. Proper spreading can be obtained by diluting a heavy oil with a sufficient amount of kerosene or a small amount of spreader. The fuel oils have the advantage of being easily inspected for continuous film, and in addition they will remain on the water surface for several days, thereby increasing the intervals between applications. What is known to the oil trade as a No. 2 diesel oil will usually be satisfactory without admixtures.

Spreading agents used are sodium lauryl sulfate (Gardinol), alkyl polyether alcohol (Triton X-100), and B-1956 [6].

Objections are sometimes raised to the oiling of some waters, such as ornamental ponds and areas where fish and waterfowl are raised or encouraged to congregate. An oil-pyrethrum larvicide has been developed by Ginsburg [1] that will be reasonably efficient wherever oil is objectionable. It is primarily an oil emulsion of the following composition: 66 per cent kerosene or similar light petroleum distillate, 0.07 per cent pyrethrins, 33.5 per cent water, and 0.5 per cent sodium lauryl sulfate. This stock emulsion can be made by the user, but it is preferable to purchase it from manufacturers, who sell it under the name of New Jersey Larvicide. In the field it is diluted with 10 parts of water before spraying. The film produced is not lasting, but there is no injury to waterfowl, fish, or plants. It is more costly than oil.

9-22. Oil Application. Oil is applied by means of spraying apparatus that will produce an even thin film over the water surface. Hand and power equipment of various sizes is used for this purpose. The conventional hand sprayer consists of a tank to hold the liquid, a nozzle for regulating the size of droplets and rate of discharge, and an internal or external liquid pump or built-in air pump to supply the force for moving the liquid through a flexible hose to the nozzle [11]. A typical power sprayer consists of a tank with an agitator to hold the liquid, an engine to supply power, a pressure regulator and relief valve, and a flexible line to carry the liquid to the discharge system, consisting of a hand-operated shutoff valve and nozzle. A relatively new type of power unit, the mist-blower machine, has been found to have wide application in mosquito-control work. This unit consists essentially of an engine-driven blower added to a low-pressure power sprayer. The spray material is discharged through nozzles or a shear plate into the air stream produced by the blower. This principle gives the machine a range effective to several hundred feet, depending on the amount of foliage, the direction and velocity of the wind, and the terrain.

The edges of reservoirs have been oiled by the Tennessee Valley Authority from flat-bottomed boats 4 to 5 ft wide, 24 ft long, 2 ft deep, and with a draft of 10 in. They are square and shallow at the ends so that approach to mudbanks is easy. Either outboard or inboard motors are installed for locomotion. If an inboard motor is used, a spray pump is powered from a friction wheel connected to the motor flywheel; otherwise, the spray pump must have a separate motor of its own. The former method is more desirable. The pump draws water from a 6-in. pipe well and also draws oil from a tank; the mixture, which contains 95 per cent or more of water, is applied through a hose for a distance of 30 to 50 ft.

The amount of oil required will depend upon conditions. Losses caused by vegetation and uneven application are likely to result in application figures of 20 to 60 gal of oil per acre of water surface covered. Addition of spreading agents mentioned above may allow use of only 5 to 10 gals/acre. The amount of oil applied by one man, using a hand sprayer, in an 8-hr day is also variable, but it should be within the limits of 40 to 80 gal/day.

In large bodies of water, oiling is necessary only along the edges or in patches of vegetation where the larvae are protected from wave action and natural enemies. Oiling should be done at frequent enough intervals to prevent emergence of a crop of mosquitoes. The interval will depend upon the type of mosquito and the weather. Inspectors in charge of oiling should check the work of oilers to ensure their efficiency.

Oiling must be done on water that cannot be drained or on streams, particularly where there are overhanging banks and quiet pools and where control by minnows cannot be obtained. Oiling should not be depended upon too greatly in streams or pools that are overgrown with vegetation which will prevent access of oil to all parts. Such sheltering vegetation must be cleared from the stream if good control is to be obtained. Poorly maintained ditches of unpaved streets need attention. The practice of allowing the discharge of waste water from residences into street ditches results in unnecessary work. A permanent remedy, either sewer connection or subsurface drainage, should be required.

Storm sewers will sometimes hold water in the sewer itself or in catch basins. Such breeding may be prevented by pouring oil into the water of the catch basin, but frequently it will be found of advantage to use one of the other larvicides mentioned later.

9-23. Chlorinated Hydrocarbon Larvicides. The most widely used of these compounds are DDT, benzene hexachloride (BHC), lindane, chlordane, heptachlor, and dieldrin. See Chap. 8. In many situations they are the cheapest, longest lasting, and most effective of the larvicides. However, they have some disadvantages. All, when used where they will leave residues on vegetation that is eaten by cattle, may later appear in meat and milk at levels above the tolerance allowed by the Food and Drug Administration. They may be destructive to fish, particularly if used above the recommended rates of application. In some areas certain

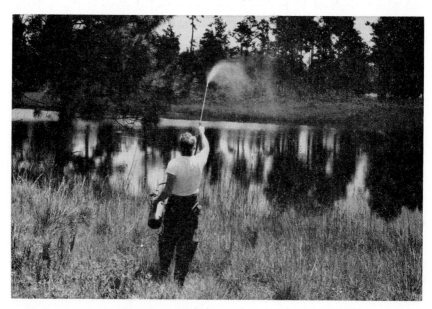

Figure 9-10 Applying DDT larvicide with a hand sprayer. (*Courtesy of Public Health Service.*)

species of *Culex, Aedes,* and *Anopheles* have become resistant to the chlorinated hydrocarbons, thus requiring the use of one of the other larvicides or adulticides. They are used as emulsions, solutions, or dusts or in pellets. Power and hand dusters and sprays are used [11].

TEMPORARY LARVICIDES. The formulations and dosages given below are recommended by the Public Health Service [7]:

DDT. Mix 1 part of 25 per cent emulsifiable concentrate of DDT with 24 parts of water. Use at 2.5 gallons per acre to obtain 0.2 pound DDT per acre.

Dissolve 0.1 pound of technical grade DDT in 1 gallon of Diesel oil. Apply 2 gallons per acre to obtain 0.2 pound DDT per acre.

In airplane application apply (*a*) 1 pint of 20 per cent DDT emulsion or solution, or (*b*) 2 quarts of 5 per cent DDT emulsion or solution per acre, to obtain 0.2 pound of DDT per acre.

Apply 4 pounds of 5 per cent DDT dust or pellets per acre, to obtain about 0.2 pound of DDT per acre.

Benzene Hexachloride, 12 per cent gamma isomer (BHC). Mix 1 part of 20 per cent emulsifiable concentrate with 19 parts of water or fuel oil.

Use at a rate of 2.5 gallons per acre, to obtain 0.2 pound per acre.

Three per cent agricultural dust. Apply at 3 to 7 pounds per acre to obtain about 0.1 to 0.2 pound BHC per acre.

Chlordane. Mix 1 part of 25 per cent emulsifiable concentrate with 24 parts of water. Apply 1¼ gallons per acre to obtain 0.1 pound of chlordane per acre.

Mix 1 part 46 per cent emulsifiable concentrate with 45 parts of water. Use 1¼ gallons per acre to obtain 0.1 pound of chlordane per acre.

Heptachlor and Dieldrin. Mix 1 part of 20 per cent emulsifiable concentrate with 39 parts of water or Diesel oil. Use 2.5 gallons per acre to obtain 0.1 pound of heptachlor or dieldrin per acre. Apply 2 pounds of pellets to obtain 0.1 pound of insecticide per acre.

Tossits. These are small plastic containers holding emulsifiable concentrates of DDT, BHC, or malathion, and a spreading agent. When tossed upon water the insecticide is released. One tossit will cover 100 to 1,000 square feet of water surface depending upon the flotage, shape of the water and its temperature. They do not always work well in cold water and they are rather expensive. They are useful for treating small puddles and inaccessible breeding places.

RESIDUAL LARVICIDES. Heavier applications of the above insecticides will give longer-lasting larvicidal action. They may be used as emulsions, solutions, or granules. The length of the effect will depend upon water depth and movement, and it may be from 5 to 52 weeks. Application rates used per acre are DDT, 1 to 6 lb; heptachlor, 6 lb; dieldrin, 1 to 3 lb; and BHC, 1 lb.

Residual larviciding with DDT or dieldrin at 1 lb or more per acre

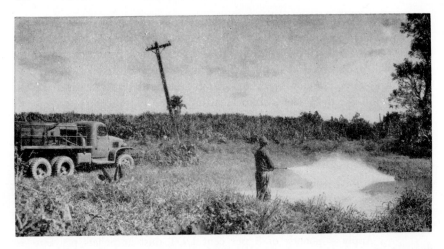

FIGURE 9-11   Applying oil solution of DDT with a power sprayer. (*Courtesy of Public Health Service.*)

is totally destructive to fish. The chlorinated hydrocarbons should always be used with caution where fish life is a matter of concern.

9-24. Organic Phosphorus Insecticides. These are sometimes called organophosphorus insecticides and are sold under various names. Malathion and parathion are much used. They have the advantages of being effective with mosquitoes resistant to the chlorinated hydrocarbons, and malathion is recommended for use in pastures or croplands producing forage [7]. Resistance to malathion has also developed in some areas. Malathion is available as 20 and 25 per cent emulsifiable concentrates which are diluted 1:19 or 1:24 with water and applied at the rate of 3 to 6 gal/acre to obtain an application of 0.25 to 0.50 lb of malathion per acre. Parathion concentrates are usually applied by airplane at a rate of about 0.1 lb of the insecticide per acre. Parathion was used in pellet form applied by airplane to treat a large salt-marsh area when freak weather conditions produced a tremendous mosquito production at Tampa Fla. [7]. Parathion is extremely toxic to humans, and precautions in its handling and use are necessary to prevent fatal poisoning. Pilots and workmen loading airplanes with parathion should wear masks and take precautions to prevent spills.

9-25. Paris Green. This arsenic compound was formerly used mixed with hydrated lime, powdered talc, or other inert materials and was blown over water to kill the surface-feeding anopheline larvae. Development of mosquitoes resistant to DDT and other insecticides has renewed interest in paris green, to which resistance apparently does not occur. A paris green–vermiculite mixture successfully used in Florida against anophelines and culicines [7] is:

53 lb of vermiculite (No. 4 Zonolite or Institute grade)

15 lb of paris green (60 per cent commercial 90 per cent paris green and 40 per cent calcium carbonate or marble dust)

30 lb of emulsifier oil sticker (Triton-101 or Tween 20)

The vermiculite and emulsifier are first mixed in a concrete mixer so that the surface of the vermiculite becomes well coated with the sticker. The paris green is then added until the mixture is uniformly green. It is blown on the water surface from the ground at the rate of 6 to 8 lb of the mixture per acre. Commercially prepared granules are also available. The granules float for several hours, during which time the poison is released through the action of the wetting agent in the sticker and is available to the surface-feeding *Anopheles* larvae. The powder settles slowly through the water, where it may be ingested by the culicines.

9-26. Natural Enemies. The mosquito has natural enemies. Dragonflies, birds, and bats prey upon the winged mosquito. Dragonfly larvae and other aquatic insects feed upon the larvae and pupae. However, of the natural enemies, only fish are useful from a practical standpoint.

The most important fish are several species of minnows. While the top-feeding minnows are not naturally present in all parts of the country, observation will probably result in the discovery of some local fish that is effective as a larvae destroyer. It is also possible to import top-feeding minnows from more favored localities for the purpose of stocking mosquito breeding places. Goldfish are of little value in keeping ornamental pools clean of larvae.

Mosquito control by fish is cheap. Fish, however, have their limitations under natural conditions, and too much reliance must not be placed upon their unaided efforts.

The top-water minnow, also known as the potbellied minnow (*Gambusia affinis*), is naturally distributed along the Atlantic Coast from Delaware to Mexico, in the Mississippi Valley from Louisiana to Illinois, and in Texas. It grows to a maximum length of approximately 3 in. Because it feeds voraciously upon larvae and pupae and multiplies rapidly, it is a particularly valuable fish to be used in stocking mosquito breeding waters. It bears its young alive in successive broods numbering up to 50 or more throughout the spring and summer. It is very hardy and is able to live equally well in brackish water, fresh water, or water with some pollution. It gets the name "top-water minnow" from its habit of surface feeding. One specimen was observed to eat 165 mosquito larvae in 1 day. The young minnows will start feeding on the larvae immediately after they are born.

Mosquito larvae seek protection in floating debris and in vegetation. Therefore, clearing the edges of bodies of water may be necessary. It is difficult to say how many fish will be necessary to prevent mosquito breeding. Few may be needed in a clean-edged pool, while great num-

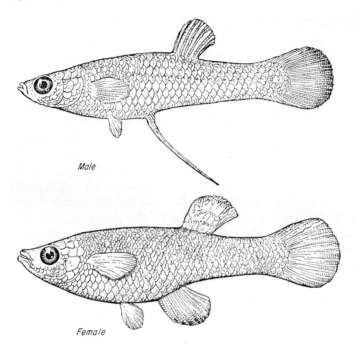

Male

Female

FIGURE 9-12   The top-water minnow, *Gambusia affinis*. (*After U.S. Bureau of Fisheries.*)

bers may be ineffective where the shores are heavily lined with vegetation. Observations must be made to determine whether control has been established or whether assistance to the fish, in the form of clearing or larviciding, may be necessary.

Gambusia is a prolific breeder, which makes it easy to establish hatcheries that will provide a supply of minnows for stocking such water as accumulates under deep culverts, watering troughs, wells, rain barrels, ponds, and streams which occasionally dry up. They may be shipped long distances in order to start a hatchery in the locality in which they are needed. The same precautions should be taken in shipping as are necessary in the transportation of live fish by government hatcheries, *i.e.*, keeping the water cool in transit.

Measures against Adults

9-27. Space Spraying. In homes and other enclosed spaces *aerosol bombs* are much used to kill mosquitoes and flies. Such "bug bombs" contain pyrethrum or allethrin to obtain a quick knockdown. These are relatively nontoxic to humans. They also contain a synergist such as piperonyl butoxide and a low-toxicity insecticide such as DDT or

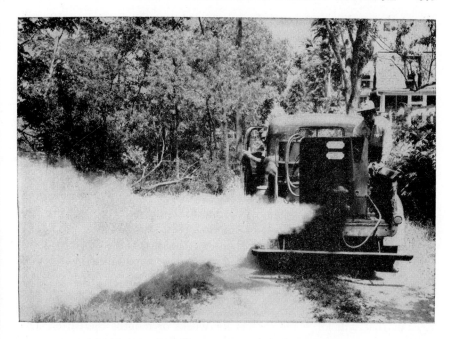

FIGURE 9-13   "Fogging" with DDT for control of adult mosquitoes.

methoxychlor to effect the final kill. The propellant is Freon, a refrigerant used in many electric refrigerators. Release of the aerosol for a few seconds will kill flying insects in an ordinary-sized room, tent, or trailer. There is no hazard to humans if the bomb is used as directed.

Fogging or misting is carried on by a number of organized mosquito-control districts in populated areas. The insecticides used against *Aedes*, *Culex*, and *Psorophora* mosquitoes are fuel-oil solutions or emulsions of DDT, chlordane, lindane, or malathion [12]. Application rates success-fully used are:

Insecticide	Pounds of technical grade insecticide per acre	Gallons of insecticide mix per lin mile with effective kill in 100–150-ft swaths
5 per cent DDT	0.3–0.5	10–15
2.5 per cent chlordane	0.1–0.2	6–12
2 per cent lindane	0.1–0.2	5–10
3 per cent malathion	0.5	8–12

Mist and fog applicators are of various types [11]. Mist is composed of particles which settle at a relatively rapid rate. Mists are therefore directed over housetops and the particles, in winds of not over 10 mph, will settle slowly enough to be effective in swaths up to 200 ft wide. Fogs have much finer particles, and they are directed as near the ground as possible. Width of swath will depend upon rate of travel and wind velocity. Particles emitted should not be smaller than 10 μ in diameter; particles of this size will settle at the rate of 1.66 ft/min. Misting or fogging should be conducted in late afternoon, early evening, at night, or in the early morning when the air is calm or winds vary from 1 to 5 mph. During this period inversions may occur that will cause fog to remain close to the ground. On a hot day rising thermal currents may disperse the insecticides into the upper atmosphere.

Where larviciding is also practiced in fogged or misted areas it is recommended that an organic phosphorus insecticide be used for one process and a chlorinated carbon for the other. It is probably preferable to use the chlorinated hydrocarbons as the larvicide. Obviously this will tend to prevent the development of a population of resistant mosquitoes.

9-28. Residual Spraying. When applied to surfaces, the chlorinated hydrocarbons and organic phosphorus insecticides will leave a film of crystals that will kill some insects for weeks or months thereafter. This method of mosquito control is well adapted to *Anopheles* mosquitoes

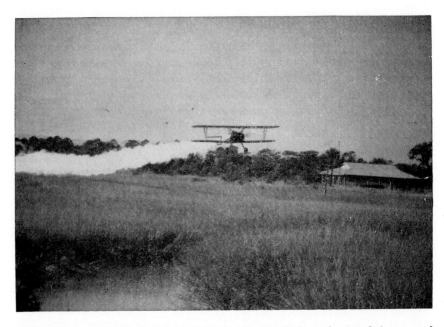

FIGURE 9-14 Spraying from an airplane with DDT thermal aerosol for control of adults and larvae of mosquitoes. (*Courtesy of Public Health Service.*)

which enter buildings and rest on surfaces. It has been very successful in reducing malaria in the worldwide campaign sponsored by the World Health Organization.

A residual-spraying campaign will prevent transmission of the disease. If medical treatment is given to persons already infected, the disease will soon be eradicated from the control area. A follow-up system should be instituted to resume spraying in the small areas where new cases are reported. Mosquitoes develop resistance to the insecticides, and this may necessitate changing from one to another; but if the work is carefully done, malaria eradication may be accomplished before resistance is established.

Residual spraying is also effective against other house-frequenting mosquitoes, including the encephalitis vectors, *Culex tarsalis, C. quinquefasciatus,* and *C. pipiens,* and the vector of yellow fever and dengue, *Aedes aegypti.*

Houseflies and other flies, and to some extent cockroaches and bedbugs, are controlled by residual spraying for mosquitoes. Chagas' disease can also be controlled or eradicated by the method since the vector (*Triatoma* sp.), which usually hides in cracks in walls in the daytime, will be killed.

In the United States the most commonly used residual spray is a 5 per cent water emulsion or solution in oil of DDT applied at the rate of 200 mg of DDT per sq ft. This is 1 gal of 5 per cent spray per 1,000 sq ft. Emulsions or solutions are preferred to suspensions since they do not leave unsightly deposits on painted walls, wallpaper, or furniture. A spraying should be effective against anophelines for one mosquito breeding season.

Where mosquitoes are DDT-resistant, sprays have been used containing 1.25 per cent dieldrin or BHC, or 2.5 per cent malathion. Malathion may require an application of only 100 mg/sq ft.

In tropical areas, suspensions which are made of wettable powder and water are used. They are absorbed to a lesser extent by surfaces, and the powdery deposit is not noticeable or objectionable on adobe, mud, or thatched walls or roofs.

The compressed-air sprayer of 1 to 5 gal capacity is much used for residual spraying. The tank is filled ⅔ to ¾ full of the liquid, and the air above is compressed by the air pump, or other source of compressed air, to a pressure of 50 psi. Spraying then proceeds until the pressure drops to about 30 psi. The pressure is then raised to 50 psi, and thus an average pressure of 40 psi is maintained. A proper combination of pressure, spray nozzle, and skill of the workman is necessary to obtain the desired coverage.

The Public Health Service [7] recommends the Teejet nozzle[1] for

¹ Manufactured by Spraying Systems, Inc., Bellwood, Ill.

spraying emulsions, solutions, and suspensions. Four Teejet nozzles have been used: 8002, 8004, 5002, and 5004. They produce flat fan-shaped sprays having an angle of 80 or 50 deg and at an average pressure will deliver either 0.2 or 0.4 gpm. The 8002 and 5002 jets have small openings and are used for emulsions and solutions, while the 8004 and 5004, with larger openings, are used for suspensions.

The worker faces the wall and moves the spray nozzle up and down to cover it in successive strips. To produce a 30-in. swath, the 8002 and 8004 nozzles are held about 18 in. from the wall, and the 5002 and 5004 are held 24 in. away. Complete coverage requires an overlap of 3 in. on each 30-in. swath. To obtain 200 mg/sq ft, 5 per cent DDT should be sprayed with an 8002 or 5002 nozzle at a rate of about 200 sq ft/min, which is approximately 1 gal per 100 sq ft in 5 min. If the 8004 or 5004 nozzle is used, concentration of the spray is reduced by one-half to compensate for the nozzle delivery rate, which is twice that of the 8002 and 5002 nozzles.

If a deposit of 100 mg/sq ft of malathion or some other insecticide is desired, 8002 or 5002 nozzles may be used with 2.2 per cent sprays or 8004 or 5004 sprays with 1.25 per cent suspension.

9-29. Protection against Mosquitoes. Screens, bed nets, protective clothing, and repellents may be necessary for protection to workers and others in malarial regions and salt-marsh areas. Bed nets and screens provide protection during sleeping hours and thus prevent infection from night-biting *Anopheles* mosquitoes.

SCREENING. Screens are made of galvanized iron, copper, bronze, aluminum, and plastics. Plastic screens are desirable near the ocean since they are not affected by the corrosive action of salt sprays. Screens should fit tightly and be kept in repair. Most screens have 16 meshes to the inch, and this will exclude most mosquitoes except the small *Aedes aegypti* and *A. taeniorhynchus*. Accordingly 20 or more meshes to the inch is recommended. Screen doors should open outward to discourage mosquitoes from entering with people. Residual sprays, preferably a 5 per cent solution of DDT in kerosene, applied on and around the screen door will be beneficial. Some solvents or emulsifiers such as xylene are corrosive to screens.

BED NETS. These are useful in camps or in the tropics. Netting of cotton or nylon with 23 to 26 meshes to the inch should be used. It should be suspended over the bed and tucked in around the mattress, and it should be large enough so that one can sit up under it. Mosquitoes which have entered the net should be killed with an aerosol bomb before retiring.

PROTECTIVE CLOTHING. This may be necessary for outdoor workers in salt marshes or irrigated fields. Head nets, gloves, knee-length boots, and clothing of closely woven material provide considerable protection. Head nets of four to six meshes to the inch will provide visibility. They should be treated with a repellent.

REPELLENTS. These are applied to the skin and clothing to repel salt-marsh, *Psorophora*, and other viciously biting and persistent mosquitoes. A number of repellents have been developed, of which a few will be mentioned. Indalone gives protection when applied to skin or clothing. Diethyl toluamide, which is also known as deet and which is sold commercially in drugstores as Det and Off, is very effective against most types of mosquitoes and is relatively long-lasting. It is applied to skin or clothing as a liquid from bottles or as a spray from pressurized cans.

Fly Control

9-30. Flies and Disease. There are many varieties of flies. Some are vicious biters, such as the biting stable fly, deerflies, horseflies, sand flies, black flies, and tsetse flies. Some of these transmit human disease, for example, the tsetse fly, which carries sleeping sickness in Africa, and a type of black fly (*Simulium*), which conveys onchocerciasis in parts of Mexico, Guatamala, Venezuela, and Africa. Biting flies as transmitters of human disease are not important in the United States.

Flies are mainly important as mechanical transmitters of human disease. The housefly is probably the most important fly in the United States in this respect. It becomes infected by feeding, crawling, and breeding in human excreta. It may then transmit pathogenic bacteria to human food from its mouth parts, by vomitus, and from its sticky foot pads and body and leg hairs. Diseases known to have been so transmitted are typhoid fever, paratyphoid fever, bacillary dysentery, amoebic dysentery, infantile diarrhea, pinworm, roundworm, whipworm, hookworm, and tapeworm [13].

Other domestic flies such as the green, bronze, and blue bottle flies; the black blowflies; and the lesser housefly may also carry the above-mentioned diseases mechanically. The eye gnat in some areas is supposed to transmit the eye disease conjunctivitis mechanically.

Some flies are capable of laying eggs or larvae on the flesh or in wounds of mammals or other animals. The larvae thus invade the flesh of the host, a condition known as myiasis. Wild animals and many domestic animals, such as cows and sheep, are frequent victims. Human cases of myiasis, although uncommon, occur in all parts of the United States. The larvae of the primary screwworm fly are able to bore into living flesh and cause considerable injury and even death to the host.

9-31. Life Cycle of Domestic Flies. In general, flies go through the stages of egg, larva, and pupa. A few species retain eggs in their bodies until hatching and produce larvae. Time of life cycle and preferred

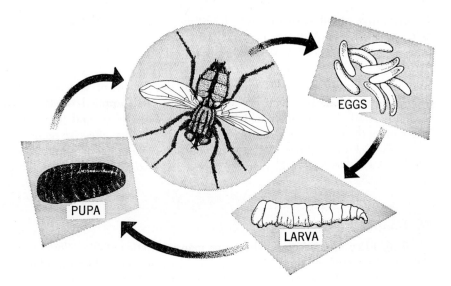

EGGS

PUPA

LARVA

Figure 9-15 Life history of the housefly. (*From H. G. Scott and K. S. Littig,* "*Flies of Public Health Importance and Their Control,*" *Public Health Service, Communicable Disease Center,* 1962.)

breeding places will vary with the species and also with the temperature and nature of the habitat.

HOUSEFLY. The housefly (*Musca domestica*) is the most numerous of the domestic flies, and because of its part in the transmission of disease and its close association with man it is considered the most important of the flies in the United States from the standpoint of human health.

The female begins laying eggs within 4 to 20 days after emerging as an adult. The eggs are white, oval, and about ⅟₂₅ in. long, and they are deposited in batches of 75 to 150. The average female will lay five or six batches in her lifetime. The eggs are usually deposited in cracks of the breeding medium away from direct sunlight. In summer temperatures, eggs hatch in 12 to 24 hr. The larvae burrow into the breeding medium, feed, and are ready to pupate in 3 to 24 days, usually 4 to 7 days. Larvae may be killed at high temperatures. They prefer temperatures from 86 to 95°F, but when ready to pupate they seek places of lower temperature and drier conditions. The pupae are shaped like elongated barrels, are about ¼ in. long, and are dark red to brown in color. They form at the dry edges of the breeding medium, or the larvae may first burrow into the soil. The pupal state usually lasts from 4 to 5 days but may be only 3 days at 95°F or several weeks at low temperatures. The adult fly emerges, burrows through soil if necessary, and crawls about until its wings unfold and its body dries and hardens.

This requires about 1 hr in summer temperatures, but 15 hr is required before complete activity is reached. Mating may take place any time after complete activity is achieved. It will be seen that the minimum period for a life cycle is about 8 days.

Houseflies will breed in almost any moist, warm organic material that will furnish nutriment to the larvae. Favorite media are manures of horses, pigs, and fowl. Somewhat less attractive is cow manure. Breeding will also occur in human excrement in privies or elsewhere, and since it may contain pathogenic organisms it is the most dangerous material. Insufficiently digested sewage sludge is also a breeding place. In populated areas, garbage stored in open containers, allowed to accumulate in piles, or placed in open dumps is an important source of houseflies.

Houseflies may fly for long distances. They rapidly disperse from breeding places and may travel as far as 6 miles within 24 hr. Flies that were tagged with radioactive materials were released and caught in baited traps placed around the releasing point. Most of the radioactive flies were caught within 1 mile, but a few were taken 20 miles away [13]. They will live 2 to 4 weeks in midsummer and longer in cool weather. They are most active at 90°F, but at 112°F they will die. They overwinter as hibernating adults and with more or less continuous breeding in protected locations, such as stables or barns.

THE LESSER HOUSEFLY. This fly (*Fannia* sp.) resembles the housefly but is markedly smaller in size. It breeds in excrement of humans and animals and also in decaying vegetable matter, such as piles of decaying grass.

THE BITING STABLE FLY. The stable fly (*Stomoxys calcitrans*) resembles the housefly in appearance, but its biting habits soon indicate a difference. It breeds in decomposing vegetable matter only, and its life cycle requires 21 to 25 days. It is not considered important as a disease transmitter to man, but it transmits several diseases of animals.

BOTTLE FLIES AND BLOWFLIES. These flies deposit eggs on meat, which they are said to "bottle" or "blow." They include the black blowfly (*Phormia* sp.), green and bronze bottle flies (*Phaenicia* sp. and others), and the blue bottle flies (*Cynomyopsis* sp. and *Calliphora*). These flies enter houses and restaurants much less frequently than houseflies. Therefore, they are not considered so great a threat to human health as the housefly. They breed preferably in decomposing animal matter but will lay eggs on any fresh or decomposing plant refuse if meat is not available. The life cycles of these flies are much the same as the life cycle of the housefly. They are also strong fliers. The larvae of many species cause human and animal myiasis.

FLESH FLIES. These belong to the *Sarcophaga* genus. They are rather large, and the abdomen has a red tip. The larvae of most species are

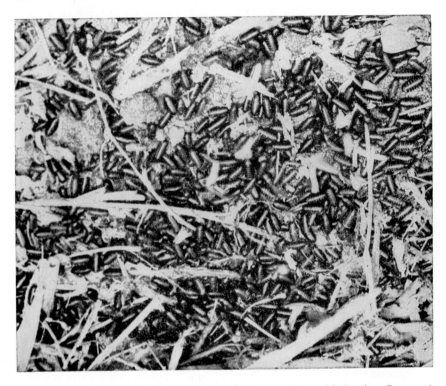

Figure 9-16   Fly pupae. (*Photograph courtesy of Public Health Service, Communicable Disease Center.*)

found in meat, but breeding also occurs in animal excrement. Some species deposit living larvae rather than eggs. They are not considered important as mechanical vectors of disease since they seldom enter houses or restaurants. They cause human myiasis.

9-32. Fly-control Measures. These include (1) environmental sanitation measures, such as a means of preventing fly breeding and also protection of food against infection by flies; (2) destruction of larvae; and (3) destruction of adults.

Fly-control work should be a part of the environmental health work of local health departments. Fly-control campaigns may be advisable as a method of arousing public interest and to get antifly measures started, particularly when permanent improvements are necessary.

9-33. The Community Fly-control Program. The program must be carefully planned and made into a cooperative endeavor since individual sanitary measures are of small value unless similar action is taken throughout the area. An initial survey of the community should be made to locate actual and potential breeding areas and principal fly densities and to determine the extent of the control area and kind of control

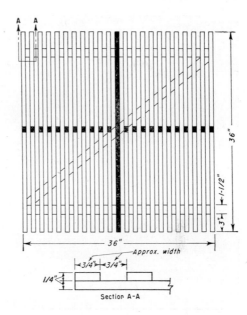

FIGURE 9-17   Fly-counting grille.

measures to be applied. Environmental-control measures should be depended upon to secure major reductions in fly populations since application of chemicals is not a substitute for sanitation.

The operation of a community-wide program should include routine checks of fly-population densities on regular schedules to determine the effectiveness of the control measures being applied and to indicate where and when operations are needed. Use of the same means for each check of fly densities will provide comparable data. This may be accomplished by using the Scudder grille (see Fig. 9-17). It is made of unplaned boards ¾ in. wide, ¼ in. thick, and 36 in. long, spaced

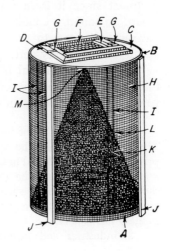

FIGURE 9-18   Conical flytrap, side view. A, hoops forming frame at bottom; B, hoops forming frame at top; C, top of trap made of barrel head; D, strips around door; E, door frame; F, screen on door; G, buttons holding door; H, screen on outside of trap; I, strips on side of trap between hoops; J, tips of these strips projecting to form legs; K, cone; L, united edges of screen forming cone; M, aperture of apex of cone. (After Bishopp, courtesy of U.S. Department of Agriculture.)

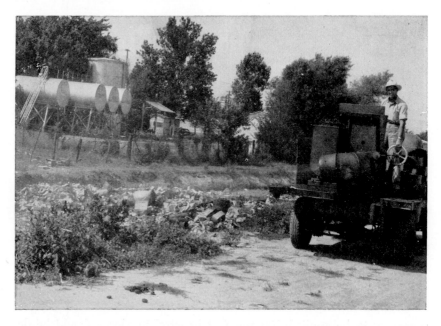

FIGURE 9-19   Treating an accumulation of refuse with a Buffalo turbine. (*Photograph courtesy of Public Health Service, Communicable Disease Center.*)

¾ in. apart on a light "z" frame. In making a count, the grille is placed over an attractant, such as garbage or manure, disturbing the flies. Those that return and alight on the slats are then counted, and species may also be noted. Baited flytraps may be used when it is desired to make surveys for species determination (see Fig. 9-18).

The fly-control program is usually operated by the local health department since it is in constant contact with many establishments in regard to sanitary conditions. The program should include educational measures directed to the public. The campaign should be continuous and not a temporary activity.

9-34. Environmental Measures. Community environmental or sanitation measures are directed toward prevention of fly breeding and prevention of fly transmission of disease. They will include the following:

1. The elimination of insanitary privies, particularly the open-back type. The requirement should be sewer connections or, if this is impossible, sanitary privies of a type described in Chap. 4.

2. Garbage should be stored in flytight containers. It and other refuse should be disposed of in such a manner that fly breeding is prevented. Incineration or sanitary fill may be used (Chap. 5). Compaction of earth over sanitary fills is necessary to prevent emergence of flies from pupae.

3. Industries and businesses which accumulate manure or other fly-

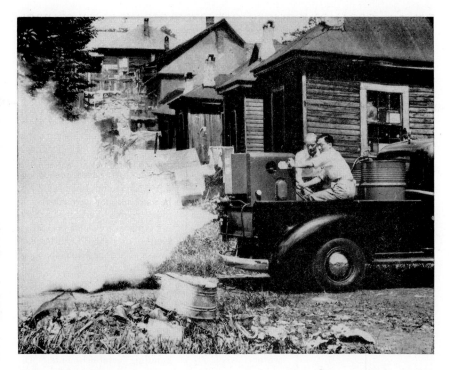

Figure 9-20 "Fogging" for fly control. (*Photograph courtesy of Public Health Service, Communicable Disease Center.*)

breeding materials should be required to store or dispose of such materials so that fly emergence will not occur. This will apply to dairies, abattoirs, chicken farms, dog kennels, and industries that have decomposable animal and vegetable wastes. Sewage treatment plants will also require scrutiny.

4. Restaurants, bakeries, and all food-processing plants should be screened, and they should also take other measures that will protect the food from flies.

5. Weeds provide cover for flies, make fogging and misting less effective, and may conceal accumulations of fly-producing material. Local health departments are justified in requiring reasonable weed control on vacant property.

9-35. Larvicidal Measures. If manure is removed daily and spread immediately upon fields or stored in flytight containers until it is spread, no fly breeding will occur. Dry conditions will kill larvae, and dry material is not attractive to flies. Heaps of manure can be treated with Diazinon or malathion emulsions or other insecticides. See Table 9-4.

9-36. Adulticidal Methods. Space sprays recommended for indoor use are of 0.1 per cent pyrethrins with synergizing agents. For outdoor use (fogging) the following are used: 5 per cent DDT, 2 per cent lindane, or 5 per cent malathion, all as emulsions or suspensions. Flies become resistant to insecticides.

Table 9-4.   ORGANOPHOSPHORUS INSECTICIDES FOR USE IN FLY CONTROL

Type of application	Toxicant	Formulations (for 50 gal finished spray)	Remarks
Residual	Bayer 29493	1.0–1.5 gal 46% EC plus water	Add sugar (25 lb) to formulation for maximum residual effectiveness. Spray surfaces at a rate of 2 or more gal per 1,000 sq ft. Maximum strength permitted for Bayer 29493, 1.5%; Diazinon, Dibrom, dimethoate, and ronnel, 1.0%; and malathion, 5.0%. Diazinon and ronnel can be used in dairy barns including milk rooms and meat-packing and other food-processing plants.* Malathion can be used in dairy barns and meat-packing establishments, but in milk rooms and other food-processing plants* it is acceptable *only* when the premium-grade material is used. Dibrom is labeled for use in dairy barns (except in milk rooms) and in food-handling establishments.* Dimethoate is accepted for treating dairy barns and poultry houses; it should not be used in milk rooms. Bayer 29493 is not labeled for use in dairies, poultry houses, or food-processing plants. None is accepted for complete interior treatment of houses. **Avoid contamination of human and animal food and of watering troughs. Do not treat milk rooms or food-processing areas while in operation.**
	Diazinon	2 gal 25% EC or 16 lb 25% WP plus water	
	Dibrom	1 gal 50% EC plus water	
	Dimethoate	1 gal 50% EC plus water	
	Malathion	2–4.5 gal 55% EC or 32–64 lb 25% WP plus water	
	Ronnel	2 gal 25% EC or 16 lb 25% WP plus water	
Impregnated cord	Parathion and Diazinon	To be prepared by experienced formulators only	Install at rate of 30 lin ft of cord per 100 sq ft of floor area. Accepted for use in dairies and food-processing plants.* Handle and install cords per manufacturer's instructions.

NOTE: EC, emulsifiable concentrate; WP, wettable powder; SP, soluble powder.

* Includes dairies, milk rooms, restaurants, canneries, food stores, warehouses, and similar establishments. As state regulations may prohibit the use of certain of these toxicants in milk rooms or at other sites, the individual should be certain that his usage conforms with local restrictions.

SOURCE: Communicable Disease Center: 1962 Report on Public Health Pesticides, *Pest Control*, vol. 30, no. 3, March, 1962.

Table 9-4.   ORGANOPHOSPHORUS INSECTICIDES FOR USE IN FLY CONTROL
(*Continued*)

Type of application	Toxicant	Formulations (for 50 gal finished spray)	Remarks
Bait	Diazinon	1 lb 25% WP plus 24 lb sugar; 2 fl oz 25% EC plus 3 lb sugar in 3 gal water	Apply 3–4 oz (dry) or 1–3 gal (wet) per 1,000 sq ft in areas of high fly concentration. Repeat 1 to 6 times per week as required. Avoid application of bait to dirt or litter. The use of permanent bait stations will prolong the efficacy of each treatment. All toxicants are available as commercial baits which are labeled for use in dairies and in food-processing plants.* None of these baits should be employed inside homes. **Do not contaminate feed or watering troughs.**
	Malathion	2 lb 25% WP plus 23 lb sugar	
	Ronnel	2 pt 25% EC plus 3 lb sugar in 3 gal water	
	DDVP	3–6 fl oz 10% EC plus 3 lb sugar in 3 gal water	
	Dibrom	1.0 fl oz 50% EC plus 2.5 lb sugar in 2.5 gal water	
	Bayer L 13/59	1 lb 50% SP plus 4 lb sugar in 4 gal water	
Larvicide	Diazinon	1 fl oz 25% EC to 1 gal water	Apply 7–14 gal per 1,000 sq ft as a coarse spray. Repeat as necessary, usually every 10 days or less. For chicken droppings, use only where birds are caged. **Avoid contamination of feed or water and drift of spray on animals.**
	Malathion	5 fl oz 55% EC to 3 gal water	
	Ronnel	1 pt 25% EC to 3 gal water	
	DDVP	2 fl oz 10% EC to 1 gal water	

Residual sprays employ the organophosphorus insecticides, malathion, ronnel, DDVP, and Bayer L 13/59. For residual use in dairies, Diazinon, ronnel, and malathion are used in the amounts and by the methods given in Table 9-4. Note that contamination of human and animal food and water must be avoided and that animals should not be sprayed.

Impregnated cords are a variation of the residual-spray method. Cords are suspended vertically from the ceiling and high enough so that persons will not make contact with them with their heads. Flies will rest on the cords, particularly at night. Parathion cords will give good control for about 10 weeks, and Diazinon cords for 7 weeks. Since parathion is extremely toxic to humans, only experienced personnel should work with it. Diazinon cord is preferable, but this should also be handled with care. In either case, the cords should be handled only with rubber or cotton gloves, and if the skin comes into contact with the cord the area must be washed with soap and water immediately. Workers should not attempt to manufacture their own cord.

Fly baits are of some value when used as indicated in Table 9-4. They are placed where flies congregate.

Control of Some Other Arthropods of Public Health Importance

9-37. Cockroaches. Cockroaches harbor in cracks and crevices of houses; they will also live in sewers. They may carry the organisms of typhoid, dysentery, and food poisoning from sewers to the human foods on which they will subsist if provided the opportunity. They impart a disagreeable odor and taste to foods which they contaminate with feces and material regurgitated while feeding. Cockroaches prefer starchy materials such as bakery goods, cereals, and book bindings but will also feed upon leather, wallpaper, and dead animals. The four common species in the United States are the American, German, brown-banded, and oriental. Adults of some species are able to fly. They are principally nocturnal in their habits.

The eggs are laid in brown capsules, or egg cases, which are attached to inconspicuous surfaces. The German cockroach, however, carries the capsule attached to its body. This insect is the most active of the cockroaches. It is sometimes called the Croton bug and is probably the commonest cockroach to be found in restaurants. It is small, about ⅝ in. long. The brown-banded cockroach is difficult to control since, instead of confining its activities to kitchen and bathroom, it roams throughout the house, frequently placing its egg capsules in furniture. It is yellowish or reddish brown in color. The American cockroach is mahogany in color. It causes damage to book bindings, clothing, glossy paper with starch sizing, and labels of bottles. The oriental cockroach is dark brown or black. It prefers damp areas and is somewhat less domestic than other species. "Wild" colonies are common in yards and outbuildings.

The eggs of all species hatch into small nymphs, which resemble the adult but do not have wings. A succession of molts occurs during growth, and mature females and males appear at the last molt. The cycle requires varying periods, from 6 to 1,000 days at room temperature, varying according to the species. Longevity of the adult varies from 3 months to 1 year.

Control is accomplished by elimination of foods, storage of foods so that they will be protected, and use of insecticides. These are chlordane, 2.5 per cent; lindane, 1 per cent; malathion, 2 per cent; and Diazinon, 0.5 per cent, and they are sprayed into cracks or other hiding places. They are used as emulsions or oil solutions. Some roaches have acquired resistance to hydrocarbons, and this may necessitate use of organophosphorus insecticides [16].

9-38. Bedbugs. Some persons are extremely sensitive to bedbug bites, and others are hardly aware of them. Immediately after feeding, the bug defecates, and this material may enter the bite injury. The bedbug, however, has not been incriminated in the transmission of any communicable disease. Man is the preferred source of food, but the bugs will also feed upon poultry, mice, rats, and other animals.

Eggs are laid, one to five per day, over a period of 2 to 10 months, until approximately two hundred have been deposited. They are cemented to bedding or in cracks of furniture, walls, and ceilings. Development occurs through a series of molts to the adult and requires 18 to 56 days. A blood meal must be taken before each molt. Adults normally live 6 months to a year. The female may live nearly a year without food, and it can withstand freezing temperature for a considerable time. The adults harbor in furniture, walls, and clothing and may also be found on poultry. Control can be obtained by spraying infested dwellings with a 5 per cent DDT emulsion, paying special attention to cracks in or near beds and upholstered furniture. If bugs have become resistant to DDT, a 5 per cent emulsion of lindane can be used.

9-39. Lice. Lice transmit louse-borne or epidemic typhus, relapsing fever, and trench fever. These diseases are likely to occur when people are crowded together as in armies, jails, and refugee camps. Epidemic typhus fever has been known as "jail fever." History has noted a number of military campaigns which were affected by this disease in one of the armies engaged. In World War I, it was common on the Eastern front and also occurred in the civilian population there. On the Western front, trench fever caused more sickness than any other disease.

There are three human lice: the body louse, the head louse, and the crab louse. All may cause dermatitis, but the body louse, apparently, is the only important vector of epidemic typhus fever, relapsing fever, or trench fever. None of these diseases occurs in the United States at the present time.

The body louse rests on clothing except when feeding, and its eggs are attached to underclothing. Hatching is reduced or prevented by temperatures under 75 and over 100°F. The eggs hatch into nymphs, which molt three times before becoming mature. The nymphal stage requires 8 to 9 days but may require 2 to 4 weeks if clothing is removed at night. If the clothes are not worn for several days, the lice will usually die. The female produces nine or ten eggs a day, with a lifetime total of 270 to 300 eggs. The eggs hatch in less than 2 weeks. When feeding, the louse may defecate, and feces may be rubbed into the skin by scratching. In this manner infection passes from the louse to the human. Lice are passed from person to person by personal contact or by putting on infested garments.

Control measures include ordinary laundering, which will kill all stages of lice on clothing. Dry cleaning will destroy lice on woolen garments. Louse powders have been used successfully: 10 per cent DDT in pyrophyllite or 1 per cent lindane in pyrophyllite. The powder should be evenly dusted on the underclothing, with special attention to seams, and seams inside the shirt and trousers should be similarly treated. About 1 oz will be required for one treatment. DDT acts slowly and does not destroy the eggs. Its long-lasting effect, however, will allow it to kill emerging lice, and thus a single application will be effective. Lindane is not long-lasting, and a second application will be required in 7 to 10 days [17].

9-40. Fleas. Fleas are important vectors of disease. They transmit the organisms of plague and murine typhus from rodents to man. In addition, fleas are intermediate hosts of some species of dog and rodent tapeworms which occasionally infest man. They may also be involved as vectors of *Salmonella* bacteria and of the bacteria causing tularemia. Fleabites are extremely uncomfortable to some persons. A number of species of fleas will attack man, and some sixty species may be important in the epidemiology of plague [18]. The oriental rat flea, *Xenopsylla cheopis,* is the important vector of plague and murine typhus. The bacteria multiply within a plague-infected flea and cause an obstruction. Such a flea is said to be "blocked," and when it attempts to feed, the blood sucked from its victim is regurgitated into the bite injury; thus it may transmit the disease. Blocked fleas soon die. The flea transmits murine typhus from its feces which are deposited near the bite. Fleas are not harmed by the typhus infection and retain it throughout their lives, but they do not transmit it to their progeny. For transmission of murine typhus fever see Art. 9-45.

Female fleas deposit their eggs among the hair or feathers of the host or in the nests of birds and rodents. The eggs normally drop from the host. The eggs, laid over a period of time and between blood meals, hatch in 2 days to several weeks, depending on temperature and humidity. The larvae are small, light-colored, and wormlike and are to be found in house floor cracks and rugs and in kennels, stables, chicken coops, animal burrows, and nests. They feed on all types of organic debris. They go through three molts, which may require 1 week to several months. Pupae are usually enclosed in a cocoon, which is encrusted with grains of sand or debris. The pupal stage may last from a week to a year. After emergence from the cocoon, the adult is usually ready to feed in 24 hr. Little is known about the length of life of fleas or how many broods they may produce.

Control of fleas on pets will not be discussed here. Premises infested with fleas may be cleared in various ways. Bedding of dog kennels should be burned or laundered in hot soapy water. Vacuum cleaning of rugs and areas containing lint and dust will remove eggs, larvae, and pupae. The premises may then be treated with a residual insecticide in emulsion or solution, such as 0.5 to 1 per cent lindane or 0.5 per cent Diazinon. Dusts may be used inside buildings where the powder will not be objectionable. Five to ten per cent DDT dust is usually used, or 2 to 5 per cent malathion if there is resistance to DDT. Control of rat fleas is discussed in Art. 9-53.

9-41. Ticks. Ticks are involved in the transmission of a number of human diseases. These include Rocky Mountain spotted fever, which has been reported in 46 of the states; Q fever, which is widespread in the United States; tularemia, which occurs throughout North America; relapsing fever (tick-borne type), which has been reported in some areas of the Western states; and Colorado tick fever, which occurs in most of the Western states. Some cattle diseases are also transmitted by ticks. Tick paralysis sometimes occurs among children. It is caused by a toxic substance in the female tick which it may inject into the human body with its bite, particularly if it is allowed to remain attached to the skin for a long period. Children are principally involved, especially girls, who may have ticks concealed in their long hair. Apparently 6 days of attachment is required. Fatalities are not uncommon.

Female hard ticks, after mating, fall from the host, lay one batch of eggs (sometimes 18,000 or more) on or near the ground, and then die. Most of the soft ticks deposit 20 to 50 eggs in a batch after each blood meal. Eggs hatch in 2 weeks to several months into larval or "seed" ticks. Seed ticks have only six legs. They may wait on vegetation for a host to pass or actively seek one. After finding a host and feeding, the larva drops to the ground, molts, and emerges as a nymph, which has eight legs. The nymph must also find a suitable host. After feeding, it drops to the ground, molts, and becomes an adult, which also seeks a host. The cycle of some hard ticks may be completed in less than a year, or it may require 2 or 3 years or longer. Multiple-host ticks are able to survive because of their great reproductive capacity and ability to survive long periods without food. Some species are more fortunate and require only one host.

Persons who have been in tick-infested areas should examine their clothing and body and remove ticks before they attach themselves. Clearing or burning brush along paths and clearing weeds and cutting grass in recreation areas will reduce the possibility of tick infestation. If a tick becomes attached, removal should be by a slow, steady pull that will not break off the mouth parts and leave them in the wound. There is no certain way of causing it to detach its mouth parts. Touching it with a lighted cigarette may accomplish this, or a drop of chloroform, ether, carbon tetrachloride, vaseline, or fingernail polish may affect it so that several minutes or ½ hr later, when the tick has removed its mouth parts, it can be removed from the skin. An antiseptic should be applied to tick bites as to other wounds.

Buildings are sometimes invaded by the brown dog tick and other dog ticks. DDT, 5 per cent; chlordane, 3 per cent; and dieldrin or lindane, 0.5 per cent, as emulsions or solutions are effective. If the ticks are resistant, 0.5 per cent Diazinon or 1 per cent malathion may be used. If oil solutions are used, they should be in deodorized kerosene. The addition of 0.2 to 0.5 per cent DDVP to these sprays is of value since its fumigant action will drive ticks from behind baseboards or from wall cracks. DDT is used over broad areas; the other insecticides are used in spot treatments to baseboards, floor and wall cracks, and other harborages [19].

Control in areas covered by vegetation can be obtained by applications of DDT, chlordane, dieldrin, or toxaphene at rates of 1 to 2 lb of the insecticide per acre, or of BHC (gamma isomer) at 0.5 lb/acre as dust, suspensions, or emulsions. BHC should be used where fish may be killed by the first four of the insecticides mentioned. Dusts are applied by airplanes or by hand or power equipment; suspensions are often applied by orchard sprayers; and emulsions are usually applied by mist blowers. It is desirable to use a high volume of the emulsion with a low percentage of insecticide, rather than a small volume of high-percentage insecticide. This will ensure better coverage with less danger of injury to vegetation.

Rodent Control and Rat Fleas

9-42. There are numerous wild rodents in the United States, and many of them are actual or potential reservoirs of disease. However, the most dangerous and destructive rodents to be dealt with are three

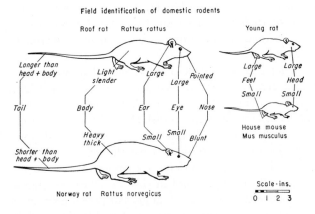

FIGURE 9-21 Characteristics of rats. (*From "Training Guide," Public Health Service, Communicable Disease Center, Rodent Control Series, Atlanta, Ga.*)

introduced domestic species: *Rattus norvegicus* (Norway rat), *Rattus rattus* (roof rat), and *Mus musculus* (house mouse). Naturalists disagree concerning the origination and dissemination of the domestic species. The Norway rat, also called the brown rat, apparently originated in western China and first appeared in Europe in about 1727. By the latter part of the eighteenth century, this species had gained a strong foothold in Europe and had migrated to America. Because of its ferocity and greater size, it is generally supposed that this species rapidly exterminates all other species with which it comes in contact. There appear to be exceptions to this rule, however, since Norway rats are occasionally seen to frequent the same buildings as roof rats. The Norway rat, whatever the reason, is the most numerous in cities, where it is sometimes referred to as the "sewer rat" or "wharf rat." It is grayish-brown and has a short tail and ears and a comparatively stocky body. It burrows and nests in the ground or under buildings and piles of rubbish. An omnivorous feeder, it consumes garbage, grain, vegetables, meat, or any food used for human consumption. Where food supplies and harborages are ample, the Norway rat breeds rapidly, producing litters of eight to twelve young four to seven times a year. Young females breed at the age of three or four months, and the gestation period averages 22 days.

The roof rat existed in Europe as early as the eleventh century and was widespread until the advent of the Norway rat curbed its further increase. It is smaller than the Norway rat and has longer ears and tail. The roof rat, as the name implies, is often found to infest the upper portions of buildings, for it climbs adroitly and can easily gain entrance to buildings through ventilators, open windows, skylights, etc., after reaching the building by traveling on trees and power lines. *Rattus rattus* (roof rat) includes three subspecies: *Rattus rattus alexandrinus* (alex or gray rat), *Rattus rattus rattus* (black rat), and *Rattus rattus frugivorus* (the fruit or tree rat). The three species have interbred to some extent, but all are commonly referred to as roof rats. Since the coloring of the roof rat varies from black to brown to gray, it is somewhat unreliable for purposes of identification. Roof rats appear to prefer grain and grain products as food but will eat other foods when grain is not available. Breeding habits are quite similar to those of the Norway rat, although roof-rat litters tend to be somewhat smaller. Whereas Norway rats predominate in urban areas, roof rats are, in general, more commonly observed in rural areas.

9-43. Rodents and Public Health. Domestic rats and other rodents, because of their wide distribution and close association with man, provide potential reservoirs of a number of important diseases. The afflictions for which rats are responsible range from discomforts caused by rodent bites to the more serious *murine typhus fever* and the often fatal *bubonic plague. Ratbite fever,* as the name indicates, is transmitted to humans by the bite of an infected animal. While only a small percentage of rat bites result in *ratbite fever,* the disease itself often becomes important in some urban areas where several hundred persons are bitten by rodents each year. Infected rats excrete the causative organism of *salmonellosis* in their urine and feces. The disease is transmitted to man from food contaminated with infected excreta. *Weil's disease,* or *hemorrhagic jaundice,* may also be transmitted to humans who ingest food contaminated with urine and feces from infected rats, who bathe in contaminated water, or who handle infected rats or excreta from infected rats. Rats have been incriminated as contributing to the transmission of various other diseases, including *amoebic dysentery, tapeworm,* and *trichinosis.* The house mouse (*Mus musculus*) has been identified as the reservoir of *rickettsialpox* in the northeastern United States and is also known to be capable of serving as a reservoir for plague. The more important rodent-borne diseases are discussed in greater detail.

9-44. **Plague.** Plague is an acute infection running a rapid, severe course. The flea is the principal vehicle of infection from rat to rat and from rat to man. The plague organism causes a mechanical stoppage in the esophagus of the flea which makes the flea regurgitate when feeding. Thus, when the flea takes blood from a host animal, the victim's blood is mixed with the plague organism within the body of the flea, which—unable to swallow normally—regurgitates the mixture back into the victim. Bubonic plague is derived from rodents in this fashion, but an especially deadly type, transmitted from man to man by nose and throat discharges, is known as *pneumonic plague.* This infection, however, is still bubonic plague; it has simply become localized in the lungs of human victims. A third term, *sylvatic plague,* is used to denote the disease in wild rodents. This infection also manifests itself as bubonic plague when transmitted to humans.

Bubonic plague in humans is essentially a disease of warm, moist climates and, having been introduced into such climates, tends to persist indefinitely. Geographically, plague is widespread and has occurred at intervals in most of the principal seaport cities of the world. With the spread of rats by ship-borne commerce, plague infections have occurred in several United States seaports. Two epidemics of flea-transmitted bubonic plague in San Francisco resulted in 281 cases, with 191 deaths, during the years 1900 and 1907. There have been a number of such outbreaks in California and elsewhere since 1900. Unfortunately, the disease in California apparently became endemic in local domestic rats and thereafter spread by means of fleas to wild rodents and other small mammals, including ground squirrels, meadow mice, deer mice, pack rats, rice rats, marmots, prairie dogs, kangaroo rats, pine squirrels, cottontail rabbits, and jack rabbits. House mice have also been found to be infected.

Plague among wild rodents has moved gradually eastward in the years since it was first introduced into California and has been observed in wild rodents in several Midwestern states. A few cases of bubonic plague in humans have been traced to contact of the victims with infected wild rodents, usually during hunting or trapping expeditions. Epidemics of human plague may result should fleas from infected wild rodents transmit the disease to the domestic rat species in heavily populated Midwestern and Eastern states.

In general, an outbreak of bubonic plague requires an abundance of infected rats, an abundance of the proper type of fleas in the rat population, and sufficient contact between the infected animals and man. Although other fleas are possible vectors of plague, the oriental rat flea (*Xenopsylla cheopis*), which is prevalent on domestic rats throughout most of the world plague belt, is accorded major responsibility for the transmission of plague from rat to rat and from rat to man. Such other fleas as *Nosopsyllus fasciatus*, the Northern rat flea, and *Pulex irritans*, the human flea, are considered of secondary importance in the infection of humans.

A vaccine has been developed that provides some immunity from plague. It is supposed, on good evidence to be the disease which was called the Black Death and which nearly depopulated Europe in the fifteenth century. At the present time, the disease remains endemic in many areas of Asia, particularly India and Arabia, and in Africa.

9-45. Typhus Fever. Two types of typhus fever have played important roles in history: *epidemic*, or the Old World type, which is transmitted from man to man by lice, and *endemic*, or the murine type, of which the rat is the reservoir and the flea is the vehicle of infection. A rather obscure ailment, which originally was erroneously called Brill's disease and which was supposed to be confined largely to Mexico, was identified only a few decades ago as murine or flea-borne typhus. Although milder, the clinical symptoms of murine typhus resemble the epidemic form, and the two diseases are caused by varieties of the same organism. Subsequent investigations have revealed that murine typhus is widespread in the rat populations of the Southern states and Texas. Approximately 90 per cent of the cases in the United States occur south of a line drawn from El Paso, Tex., to Norfolk, Va.

Murine typhus is far less fatal than plague, or epidemic typhus, but its incidence in many sections of the Southern United States justifies the use of preventive measures against both the rat and the vector, the flea. As in the case of plague, the principal vector is the oriental rat flea (*Xenopsylla cheopis*). The infected *X. cheopis* deposits feces while feeding on its victim, who then scratches a portion into the bite or other

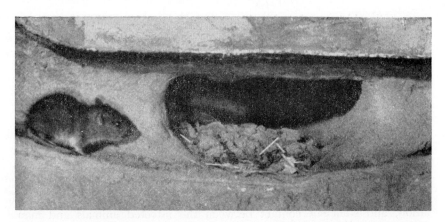

FIGURE 9-22   Harborage of a Norway rat. (*Photograph courtesy of Public Health Service, Communicable Disease Center.*)

abraded part of his skin. The flea transmits the disease from rat to rat and from rat to man. Murine typhus is not known to be transmissible from man to man.

9-46. Rodents as an Economic Factor. The toll taken by rats is enormous. Estimates indicate that the rat population equals the human population in the United States and that each rat can be expected to consume at least 1 oz of food per day. Rodents may eat practically anything used as food by humans or livestock. If the rat population lived only on wheat, they would need a daily food supply of almost 5,000 tons, which would amount to an annual food bill of over 100 million dollars.

Other rat damages and resulting economic losses occur in food-processing establishments, where hair, droppings, and urine stains in foods necessitate condemnation and disposal. It has been estimated that rats and mice waste or render unfit for human consumption several times as much food as they actually eat. Gnawing damage, fires, and poultry losses are also attributable to domestic rat populations. With these indictments of the rat, it is difficult to account for the tolerance with which its depredations are regarded.

9-47. Rodent-survey Techniques. The presence of rats may be detected in a number of ways, the most common being the discovery of damaged materials. Reasonably accurate determinations of the severity of rat infestations can be obtained by observing feeding or nesting activity and signs of movement between nesting and feeding areas. Although rats will nest as close as possible to the food supply so as to minimize exposure to predators, it is not unusual for a rat to range up to approximately 100 ft from its nest. The house mouse is normally limited to a range of not more than 30 ft.

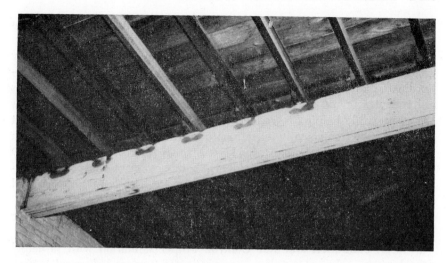

FIGURE 9-23 Interior of a building showing marks left by rats running along ceiling beams. Rat runs are used in determining the location of traps. (*Photograph courtesy of Public Health Service, Communicable Disease Center.*)

The following signs can be observed in evaluating the extent of rat infestations:

1. Gnawing. Rats gnaw continually during active hours so that their rapidly growing front teeth can be kept short. In order that food supplies may be obtained, rats gnaw doors, boxes, bags, and other storage containers.

2. Burrows. Burrows will frequently be observed along fences, near foundations, near garbage containers, and under concrete slabs or walks. Fresh burrows will have a clean, slick appearance.

3. Droppings. Rat droppings will be noticed along runways, near food and water sources, and in harborages. Rat droppings are up to ¾ in. long and may be easily distinguished from mice droppings, which are about the size of a grain of wheat.

4. Runways. Rats follow a specific pathway in their movements from burrows or nests to sources of food and water. Active runways have a shiny, slick, dust-free appearance and, if outside, will be almost free of vegetation.

5. Footprints and tail marks. Tracks will often be noticed in dust, in mud, and in some food products, such as flour.

6. Rub marks. Roof rats commonly climb posts and studs leading to a ceiling and then travel along the plate where the rafters and joists join. When rats travel these routes, they usually have to swing under the rafters on joists. Grease and dirt from the body of the rat will soon begin to accumulate on the rubbed surfaces to form black "swing" marks. Such marks are also noticed on pipes and ducts which have been utilized for runways.

7. Miscellaneous signs. Rat odor, urine stains, live rats, dead rats, nests, and stored food may also be encountered in the course of rat-infestation inspections.

9-48. General Methods of Control. The principal means of rodent control are poisoning; trapping; fumigation; ratproofing; the elimination of food, water, and harborages; and to some extent, destruction by natural enemies. Rodent-control activities are more effective when coordinated into organized community-wide campaigns. Natural enemies of rodents, among which may be counted cats, dogs, snakes, and birds of prey, while helping to reduce the number of rats and mice, will not usually prove sufficiently effective to exterminate these pests from a given area without human aid. Hawks, owls, and other birds of prey destroy wild species of some rodents, but because of the popular misconception that all these birds are injurious to the interests of man and because of the consequent war on them, this method of control is reduced in value. The important methods are discussed in the following articles.

9-49. Sanitation and Rat Control. Proper sanitation with principal emphasis on adequate garbage storage, collection, and disposal is considered the most effective rat-control measure available. In any given rat-infested area, there is a more or less constant population of rats whose number is determined largely by the amount of food, water, and harborage available. As more food becomes available, the rat population increases rapidly. As the food supply diminishes, the rat population rapidly decreases. To a lesser degree, rat-population fluctuations are dependent upon the availability of suitable harborage or nesting places. Rats require three things for propagation: food, water, and harborage. If insanitary conditions which provide the rat with these necessities can be eliminated, the problem of rat control can likewise be eliminated.

9-50. Poisoning. In general, poisoning, where it can be used without danger to man or domestic animals, is an efficient method of destroying rats. The poisons commonly used in the past were arsenic, strychnine, phosphorus, red squill, barium carbonate, and compounds containing one or more of these. In ordinary use, these rodenticides did not always give satisfactory results. Newer poisons are 1080, Antu, Warfarin, and Pival. A brief discussion of some of the more satisfactory rodenticides follows.

ANTICOAGULANTS. The anticoagulants, when ingested at intervals for a period of days, cause sufficient internal bleeding to result in death. The common types are Warfarin and Pival, which are formulated into solid baits, and Warficide and Pivalyn, which are formulated into liquid baits. Continuous feeding from a constant supply of poison bait is necessary to produce the desired results. For this reason, it is recommended that frequent checks be made of bait containers during the first few days the poison is made available to ensure that adequate supplies of bait are kept accessible. Occasionally dead rats are noticed within 4 to 7 days after the baits have been established. However, in some instances rats die in their nests, and bait effectiveness becomes apparent only by the odor produced by dead rats or by the continued absence of rats from bait locations.

The toxic action of Warfarin and Pival is considerably slower than that of 1080. Antu, red squill, and other rodenticides; however, an advantage of the retarded action is that rats do not develop an aversion to these materials and will continue to feed from both liquid and solid baits until they die or until the baits are exhausted. While the anticoagulant action of Warfarin and Pival is also effective in other warm-blooded animals and humans, these poisons are not considered as hazardous as other types because an efficient antidote, vitamin D, is readily available and because repeated feedings in liberal quantities of the concentration recommended for rodent control are necessary to endanger human beings. Both Warfarin and Pival are usually purchased in concentrates of 0.5 per cent. This material is diluted 1 part poison to 19 to 49 parts bait for Norway rats, and 1 part poison to 19 parts bait for roof rats and house mice. Common bait materials include cornmeal, rolled oats, bread crumbs, nut crumbs, sugar, and corn or peanut oil. Warficide and Pivalyn are obtainable in preformulated units, with each unit containing sufficient toxicant to produce an effective bait when mixed with 1 qt of water. Effective bait stations utilizing the liquid baits have been prepared by inverting a quart or pint jar containing the poison into chick fountains and placing them where they are accessible to rats.

The development of anticoagulant poisons has enabled a new approach to rodent control in that complete control in a given building is possible and reinfestation can be limited by making the baits constantly available. The relative safety and convenience of the materials enable them to be used by individuals not trained in rodent control, thus making possible community-wide efforts in rodent control. While safety precautions are inherent in both liquid- and solid-bait formulations, it is recommended that the poisoned baits be considered hazardous to humans and warm-blooded animals and that steps be taken to prevent exposure of the materials to accidental ingestion.

RED SQUILL. Powdered red squill has proved a useful rodenticide and is commonly used in the proportion of 1 part squill to 9 parts bait. While red squill was one of the earliest poisons utilized in organized rodent-control activities, its popularity has remained, chiefly because it has the advantage of being relatively safe for human beings, cats, dogs, and fowls. The substance is a natural emetic which, when taken by most warm-blooded animals, results in immediate regurgitation and evacuation of the poisonous material. The emetic action of red squill provides an almost specific poison for Norway rats, since they are unable to regurgitate. Squill baits are bitter and have the disadvantage of creating an aversion in rat populations, and some rats appear always to avoid baits containing red squill, especially if they have observed its poisonous effects on other rodents.

1080. This is the common name for sodium fluoroacetate, a very efficient poison for rodents. Its great disadvantage is that it is highly poisonous to man and domestic animals, and there is no known antidote for the material. It is, therefore, recommended for use only by qualified responsible persons who are obligated to protect poisoned premises and to remove unused baits, bait containers, and poisoned rodents prior to public admittance. Water is probably the most effective bait, and $\frac{1}{2}$ oz of 1080 in 1 gal of water is the recommended formulation.

ANTU. This poison, which has the chemical name alpha naphthylthiourea, is an effective poison against the brown or Norway rat but is not recommended for use against any other species of rat or rodent. A disadvantage of the poison is that a tolerance is quickly built up by rats which have eaten a less than lethal amount. In practice, therefore, it has been found that Antu cannot be effectively used at closer intervals than 4 to 6 months in the same locality. Antu may be utilized in preparing food baits containing 0.75 to 3.0 per cent Antu by weight. Also, considerable success has been achieved by placing 20 per cent Antu powder near rat burrows or in runways, making it necessary for the rat to walk through the material, a portion of which adheres to the feet. The rats then lick the feet in the process of preening and consume toxic amounts of Antu in this manner.

9-51. Trapping. Another method of reducing rat populations is through the use of a well-planned trapping program. Among the many traps on the market, the simple inexpensive "snap" or "guillotine" trap is usually found to be best adapted for all-round usage. Cage traps and unbaited steel traps are sometimes utilized if it is desired to capture live rats for inspection of their ectoparasites. Traps should be set in runways, behind boxes, along walls, or in other sheltered places where concealment is easy and rodents are moving. For good results a great many traps must be used. A dozen or more traps are needed for a heavily infested dwelling, and 50 to 100 or more for a large building or farm. The trapping campaign must be short and decisive, or the rats become wary and avoid the traps no matter how well they have been placed. Trapping activities are usually most successful when utilized following a rat-poisoning campaign that did not achieve complete control.

9-52. Fumigation. Fumigation may be effectively employed in places fitted for such an undertaking. Fumigation is recommended and extensively used to free ships from rodents and other vermin. Hydrocyanic acid gas is perhaps the most effective fumigant, but since it is extremely dangerous to man, great care must be exercised where this method is employed. Its principal use is in the fumigation of ships under the

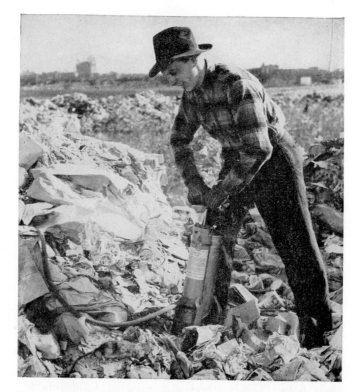

FIGURE 9-24 Dusting with Cyanogas to kill domestic rats. (*Photograph courtesy of Public Health Service, Communicable Disease Center.*)

supervision of the Public Health Service. A disadvantage to the use of fumigants in buildings is the possibility of unpleasant odors resulting from dead rats in walls, under floors, and in other obscure places.

Approximating fumigation is the use of calcium cyanide, which is sold under the name of Cyanogas A-Dust and other proprietary names. The poison can be obtained in granular or powdered form, and it can be introduced into rat burrows by means of a pump devised by the poison manufacturer. When exposed to the atmosphere, calcium cyanide gives off hydrocyanic acid gas, which will spread through any enclosed space. In using this material and other fumigants in buildings or other indoor areas, it is necessary that the premises be tightly closed, with door and window cracks sealed with paper. The fumigant should be allowed to remain in the building for at least 4 hr, at the end of which time the treated building should be thoroughly ventilated. This method of using hydrocyanic acid gas is fairly safe, but during actual application inside buildings the workman should wear an appropriate gas mask.

Where convenient and safe in exterior places, a hose may be con-

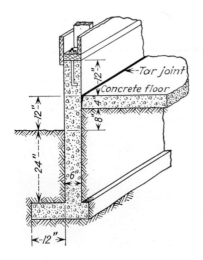

FIGURE 9-25 Floor and foundation construction of a new building without a basement. This type of construction should be used for buildings where food will be handled or stored.

nected to the exhaust of a tractor or an automobile, and the burned gases will serve effectively in destroying rats, provided that all openings to burrows are tightly closed to prevent the entrance of fresh air and dilution of the toxic gases. In shallow burrows under buildings and in similar places, a wad of cotton the size of an orange saturated with carbon bisulfide ("high life") may be stuffed into the mouth of the burrows, the entrance further closed by filling with earth, and the rats suffocated in their holes. This method was used in California to destroy ground squirrels during antiplague activities.

9-53. Ectoparasite Control. Obviously, if the number of fleas can be reduced, there is a corresponding reduction in disease transmission both from rat to rat and from rat to man. This line of attack, called ectoparasite control, has achieved good results. Common methods of rat ectoparasite control include the application of 10 per cent DDT dust to rat runways and burrows in amounts of approximately 2.5 lb of dust or 0.25 lb of technical DDT per premises, depending on the extent of rat infestation and the area to be treated. In normal activity, rats will pass through the DDT and eventually spread particles of the toxicant throughout the fur. Fleas and other external parasites are killed in this manner. The dust is sometimes blown into burrows by some type of dust gun, usually a rotary type or a simple garden duster. Dust is best distributed on interior runways by spooning small piles at intervals along rat runways. Sifters, made from jars, cans, or boxes, are also conveniently used for dust distribution when metal lids can be provided and punctured with several ⅛-in. holes. Handles are sometimes attached to sifters for convenience in reaching high runways.

In those areas of the world where typhus in rat populations has become endemic. it is recommended that DDT dusting for control of rat

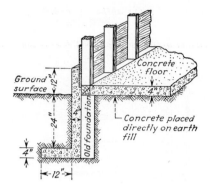

FIGURE 9-26   Old building made ratproof by placing concrete curtain wall around old foundation.

fleas be routinely practiced. Also, where any threat of plague is imminent, ectoparasite control should precede or accompany rodent-poisoning activities. If one of the rapidly effective poisons, such as red squill or 1080, is utilized as the rodenticide, flea extermination with DDT dust should precede the placing of poison baits by 3 or 4 days. However, if one of the slow-acting rodenticides, such as Warfarin or Pival, is employed, dusting can be carried out simultaneously with the placing of baits. Rodent poisoning without adequate provision for flea control often results in fleas leaving their dead rat hosts, where blood is no longer available, and seeking blood meals from man.

9-54. **Ratproofing.** Rats tend to breed and multiply proportionately to the food supply available for them. Unless carried on continuously, other control measures provide only temporary relief unless rats are starved out by being excluded from food. The ratproofing of buildings is, therefore, considered an effective means of rat control. It is a simple matter to erect buildings of ratproof construction, and an ordinance requiring such construction, properly enforced, will result in a practically rat-free city. It is necessary to exercise vigilance at all times, however, to maintain a building in ratproof condition.

The ratproofing of new buildings involves both interior and exterior ratproofing as well as the elimination of interior structural harborage. Ratproof construction of new buildings provides for the complete absence of nonessential openings through which rats may enter buildings. The liberal use of ratproof materials, such as 19-gage or heavier ½-in. mesh hardware cloth, 24-gage or heavier galvanized sheet metal, and portland cement mortar, will prohibit rat entry through essential openings of ½ in. or larger. Buildings should be constructed of materials impervious to rat attack, and approved methods of construction should be utilized. An approved design that fundamentally eliminates all unnecessary enclosed places, such as double floors and walls, should be employed.

Buildings in which food is handled or stored should have floors of

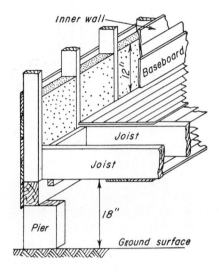

FIGURE 9-27 When buildings are supported on posts or piers, they are made ratproof by raising them 18 in. or more above the ground level and by placing concrete between inner and outer walls above sill. (*Courtesy of Portland Cement Association.*)

ratproof material or of concrete not less than 4 in. thick poured directly upon the ground or earth fill. The floor should be sealed into the walls, and the walls must be of ratproof material, such as concrete, stone, brick, or tile, not less than 6 in. thick. To prevent burrowing beneath the building, the foundation walls should extend at least 2 ft into the ground to a horizontal offset of 12 in. and must extend at least 1 ft above the floor.

Other buildings may be ratproofed by being elevated on pillars at least 18 in. above the ground and having the underlying ground kept free of rubbish and other rat-harboring material; or a curtain wall may be constructed at least 4 in. thick and extending at least 2 ft into the ground to a 12-in. horizontal offset at least 4 in. thick.

9-55. Rat Stoppage. Rat stoppage is a modified method of the orthodox ratproofing procedure which is applicable to existing buildings. It involves some inexpensive construction alterations designed to prevent rats from entering buildings by blocking off or stopping up all actual and potential passages by which they might gain entry. Essentially, it is the closing of openings in exterior walls with materials through which rats cannot penetrate, together with such interior rat stoppage, harborage removal, and cleanup as may be necessary to reduce or eliminate rat breeding places.

Rat stoppage is accomplished, in part, by sealing all holes or cracks in foundations and walls and around pipes passing through walls with bricks or portland cement mortar. Holes in wood floors or walls are stopped with fitted sheet metal. The lower edges of doors, the door casings, and the thresholds are covered with 24-gage galvanized sheet iron. Preferably this should be "channeled" or bent around the edge of

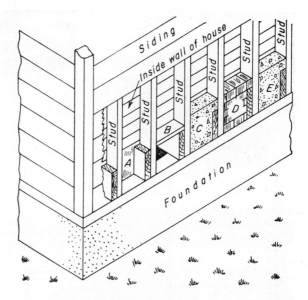

FIGURE 9-28 Methods of excluding rats from double walls. *A*, metal plate; *B*, wood stop; *C*, cinder concrete; *D*, bricks; *E*, ordinary concrete.

the door. The channels or plates at the vertical edges should extend at least 6 in. above the bottom of the door. Cellar and basement windows and other windows and ventilators allowing access by rats from the ground, roof, or trees are protected with galvanized 19-gage metal screen or ⅜-in. or smaller hardware cloth that is securely fastened. Metal guards or other means are used to prevent rats from climbing pipes, rainspouts, or wires and using them as a means of entrance. Sheet aluminum is not satisfactory for stopping rats, as they are able to gnaw through it. If foundations are less than 24 in. deep, a curtain wall is installed outside in contact with the original wall to a depth of at least 24 in. with a 12-in. horizontal extension. The curtain wall may be of good concrete, 3 to 4 in. thick, or of 24-gage galvanized metal. Well-poured concrete floors will prevent the entrance of rats into buildings with foundations extending at least 24 in. into the ground, and they are superior to curtain walls in that they increase the value of the property.

After all avenues of rat entry have been stopped, poisoning or fumigation and trapping should be employed to kill the rats already within the building. Continuous maintenance of the rat-stoppage alteration is required if they are to retain their efficiency.

9-56. Port Regulations. Since seaports are the usual points of entrance for plague, health authorities are especially careful to prevent

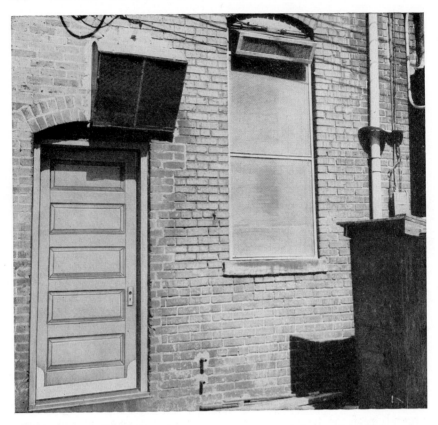

FIGURE 9-29   Ratproofing details. Note screens over window and ventilators, door plates, guards at downspouts and wires, and mortar around pipes. (*Courtesy of Public Health Service, Communicable Disease Center.*)

rats from leaving ships. The Texas State Board of Health issued the following regulations governing this matter during a threatened plague epidemic:[1]

1. All ships docking at Texas ports, both foreign and coastwise, must fend off a minimum of 8 feet from wharf, using submerged fender or raft to hold ship away from wharf or dock.

2. All lines, hawsers, cables, etc., from ship to dock must be equipped with circular rat guards 36 inches in diameter equipped with a sleeve to hold same in proper position a maximum of three feet from vessel. All rat guards must be approved by the Texas State Board of Health.

3. All hawse pipes must be plugged with tarred fabric. All hawse lines too small to hold rat guards or too close to side of vessel to use rat

[1] These regulations are no longer enforced but served their purpose well at the time.

guards, must be covered with fabric and tarred a distance of 3 lineal feet—must be tarred daily before 6:00 P.M.

4. All gang planks and ship ladders must be removed at sunset and not be replaced until sunrise, except when during actual loading or unloading and then a guard must be placed at each gang plank or ladder to see that rats neither leave nor enter vessel.

5. Ropes, cables, swinging stages, ladders, hose, or any object upon which a rat may leave vessels must be taken aboard by sunset and may not be replaced before sunrise of each day.

In addition to such regulatory measures as the above enacted by the national and state health authorities, there is a movement toward the ratproofing of docks and wharves in many ports, and some ratproof structures have actually been constructed. Ratproofing of ships is also recommended.

9-57. Community Efforts in Rat Control. The local health department should accept responsibility for rat control. One or more sanitarians or inspectors should understand the techniques and be able to apply them should an emergency arise. The city council should be urged to pass an ordinance requiring that all new buildings, or those which are extensively altered, be made of rodentproof construction. Building inspectors should be required to enforce this requirement. Education of the public should be continuous, and owners of warehouses, food-handling establishments, etc., should be encouraged to complain of rat infestations so that they may be assisted or given advice in obtaining control on their premises. Dealers in poisons may be encouraged to stock the rodenticides recommended.

Bibliography

1. Russell, P. F., et al.: "Practical Malariology," 2d ed., Oxford University Press, New York, 1963.
2. Pratt, H. D., et al.: "Introduction to Arthropods of Public Health Importance," Public Health Service, Communicable Disease Center, 1960.
3. Pratt, H. D., et al.: "Mosquitoes of Public Health Importance," Public Health Service, Communicable Disease Center, 1960.
4. Boyd, M. F.: "Malariology," W. B. Saunders Company, Philadelphia, 1949.
5. Soper, F. L.: The 1957 Status of Yellow Fever in the Americas, *Mosquito News*, vol. 18, no. 3, September, 1958.
6. Pratt, H. D., and R. C. Barnes: "Identification Keys for Common Mosquitoes of United States," Public Health Service, Communicable Disease Center, 1959.
7. Pratt, H. D., et al.: "Survey and Control of Mosquitoes of Public Health Importance," Public Health Service, Communicable Disease Center, 1960.
8. Magoon, E. H.: "Drainage for Health," Rockefeller Foundation, International Health Division, New York, 1945.

9. "Malaria Control on Impounded Waters," Public Health Service and Tennessee Valley Authority, U.S. Government Printing Office, 1947.
10. Herms, W. B., and H. F. Gray: "Mosquito Control," 2d ed., Commonwealth Fund, New York, 1944.
11. Scott, H. G., and K. S. Littig: "Insecticidal Equipment for the Control of Insects of Public Health Importance," Public Health Service, Communicable Disease Center.
12. Pratt, H. D., and K. S. Littig: "Insecticides for the Control of Insects of Public Health Importance," Public Health Service, Communicable Disease Center, 1962.
13. Scott, H. G., and K. S. Littig: "Flies of Public Health Importance and Their Control," Public Health Service, Communicable Disease Center, 1962.
14. Communicable Disease Center: 1962 Report on Public Health Pesticides, *Pest Control*, vol. 30, no. 3, March, 1962.
15. Herms, W. B.: "Medical Entomology," The Macmillan Company, New York.
16. Scott, H. G.: "Household and Stored-food Insects of Public Health Importance," Public Health Service, Communicable Disease Center, 1960.
17. Pratt, H. D., and K. S. Littig: "Lice of Public Health Importance and Their Control," Public Health Service, Communicable Disease Center, 1960.
18. Pratt, H. D., and J. S. Wiseman: "Fleas of Public Health Importance and Their Control," Public Health Service, Communicable Disease Center, 1962.
19. Pratt, H. D., and K. S. Littig: "Ticks of Public Health Importance and Their Control," Public Health Service, Communicable Disease Center, 1962.
20. Bjornson, B. F., and C. V. Wright: "Control of Domestic Rats and Mice," Public Health Service, Communicable Disease Center, 1960.
21. Scott, H. G.: Rodent-borne Disease Control through Rodent Stoppage, Pts. I and II, *Pest Control*, vol. 31, nos. 8 and 9, August and September, 1963.
22. Chandler, A. C., and A. P. Read: "Introduction to Human Parasitology," 10th ed., John Wiley & Sons, Inc., New York, 1961.

10

VENTILATION AND AIR CONDITIONING

10-1. Ventilation is defined as the process of supplying air to, or removing it from, any enclosed space by natural or mechanical means. Such air may or may not be conditioned. Complete air conditioning is the control of all those factors affecting both physical and chemical conditions of the atmosphere within any structure. These factors include temperature, humidity, motion (air movement), distribution, dust, odors, toxic gases, and bacteria, most of which affect in greater or lesser degree human health or comfort.

Successful ventilation and air conditioning require the services of an engineer who is a specialist in the subject, or money may be wasted. The basic principles that should be understood by the sanitary engineer and sanitarian are discussed here.

10-2. Composition of the Earth's Atmosphere. The air envelope overlying the earth's surface is a composition of various elements, present in the following proportions by volume: nitrogen, 78.1 per cent; oxygen, 20.9 per cent; carbon dioxide, 0.03 per cent; and argon, 0.9 per cent. The balance is made up of other inert gases and a varying proportion of water vapor. The nitrogen, argon, and other inert gases occur in practically the same proportions. The others vary somewhat, although not to any great extent. Other contaminants frequently or occasionally encountered are organic matter from human or animal bodies; smokes, fumes, mists, and gases produced by various industrial processes; and pollens from various plants, some of which cause hay fever or asthma.

10-3. Effects of Occupancy. There are five effects resulting from human occupancy of unventilated or poorly ventilated rooms: (1) The oxygen content is reduced; (2) the amount of carbon dioxide present is increased; (3) organic matter and odors are given off from the skin, clothing, and mouths of the occupants; (4) the temperature is raised by heat generated in the body processes; and (5) the humidity is increased by the moisture in the breath and the evaporation from the skin. All these effects are greatly increased if the vital processes are speeded up through physical exertion.

The consumption of oxygen in breathing, of course, results in a reduction of the amount in the atmosphere of a closed room and a proportional increase in the amount of carbon dioxide. In breathing, an adult contributes about 0.7 cu ft of carbon dioxide per hr to the atmosphere. Children contribute somewhat less; the average in mixed groups can be taken at about 0.6 cu ft/hr. The reduction of oxygen and the increase of carbon dioxide, except in tightly closed rooms and for long periods, are of no importance, probably requiring only a slightly increased rate of respiration. According to the *U.S. Bureau of Mines Circular* 33, 0.5 per cent of carbon dioxide, at the expense of oxygen, would require a slight increase of lung ventilation, while 10 per cent cannot be endured for more than a few minutes.

The early belief that carbon dioxide was poisonous led to ventilation codes calling for new fresh air per person per minute that would keep the carbon dioxide content at a low level. These requirements were as high as 30 cu ft per person per min. At present, however, the carbon dioxide content is not considered a reliable index for new fresh air or for prevention of odors. The abandonment of this requirement has led to requirements nearer to 10 cu ft of new fresh air per min. Local codes, however, still specify the old code of ventilation and air conditioning.

In nature the carbon dioxide produced by animals or otherwise in combustion is used by green plants, which take up the carbon and release the oxygen.

10-4. Air Contaminants. Air contaminants and their sources are discussed in Chap. 3. They include carbon monoxide, a poison which results from incomplete combustion of fuel; various mists, fumes, gases, and vapors which are produced in certain industrial processes; dusts, which are produced in city streets and in nature but which also accompany industrial processes; pollens, which are released into the air by certain plants and which may cause hay fever or asthma; and bacteria, which may cause disease. Air conditioning may have to eliminate or prevent any or all of these impurities.

10-5. Bacteria in Air. It is supposed that bacteria are not suspended in the air alone but are carried by particles of dust, organic matter, or moisture. According to Winslow [5], street dust may contain 50 million bacteria per gram, and indoor dust up to 5 million per gram. Of these, 1 in 1,000 of the street bacteria and 1 in 4,000 of the indoor bacteria are of the intestinal type. Except during high winds outdoors and dry sweepings indoors, little of the dust gets into the air, and consequently it is of little importance. The number of bacteria in indoor air may vary from 1 to 1,000 per cubic foot. Infection of open wounds from air is possible, and infections of other sorts, particularly of respiratory diseases, may occur by means of bacteria attached to droplets discharged into the air during coughing, sneezing, and talking. They may be carried to other persons or to food by air currents, or they may settle and be incorporated in dust.

10-6. Organic Matter and Odors. The odors which can sometimes be detected in crowded or poorly ventilated rooms are due to perspiration mingled with organic compounds from skin and clothing and also to decomposition taking place in mouths. They must be prevented by an addition of fresh air sufficient to keep down the concentration of organic matter, as indicated in a preceding article. These noticeable body odors were formerly supposed to be the cause of disease and to be generated in direful amounts wherever crowds were assembled. Years ago the term "crowd poison" was in common use, and delicate ladies were frequently known to faint from its effects. The idea that vitiation of the atmosphere by decomposing organic matter in general is responsible for disease has been definitely discredited. While no specific disease results even from long exposure to vitiated air and unpleasant odors, bad effects such as nausea, loss of appetite, and perhaps aggravation of certain illnesses may result. In this connection, Prof. C.-E. A. Winslow, of the Yale School of Medicine, reports that the exposure of young guinea pigs to the odors from decomposing organic matter quite definitely retards their growth [5]. An exception must be made in the case of poisoning of air by carbon monoxide, the fumes of lead, and other poisonous substances which may have very serious results.

10-7. Heat Loss. Air conditioning is primarily the control of the air environment by addition or removal of heat and secondarily the removal of dust, fumes, and odors. For comfort, air conditions should be so maintained that necessary heat loss from the body can take place without unnecessary strain to the occupants of the space. Body heat is lost by conduction, convection, and radiation. By conduction, air in contact with the heat source becomes warmed. The greater the difference in temperature, the more rapidly loss by conduction proceeds. By convection, currents are set up, removing the warmed air and replacing it with cool air, and conduction continues. By radiation, heat is lost from the warm body to the cool body without warming the intervening air. In the human body, there is also a loss of heat through evaporation of perspiration.

Loss of heat from the body will be rapid (1) when there are cold objects in the room—walls, for example—so that radiation is high; (2) when the air temperature is low and conduction loss is high; (3) when there is enough air movement to prevent a blanket of warm air from enveloping the body; (4) when the skin surface is moist and cooling by evaporation is in process; and (5) when the relative humidity of the air is low and evaporation is speeded up. In still air, radiation accounts for about 45 per cent of the total heat loss, convection for 30 per cent, and evaporation for 25 per cent. Evaporation losses consist of about 11 per cent from the lungs and 14 per cent from the skin. These percentages will vary, however, according to air conditions and type of work.

10-8. Effective Temperature. Effective temperature is defined by the American Society of Heating, Refrigerating and Air-Conditioning Engineers (ASHRAE) as an arbitrary index of the degree of warmth or cold felt by the human body in response to the combined effects of temperature, humidity, and air movement. The numerical value of the effective temperature for any given air condition is fixed by the temperature of moisture-saturated air which, at a velocity of 15 to 25 fpm (feet per minute), or practically still air, induces a sensation of warmth or cold like that of the given condition. Thus any air condition has an effective temperature of 65°F when it induces a sensation of warmth like that experienced in practically still air at 65°F and saturated with moisture. But the same degree of comfort is not always experienced all along the line of a constant effective temperature, for discomfort may be felt at excessively high and low relative humidities, although this is less important than temperatures. The most comfortable effective temperatures in summer and winter are given in Fig. 10-1. Effective temperatures can be calculated from charts prepared by manufacturers of air-conditioning equipment.

10-9. Air Motion. The cooling power of air is highly important and mainly dependent upon its temperature and motion. Anemometers with rotating or deflecting vanes are used for rough measurements of air motion. New thermoanemometers have been developed which are quite accurate in the low ranges. The ASHRAE Guide [1] suggests air velocities of 20 to 50 fpm, with the lower values applying to heating systems and the higher to cooling.

10-10. Humidity. The amounts of moisture occurring in the air are small but important in effect. The amount of moisture which the air can carry varies with its temperature. At 0°F it will hold only 0.5 grain of water vapor per cubic foot. At 32°F it will hold 2.1 grains, and at 98°F it will hold 18.7 grains. At the above values the air is saturated and can hold no more. If the temperature is lowered, the excess moisture condenses to the saturation point for the lower temperature. This is known as the dew point. For any humidity, therefore, the temperature may be lowered so that the air becomes saturated. Conversely, cold air after being heated and with its moisture-carrying power increased has a much lower humidity at the higher temperature and hence becomes drying in its effect. The percentage of moisture which air at any temperature contains when compared with the amount which it could contain if saturated is the relative humidity. Relative humidity is measured by a comparison of wet-bulb and dry-bulb thermometers. The bulb of one thermometer is covered with damp wicking or cloth. The evaporation from the cloth lowers the temperature of the mercury in the thermometer. The drier the air, the quicker the evaporation and the lower the wet-bulb temperature. The difference between this temperature and that of the ordinary dry-bulb thermometer is a measure of the relative humidity. For instance, at a dry-bulb temperature of 80°F, the wet-bulb temperature may show 73°F; the difference at this particular dry-bulb temperature indicates a relative humidity of 60 per cent. Tables or charts are used to obtain both the relative humidities when the dry-bulb temperatures are known and the difference between wet-bulb and dry-bulb readings. The sling psychrometer, or hygrometer, is a convenient means of measuring relative humidity. It consists of two thermometers—a wet-bulb and a dry-bulb—mounted on a handle so that they may be twirled through the air. The cover of the wet-bulb thermometer is moistened, and the thermometers are twirled until the difference in temperatures is uniform.

10-11. Comfort Standard of Ventilation. Our present knowledge of air conditioning allows drawing no definite conclusions as to relationships between air condition and health. So far as known, air conditions that give a feeling of well-being or comfort are those which are most conducive to health. The feeling of comfort must be induced by proper control of temperature, humidity, and air movement together with precautions against accumulations of body odors, fumes, and dusts.

Exertion increases the metabolism rate of the body and raises body temperature. Therefore, conditions where exercise or strenuous work is in progress must be different from those in rooms where occupations are sedentary. Character of clothing is also important. The American

Society of Heating, Refrigerating and Air-Conditioning Engineers has conducted many experiments to determine the comfort zones at various combinations of relative humidity, temperature, and air movement. Figure 10-1 is the ASHRAE comfort chart [1] for air movement of 15 to 25 fpm with persons normally clothed and not strenuously active. Curves marked "summer" and "winter" indicate that nearly 100 per cent of all persons will feel comfortable at an effective temperature of 71°F in summer, and 68°F in winter. Curves marked "slightly cool," "comfortable," etc., represent sensations felt by the subjects after 3 hr in the air-conditioned space and adaptation to the conditions, including moisture accumulations on skin and clothing. For example, a comfortable

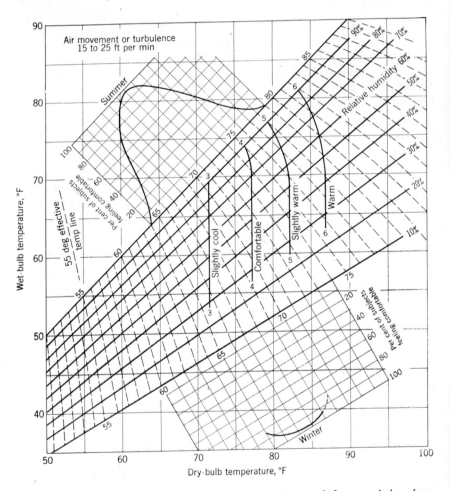

FIGURE 10-1   Revised ASHRAE comfort chart. (*Reprinted by permission from "ASHRAE Guide and Data Book," American Society of Heating, Refrigerating and Air-Conditioning Engineers, Inc., New York, 1963.*)

feeling was attained at an effective temperature of 72°F, relative humidity of 50 per cent, dry-bulb temperature of 77°F, and wet-bulb temperature of 65°F. Note that relative humidities have only a slight effect upon comfort, and then only at humidities above 50 to 60 per cent, at which points the curves turn slightly toward lower dry-bulb and effective temperatures.

10-12. Physiological Effects of Heat. In order to maintain itself at the proper temperature, the body is continually adjusting to the effective temperature of the air. Although in cold weather somewhat more heat is generated, most of the changes involve the skin and the blood vessels that are directly beneath. If the air is cold, the blood is withdrawn from the skin to the inner parts, thereby tending to prevent too great a loss of body heat. If the air is warm, but still cooler than the blood, the capillaries or small blood vessels beneath the skin expand, thereby bringing blood near the surface and allowing the excess heat of the body to flow to the air. The greater the difference between the temperatures of body and air, the more rapid the heat flow. Perspiration is secreted by the skin, and its evaporation lowers the body temperature. It is apparent, therefore, that with high air temperature and high humidity occurring together, evaporation is retarded, and the heat is more oppressive. Considerable air movement aids evaporation and results in cooling of the body. Low air temperature combined with high humidity is likely to cause discomfort because the accumulation of moisture in small amounts in the clothing lessens its efficiency as a nonconductor of heat. Regardless of the relative humidity, however, moisture on the skin will cause chilliness [9].

In a hot room the mucous membranes of the nose normally show swelling, redness, and moisture, while cold results in opposite effects. Drafts or currents of cold air on the face or sudden temperature changes cause contraction of the blood vessels with resulting local anemia, without, however, diminishing the swelling or loss of moisture. This loss of the protecting blood supply allows an increase of bacteria and may result in the development of colds or other respiratory infections. Continual exposure to overheated air increases the liability to the abnormal condition mentioned above. Those people who are habitually in still, overheated air are most susceptible to the bad effects of chilling drafts. High temperatures combined with high humidity, as in the case of laundry workers, may result in chronic respiratory diseases.

Methods

10-13. Ventilation is a problem for dwellings, schools, hospitals, industrial plants, office and business buildings, and such places of public assembly as theaters. Originally, ventilation consisted simply in furnishing sufficient "fresh" air, at as comfortable a level of temperature as was obtainable, and in keeping out noticeable odors and drafts. In the winter this was accomplished by heating with stoves, and in summer it depended upon windows, natural air currents, and fans. In industrial plants, dusts and fumes were removed by exhaust systems, and where required by certain processes, the air was humidified. Of late years a more positive attitude has been taken toward ventilation, with the result that it is now required not merely to furnish warm air but also to cool it, dry or moisten it, or otherwise condition it so that it will be comfortable at all times of the year. Air conditioning has been found to be profitable. It makes theaters and stores more attractive in warm weather and, more important, increases the output of industrial and office workers by increasing efficiency and by reducing lost time and labor turnover.

Ventilation, with heating as the only air treatment, is still all that is applied in most homes and in the smaller schools, although it is highly desirable that during the heating season other air conditions be controlled. As the cost of summer air conditioning or cooling is being reduced, however, it is being applied more and more not only to commercial buildings but also to moderately priced residences.

10-14. Methods of Heating. The methods of heating buildings may be classified as follows: (1) Direct heating places the source of heat within the room—the source may be a radiator or stove; (2) indirect heating employs a central heating unit, which may be an ordinary furnace or steam coils over which the air passes, and the heated air is furnished to the rooms through ducts by fans or gravity; and (3) the direct-indirect system employs heat sources in the rooms and also introduces warm air from a central furnace.

In so-called "radiant heating," which is an indirect method, rooms are heated by circulating hot water through coils of pipe within the floors, ceilings, or walls. The advantages claimed for this method are the following: (1) No radiators or ducts interfere with floor area or decoration; (2) air currents are absent, so that curtains remain clean; and (3) greater comfort is obtained, particularly near the floor, as heat is supplied where it is most needed. Electric coils and new glass-covered electrically heated radiant panels are also available for installation near baseboard level or in ceilings.

All the above systems may be controlled automatically by means of thermostats which operate the valves of radiators or dampers placed in ducts for the purpose of keeping rooms at a desired temperature. Since thermostats have been known to get out of order, they should be checked occasionally by accurate thermometers. As a matter of fact, rooms occupied for any purpose should have thermometers, although it should be recognized that temperature is only one factor in air quality.

10-15. Air Interchange. As previously mentioned, the earlier notion as to the requirement for good ventilation was based upon an erroneous belief about the effect of carbon dioxide, particularly if the concentration of that gas exceeded 0.06 per cent. In spite of proof to the contrary, this requirement, which necessitates the furnishing of 30 cu ft of fresh air per person per min, is still specified by some state and city laws, ordinances, and regulations governing schools and factories. An objection to such a high air change is the increase it causes in the heating or cooling load. An air velocity of 15 to 25 fpm is preferred in occupied areas of rooms, but as long as anemometer readings are below 50 fpm, drafts are not felt by occupants. Table 10-1 gives recommended air interchanges for various occupied spaces. Note that they are related to smoking and that the amounts of air suggested should prevent stinging of the eyes.

Table 10-1. VENTILATION STANDARDS

Application	Smoking	CFM of air per person		CFM per sq ft of floor, minimum
		Recommended	Minimum	
Apartment, average.	Some	20	15	....
Apartment, deluxe	Some	30	25	0.33
Barber shops.	Considerable	15	10	....
Beauty parlors	Occasional	10	25	....
Cocktail bars.	Heavy	30	25	....
Corridors.	....	....	....	0.25
Department stores	None	7.5	5	0.05
Directors' rooms.	Extreme	50	30	....
Drugstores*	Considerable	10	7.5	....
Factories.	None	10	7.5	0.10
Hospitals, operating rooms†,‡.	None	....	....	2.0
Hospitals, private rooms	None	30	25	0.33
Hospitals, wards.	None	20	15	....
Hotel rooms	Heavy	30	25	0.33
Kitchen, restaurant.	....	....	....	4.0
Kitchen, residence	....	....	....	2.0
Office, general	Some	15	10	....
Office, private	Considerable	30	25	0.25
Restaurant, cafeteria*	Considerable	12	10	....
Restaurant, dining room*	Considerable	15	12	....
Schoolrooms‡	None	....	....	....
Shop, retail	None	10	7.5	....
Theater‡.	None	7.5	5	....
Theater	Some	15	10	....
Toilets (exhaust)‡	....	....	....	2.0

* May be governed by exhaust.
† All outside air recommended to overcome explosion hazard.
‡ Local codes may govern.
SOURCE: W. H. Carrier *et al.*, "Modern Air Conditioning, Heating and Ventilating," 3d ed., Pitman Publishing Corporation, New York, 1959. Reproduced by permission of the publisher.

Sufficient air change is not a problem for the residence. For the small school, the system of window ventilation described in Art. 10-16 is satisfactory if complete mechanical air conditioning is unobtainable. In theaters and possibly in factories where heat loss is small in proportion to the large number of people present, large volumes of air or cooled air must be provided. It should be recognized that a man loses 400 Btu/hr when seated at rest at effective temperatures from 70 to 88°F and that this increases greatly when movement occurs. Some of the heat loss is sensible loss, *i.e.*, due to radiation, and the rest is lost by evaporation (latent heat). It varies as shown in the following table:

Type of heat loss	At 70°F, Btu	At 88°F, Btu
Sensible loss (radiation) per hour	300	90
Evaporation loss per hour	100	310
Total	400	400

10-16. Natural Ventilation. This depends upon windows, doors, skylights, and roof ventilators. Natural ventilation cannot be used successfully in theaters, auditoriums, large schools, or large churches, but it must be depended upon in homes and small offices. Most newly constructed schools depend upon artificial ventilation. Normally, natural ventilation supplies an ample amount of air for a dwelling. It should be kept in mind that air movement into rooms through windows and walls depends upon winds and temperature differences between inside and outside air. Roof ventilators are actuated by wind forces, and their efficiency depends upon their resistance to air flow, height of draft, their ability to utilize wind energy, and their location on the roof. Ventilation by windows and transoms requires judgment. For instance, merely opening a window at the bottom may produce no air movement and no entrance of fresh air. Windows open at top and bottom or a window open at the bottom together with an open transom may give good results. The disadvantages of this type of ventilation are the dependence upon wind direction and the difficulty of control, including the possibility of entrance of smoky, dusty, and generally undesirable air.

10-17. Artificial Ventilation. In the exhaust system of ventilation, the air is exhausted to the outside by a fan or blower, thereby causing a lower pressure inside and a leakage inward through windows, doors, and walls. This method is largely used in kitchens to remove odors; in industrial plants to remove dusts and fumes, the inlets to the ducts being placed near the point of their production; and in other circumstances where local ventilation is required.

The plenum system forces air into the room and causes a leakage outward, although exhaust ducts may also be provided. The forcing is accomplished by centrifugal fans, which operate in a manner similar to that of the centrifugal pump or by impeller fans, which are larger editions of the ordinary small electric fan. The former are more generally used in ventilation by ducts. The plenum system has the advantage of allowing control of the amount of air furnished, its source, and the treatment it may require. This is the method used for supplying air to air-conditioned buildings.

The ducts of a plenum system require careful design. Each room should be governed by separate dampers, and a small branch duct rather than merely an opening in the main duct should supply the air. To prevent the entering air from causing drafts, its velocity at the outlet grille should not exceed 500 fpm. In the duct it may be up to 3,000 fpm if the noise is not objectionable. The air usually enters at ceiling height, except where the problem is to remove heat generated by large numbers of people, as in a theater, in which case the air is applied through many outlets located under the seats.

Since the temperature of the room air is lower than that of outside air during the cooling season and higher during the heating season, it is economical to recirculate air, and accordingly most air-conditioning systems are arranged to recirculate a large part of the air from the occupied space and to take from the outside the quantity necessary to prevent concentration of odors. The total amount of air handled depends upon the amount of heat to be added or removed and upon the permissible difference between the temperature of the air as it enters the occupied rooms and the air already present. Great differences are undesirable because of the discomfort they may cause, although good mixing as the air leaves the duct is beneficial. For comfort ventilation during the cooling season, the entering air is introduced into occupied rooms at a temperature 2° cooler than that to be maintained in the room for every foot the center of the grille is above the floor.

Health officers of some cities have expressed concern about the possible effect, during very hot weather, of entering and leaving buildings which have been cooled. It is thought that too great a difference in temperature may be injurious, but investigation has established that this fear is unfounded.

10-18. Air Conditioning. Figure 10-2 shows the various devices that are used in air-conditioning systems. This article briefly describes these devices and explains what they accomplish. Figure 10-3 shows one type of air-conditioning unit.

FILTERS. Filtration removes soot and dust from the air. Dry filters are most commonly used. They are discarded when they are dirty, while others are cleaned by vacuum-cleaning methods. Viscous filters use mats of crimped metal ribbon or glass wool that are coated with a viscous

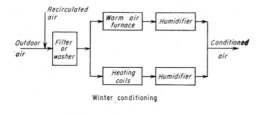

Winter conditioning

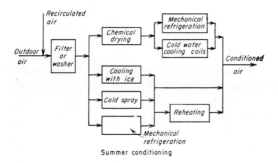

Summer conditioning

FIGURE 10-2 Various combinations of air treatments used in air conditioning.

nondrying oil. When the mats are dirty, they are washed and reoiled,
although some inexpensive types are discarded. Automatic filters are
self-cleaning and may be of higher capacity. They have filtering mats
or panels moving over endless chains, and at the low point of their
path they pass through a bath of oil for cleaning and reoiling. The water
spray also has cleaning ability. Many of the dust particles are carried
down by the drops of water, while others are caught on the plates,
which eliminate droplets from the air (Fig. 10-2). Electrostatic methods
have also been used. Electric precipitators are used where exceptionally
dust-free air is required, as in hospitals, or in collection systems where
valuable chemical or mineral dusts are recovered. They consist of a
high-intensity ionizing field and a secondary field where the dust is
precipitated. They are very expensive but low in operating cost.

HEATING. In air-conditioned buildings some of the heat loss from the
building during cold weather may be provided by radiators in the
rooms. The outside air introduced by the forced-draft, or plenum, system
must then be heated, either by a warm-air furnace or by coils through
which steam or hot water circulates.

HUMIDIFYING AND DEHUMIDIFYING. Humidifying may be done by
passing air over pans of water having a very large surface or over
cloth strips which are kept wetted by capillary action. If large amounts
of air are to be moistened, spray humidifiers are generally used. The
simplest spray system passes water directly from the city water system

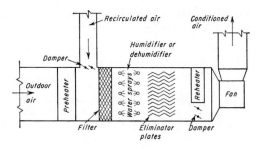

FIGURE 10-3   Spray-type air conditioner.

through spray nozzles which break the water up into very small drops. Another method is to impinge water jets against flat surfaces to form the spray. In either case the water may be wasted, or in large installations it may be more economical to re-use the spray water by means of a tank and pump. In this case the principal water loss is caused by evaporation. The spray humidifiers are followed by elimination plates so arranged that the air must follow a tortuous path between them. This removes droplets from the air.

Humidification of the air in the winter is important and at times very necessary. The hotter the air, the more water it evaporates and carries. Although the cold outside air may have a high relative humidity, when it is heated the relative humidity is very low. Although the drying has no definite harmful effects on people, it can make them very uncomfortable and may cause a dermatitis in the form of flaking or scaling of the skin. If the air is humidified too much, condensation takes place on the windows, although this can be prevented or reduced by the use of double glass windows. The control of humidity is probably most important to human comfort in the summer, when a high humidity may cause discomfort.

Dehumidification can be obtained by first lowering the temperature of the air below the dew point and condensing out the necessary amount of moisture and then reheating with a dry heat to the desired temperature. The cooling of the air may be done in several ways, but the most dependable is mechanical refrigeration of a type similar to that used in a household refrigerator. The "frost" on a household box shows the moisture that has been removed by cooling. When warm air is passed through a water spray, evaporation takes place and cools the air. In a very dry climate this is satisfactory, particularly if a source of very cold water is available. Frequently, mechanical refrigeration, and at times ice, is used to cool the spray water. In wet or humid climates there is little or no evaporation, but some cooling of the air is still obtained. Usually a water spray humidifies rather than dehumidifies. Whenever the air is dehumidified by refrigeration, it is usually necessary to reheat the air. If this is not done, there is a sensation of clamminess caused by the high humidity.

Dehumidification is also accomplished by means of chemicals which absorb moisture, used either as a liquid spray or as a solid made into filters. There are numerous substances now used that are considered equally acceptable, although they differ in cost and efficiency, some being much easier to reactivate than others. After chemical dehumidification, the air must still be cooled, so the air is frequently cooled first. This at times relieves the dehumidifier of some of its load.

COOLING. Cooling by a water spray—through its evaporative effect or the use of cold water, or both—has already been mentioned. Ice is sometimes used to cool the spray water, but this is expensive and is generally used for buildings such as auditoriums which are used only occasionally. Spray cooling is not advisable in humid climates since the humidity is raised. The air may be passed over coils containing cool water if there is a supply available. This is sometimes possible in residential installations that have their own well-water supplies. Mechanical refrigeration is frequently employed. It uses a refrigerant which is compressed, cooled, allowed to expand, and then passed through coils where it can absorb heat from the air.

THE HEAT PUMP. The heat pump is used for heating and cooling, particularly for residences in areas with mild winters. A compressor circulates a vapor refrigerant; its condensation, in which heat is released, is used for heating, and its evaporation after expansion, in which heat is absorbed, is used for cooling. On the heating cycle, heat from the atmospheric air, small though it is, is absorbed by the expanded refrigerant in the evaporator. Thus it increases the heat of the refrigerant after compression. In the condenser, heat is transferred to the coolant, which is the air to be heated. On the cooling cycle, heat is absorbed from the air to be cooled at the evaporator. At the condenser, air is used as the coolant to absorb heat and is then wasted. Water, if it is available at suitable temperature, can be used instead of air to receive or remove heat. In this case the water is then used to heat or cool the air of the residence.

10-19. Insulation of Buildings. An economical method of attaining comfort is through the insulation of buildings and the stoppage of drafts from doors, windows, and fireplaces. Weather stripping of exposed doors and windows may result in a 20 per cent saving in fuel, while complete house insulation, which includes wall and roof insulation in addition to weather stripping, may save as much as 60 per cent of fuel. This improvement greatly increases comfort by preventing unduly cold walls and ceilings, to which the warmer bodies of occupants radiate heat, and in the summer the cooler ceilings and walls do not radiate so much heat to the occupants.

10-20. Disinfection of Air in Occupied Rooms. While there has been a tendency to minimize the importance of air as a transmitter of disease, it is recognized that it may play a significant role in the spread of many diseases, including influenza and pneumonia, and such childhood diseases as mumps, measles, chicken pox, scarlet fever, and whooping cough. Possibly it also plays a part in the spread of staphylococcal infections in hospitals.

Such diseases, as previously explained, are also spread by direct and indirect contact, and it is difficult to say how important airborne infection is in relation to the other methods. It is known, however, that bacteria and viruses of human origin occur in the air in droplets, in droplet nuclei, and in dusts. Droplets originate from secretions of the nose, throat, and mouth. When they are expelled during talking, coughing, sneezing, or spitting, some may be inhaled by nearby persons, or they may fall upon food or objects which are handled in such a manner that the infection is quickly spread to other persons. Transmission of this type is considered direct or indirect contact. The larger droplets quickly settle and dry on nearby surfaces, such as floors, tables, clothing, and bedding. The smaller droplets evaporate in the air, and their dried residues, called "droplet nuclei," float about in the air and drift with currents. Dust in the air, therefore, may be contaminated by droplets and droplet nuclei or by contact with infected handkerchiefs, bandages and dressings of infected wounds, bedding, and clothing.

Investigations and experiments in air disinfection have not produced consistent results. In some cases disinfection appeared to be beneficial, and in others there was no appreciable effect. According to present knowledge, it is justifiable only in hospitals and research laboratories. Further research may indicate its value in schools and barracks but probably not in any other buildings.

Four measures are used to control or prevent infection of air in rooms: (1) ventilation, (2) ultraviolet irradiation, (3) use of disinfectant vapors, and (4) dust suppression. The value of these methods has been tested by noting the reduction they effect in the total bacterial count of the air or in the number of test organisms added, such as certain microorganisms usually found in the nasopharyngeal tract and certain specific pathogens, such as beta hemolytic streptococci or influenza virus A. To obtain even more knowledge, records have been kept of disease incidence among persons living and/or sleeping in buildings where air has been treated. These records have been so contradictory as to throw doubt upon the value of air disinfection for general use.

VENTILATION. This consists in opening windows or using fans, with or without washing of air, so that there is a considerable air interchange. Within practical limits of air interchange, there is no apparent effect upon disease incidence. This, however, does not apply to hospital operating rooms and nurseries, where a high dilution of room air with filtered and conditioned new air prevents infection.

ULTRAVIOLET IRRADIATION. Ultraviolet light is well known for its bactericidal effect; under test conditions it greatly reduces the number of bacteria in air, although under field conditions equal results are not always obtained. Fixtures are now available which, with the use of photometers, allow economical and safe use of ultraviolet light. Its use, however, requires installation and supervision by competent engineers. It must be recognized also that the ultraviolet ray, if not properly controlled, is uncomfortable for the eyes and may cause "sunburn" to the skin. It has no effect upon bacteria in dust.

Irradiation of upper air has been tried in military barracks, in schoolrooms, and in hospital wards and operating rooms. The results obtained have not been encouraging.

USE OF DISINFECTANT VAPORS. Various disinfectants have been investigated for this purpose, but triethylene glycol appears to be the most useful because of its high bactericidal effect, its reasonable cost, and its freedom from odors, toxicity, and corrosiveness to metal surfaces. If air temperatures are high, complaints of stuffiness may result, and since its volatility is low, the concentration required for killing bacteria may be exceeded, and fogging may result. The glycol, on the other hand, effectively permeates all parts of a room. Its bactericidal effect depends upon its relative saturation rather than the total concentration. It has been found to be most efficient when combined with dust-suppressive measures. Methods of vaporizing triethylene glycol and maintaining its relative saturation in the air have been developed on an experimental basis and may in the future be standardized for practical use. Perhaps when these technical problems have been worked out, this method will prove of greater usefulness.

DUST-SUPPRESSIVE MEASURES. A simple and effective measure for laying dust in military barracks which have wood floors is to apply light paraffin oil or spindle oil. A saturation application to soft unvarnished wood is effective for 3 months or longer. If the floor is of hardwood, more frequent treatments are needed. The method is not applicable to concrete, linoleum, or waxed surfaces, but daily use of oiled mops or oiled sawdust during sweeping is equally effective. For treatment of hospital floors see Art. 15-15.

Not all dust comes from floors. Much is discharged into the air from bedclothing, especially during bed changing, and accordingly various methods have been developed to impregnate blankets, bedding, and certain types of clothing with oil. A simple method which can be used in any well-equipped laundry is as follows: A stable oil-water emulsion, made with a neutral detergent, triton NE, is added at the time of the final rinse in the laundry process. This treatment causes the clothing to retain its dust and bacteria. The effect remains after many months and after subsequent washings.

Dust-suppressive procedures are to be recommended as a hygienic measure. They result in a great reduction in the bacterial content of the air, and they are practical of application. There is insufficient evidence as yet, however, to establish their value in the control of respiratory disease.

10-21. Heating Appliances and Carbon Monoxide. The increased use of natural and artificial gas for heating purposes has caused a hazard which has frequently resulted in deaths. The National Safety Council reports that in 1961 there were 700 deaths caused by gas heating and cooking appliances and standing vehicles [6]. While many state and city health departments have launched educational campaigns on the subject, the public still requires further instruction.

Carbon monoxide (CO) poisoning from gas heating appliances is generally due to the fact that they are unvented (space heaters and hot-water heaters), to "plugged-up" or faulty flues, or to lack of sufficient makeup air to support combustion and life. While faulty appliances previously caused great carbon monoxide production, a more common cause of deaths at present is improper vents and lack of fresh air. The danger is increased by the fact that carbon monoxide is odorless and nonirritating. When breathed, it first causes headache, weariness, and dizziness, then nausea, vomiting, and finally death. The symptoms are caused by the fact that the carbon monoxide has a chemical affinity for the hemoglobin, thereby interfering with the normal oxygen-carrying power of the blood. Serious results may be caused by long exposure to low concentrations or by short exposure to high concentrations. According to Webster [7], a blood saturation of 20 to 30 per cent of carbon monoxide produces headache and throbbing of the temples, and this result is noticed after exposure for $3\frac{1}{2}$ to 5 hr in a concentration of 200 ppm of carbon monoxide (0.02 per cent by volume) in room air. At 400 ppm the same result is noted in $1\frac{1}{2}$ to $3\frac{1}{4}$ hr. At 2,000 ppm death occurs in 1 to 2 hr, while 5,000 ppm causes death in 20 min.

Carbon monoxide is a common constituent of manufactured gas, which, when burned under proper conditions, is transformed into harmless products. Burning of any fuel with an insufficient air supply, however, results in more or less carbon monoxide being produced. The so-called coal-gas poisoning, due to coal fires having their drafts cut off by dampers or soot accumulations, is essentially carbon monoxide poisoning. In connection with the use of gas, carbon monoxide may be given off by hot-water heaters, cooking stoves, some makes of solid-top gas ranges, radiant heaters, and gas lights with mantles. Poorly adjusted and dirty burners are dangerous, as are homemade contrivances and amateur adjustments of appliances. According to the standards of the

American Gas Association, gas-burning appliances should not produce over 0.02 per cent carbon monoxide in the air-free products of gas combustion. In actual use this is frequently exceeded, and probably carbon monoxide poisoning in its less severe forms is more prevalent than is generally recognized.

Prevention of poisoning may be accomplished by simple precautions. Proper venting to flues carries off the products of combustion and is effective for ovens, water heaters, and room heaters. For ranges, a hood is necessary. Restrictions or dampers in the vents are dangerous. Under no circumstances should an unvented heater be used in a bedroom during sleeping hours. Radiant heaters [8], the most frequent cause of fatalities, should be given special attention. If they are of the non-luminous-flame, or blue-flame, type and are turned on only enough to cause glowing of three-fourths of the radiant material from bottom to top, and if the air supply into the gas feed pipe is sufficient, the heater may be used without a vent in a well-ventilated room that is not a bedroom. If the radiant material is glowing over its entire height or if insufficient air is being mingled with the gas, carbon monoxide may be generated. Broken radiants resting upon the burner openings are also dangerous. Enlarging the perforations in the pipe so that more gas escapes is an exceedingly dangerous practice, as the proper relation between air supply and gas is destroyed. Luminous, or yellow, flames are produced by gas jets which derive their air supply from the surrounding air and not from an air hole in the pipe. Luminous flames should not be permitted to come into contact with metal surfaces, or carbon monoxide will be given off. Should a gas-burning apparatus produce a luminous flame when it normally should have a blue flame, the opening which supplies air to the gas feed pipe should be examined. Not infrequently dust or dirt clogs these openings. Adjustments of all appliances should be frequently checked by skilled employees of the gas company.

New York City, in which only natural gas is used, has established regulations to control heaters. Those in bedrooms must be of the sealed combustion type, that is, the type that draws air for combustion from outside and vents combustion products to the outside. Devices are also required that automatically shut down the heater if a vent or flue is blocked [10].

10-22. Automobile Exhausts. Many deaths have resulted from automobile exhaust gases in garages. These gases include carbon monoxide, and the concentration in small individual garages may be expected to become dangerous after a motor has been running for 5 to 10 min. Motors should be kept tuned up and the exhaust system tight. Sleeping in a closed running automobile is dangerous. Because of the danger of exhaust gases entering closed cars, some cities are requiring by ordinance special safeguarding of closed buses. Many state health departments require adequate ventilation and tail-pipe exhaust systems for repair garages. Adequate ventilation is the most effective method for control of the carbon monoxide hazard in garages. The amount of carbon monoxide exhausted is directly proportional to the richness of the mixture, and the so-called "wet" or "dry" mixtures have no bearing on the matter.

Ethyl gasoline contains tetraethyl lead, a highly poisonous compound which has been responsible for fatalities in laboratories and factories in connection with the manufacturing of the gasoline. There appears to be no danger in the proper use and dispensation of ethyl gasoline, but it should be used only as a fuel and for no other purpose.

Bibliography

1. "ASHRAE Guide and Data Books," American Society of Heating, Refrigerating and Air-Conditioning Engineers, Inc., New York, 1961, 1962, 1963.
2. Carrier, W. H., *et al.:* "Modern Air Conditioning, Heating and Ventilating," 3d ed., Pitman Publishing Corporation, New York, 1959.
3. Severns, W. H., and J. R. Fellows: "Air Conditioning and Refrigeration," John Wiley & Sons, Inc., New York, 1958.
4. Jennings, B. H.: "Heating and Air Conditioning," International Textbook Company, Scranton, Pa., 1956.
5. Winslow, C.-E. A.: "Fresh Air and Ventilation," E. P. Dutton & Co., Inc., New York.
6. "Accident Facts," National Safety Council, Chicago, 1962.
7. Webster, R. W.: "Legal Medicine and Toxicology," W. B. Saunders Company, Philadelphia.
8. Jones, G. W., *et al.:* Incomplete Combustion in Natural Gas Heaters, *U.S. Bur. Mines Tech. Paper* 362.
9. Lee, D. H. K.: "Heat and Cold Effects and Their Control," Course Manual, Public Health Service.
10. Cohen, R., and E. Sineno: A New Method for the Prevention of Carbon Monoxide Poisoning, *Sanitarian*, vol. 24, no. 6, May–June, 1962.

11

PLUMBING

11-1. An important factor in control of the environment for health is the provision of safe methods of sewage collection and disposal. One of the links in this chain is the house-drainage system—in other words, the plumbing. Its importance is enhanced by the fact that it is in far closer contact with the everyday life of the citizen than the common sewer or sewage treatment plant. The sewage which the plumbing system carries is potentially dangerous in that it frequently contains disease-producing bacteria. Leakage in plumbing systems, therefore, is a menace to health, whether it occurs in the house, where infection of food is possible, or in the ground outside the house, where water supplies may be contaminated. In either case an offensive condition will result. Even more important is the fact that defective plumbing may allow wastes to enter the water-supply pipes. A further danger is the possible entrance into the house of insects and rats from the drainage system, possibly bearing upon their feet and bodies the germs of disease. Sewer air may also make its way into buildings through defective plumbing. The nature of sewer air will be discussed further below.

Important also is the provision of water to the home. Physical cleanliness, particularly of infants and small children, is a significant factor in the prevention of diarrhea and dysentery. The well-designed plumbing system will provide water in adequate amounts to the home and to each water-using fixture.

A knowledge of good practice in plumbing is valuable in many ways to the sanitarian, the sanitary engineer, and also the city engineer. In municipalities which require licenses for plumbers, one or more may be members of the examining board. In smaller cities, very frequently the city engineer or sanitarian is the plumbing inspector. He encounters defective plumbing in the investigation of nuisances and occasionally in the study of epidemics.

11-2. Legal Control. Public regulation of plumbing is based upon the police power of government, the principle of which is that government has the right to provide for the safety, health, and morals of the people. Plumbing codes, therefore, are or should be designed to protect, with reasonable provisions, the health, welfare, and comfort of the public. The police power is delegated to the individual states, but not all of them have yet attempted to apply it to plumbing. Some states have no laws regulating plumbing, although there are local codes in force in the larger cities and in many of the smaller ones. Others have laws that prescribe statewide regulations. Some have laws that are applicable only to cities of a certain size, while still others require the licensing of plumbers with or without making it obligatory for cities to adopt plumbing ordinances. Other states have recommended a state plumbing code which is offered to the communities for adoption. The "Revision of the National Plumbing Code ASA A40.8-1955" [1] includes a plumbing ordinance which may be adopted by cities. By reference or inclusion, it makes the National Code a part of the Ordinance. Uniformity of codes, throughout a state at least, is desirable.

11-3. Plumbing Codes. As may be imagined, there is little or no uniformity of principles or practice in plumbing codes. Furthermore, there is a regrettable tendency on the part of officials, particularly in the smaller cities, to neglect the enforcement of regulations. Occasionally the attitude is encountered that the only purpose of codes is to make plumbing more elaborate, to the greater profit of the plumber. The price of plumbing may be increased insofar as plumbing codes eliminate the incompetent workman who is competing with responsible master plumbers. The work of the incompetent, however, is expensive at any price. Well-designed plumbing regulations, properly enforced, result in no increase in plumbing costs when the work is done by conscientious and skilled plumbers. In general, however, plumbing codes make provisions for the examination and licensing of plumbers; regulate the sizes and kinds of pipes and fittings, placing of traps and vents, and grades of horizontal lines; and require inspections and tests of new work before approval. As space does not allow discussion of all details of a comprehensive plumbing code, the following articles emphasize only the points in which sanitation is particularly involved and the more important matters concerned with adequacy and good workmanship.

In 1951, the Coordinating Committee for a National Plumbing Code published its Report [1], which represents a consensus of the members of the Coordinating Committee and of its advisory committee. This Report reflects the experience and conclusions reached from research in the field of plumbing conducted by laboratories, including those of the National Bureau of Standards, the University of Iowa, the University of Illinois, and the Public Health Service. It is an attempt to attain national uniformity, and to this end it is soundly conceived and suitable for general acceptance. The American Standards Association accepted the recommendations of this committee, and they were published as the National Plumbing Code in 1955 [2], sponsored by the American Society of Mechanical Engineers and the American Public Health Association. Periodic revision of codes is desirable, and after a study by the Technical Committee on Plumbing Standards, established by the Public Health Service at the request of the sponsors, a report was issued by the Service in 1962 [1]. Plumbing practice, which can only be outlined in this chapter, follows in general the recommended requirements contained in the Code and the 1962 Report.

11-4. Enforcement. In the smaller cities, enforcement of plumbing regulations may present some difficulties. Two possibilities present themselves: either placing enforcement within the jurisdiction of the city engineer or placing it within the jurisdiction of the waterworks division. The city engineer, if one is retained by the city, is probably the logical enforcement officer, as he has the maps showing sewer locations and is also concerned with street openings. If no city engineer is available, some qualified member of the waterworks staff may be selected for this work. The employment of a plumber on a part-time basis is unsatisfactory, since he must inspect and pass upon work of his competitors. In the larger cities, full-time plumbing inspectors are essential. Practice varies as to the placing of the plumbing division within the city government. In some cities it is a division of the health department; in others, of the bureau of building inspection or the public works department. If the health department has a division of sanitary engineering, plumbing inspection should be placed in it.

Plumbers are required to obtain permits to make sewer connections or to install or construct plumbing fixtures. Fees are charged according to the number of fixtures placed. Permits for opening streets or alleys to make connections with sewers are also required. Before the work is approved, two tests are applied: the first, after the "roughing in" is completed; the final, after all fixtures have been placed and trap seals filled. No work is covered before the inspector has seen it. Certificates of approval are issued, and in many cities the certificate must be presented by the property owner or agent when application is made for turning on the city water.

11-5. Scope of Plumbing. Plumbing has two objects: (1) to furnish water to the various parts of a building and (2) to remove the liquid wastes and discharge them into the sewer or private disposal plant.

The water system must accomplish two objects: (1) There must be provided a sufficient amount of water to serve each fixture; (2) there must be no opportunity for backflow of used water into the water pipes. The waste system must also accomplish (1) quick removal of the wastes with minimum chance for stoppage of drains or leakage and (2) prevention of entrance into the house of vermin and "sewer gas," or foul-smelling air from the plumbing system or sewer.

11-6. Sewer Gas. A few words as to the character of the so-called "sewer gas" will be appropriate here. Strictly, it is not a gas of definite chemical composition but air that has come into contact with decomposing organic matter. The sewer air may contain some of the gases which are the results of decomposition, such as hydrogen sulfide and carbon dioxide, and which, under some circumstances, as in unventilated sewers or in sewer manholes, may overcome workmen. Numerous bacteriological tests have shown that sewer air is as free from bacteria as ordinary air, so that no disease infection need be feared from sewage bacteria floating into houses with sewer gas. The matter should not be dismissed so lightly, however. No one can say with certainty that long exposure to sewer air will not have some harmful physiological effect other than the causing of a specific disease. Hence, safe practice and good sense dictate that sewer air be prevented from entering buildings. On the other hand, since it is established that occasional small amounts of sewer air are not dangerous, heavy expense is uncalled for in cases where possible entrance of offensive air is problematical and where such entrance would be likely to occur only at widely spaced intervals.

11-7. Definition of Terms. Following are definitions of the more important plumbing terms. They are extracted from the American

Standard National Plumbing Code (ASA A40.8-1955) with the permission of the publisher, the American Society of Mechanical Engineers.

Air Gap. An air gap in a water-supply system is the unobstructed vertical distance through the free atmosphere between the lowest opening from any pipe or faucet supplying water to a tank, plumbing fixture, or other device and the flood-level rim of the receptacle.

Backflow. Backflow is the flow of water or other liquids, mixtures, or substances into the distributing pipes of a potable supply of water from any source or sources other than its intended source. (See back-siphonage.)

Backflow Preventer. A backflow preventer is a device or means to prevent backflow into the potable water system.

Back-Siphonage. Back-siphonage is the flowing back of used, contaminated, or polluted water from a plumbing fixture or vessel into a water-supply pipe due to a negative pressure in such pipe. (See backflow.)

Battery of Fixtures. A "battery of fixtures" is any group of two or more similar adjacent fixtures which discharge into a common horizontal waste or soil branch.

Branch. A branch is any part of the piping system other than a main, riser, or stack.

Branch Interval. A branch interval is a length of soil or waste stack corresponding in general to a story height, but in no case less than 8 feet within which the horizontal branches from one floor or story of a building are connected to the stack.

Branch Vent. A branch vent is a vent connecting one or more individual vents with a vent stack or stack vent.

Building Drain. The building (house) drain is that part of the lowest piping of a drainage system which receives the discharge from soil, waste, and other drainage pipes inside the walls of the building and conveys it to the building (house) sewer beginning 3 feet outside the building wall.

Building Sewer. The building (house) sewer is that part of the horizontal piping of a drainage system which extends from the end of the building drain and which receives the discharge of the building drain and conveys it to a public sewer, private sewer, individual sewage-disposal system, or other point of disposal.

Building Trap. A building (house) trap is a device, fitting, or assembly of fittings installed in the building drain to prevent circulation of air between the drainage system of the building and the building sewer.

Circuit Vent. A circuit vent is a branch vent that serves two or more traps and extends from in front of the last fixture connection of a horizontal branch to the vent stack.

Combination Fixture. A combination fixture is a fixture combining one sink and tray or a two- or three-compartment sink or tray in one unit.

Combination Waste and Vent System. A combination waste and vent system is a specially designed system of waste piping embodying the horizontal wet venting of one or more sinks or floor drains by means of a common waste and vent pipe adequately sized to provide free movement of air above the flow line of the drain.

Common Vent. A common vent is a vent connecting at the junction of two fixture drains and serving as a vent for both fixtures.

Continuous Vent. A continuous vent is a vertical vent that is a continuation of the drain to which it connects.

Continuous Waste. A continuous waste is a drain from two or three fixtures connected to a single trap.

Cross-Connection. A cross-connection is any physical connection or arrangement between two otherwise separate piping systems, one of which contains potable water and the other water of unknown or questionable safety, whereby water may flow from one system to the other, the direction of flow depending on the pressure differential between the two systems. (See Backflow and Back-Siphonage).

Dead End. A dead end is a branch leading from a soil, waste, or vent pipe, building drain, or building sewer, which is terminated at a developed distance of 2 feet or more by means of a plug or other closed fitting.

Developed Length. The developed length of a pipe is its length along the center line of the pipe and fittings.

Drainage System. A drainage system (drainage piping) includes all the piping within public or private premises, which conveys sewage, rain water, or other liquid wastes to a legal point of disposal, but does not include the mains of a public sewer system or private or public sewage-treatment or disposal plant.

Dual Vent. See Common Vent.

Effective Opening. The effective opening is the minimum cross-sectional area at the point of water-supply discharge, measured or expressed in terms of (1) diameter of a circle, (2) if the opening is not circular, the diameter of a circle of equivalent cross-sectional area. (This is applicable to air gap.)

Fixture Branch. A fixture branch is a pipe connecting several fixtures.

Fixture Drain. A fixture drain is the drain from the trap of a fixture to the junction of that drain with any other drain pipe.

Fixture Supply. A fixture supply is a water-supply pipe connecting the fixture with the fixture branch.

Fixture Unit. A fixture unit is a quantity in terms of which the load-producing effects on the plumbing system of different kinds of plumbing fixtures are expressed on some arbitrarily chosen scale.

Fixture-Unit Flow Rate. Fixture-unit flow rate is the total discharge flow in gpm of a single fixture divided by 7.5 which provides the flow rate of that particular plumbing fixture as a unit of flow. Fixtures are rated as multiples of this unit of flow.

Flush Valves. A flush valve is a device located at the bottom of the tank for the purpose of flushing water closets and similar fixtures.

Flushometer Valve. A flushometer valve is a device which discharges a predetermined quantity of water to fixtures for flushing purposes and is actuated by direct water pressure.

Frostproof Closet. A frostproof closet is a hopper that has no water in the bowl and has the trap and the control valve for its water supply installed below the frost line.

Grade. Grade is the slope or fall of a line of pipe in reference to a horizontal plane. In drainage it is usually expressed as the fall in a fraction of an inch per foot length of pipe.

Grease Trap. See Interceptor.

Horizontal Branch. A horizontal branch is a drain pipe extending laterally from a soil or waste stack or building drain, with or without vertical sections or branches, which receives the discharge from one or more fixture drains and conducts it to the soil or waste stack or to the building (house) drain.

Horizontal Pipe. Horizontal pipe means any pipe or fitting which makes an angle of more than 45 deg. with the vertical.

House Drain. See Building Drain.

House Sewer. See Building Sewer.

House Trap. See Building Trap.

Interceptor. An interceptor is a device designed and installed so as to separate and retain deleterious, hazardous, or undesirable matter from normal wastes and permit normal sewage or liquid wastes to discharge into the disposal terminal by gravity.

Leader. A leader (downspout) is the water conductor from the roof to the building storm drain, combined building sewer, or other means of disposal.

Liquid Waste. Liquid waste is the discharge from any fixture, appliance, or appurtenance, in connection with a plumbing system which does not receive fecal matter.

Local Ventilating Pipe. A local ventilating pipe is a pipe on the fixture side of the trap through which vapor or foul air is removed from a room or fixture.

Loop Vent. A loop vent is the same as a circuit vent except that it loops back and connects with a stack vent instead of a vent stack.

Main. The main of any system of continuous piping is the principal artery of the system, to which branches may be connected.

Main Sewer. A sewer directly controlled by public authority.

Main Vent. The main vent is the principal artery of the venting system, to which vent branches may be connected.

Plumbing Fixtures. Plumbing fixtures are installed receptacles, devices, or appliances which are supplied with water or which receive or discharge liquids or liquid-borne wastes, with or without discharge into the drainage system with which they may be directly or indirectly connected.

Plumbing System. The plumbing system includes the water-supply and distribution pipes; plumbing fixtures and traps; soil, waste, and vent pipes; building drains and building sewers including their respective connections, devices, and appurtenances within the property lines of the premises; and water-treating or water-using equipment.

Relief Vent. A relief vent is a vent the primary function of which is to provide circulation of air between drainage and vent systems.

Revent Pipe. A revent pipe (sometimes called an individual vent) is that part of a vent pipe line which connects directly with an individual waste or group of wastes, underneath or back of the fixture, and extends either to the main or branch vent pipe.

Riser. A riser is a water-supply pipe which extends vertically one full story or more to convey water to branches or fixtures.

Roughing-In. Roughing-in is the installation of all parts of the plumbing system which can be completed prior to the installation of fixtures. This includes drainage, water-supply, and vent piping, and the necessary fixture supports.

Side Vent. A side vent is a vent connecting to the drain pipe through a fitting at an angle not greater than 45 deg. to the vertical.

Soil Pipe. A soil pipe is any pipe which conveys the discharge of water closets or fixtures having similar functions, with or without the discharge from other fixtures, to the building drain or building sewer.

Stack. A stack is the vertical main of a system of soil, waste, or vent piping.

Stack Group. Stack group is a term applied to the location of fixtures in relation to the stack so that by means of proper fittings, vents may be reduced to a minimum.

Stack Vent. A stack vent (sometimes called a waste vent or soil vent) is the extension of a soil or waste stack above the highest horizontal drain connected to the stack.

Stack Venting. Stack venting is a method of venting a fixture or fixtures through the soil or waste stack.

Trap. A trap is a fitting or device so designed and constructed as to provide, when properly vented, a liquid seal which will prevent the back passage of air without materially affecting the flow of sewage or waste water through it.

Trap Seal. The trap seal is the maximum vertical depth of liquid that a trap will retain, measured between the crown weir and the top of the dip of the trap.

Vacuum Breaker. See Backflow Preventer.

Vent Stack. A vent stack is a vertical vent pipe installed primarily for the purpose of providing circulation of air to and from any part of the drainage system.

Vent System. A vent system is a pipe or pipes installed to provide a flow of air to or from a drainage system or to provide a circulation of air within such system to protect trap seals from siphonage and back pressure.

Vertical Pipe. A vertical pipe is any pipe or fitting which is installed in a vertical position or which makes an angle of not more than 45 deg. with the vertical.

Waste Pipe. A waste pipe is a pipe which conveys only liquid waste, free of fecal matter.

Water-Distributing Pipe. A water-distributing pipe in a building or premises is a pipe which conveys water from the water-service pipe to the plumbing fixtures and other water outlets.

Water-Service Pipe. The water-service pipe is the pipe from the water main or other source of water supply to the building served.

Water-Supply System. The water-supply system of a building or premises consists of the water-service pipe, the water-distributing pipes, and the necessary connecting pipes, fittings, control valves, and all appurtenances in or adjacent to the building or premises.

Wet Vent. A wet vent is a vent which receives the discharge from wastes other than water closets.

11-8. Plumbing Fixtures Required. The types and minimum number of plumbing fixtures that will be required in a building will depend upon the type of occupancy and the number of persons that must be served. Table 11-1 gives some types of buildings and their minimum requirements. For a more complete list, the reader is referred to the Revision of the National Plumbing Code [1].

11-9. Water Supply. The water-service pipe of any building should be of sufficient size to permit a continuous ample flow of water at any time and never less than ¾ in. If flush valves or other devices requiring high flow rates are used, the water-service pipe must be designed to meet this flow. It may be of asbestos cement, brass or copper pipe, copper tubing, wrought iron, open-hearth iron, lead, plastic, or steel. Ferrous threaded pipe must be galvanized or cement-lined.

Pipe of the distribution system may be of brass or copper pipe, copper tubing, galvanized wrought iron, galvanized open-hearth iron, galvanized steel, or exposed plastic cold-water pipe.

The plumbing fixtures should be provided with a sufficient supply of water for flushing purposes. Water closets or urinal bowls should not be supplied directly from the water system through a flushometer or other valve unless such valve has an approved vacuum breaker that will prevent siphonage of water back into the water pipes. This requirement applies to all fixtures having under-rim water inlets. Backflow preventers should also be provided with lawn sprinkler systems and fixtures with hose attachments. For sprinkler systems the backflow preventer should be placed at least 6 in. above the highest sprinkler head and never less than 6 in. above the surrounding ground. A cutoff in the water-service pipe should be provided at the curb, and if the building is divided into apartments, cutoffs should also be placed in the individual supply lines just inside the foundation walls. Good practice also calls

Table 11-1. MINIMUM NUMBER OF PLUMBING FIXTURES

Type of building	Water closets	Urinals	Lavatories	Bathtubs or showers	Drinking fountains	Other fixtures
Dormitories—school or labor, also institutional	Men: 1 per 10 persons Women: 1 per 8 persons	1 per 25 men. Over 150, add 1 fixture for ea. 50 men.	1 per 12 persons. (Separate dental lavatories should be provided in community toilet rooms. A ratio of 1 dental lavatory to ea. 50 persons is recommended.)	1 per 8 persons. For women's dormitories, additional bathtubs in the ratio of 1 per 30 women. Over 150 persons, add 1 fixture for ea. 20 persons.	1 per 75 persons	Laundry trays, 1 per 50 persons Slop sinks, 1 per 100 persons
Dwellings—one- and two-family	1 per dwelling unit		1 per dwelling unit	1 per dwelling unit		Kitchen sink, 1 per dwelling unit
Dwellings—multiple or apartment	1 per dwelling unit or apartment		1 per dwelling unit or apartment	1 per dwelling unit or apartment		Kitchen sink, 1 per dwelling unit. For multiple units in excess of 10, 1 double laundry tray per 10 units or 1 automatic washing machine per 20 units

SOURCE: "A Revision of the National Plumbing Code ASA A40.8-1955," Report of the Public Health Service Technical Committee on Plumbing Standards, 1962.

Table 11-1. MINIMUM NUMBER OF PLUMBING FIXTURES (Continued)

Type of building	Water closets	Urinals	Lavatories	Bathtubs or showers	Drinking fountains	Other fixtures
Industrial—factories, warehouses, foundries, and similar establishments	No. of ea. sex / No. of fixtures: 1–10, 1; 11–25, 2; 26–50, 3; 51–75, 4; 76–100, 5. 1 fixture for ea. additional 30 employees	Where more than 10 men are employed: No. of men / No. of urinals: 11–30, 1; 31–80, 2; 81–160, 3; 161–240, 4	No. of persons / No. of fixtures: 1–100, 1 per 10 persons; Over 100, 1 per 15 persons	1 shower per 15 persons exposed to excessive heat or to hazard from poisonous, infectious, or irritating material	1 per 75 persons	
Public buildings, offices	No. of ea. sex / No. of fixtures: 1–15, 1; 16–35, 2; 36–55, 3; 56–80, 4; 81–110, 5; 111–150, 6. 1 fixture for ea. additional 40 employees	Urinals may be provided in men's toilet rooms in lieu of water closets, but for not more than ⅓ of the required number of water closets.	No. of employees / No. of fixtures: 1–15, 1; 16–35, 2; 36–60, 3; 61–90, 4; 91–125, 5. 1 fixture for ea. additional 45 persons			
Schools—elementary and secondary	Boys / Girls: 1 per 40 / 1 per 35; 1 per 75 / 1 per 45	1 per 30 boys; 1 per 30 boys	1 per 50 pupils; 1 per 50 pupils	In gym or pool shower rooms, 1 per 5 pupils *of a class*	1 per 100 pupils, but at least 1 per floor	Slop sinks, 1 **per** floor

for cutoffs for each closet, lawn sprinkler, and hot-water tank. A check valve, to prevent the backing up of hot water, should be placed in the cold-water pipe which supplies the hot-water tank. This will also necessitate a relief valve in the hot-water system. The entire water distribution system should be protected against freezing. (See Table 11-2 for recommended minimum sizes of water-supply pipes, and Table 11-3 for fixture units per fixture or group.)

11-10. Building Sewer. The line from the public sewer to within 3 ft of the foundation wall of the building is known as the building sewer and is of cast iron, vitrified clay, concrete, bituminized fiber, or asbestos cement. The required size of the building sewer will vary according to the number of fixtures drained by it. Some ordinances prescribe a minimum of 6 in. However, 4 in. will probably be sufficient for the ordinary residence having one closet and the usual number of other fixtures, provided that a slope of ⅛ to ¼ in./lin ft can be obtained. This pipe is laid in the same manner as public sewers are. The spigot of the pipe is the downstream end of each length. Care must be taken that the bottom of the trench is hollowed at each joint sufficiently to allow for the excess diameter caused by the bell and also that the trench bottom is shaped to the pipe so that one-third of the pipe surface will have a bearing area. In backfilling the trench, fine earth must be carefully tamped around the pipe until it is covered. In completing the backfilling, no heavy stones should be dropped in the trench until the pipe is covered to a depth of at least 1 ft. The method of making joints is described in Art.

Table 11-2.   MINIMUM SIZE OF FIXTURE-SUPPLY PIPE

Type of fixture or device	Pipe size, in.
Bathtub	½
Combination sink and tray	½
Drinking fountain	⅜
Dishwasher, domestic	½
Kitchen sink, residential	½
Kitchen sink, commercial	¾
Lavatory	⅜
Laundry tray, 1, 2, or 3 compartments	½
Shower, single head	½
Sinks, service slop	½
Sinks, flushing rim	¾
Urinal, flush tank	½
Urinal, direct-flush valve	¾
Water closet, tank type	⅜
Water closet, flush-valve type	1
Hose bibs	½
Wall hydrant	½

SOURCE: "Report of the Coordinating Committee for a National Plumbing Code," U.S. Department of Commerce, Domestic Commerce Series, no. 28.

Table 11-3. FIXTURE-UNIT VALUES AND TRAP SIZES FOR VARIOUS PLUMBING FIXTURES

Type of fixture or group of fixtures	Fixture-unit value	Trap size, in.
Automatic clothes washer (2-in. standpipe) . . .	3	. . . .
Bathroom group consisting of a water closet, lavatory, and bathtub or shower stall:		
Flushometer valve closet	8	. . . .
Tank-type closet	6	. . . .
Bathtub* (with or without overhead shower) . .	2	1½
Combination sink and tray with food disposal unit .	4	separate traps 1½
Combination sink and tray with one trap . . .	2	1½
Combination sink and tray with separate trap. . .	3	1½
Dental unit or cuspidor	1	1¼
Dental lavatory	1	1¼
Drinking fountain	½	1
Dishwasher, domestic (gravity drain)†	2	1½
Floor drains with 2-in. waste.	3	2
Kitchen sink, domestic, with one 1½-in. waste . .	2	1½
Kitchen sink, domestic, with food-waste grinder . .	2	1½
Lavatory with 1¼-in. waste	1	1¼
Laundry tray (1 or 2 compartments)	2	1½
Shower stall, domestic.	2	1½
Showers (group)†	2	. . . .
Sinks:		
Surgeon's.	3	1½
Flushing rim (with valve)	6	3
Service (trap standard)	3	3
Service (P-trap)	2	2
Pot, scullery, etc.†	4	2
Urinal, pedestal, syphon-jet blowout	6	3
Urinal, wall lip.	4	1½
Urinal, stall, washout	4	2
Urinal trough† (each 6-ft section)	2	. . . .
Wash sink† (circular or multiple):		
Each set of faucets	2	. . . .
Water closet, tank-operated	4	3
Water closet, valve-operated.	6	3
Unlisted fixture drain or trap size:		
1¼ in. or less	1	. . . .
1½ in.	2	. . . .
2 in.	3	. . . .
2½ in.	4	. . . .
3 in.	5	. . . .
4 in.	6	. . . .
Fixtures with continuous or semicontinuous flows‡ .	. . .	. . . .

* A shower head over a bathtub does not increase the fixture value.

† See [1] for a method of computing unit value of devices with continuous or semicontinuous flows.

‡ Fixture-unit values for continuous or semicontinuous flow into a drainage system, such as from a pump, sump ejector, air-conditioning equipment, or similar device, shall be computed on the basis of one fixture unit for each gallon per minute of flow.

SOURCE: "A Revision of the National Plumbing Code, ASA A40.8-1955," Report of the Public Health Service Technical Committee on Plumbing Standards, 1962.

11-14. Table 11-4 gives recommended sizes of house sewers and drains (column 1), together with the slope required and the number of fixture units connected.

Careless construction of house sewers has resulted in much infiltration of water into them from the ground after rains. This has resulted in overloading of the public sanitary sewers, with flooding of some buildings and considerable expense to the city for relief measures. It is extremely important that house sewers be carefully inspected before they are covered and that the joints described in Art. 11-14 be used instead of the inadequate mortar joint. Care must also be taken that leaders (rain leaders) are not connected to the house sewer if the latter discharges into a public sanitary sewer.

11-11. Building Drains and Branches. The building drain is of cast-iron pipe of a size conforming to the specifications given in Table 11-4. It should be laid or supported so that there will be no sags. Special precautions should be taken where it runs through the foundation wall. It is common practice to leave an opening around the pipe. This is justified by the fact that settlement of the foundation wall may damage the pipe. It is felt, however, that protection from this possible damage is more than offset by the certainty that rats and mice will find easy entrance through such an opening. Accordingly, many codes recommend that all

Table 11-4. MAXIMUM LOADS IN FIXTURE UNITS FOR HORIZONTAL DRAINS AND SOIL AND WASTE HAVING ONE OR TWO BRANCH INTERVALS

Diameter of drain or stack, in.	Horizontal fixture branch	Building drain or building sewer slope				Maximum load on stack
		$\frac{1}{16}$ in./ft	$\frac{1}{8}$ in./ft	$\frac{1}{4}$ in./ft	$\frac{1}{2}$ in./ft	
1¼	1	.....	......	....	....	2
1½	3	.....	......	....	....	4
2	6	.....	......	21	26	8
2½	12	.....	......	24	31	20
3 (waste)	32*	.....	36*	42*	50*	48†
4	160	.....	180	216	250	240
5	360	.....	390	400	575	540
6	620	.....	700	840	1,000	930
8	1,400	1,400	1,600	1,920	2,300	2,100
10	2,500	2,500	2,900	3,500	4,200	3,750
12	3,900	3,900	4,600	5,600	6,700	5,850
15	7,000	7,000	8,300	10,000	12,000	10,500

* Not more than two water closets or two bathroom groups.

† Not more than two water closets or bathroom groups within each branch interval, nor more than four water closets or bathroom groups on each stack.

SOURCE: "A Revision of the National Plumbing Code, ASA A40.8-1955," Report of the Public Health Service Technical Committee on Plumbing Standards, 1962.

exterior openings provided for the passage of piping be properly sealed with snugly fitting collars of metal or other ratproof material securely fastened in place. Interior openings should likewise be ratproofed.

Horizontal branch drains carrying waste from a water closet must be not less than 3 in. in size. All horizontal branch drains should be laid on a uniform grade and at no lesser slopes than $\frac{1}{4}$ in./ft for 3-in. size or smaller, and $\frac{1}{8}$ in./ft for larger pipes. Dead ends are prohibited.

Soil and waste pipes for drainage in a building should be of cast iron, galvanized wrought iron, galvanized open-hearth iron, galvanized steel, brass, copper, or lead. All drains which are underground should be of cast-iron soil pipe, service weight for buildings of not over four stories and extra heavy for higher buildings.

11-12. The Building Trap. The building trap, if used, is placed in the building drain just within the foundation walls. It is a running trap and should have at least one cleanout hole. The purpose of this trap is to isolate the house-drainage system from the sewer, particularly to prevent passage of sewer air into the house system. If it is used, a fresh-air inlet is necessary, running from the house side of the building trap to the outer air. The fresh-air inlet allows circulation of air through the building drain into the stacks and vent pipes.

The building trap was formerly much used. That there are advantages has already been noted, but it is doubtful whether such isolation is necessary. It is an advantage to have the sewer system ventilated through the house stacks, and there should be no excessive amount of odorous sewer air at any particular point if the sewer system is properly designed and constructed. The building trap is likely to clog and in cold weather may freeze, particularly if the fresh-air inlet is close to the trap. The general opinion at present is that the building trap can be safely dispensed with.

11-13. Changes of Direction. Changes in direction are made by the use of 45-deg wyes; short- or long-sweep quarter bends; sixth, eighth, or sixteenth bends; or combinations of the same or equivalent fittings. See Fig. 11-1. Single and double sanitary tees may be used on vertical stacks, and short quarter bends may be used in soil and waste lines when the change in direction of flow is from the horizontal to the vertical. Tees, crosses, and short quarter bends may be used in the vent pipes.

11-14. Joints. Joints in cast-iron soil pipe known as calked joints are made by firmly packing the opening between the bell and spigot with oakum or hemp and then filling with molten lead in a single pouring to a depth not less than 1 in. and not to extend more than $\frac{1}{8}$ in. below the rim of the hub. The lead is then tamped or calked so that the joint will be tight. No paint, varnish, or putty is permitted until after the joint is tested. In joining wrought iron, steel, or brass to cast iron, either screwed or calked joints are used. When joining lead pipe to cast iron,

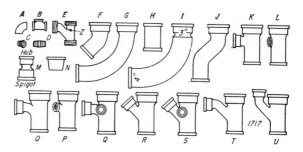

FIGURE 11-1 Fittings. A, plain elbow or ell, turns one-quarter of a circle, or 90 deg; B, beaded tee branch; C, shoulder bushing; D, shoulder nipple (these four are typical wrought water-pipe fittings); E, section of 90-deg long-turn Y-branch or TY drainage fitting recessed and threaded for wrought pipe (note that the point Z is below the center line of the inlet pipe, an important feature in soil and waste lines); F, eighth, or 45-deg bend—cast-iron, hub, and spigot type; G, long-sweep quarter bend; H, sleeve, sometimes used for joining two spigot ends on repair work; I, long-sweep reducing quarter bend, 4-in. spigot, 3-in. hub, often used at the bottom of 3-in. soil stacks; J, offset; K, T-branch; L, T-branch tapped for wrought pipe; M, reducer (an increaser has the spigot on the smaller end); N, plug; O, sanitary T-branch; P, sanitary T-branch tapped for wrought pipe; Q, sanitary T-branch with right-hand side inlet; R, Y-branch; S, Y-branch with right-hand side inlet; T, combination Y- and eighth bend or TY fitting; U, upright Y-branch. (*Courtesy of U.S. Department of Agriculture.*)

steel, or wrought iron, the joint should be made by means of a ferrule, soldered nipple, or bushing (see Fig. 11-2). Joints in lead pipe, or between lead pipe and ferrules, or in brass or copper pipe should be wiped joints, with an exposed surface of the solder to each side of the joint of not less than ¾ in. and at least as thick as the material being joined.

Threaded joints should have all burrs removed, and pipe ends should be reamed or filed so that the interior of the pipe is unobstructed. Pipe-joint cement and paint are permitted only on the male threads. For soft copper tubing, flared joints are permissible when made with proper fittings. The tubing must be expanded with a proper flaring tool. When such joints are concealed either in a building or underground, they should also be soldered. Soldered or sweat joints are used for joints between tubing and appropriate types of brass fittings. Joints in plastic pipe are made with approved fittings which are solvent-welded or fusion-welded or with insert fittings and corrosionproof metal clamps and screws.

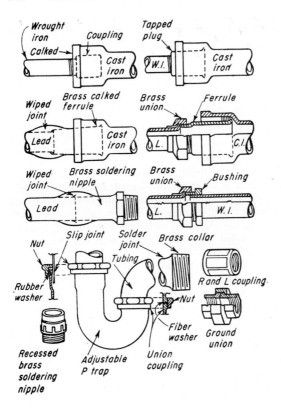

FIGURE 11-2 Methods of joining different kinds of pipe. The right and left coupling and ground union are used to join threaded male ends on water and vent pipes. (*Courtesy of U.S. Department of Agriculture.*)

Where slip joints are used, they should be installed only on the inlet side of a trap, or in the trap seal, and on the exposed fixture supply.

When hot poured joints for clay or concrete sewer pipe are made, all surfaces joined must be cleaned and dried, or a suitable primer should be applied. Approximately 25 per cent of the joint space in the base of the socket should be filled with jute or hemp. A pouring collar of rope or other device should be used to hold the hot compound during the pouring. A better joint for clay or concrete house sewers uses collars of plastic material placed on spigots and bells in the factory. A combined lubricant and cementing compound is then brushed on the spigot, which is then forced into the bell. The use of cement-mortar joints is discouraged. Asbestos-cement pipe joints are made with sleeve couplings of the same composition as the pipe sealed with rubber rings. Bituminized-fiber pipe joints are made with tapered-type couplings of the same material as the pipe.

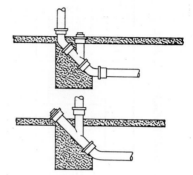

FIGURE 11-3 Methods of supporting stacks.
(*From New York Standard Plumbing Code.*)

11-15. Stacks. At least one of the stacks of the plumbing system must extend full size through the roof for the following purposes: to ventilate and carry off the sewer air above the roof; to prevent the siphoning of the traps by suction; and to prevent the possibility of a back pressure forcing the seals of the fixture traps. Stacks that receive wastes from fixtures only are known as waste stacks; those receiving wastes from fixtures and also from water closets are known as soil and waste stacks. The sizes of soil and waste stacks with number of fixtures contributing are given in Table 11-4. Many plumbing ordinances require that no water closet discharge into a stack less than 4 in. in diameter. However, the Revised National Plumbing Code [1] states that no soil or waste stack shall be smaller than the largest horizontal branch connected thereto, except that a 4- by 3-in. water-closet connection is not to be considered a reduction in pipe size. Any structure on which a building drain is installed must have at least one stack vent or vent stack which is carried full size through the roof for at least 12 in. and which is not less than 3 in. in diameter or is the size of the building drain, whichever is smaller. When the roof is used for purposes other than weather protection, the extension should be not less than 7 ft above the roof.

11-16. Pipe Supports. Since cast-iron stacks and soil pipes are jointed with lead, it is important that they be properly supported; otherwise changes in alignment may occur that will cause leaks. Vertical stacks should be supported at their bases by brick or concrete piers, and at each floor a wrought-iron strap should be placed just below the bell of the joint or branch of a fitting, securely fastening the pipe to a rafter or vertical timber. Wherever possible, the stack support should be built integrally with the foundation so that there will be uniform settlement. Unequal settlement may cause breakage of branch waste pipes and even raising of fixtures off the floors. Vertical piping must be supported as follows: cast-iron soil pipe, at not less than every story height and at its base; screwed pipe, at not less than every other story; copper tubing, at every story but not at more than 10-ft intervals; and lead and plastic

Table 11-5. MAXIMUM LOADS IN FIXTURE UNITS FOR ANY ONE BRANCH INTERVAL ON MULTISTORY SOIL AND WASTE STACKS*

Diameter of stack, in.	Number of branch intervals													Load limit for tall stacks
	3	4	5	6	7	8	9	10	11	12	13	14	15	
	fixture units	fixture units	fixture units	fixture units	fixture units	fixture units	fixture units	fixture units	fixture units	fixture units	fixture units	fixture units	fixture units	fixture units
2	3	.....	.....	.....	.....	.....	.....	.....	.....	.....	.....	.....	.....	10
2½	8	7	.....	.....	.....	.....	.....	.....	.....	.....	.....	.....	.....	28
3†	20	18	17	16	.....	.....	.....	.....	.....	.....	.....	.....	.....	102
4	100	90	84	80	77	75	73	72	71	70	69	68	68	530
5	225	205	190	180	175	170	165	162	159	157	156	154	153	1,400
6	385	350	325	310	300	290	285	280	275	271	268	266	263	2,900
8	875	785	735	700	675	655	640	630	620	612	606	600	594	7,600
10	1,560	1,405	1,310	1,250	1,205	1,170	1,140	1,125	1,110	1,095	1,080	1,075	1,062	15,000
12	2,435	2,195	2,045	1,950	1,800	1,825	1,790	1,755	1,730	1,705	1,685	1,670	1,655	26,000
15	4,375	3,935	3,675	3,500	3,380	3,280	3,210	3,150	3,110	3,060	3,030	3,000	2,975	50,000

* These limits are applicable only when the maximum load within any one branch interval is not greater than $N\left(\dfrac{1}{2n}+\dfrac{1}{4}\right)$, where N is the permissible load on a stack of one or two branch intervals, and n is the number of branch intervals of the stack under consideration.

† Not more than two water closets or bathroom groups within each branch interval, nor more than six water closets or bathroom groups on the stack.

SOURCE: "A Revision of the National Plumbing Code, ASA A40.8-1955," Report of the Public Health Service Technical Committee on Plumbing Standards, 1962.

pipe, at intervals not exceeding 4 ft. Horizontal piping must be supported as follows: cast-iron soil pipe, at not more than 5-ft intervals, except when 10-ft lengths are used, in which case supports at 10-ft intervals are acceptable; screwed pipe, at approximately 12-ft intervals; copper tubing, at 6-ft intervals for sizes $1\frac{1}{2}$ in. and smaller and at 10-ft intervals for sizes 2 in. and larger; and plastic and lead pipe, for the entire length on metal or wood strips.

11-17. Fixture Traps and Trap Venting. The pipes that carry off the waste from various plumbing fixtures would allow the entrance of air from the plumbing system into rooms if traps were not placed in the waste-pipe lines. The trap seal should be not less than 2 or more than 4 in. There are several varieties of plain traps. These are known as the S-, $\frac{3}{4}$S-, and $\frac{1}{2}$S- or P-traps. The plain traps are subject to siphonage, which results in the removal of the water in the trap, thereby allowing free passage of sewer air. This may be prevented by venting the trap. Nonsiphoning traps have been devised which are supposed to resist siphoning without the necessity of venting. These traps usually depend upon some form of ball within the trap or some mechanical device to prevent loss of the seal. They do not usually have the same scouring power, however, as the plain traps, and also, in the course of time, the division wall or mechanical device may become so corroded that the seal can no longer be held. The unrestricted use of nonsiphoning traps without vents is therefore recommended only under exceptional conditions, and many codes forbid them. Bell traps are also prohibited.

Ordinary traps are vented in various ways as indicated in Figs. 11-4 and 11-5. S-traps must be vented from the upper part of the curve. This is known as crown venting and is prohibited by most codes. A particular danger arises in crown venting which may also be present in the venting of other trap fixtures. This is the accumulation of lint and grease in the vent pipe, particularly if, as the waste water is drained from the fixture, the water level rises into the vent pipe during the early periods of flow. This in time will surely cause stoppage; consequently the trap will be unvented, and siphonage may

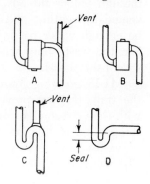

FIGURE 11-4 *A,* drum trap with crown vent; *B,* drum trap as usually placed, allowing easy cleaning but possible leakage of sewer air at cleanout; *C,* the S-trap with crown vent; *D,* the P-trap.

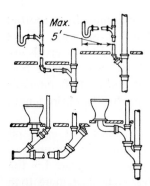

FIGURE 11-5 Approved forms of venting single fixtures. (*From New York Standard Plumbing Code.*)

result. For this reason the P-trap is probably the best trap for all-round use for washbowls, sinks, and similar fixtures. The P-trap may be used safely without a vent if it is within permissible distance (Table 11-6) of the waste stack into which the waste pipe discharges and if the nominally horizontal waste pipe does not join the stack at a point lower than the dip of the trap. Some codes allow venting by a stack or otherwise if the trap is not over 5 ft from the vent or stack used as a vent. This is permissible only if no fixture or only a minor fixture discharges into the stack used as a vent. See Fig. 11-8 for an illustration of stack venting.

Drum traps have been widely used, particularly in connection with the waste pipes from bathtubs. They are somewhat more resistant to siphonage than S- or P-traps but do not give so good a scouring velocity. When used, they should be placed as shown in Fig. 11-4 so that the cleanout at the bottom will be covered by the trap seal; otherwise leakage around the opening may allow the escape of sewer air. The vents of drum traps are subject to the same dangers of stoppage as those of S-traps. There is no reason why P-traps should not be used in place of drum traps.

Trap seals may be broken by back pressure resulting from a large mass of liquid compressing air as it moves down a nearby stack, by evaporation of the water in the trap, or by capillary attraction working through lint or threads partly in the trap. The first-named can be prevented by venting, and the last two by ensuring that there will always be enough water passing through to keep the seal intact. Vents should join the waste lines within certain prescribed distances from the traps (see Table 11-6).

11-18. Venting Systems. Trap venting is necessary to supply air to the trap, thereby preventing siphonage. The trap vent must connect with the vent stack or main stack in such a manner that there will be no stoppage of circulation of air and, in addition, no danger of backing up of wastes into the vent pipes. No vents are less than 1¼ in. in diameter. The size is based upon the size of the waste or soil stack, the number of

Table 11-6. PERMISSIBLE DISTANCE OF TRAP
FROM VENT

Size of fixture drain, in.	Distance from trap to vent, ft
1¼	2½
1½	3½
2	5
3	6
4	10

SOURCE: "Report of the Coordinating Committee for a National Plumbing Code," U.S. Department of Commerce, Domestic Commerce Series, no. 28.

fixtures or closets connected, and the actual length of the vent or vent stack (see Table 11-7). Branch vents are restricted in the same manner as the main vents. Vent pipes should have uniform grades without sags or depressions so that moisture will drip back to the soil or waste pipe. Vent pipes that are connected to horizontal soil and waste pipes should branch off above the center line of the pipe and extend vertically or at an angle of 45 deg to the vertical for at least 6 in. above the fixtures they are venting before changing to a horizontal direction or connecting with a branch vent. This latter precaution is necessary to prevent flow through the vent pipe due to stoppage in the waste line.

In houses of two or more floors, a venting system like that shown in Fig. 11-6 is used. In this connection it should be noted that the vent stack should connect with the main stack at the bottom at an acute angle. This prevents clogging of the bottom with rust and scale. The top of the vent stack may go through the roof in the same manner as the main stack but is usually connected with the main stack. This connection, of course, must be made above the highest fixture.

Wet vents are shown in Fig. 11-6. They are permitted only on the waste pipes from lavatories, kitchen sinks, or a combination fixture. A wet vent may be used to vent a bathtub, shower trap, water closet, or bathroom group, provided that not more than one fixture unit discharges into a 1½-in. wet vent, and not more than four fixture units into a 2-in. wet vent, and provided also that the horizontal branch connects to the stack at the same level as the water-closet drain or below the water-closet drain when installed on the top floor. It may also connect to the water-closet bend. For further uses of wet vents, the reader is referred to the Code [2]. Figure 11-6 also shows common vents.

Figure 11-7 illustrates circuit venting and loop venting.

Where crown venting is used, the vent pipes are run from the crowns of the individual traps to the vent stack. Owing to the possibility of stoppage of the vents in this case, most plumbing codes prohibit this practice.

Venting may be dispensed with in the case of rain-leader traps, floor drains, and subsoil drains. Individual fixture vents may be dispensed

Table 11-7. SIZE AND LENGTH OF VENTS

Size of soil or waste stack, in.	Total fixture units connected to stack	Diameter of vent, in.										
		1¼	1½	2	2½	3	4	5	6	8	10	12
		Maximum length of vent, ft										
1¼	2	30	...	...	...	......	...	...	......	...	...	...
1½	8	50	150	...	...	...	...	...	......	...	...	...
1½	10	30	100	...	...	......	...	...	......	...	...	...
2	12	30	75	200	...	......	...	...	......	...	...	...
2	20	26	50	150	...	......	...	...	......	...	...	...
2½	42	...	30	100	300	......	...	...	...	...	...	...
3	10	...	42	145	355	1,040	...	...	...	...	...	...
3	21	...	32	110	270	805	...	...	......	...	...	...
3	53	...	27	94	230	680	...	...	...	...	...	...
3	102	...	25	86	210	620	...	...	...	...	...	...
4	43	...	...	35	85	250	975	...	...	...	...	...
4	140	...	...	27	65	195	750	...	......	...	...	...
4	320	...	...	23	55	165	635	...	...	...	...	...
4	530	...	...	21	50	150	580	...	......	...	...	...
5	190	...	...	...	28	82	320	985	......	...	...	...
5	490	...	...	...	21	63	245	760	......	...	...	...
5	940	...	...	...	18	53	207	670	......	...	...	...
5	1,400	...	...	...	16	49	189	585	......	...	...	...
6	500	...	...	...	...	33	130	400	1,000	...	...	...
6	1,100	...	...	...	...	26	100	310	775	...	...	...
6	2,000	...	...	...	...	22	84	260	655	...	...	...
6	2,900	...	...	...	...	20	77	240	595	...	...	...
8	1,800	...	...	...	...	......	31	95	240	940	...	...
8	3,400	...	...	...	...	......	24	73	185	720	...	...
8	5,600	...	...	...	...	......	20	62	155	610	...	...
8	7,600	...	...	...	...	......	18	56	140	555	...	...
10	4,000	...	...	...	...	......	...	31	78	305	960	...
10	7,200	...	...	...	...	......	...	24	60	235	735	...
10	11,000	...	...	...	...	......	...	20	51	200	625	...
10	15,000	...	...	...	...	......	...	18	46	180	570	...
12	7,300	...	...	...	...	......	...	...	31	120	380	940
12	13,000	...	...	...	...	......	...	...	24	94	295	720
12	20,000	...	...	...	...	......	...	...	20	79	250	610
12	26,000	...	...	...	...	......	...	...	18	72	225	555
15	15,000	...	...	...	...	......	...	...	......	40	125	305
15	25,000	...	...	...	...	......	...	...	......	31	96	235
15	38,000	...	...	...	...	......	...	...	......	26	81	200
15	50,000	...	...	...	...	......	...	...	......	24	74	180

SOURCE: "A Revision of the National Plumbing Code, ASA A40.8-1955," Report of the Public Health Service Technical Committee on Plumbing Standards, 1962.

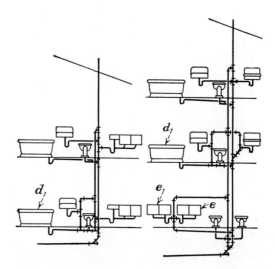

FIGURE 11-6   Continuous venting in buildings of two or more stories. Bathtubs, *d*, have wet vents. The fixtures marked *e* have a common vent. Note that the top-story fixture groups are stack-vented and that the vent stack in each case has one or more fixtures discharging into it at the ground floor.

with for a group of fixtures consisting of one bathroom group and a kitchen sink in a one-story building, or on the top floor of a building, provided that each fixture drain connects independently to the stack and that each enters the stack at the same level, except the lavatory. See Fig. 11-8.

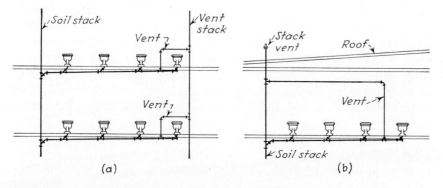

FIGURE 11-7   (*a*) Circuit venting of a group of toilets; (*b*) loop venting, which is permitted if there are no other fixtures discharging into the stack above where the vent joins.

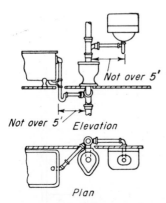

Not over 5'

Not over 5' *Elevation*

Plan

Figure 11-8 Approved design for a stack-vented bathroom group of fixtures. (*From Report of Subcommittee on Plumbing, U.S. Department of Commerce.*)

11-19. Inspection. Building plans submitted for approval by building control authorities should have their plumbing layouts inspected. The first inspection of a drainage and vent system is made after the roughing in. Plumbing work is said to be roughed in when all the work has been done up to the setting of the fixtures and with all piping open to view. Usually at this time the water test is given. All the openings except the top of the stack are closed by caps, soldering, or special plugs, and the complete system is filled until water flows from the top of the stack. The water is then allowed to stand in the pipes for a period of at least 15 min. Every part of the system should be tested with at least a 10-ft head of water, except the top 10 ft. All joints should then be examined for leakage. The air test is made by attaching an air compressor or testing machine to any suitable opening, closing all other openings, and forcing in air until there is a gage pressure of 5 psi. This pressure is held for a period of at least 15 min. Joints are sometimes tested by applying soapsuds to them with a brush. In the case of a very high building, it may be necessary to test the system in 75-ft sections of stack.

Smoke or peppermint is used for the final test, which is made after the work is completed and the traps have their seals. When smoke is used, a machine for generating it and producing a small air pressure is connected to the system, and smoke is forced in. After smoke appears at stack openings, they are closed, and a pressure equivalent to 1 in. of water column is reached and maintained for 15 min. before inspection starts.

The peppermint test is an old favorite, but because of its disadvantages it is falling into disuse. A mixture of 2 oz of oil of peppermint to 10 qt of water at 160°F or higher, sufficient for testing the plumbing of an ordinary house, is poured down the stack from the roof. The man who does the pouring must then efface himself until the joints have been inspected, as the odor of peppermint may cling to his clothes sufficiently

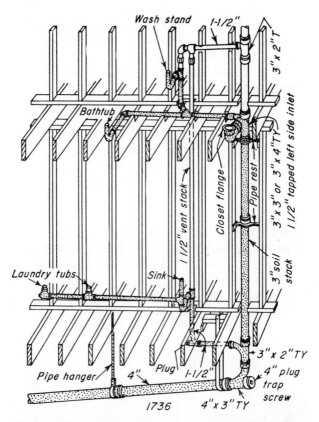

FIGURE 11-9   A job roughed in. Waste and soil pipes are stippled, and vent pipes are outlined. (*Courtesy of U.S. Department of Agriculture.*)

to make it impossible to detect a leak. There is also the possibility of one leak in the system causing sufficient odor to conceal other leaks.

It is possible to make simple tests to discover whether traps are sealed. If knocking on the pipe at the trap results in a hollow sound, it will probably mean that the trap seal has been lost. A still better method is to hold a match at the entrance to the waste pipe. Flickering will indicate a loss of the trap seal.

The building sewer must also be tested. This is done by plugging the end of the sewer at the point of connection to the public sewer and applying a head of at least 10 ft of water.

The water system is tested by filling it with water from the source of supply at a pressure not less than the normal working pressure.

Whenever it is suspected that the plumbing system of any building has become defective, it should be inspected and defects found ordered to be corrected.

11-20. Grease Traps. Traps are installed for the purpose of removing grease from waste water. These are also known as interceptors. Figure 11-10 shows one type. They can also be purchased ready-made, and they should be placed as near as possible to the fixture which they are serving. Also, they should be frequently cleaned. They are especially desirable in waste lines from the sinks of kitchens in restaurants and hotels.

11-21. Fixtures. Many of the older types of fixtures tended to become offensive because of their unsightliness and their odors. These conditions were frequently due to the use of absorbent material or construction which resulted in joints that tended to accumulate organic matter. For this reason, modern plumbing codes require that porcelain or vitrified earthenware, white-enameled cast iron, or hard natural stone be used in fixtures for excreta disposal. Water closets are required to be molded in one piece, to hold sufficient water between flushes so that surfaces will not be fouled, and to have a flushing rim that will ensure complete cleansing of the inside of the bowl. Closets of the pan type or of the long-hopper or frostproof and washout varieties are no longer considered desirable.

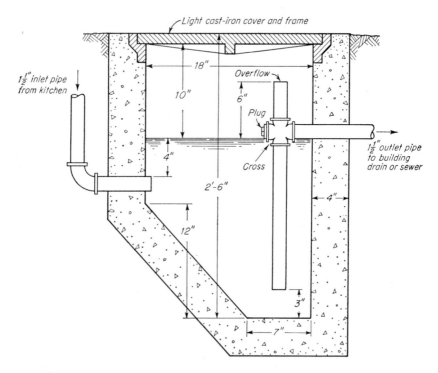

FIGURE 11-10 Cross section of a grease trap. It may be circular or square in plan.

All fixtures should be so installed as to allow ease of cleaning. The overflows from washbowls, bathtubs, and similar fixtures should enter the waste pipes on the inlet side of the trap and should be arranged for ease of cleaning. Good practice requires that all fixture pipes run directly into the wall and that no lead pipes or traps be within 12 in. of the floor unless protected. Strong metal strainers are required at the outlets of all fixtures except closets and pedestal urinals.

11-22. Cross-connections in Plumbing Systems. A *cross-connection* is defined as any physical connection or arrangement between two otherwise separate piping systems, one of which contains potable water and the other either water of unknown or questionable safety or steam, gas or chemical, whereby there may be a flow from one system to the other, the direction of flow depending on the pressure differential between the two systems [6]. *Backflow* is the flow of water or other liquids into the distributing pipes of a potable supply of water from any source or sources other than its intended source. *Back siphonage* is the backflow of used, contaminated, or polluted water from a plumbing fixture or vessel or other source into a water-supply pipe due to a negative pressure in such pipe. A negative pressure is sometimes called a vacuum or, more properly, a partial vacuum.

Cross-connections have caused numerous outbreaks of typhoid fever, dysentery, infectious hepatitis, and gastroenteritis. They should be avoided by intelligent design of water and drainage systems, and their existence should be checked and reported by plumbing inspectors and sanitary inspectors.

The cross-connection requires a physical link between the two systems. Such connections result from (1) direct connections between two water supplies, such as an auxiliary or fire-fighting supply of an industrial plant connected to the potable public supply or potable supplies of industries or business buildings with connections to the public supply for emergency use, and (2) plumbing fixtures or tanks of various types with under-rim water inlets. Under-rim plumbing fixtures are less numerous than they were, but many of the older lavatories, bathtubs, etc., had their faucets or faucet outlets beneath the rims. Much in use, however, are flush valves for water closets and urinals, and these are dangerous unless some form of backflow preventer is used. In industrial plants tanks are frequently used for various purposes, and they may have under-rim water inlets. Laboratories often have water outlets well above a sink, but the outlet may be used as a hose connection, and the hose end may be submerged in the sink or other liquid container. Table 11-8 is a partial list of hazards an inspector may encounter.

PREVENTION OF BACKFLOW. The best safeguard against contamination of a potable water supply is to place an air gap between it and the

Table 11-8. PARTIAL LIST OF PLUMBING HAZARDS

Fixtures with direct connections	*Fixtures with submerged inlets*
Air conditioning, air washer	Baptismal fount
Air conditioning, chilled water	Bathtub
Air conditioning, condenser water	Bedpan washer, flushing rim
Air line	Bidets
Aspirator, laboratory	Brine tank
Aspirator, medical or dental	Cooling tower
Aspirator, weedicide or fertilizer sprayer	Cuspidor, dental
Autoclave and sterilizer	Drinking fountain
Auxiliary system, industrial	Floor drain, flushing rim
Auxiliary system, surface water	Garbage-can washer
Auxiliary system, unapproved well	Ice maker
supply	Laboratory sink, serrated nozzle for hose
Boiler system	Laundry machine
Chemical feeder, pot type	Lavatory
Chlorinator	Lawn sprinkler system
Coffee urn	Photo laboratory sink
Cooling system	Sewer flushing manhole
Dishwasher	Slop sink, flushing rim
Fire standpipe or sprinkler system	Slop sink, threaded supply
Fountain, ornamental	Steam table
Hydraulic equipment	Urinal, siphon-jet blowout
Laboratory equipment	Vegetable peeler
Lubrication, pump bearings	Water closet, flush tank, ball cock
Photostat equipment	Water closet, flush valve, siphon jet
Plumber's friend, pneumatic	
Pump, pneumatic ejector	
Pump, prime pipe	
Pump, water-operated ejector	
Sewer, sanitary	
Sewer, storm	
Swimming pool	

SOURCE: "Plumbing Inspectors' Handbook," Texas State Board of Plumbing Examiners, Austin, Tex., 1957.

polluted water. For plumbing fixtures the required air gap between the faucet or pipe inlet and the rim will depend upon the effective size of the opening of the inlet pipe or faucet and the presence of vertical walls or ribs near the pipe or faucet. The minimum gap is prescribed because a vacuum or strong suction in the pipe or open faucet sets up air currents which will carry water from a full bowl or tank for a short distance vertically into the opening. Nearby walls which tend to channelize air flow tend to increase the effect. Table 11-9 gives the air gaps required for safety. A "near" wall or rib is one that is located within three times the effective opening if it is only one wall, or four times the effective opening when there are two walls. The effective opening is the minimum cross-sectional area at the point of water discharge and is

Table 11-9. MINIMUM AIR GAPS FOR PLUMBING FIXTURES

Fixture	Minimum air gap	
	When not affected by near wall, in.*	When affected by near wall, in.†
Lavatories and other fixtures with effective opening not greater than ½ in. in diameter	1.0	1.50
Sink, laundry trays, gooseneck bath faucets, and other fixtures with effective openings not greater than ¾ in. in diameter . . .	1.5	2.25
Over-rim bath fillers and other fixtures with effective openings not greater than 1 in. in diameter	2.0	3.0
Drinking-water fountains, single orifices ⁷⁄₁₆ (0.437) in. in diameter or multiple orifices having total area of 0.150 sq in. (area of circle ⁷⁄₁₆ in. in diameter)	1.0	1.50
Effective openings greater than 1 in. . . .	2 × diameter of effective opening	3 × diameter of effective opening

* Sidewalls, ribs, or similar obstructions do not affect air gaps when spaced from inside edge of spout opening a distance greater than three times the diameter of the effective opening for a single wall, or a distance greater than four times the diameter of the effective opening for two intersecting walls.

† Vertical walls, ribs, or similar obstructions extending from the water surface to or above the horizontal plane of the spout opening require a greater air gap when spaced closer to the nearest inside edge of spout opening than specified in footnote above. The effect of three or more such vertical walls or ribs has not been determined. In such cases, the air gap shall be measured from the top of the wall.

SOURCE: "A Revision of the National Plumbing Code, ASA A40.8-1955," Report of the Public Health Service Technical Committee on Plumbing Standards, 1962.

measured in terms of the diameter of a circle or, if the opening is not circular, the diameter of a circle of equivalent cross-sectional area.

For tanks with under-rim inlets, overflows may be considered to provide safety if the arrangement is as illustrated in Fig. 11-11. A safe method of providing dual water supplies for an industrial plant using the air-gap method is shown in Fig. 2-13. The use of a float-controlled valve in a supply line which terminates above the rim of a tank is a frequently used device. The tank may be used in industrial processes, or it may supply a pump.

Connections between public or potable supplies and private supplies are sometimes safeguarded by check valves. Check valves frequently leak, however, and such an installation cannot be approved. An assembly of two check valves and two gate valves with test hose bibbs, between the gates and checks, known as the factory-mutual assembly, has been

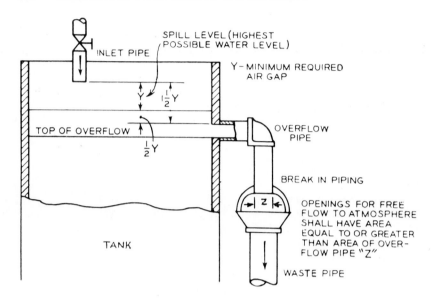

FIGURE 11-11   Air gap in open tank with overflow. (*From "American Standard National Plumbing Code," American Society of Mechanical Engineers, New York, 1955.*)

permitted in some jurisdictions. The test hose bibbs or faucets allow testing to determine whether the check valves, and gate valves also, are leaking [6].

Backflow preventers that will prevent back siphonage are placed in flush-valve lines to water closets and urinals, hose supply lines, garden sprinkling systems, etc. Figure 11-12 shows one type of nonpressure vacuum breaker. The flush valve is placed above the vacuum breaker, which is located at least 6 in. above the flood line or rim of the water closet. When the flush valve is operated the flow of water is downward, and the disk is in the normal seated position. If a negative pressure or partial vacuum develops, the atmospheric pressure exerted on the disk closes it into the vacuum-breaking position, and back siphonage from the closet is prevented.

HOW A VACUUM MAY OCCUR. How this may happen is illustrated in Fig. 11-13, which shows a water-supply system that is fed upward from the public supply. The toilet is of the siphon-jet type and has a flush valve. The siphon jet is formed at the opening C when the toilet is flushed. The chamber D is filled with water at all times. With valve A closed and faucet B opened, water may be siphoned back from the toilet bowl down in the water pipe. There are small openings in the flushing rim of the bowl, and these may prevent a vacuum from forming between D and the flushometer, but they are likely to clog and even when open

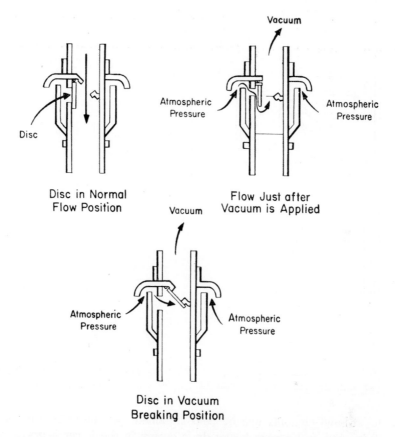

Disc in Normal
Flow Position

Flow Just after
Vacuum is Applied

Disc in Vacuum
Breaking Position

FIGURE 11-12   Vacuum breaker, nonpressure type. It is not designed for protection against backflow due to back pressure. (*From "Water Supply and Plumbing Cross-connections," Public Health Service, 1963.*)

may not furnish sufficient air to break the vacuum. If there is a stoppage at E, water will rise to the rim of the toilet bowl, and siphonage is even more likely. A stoppage in the drain of washbowl F will cause the faucet outlets to be submerged, and siphonage may again occur. With valve A open, a heavy usage at B or a fire demand outside the building may cause a partial vacuum in the riser pipe and cause siphonage.

Figure 11-14 shows how a vacuum may occur in a downfeed layout of the water-supply system. This method is used in large buildings where the pressure in the public supply is insufficient to raise water to the upper floors. A booster pump is installed to raise the water to the supply tank. The supply pipe should terminate above the overflow or preferably above the top of the tank; otherwise it would constitute a cross-connection. From Fig. 11-14 it is seen that if valve A is closed and the toilet on the upper floor is clogged and if any fixture below is opened, the

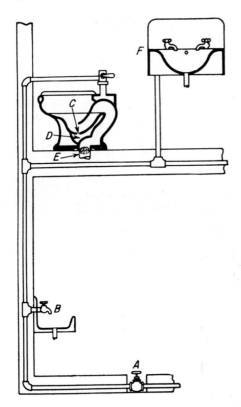

FIGURE 11-13   How back siphonage occurs in water-supply pipes.

toilet-bowl contents will be back-siphoned into the water pipe. If valve *A* is open and a very heavy draft occurs in the lower floors, a vacuum may occur in the upper part of the downfeed pipe, and the closet-bowl contents will be back-siphoned. Another hazard may occur in a layout similar to that shown in Fig. 11-14. The booster pump may be located in the building basement with supply pipes to the lower floors taking off from the suction side of the pump. Low pressure in the public water main may result in a negative pressure in the line to the pump and possible back siphonage from some fixtures.

WATER CLOSETS. Figure 11-15 is a cross section of the ordinary jet-type closet generally used with flush valves. Water enters the bowl at the top and in the rear top chamber divides, one part going to the flushing rim through port *A* and the rest going to the submerged jet *B*. With the water at the normal level, if a vacuum tends to occur in the water-supply line it will be broken by air entering through the rim ports and port *A*, and no back siphonage will occur. If the port *A* and the rim ports are too small, if the latter are completely or partly clogged or "limed up," or if they are submerged as a result of a stoppage in the toilet or at some point in the soil pipe below, air cannot enter, and the

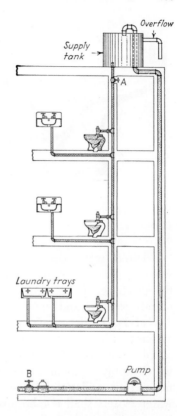

Figure 11-14 How back siphonage occurs in water-supply pipes. Downfeed layout. (*Courtesy of Wisconsin State Board of Health.*)

vacuum will siphon water from the bowl back into the water-supply line.

Pan, valve, plunger, offset, frostproof, and side or rear spud water closets are prohibited. Those which have an invisible seal, an unventilated space, or walls which are not thoroughly washed at each flush and any type which might permit back siphonage of the bowl contents into the flush tank are also prohibited.

Flush valves should be protected by placing the valve about 6 in. above the overflow rim of the bowl and using a vacuum breaker between the flush valve and the bowl at least 4 in. above the bowl top. A check valve may be combined with the stop valve to the toilet as an added protection.

There is no danger of water contamination from the commonly used closet tank with a water-supply float valve if the tank is high above the toilet bowl or is elevated only a short distance. There is a possible cross-connection between the usual water-closet flush tank and the water supply should the air inlet to the valve be clogged. Hence filling the flush tank with unsafe water for flushing purposes during a water-supply interruption is dangerous.

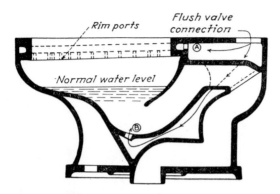

FIGURE 11-15 Cross section of jet-type closet.
(*Courtesy of Wisconsin State Board of Health.*)

Direct water connections to waste pipes should be cut off and the water discharged into a funnel or pipe that is properly trapped, with the discharge point above the funnel rim. This applies also to drains of refrigerators and potable water systems (see Fig. 11-16).

11-23. Trailer-coach and Trailer-camp Standards. The water-supply systems of trailer coaches are frequently connected to public or camp supply systems. The Code [2] therefore suggests plumbing standards which apply to them. Some special features are that water closets shall not permit spillage of trap-seal contents during transit; that flushing of water closets shall not be possible except when the trailer is connected to a water-supply and sewage disposal system; and that an approved backflow preventer or vacuum-breaker device shall be provided for each water closet. In general the plumbing system must be designed to withstand shocks and vibration.

Trailer-park plumbing standards are also given in the Code. Sewage disposal into a public sewer is recommended, but if not available a private system will be necessary, complying with the requirements of the local health authorities and those of the state. The following suggestions are made: up to 75 trailers, septic tank and either tile absorption field or sand filter; 75 to 150 trailers, septic tank and sand filters or, if space is available, an Imhoff tank followed by a trickling filter; over 150 trailers, Imhoff tank and trickling filters, with the additional requirement of chlorination to prevent odors. Activated sludge, including sedimentation and separate sludge digestion, is recommended only where space is restricted. There are a number of compact "package" sewage treatment plants available for trailer camps and fabricated by various manufacturers. They usually employ activated sludge, contact aeration, or some variation thereof. They should not be used unless approved by state health authorities.

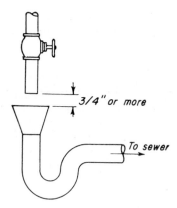

3/4" or more

To sewer

FIGURE 11-16 Method of placing an air break in lines draining water systems, refrigerators, etc.

Each trailer sewer outlet is connected to a 3-in. lateral that terminates in a P-trap, extended to grade and then through a riser to 4 in. above grade. The extension to the ground must be protected by a metal casing or concrete mount. A flexible connector must be provided by the camp operator. It clamps to the trailer outlet but is so arranged that in case of emergency the coach may pull out and the connection will automatically disconnect without damage to coach or piping.

Potable water satisfactory to the health authorities must be furnished. Each trailer outlet must be provided with a ¾-in. control valve, so located that backflow cannot occur from surface-contaminated water or from any other source. A flexible connector is required of a type that is automatically disconnected should a coach pull out in an emergency.

11-24. Hospital Plumbing. The plumbing of hospitals requires special care because of its relationship to provision of adequate medical care and the need to protect patients and personnel from health hazards. The hospital system should comply with the provisions of a comprehensive and adequate code, but the numerous specialized fixtures and equipment used in the modern hospital require special mention and special safeguards. Appendix C of the Revision of the National Code [1] sets forth the special measures necessary to prevent backflow or back siphonage from aspirators, sterilizers, vacuum systems, bedpan washers, and steamers; the principles involved have been stated in Art. 11-22. A dual water-supply system is recommended for hospitals to prevent interruption in water service.

11-25. Storm-water Drainage. Storm water from roofs and paved areas should not be discharged into a sewer system designed for domestic sewage only. Connection should be made with the storm sewers if available. If the storm-water drains are discharged into a combined sewer system, i.e., one designed to carry both domestic and storm water, the pipes should be trapped unless the roof gutter or opening is more than 12 ft from a door, window, or air shaft. No soil, waste, or vent pipes should be used as storm-water conductors, nor should vent connections to the conductors be permitted.

Bibliography

1. "A Revision of the National Plumbing Code ASA A40.8-1955," Report of the Public Health Service Technical Committee on Plumbing Standards, 1962.
2. "American Standard National Plumbing Code," American Society of Mechanical Engineers, New York, 1955.
3. Babbitt, H. E.: "Plumbing," 3d ed., McGraw-Hill Book Company, New York, 1960.
4. Day, L. J.: "Standard Plumbing Details," John Wiley & Sons, Inc., New York.
5. "Cross-connections in Plumbing and Water Supply Systems," Wisconsin State Board of Health, Madison, Wis.
6. "Water Supply and Plumbing Cross-connections," Public Health Service, 1963.
7. "Plumbing Inspectors' Handbook," Texas State Board of Plumbing Examiners, Austin, Tex., 1957.

12

PUBLIC BATHING - PLACE SANITATION

12-1. Swimming pools and bathing places are acquiring ever-increasing popularity for recreation. They were formerly considered to be in the category of a municipal, YMCA, institutional, or country-club installation, but they are now becoming essential features of motels, hotels, and even apartment houses, subdivisions, and residences. The technology of plastics has been utilized in this field to make more widespread the installation of a personal swimming pool for the average backyard. Not only have pools been built of concrete, fiber glass, and steel, but a vinyl liner has been developed which can be laid over a basin formed or constructed of sand or similar material. In 1962, it was estimated that there were at least 100,000 commercial and public pools and 250,000 backyard installations.

Supervision of these large numbers and types of pools, from a public health standpoint, is attaining more importance, although the problem is primarily one of public health education and training. Municipal pools are usually operated by the city park or recreation department, and cooperation between it and the health department is necessary to maintain sanitary standards. The close association of many persons, with the water as a vehicle of infection, presents a problem for the sanitarian. There is no reason, however, for the public to fear patronizing a swimming pool at which the recognized sanitary precautions are employed. Sanitary control of small private and backyard pools may be applied by city ordinances or by regulations of state health departments. The building-permit system used in municipal practice affords a means of control over design of pools, but liaison between public health agencies and the office issuing such permits is required to assure the upholding of sanitary standards.

Widespread interest in this phase of the recreation industry has led to new developments in basic techniques of design and operation. The shock hazard of underwater lights and other electrically operated fixtures with submerged parts has been recognized in new standards for wiring. New disinfectants have been added to the market. The rigid and durable plastics are now being employed in piping and manufacture of pumps and other accessories. The automatically operated swimming pool is now economically feasible for commercial installations.

12-2. Bathing Waters and Health. Disease may be transmitted to bathers from waters contaminated by sewage or by the bathers themselves. Because of the close association of people in pools, a wide spectrum of diseases has been associated with bathing. Among the illnesses cited are the intestinal disorders, such as typhoid and paratyphoid fevers, leptospirosis, and dysentery; eye, ear, nose, and throat infections, including the respiratory diseases; skin disorders, such as ringworm, scabies, impetigo, granuloma, and "swimmer's itch"; and the venereal diseases. Poliomyelitis may possibly be transmitted in swimming pools, but epidemiological evidence is lacking. In fact there is little confirmed epidemiological evidence of any kind incriminating pools, except a few instances of outbreaks of intestinal disease, granuloma, and "swimmer's itch." However, despite the absence of any great danger, decency requires that the water of public bathing places be kept as clean as possible and as free as practical from organisms causing disease. Public bathing beaches can present more of a hazard, especially from the standpoint of transmission of intestinal diseases. As late as 1958, 10 cases of typhoid fever out of a total outbreak of 15 were epidemiologically traced to a beach at Perth in western Australia, where the water was contaminated from the outfall of a primary sewage treatment plant a mile distant.

Some of the dangerous bacteria, particularly those causing respiratory diseases, do not survive long in the presence of adequate disinfecting residuals. Hence the greatest danger of contracting such diseases will be during periods when the pool is crowded. The intestinal bacteria are able to survive for a longer period. As in the testing of water supplied for public use, therefore, the presence of the coliform group of organisms is ascertained in investigating the quality of the pool water. If the coliforms have been removed or killed, it is considered good evidence that all disease bacteria have been eliminated. Examination of the water for the presence of hemolytic streptococci is also helpful in gaging the sanitary condition of a swimming pool. Mallmann [4] suggests the use of a "coccus test," in which a special medium can be employed to culture a mixture of streptococci and staphylococci of respiratory and intestinal origin. The bacterial standards of swimming-pool water are similar to, but not quite so stringent as, those governing drinking water. By the regulation of bathing loads, or the proportioning of the allowable number of patrons to the size of the pool, an attempt is made to reduce water contamination and eliminate the hazards caused by overcrowding.

Certain skin infections are associated with swimming pools, the commonest being a form of ringworm or fungus infection known as "athlete's foot." This disease is not spread by the pool water, however, but by contact with the floor surface of dressing rooms, locker rooms, runways, etc. The infection may also be acquired at gymnasiums and other places where persons go barefoot over damp wood or other surfaces which are favorable to growth of the organism. Prevention is a serious problem because about 50 per cent of the population of this country is infected. Eliminating wooden walkways and mats and maintaining the cleanliness of all walking surfaces around the pool and bathhouse are important. Application of a 0.3 to 0.6 per cent solution of hypochlorite is considered an acceptable method of disinfecting floors. Personal measures include having patrons wear foot coverings in the bathhouse and toughen their feet on a pad soaked in a 10 per cent salt solution.

Outbreaks of granuloma, or "sore elbow," have been reported in Sweden, the United States, and Canada. Granuloma is caused by a specific organism, *Mycobacterium balnei*. The clinical manifestation is a lesion, commencing as a small reddish papule 3 or 4 weeks after swimming and later becoming enlarged and hardened and covered with brownish crusts or scales. It appears to be associated with a skin abrasion acquired from rough surfaces on the walls of pools.

A disease contracted by bathing in natural waters, particularly in weedy lakes and ponds, is schistosome dermatitis. Most cases have been reported in Minnesota, Michigan, and Wisconsin. It is caused by a small parasite, derived from birds, that spends a part of its life cycle in certain species of water snails. These release the larval organisms in the water.

In their search for a second host, they enter the skin of human bathers, where they cause a rash and intense itching which may last for several weeks, until the organisms die. They do not produce any other ill effects. Preventive methods are directed against the snails. Application of 2 lb of copper sulfate and 1 lb of copper carbonate for 1,000 lin ft of shoreline will kill the snails for a season or longer. The treatment should be applied to at least 1,000 ft of shoreline. A solution of the two chemicals is made and applied by means of a garden hose dragged on the bottom from a boat, or two hoses may be used, with one on each side of the boat. Sodium arsenite has been used to kill the rooted aquatic plants to which the snails attach themselves. In any area used for swimming, however, this chemical must be used with extreme caution because of its high toxicity. It is difficult to secure uniform distribution of the chemical in natural waters; consequently, after its application, tests for arsenic should be conducted throughout the area at varying depths to ascertain, before swimming is permitted in the area, that at no point does there exist a lethal concentration. Sampling might also include bottom sediments. It is reported that BHC, or Gammexane (Chap. 8), is effective against snails when applied as a dust to water containing them to produce a concentration of 5 to 6 mg/l.

The natural bathing beaches at lakes, on streams, or at the seashore are somewhat more difficult to control as to water quality than artificial pools. The most important consideration is that the beaches be located where there is no possibility of pollution by sewage from sewer outlets.

Also important from the public health standpoint in connection with pools and beaches is protection from drowning and mechanical injury. This calls for such measures as the stationing of lifeguards, avoidance of overcrowding, careful adherence to electrical standards in wiring, and placing of the deep portion of the pool on the side opposite to the entrance.

The proper grounding of all electrical apparatus or metal parts even remotely connected with electrically operated accessories is considered of sufficient importance to warrant a special section in the 1962 National Electrical Code. This is discussed in Art. 12-14.

12-3. Bathing-place Standards. Standards for the sanitation of swimming pools have been developed by the Conference of State Sanitary Engineers and the Public Health Engineering Section of the American Public Health Association. Their latest joint report was made in 1957. Certain important portions are directly quoted as follows:

24. CHEMICAL AND PHYSICAL QUALITY OF SWIMMING POOL WATER

A. *Excess Chlorine*—Whenever chlorine, calcium hypochlorite, or other chlorine compounds, without the use of ammonia, are used for swimming pool disinfection, the amount of available or excess chlorine in the water at all times when the pool is in use shall not be less than 0.4 ppm or more than 1.0 ppm except where high–free residual chlorine is used as described below. Available data indicate that for most effective results this should be present as free available residual chlorine. Whenever chlorine or chlorine compounds are used with ammonia effective results have been reported where the amount of available or excess chloramine is between 0.7 ppm and 1.0 ppm, but recent reports suggest the desirability of operating with higher chloramine residuals such as 2.0 ppm and there is a trend away from chlorine and ammonia disinfection in properly designed pools, inasmuch as less reliable disinfection is accomplished. Attention is directed to the possibility of interference by nitrites with the orthotolidine test particularly when chlorine-ammonia disinfection is employed. If readings are made on the water to be tested within 5 to 10 minutes after the orthotolidine is added, and samples are kept away from the light during this period, the nitrite interference will be decidedly lessened. Standards for determining chlorine residuals shall be prepared and used according to the recommendations in *Standard Methods for the Examination of Water, Sewage, and Industrial Wastes*[1] of the American Public Health Association. Standardized color discs and comparators may be used.

B. *High–Free Residual Chlorine*—A new development in the United States, "High–Free Residual Chlorine," has been based on successful English practice whereby advantages have been cited in maintenance of relatively high concentrations of free available chlorine (1.0 ppm or above) with accompanying high alkalinity (usually pH 8.0 to 8.9), as compared with lower chlorine residuals and pH of 7.0 to 7.5 as generally practiced in the United States. Advantages claimed are: more consistent satisfactory bacteriologic conditions, especially in outdoor pools, clearer pool water, and less irritation of the eyes of swimmers. A disadvantage is the higher cost of chlorine. This development is looked upon with considerable favor by some who have observed it in the United States and its progress will merit watching.

C. *Acidity-Alkalinity*—Whenever alum or sulfate of alumina is used during purification or repurification of swimming pool waters, the water at all times when pool is in use shall show an alkaline reaction. This means that the hydrogen ion content of the pool water shall not fall below 7.0.

D. *Clearness*—At all times when the pool is in use the water shall be sufficiently clear to permit a black disc 6 inches in diameter on a white field, when placed on the bottom of the pool at the deepest point, to be clearly visible from the side walks of the pool at all distances up to 10 yards measured from a line drawn across the pool through said disc. This is a minimum standard and most pools with modern filtration systems produce water far clearer than this minimum safety standard.

---

[1] Now entitled "Standard Methods for the Examination of Water and Wastewater."

Accident prevention is an important reason for maintaining clear water and very clear water adds greatly to the pool attractiveness.

E. *Temperatures*—The water in any swimming pool should not be artificially heated to a temperature above 78°F. The temperature of the air at any artificially heated swimming pool must not be permitted to become more than 8°F warmer nor more than 2°F colder than the water in the pool at any time when the pool is in use. For best results it is desirable that air temperatures shall be about 5°F warmer than the pool temperature.

25. BACTERIAL QUALITY OF SWIMMING POOL WATERS

A. *Bacteria Count on Standard Nutrient Agar—24 Hours—37°C¹—and Confirmed Test*—Not more than 15 per cent of the samples covering any considerable period of time shall contain more than 200 bacteria per ml or shall show positive test (confirmed test) in any of five 10 ml portions of water at times when the pool is in use. All primary fermentation tubes showing gas should be confirmed.

B. All chemical and bacterial analyses should be made in accordance with the procedures recommended in the *Standard Methods for the Examination of Water, Sewage, and Industrial Wastes* of the American Public Health Association in so far as these methods are applicable to swimming pool waters. In order to secure a true picture of the condition of the swimming pool water at the time of sampling, it is recommended that sodium thiosulfate be employed to neutralize the chlorine residual in the water sample bottle during transportation to the laboratory.

C. The part played by the various strains of streptococci in the respiratory diseases and their prevalence in the intestinal, buccal, and nasal discharges make the presence of streptococci in bathing water very undesirable. Yet to eliminate them from swimming pools would mean decidedly smaller bathing loads and decided increases in chlorine residuals, either or both of which would hamper the usefulness of the pool. The committee calls attention to the fact that streptococci tests are of value in passing on the conditions of swimming pool water but does not recommend any uniform standard limit for their presence.

D. 1. *Preparation of bottle for sampling*—All samples of chlorinated swimming pool water shall be collected in bottles treated with sodium thiosulfate. The purpose of using water sample bottles containing sodium thiosulfate is to reduce the chlorine present in a treated water at the moment the sample is collected to prevent a continuance of the killing action of the chlorine on the bacteria while the sample is being transported to the laboratory. The bacteriological examination then shows the true sanitary quality of the water at the time the sample was collected.

2. Several procedures for preparing the bottles are presented.

---

[1] Incubation temperature now recommended is $35 \pm 0.5°C$. The membrane filter test (see Chap. 2) is now applicable to bacteriological examination of swimming-pool water.

For Moist Heat Sterilization

Option 1—The sodium thiosulfate solution is prepared by dissolving 1.5 gm of sodium thiosulfate in 100 ml of distilled water. One-half ml of this solution is placed in each clean bottle. (This amount has been found sufficient to reduce completely residual chlorine in an amount up to 2.0 ppm in a sample of 130 ml of water.) After the introduction of the sodium thiosulfate solution, the bottle is stoppered and capped. The bottles are then placed in an autoclave and sterilized for 15 minutes at a pressure of 20 pounds per square inch.

Option 2—Into clean wet bottles, add approximately 0.02 to 0.05 gm of powdered sodium thiosulfate. The amount need not be weighed. An estimated amount on the tip of a spatula is sufficiently accurate. The bottles are sterilized as in *Option 1*.

For Dry Heat Sterilization

Into clean dry bottles is added from 0.02 to 0.05 gm of powdered sodium thiosulfate as in *Option 2*. The bottles are stoppered, capped, and sterilized at 180°C for 10 minutes. The temperature of sterilization must not approach 220°C as sodium thiosulfate decomposes at this temperature.

E. *Collection of Samples*—The samples should be collected by plunging the open bottle beneath the surface, sweeping the bottle forward until filled. The bottle should not be rinsed in the pool or the sodium thiosulfate will be removed. Samples should be collected only when the pool is in use and preferably during periods of heaviest bathing loads during the day. The hour of the day, the day of the week, frequency of collection, and the location of the point of sampling shall be varied in order to obtain over a period of time a representative cross-section of the sanitary quality of the pool. It is desirable wherever facilities permit, to collect one or more samples weekly from swimming pools.

26. CLEANING POOL

A. Visible dirt on the bottom of a swimming pool shall not be permitted to remain more than 24 hours.

B. Any visible scum or floating matter on the surface of pool shall be removed within 24 hours by flushing or other effective means.

. . . .

28. OPERATING CONTROL

A. *Trained Operators*—Each swimming pool should be operated under the close supervision of a well-trained operator with common sense and good judgment. Operator training courses have been of aid in promoting good operation.

B. *Tests for Excess Chlorine*—At any pool where chlorine, hypochlorite of lime or other chlorine compound is used for disinfection, the operator must be supplied with a proper outfit for making the orthotolidine test for excess chlorine and with permanent standards showing maximum and minimum permissible chlorine in the water.

Tests for excess chlorine in the water shall be made as frequently as experience proves to be necessary to maintain adequate residuals.

C. *Tests for Acidity*—At any pool where alum or sulfate of alumina is used or where artificial alkalinity is added to the water, the pool operator must be equipped with a hydrogen ion testing outfit and must take hydrogen ion tests on the water every day that the pool is in use, and more often if necessary.

D. *Operating Records*—Every pool operator must be supplied with a proper note book or with blank forms on which shall be recorded every day the number of persons using the pool, peak bathing loads handled, the volume of new water added, the temperature of the water, and the temperature of the air. Wherever a pool is used by both males and females the number of each and whether adults or children should also be recorded. At all pools where artificial circulation, filtration, or any chemical treatment is used, a full daily record must also be kept of the actual time pumps and filters are in operation, of the time each filter is washed or cleaned, of the time and amount of each chemical used or added, of the time the bottom and sides of pool are cleaned, and the results of all hydrogen ion, excess chlorine, or other tests.

12-4. Types of Pools. Pools are classified according to the manner in which they are operated. Fill-and-draw pools are filled with fresh water, used, drained, cleaned, and refilled. Other pools operate with a continuous flow of water passing through them, either fresh water from the source of supply or water which has been filtered and recirculated. Discussion of the area-load requirement will be found in Art. 12-14, "Safety Provisions."

The purpose of recirculation of water is to remove suspended material and to carry chlorine into the pool and thus maintain the required chlorine residual. The presence of much suspended material will reflect upon the safety of the pool water since it will reduce the disinfection efficiency of the chlorine residual. Experience indicates that the rate of turnover should be at least three times daily and preferably four times where the recirculation system is kept operating continuously, as it should be. Also, the chlorine residual should be maintained at all times.

Fill-and-draw pools are not recommended since they are more difficult to keep clean and to disinfect. Where used, however, they should supply at least 500 gal of water per person using the pool between complete changes of pool water. Chlorine residuals must be maintained within the limits already specified.

For outdoor pools which are partly artificial and partly natural, such as a pool created by building a dam across a stream and making other improvements, and for other situations where dependence is placed upon a continuous flow of water from a clean, unpolluted stream, a safe well, or a spring, the 500-gal requirement should be applied, although bacteriological conditions should rule. If cleansing baths are not required prior to using such pools, reductions in bathing loads will be found necessary to maintain safe bacteriological conditions, even with high chlorine residuals. Cleansing baths should, of course, be required at all pools.

12-5. Bacteriological Control. The swimming-pool standards given above require that the total bacterial count be no more than 200 per milliliter (standard plate count) after incubation of nutrient agar plates for 24 hr at $35 \pm 0.5°C$ in at least 85 per cent of the samples and that not more than 15 per cent of the standard samples for determination of coliform organisms show gas in any of the five 10-ml portions. If the membrane-filter technique is used, the arithmetic mean density of all standard samples examined per month should not exceed one coliform organism per 100 ml. The statistical limits on the extent to which occasional samples may exceed the mean are three coliforms in a 50-ml sample, four in 100 ml, seven in 200 ml, 13 in 500 ml, and 22 in 1,000 ml. These are permissible provided they do not occur in consecutive samples, in more than 5 per cent of the samples when 20 or more samples per month are analyzed, or in more than one sample when less than 20 per month are examined.

Frequent bacteriological tests are necessary, and steps should be taken by pool owners to have them made at a laboratory. If no commercial laboratory is available, arrangements can sometimes be made with instructors at schools or colleges who have the necessary technical training. Daily testing should be the rule, in addition to the occasional check tests made by the public health authorities.

Among the causes of failure of a pool water to meet the bacteriological standards are (1) inadequate disinfection procedure or presence of algae, leaves, and organic matter creating a high chlorine demand; (2) rough pool surfaces that permit harborage of organic growths; (3) improper rate of filtration or poor filter condition; (4) lack of use of shower facilities by swimmers; (5) inadequacy of surface skimming (the highest concentrations of bacteria are at the pool surface); and (6) improper sampling techniques.

12-6. Recirculation Systems and Their Control. The most acceptable practice in swimming-pool design and operation, from standpoints of both water conservation and sanitation, is the re-use of pool water, filtering it continuously, with three or four complete turnovers a day.

There are two types of filter systems employed, the "rapid sand and gravel" type, operating on the same principles as filters applied in drinking-water treatment systems, and the diatomaceous earth filters.

Where rapid sand filters are used, nearly all are of the pressure variety. Open gravity filters are seldom used. A pressure-filter installation requires little space, and since the filter assembly is enclosed in a steel

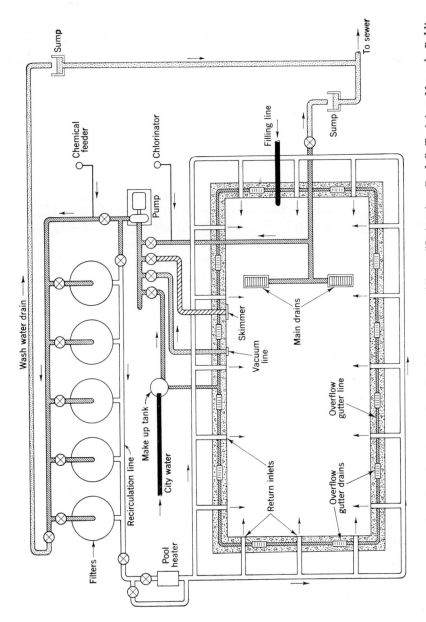

FIGURE 12-1 Plan of swimming pool and piping system. (*From "Swimming Pools," Training Manual, Public Health Service, Communicable Disease Center.*)

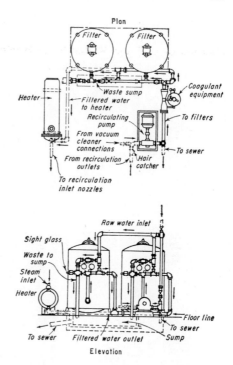

FIGURE 12-2 Typical arrangement of pressure filters used in recirculating water of swimming pools.

tank, one recirculating pump can force the water through the whole system. Figure 12-1 shows a typical layout of the piping system, filters, etc. Preferably two or more filters are used in parallel with the cylinders placed vertically or horizontally. Figure 12-2 shows piping details of two filters.

The water is pumped from the pool, and prior to entering the filter, it receives a dose of chemical coagulant. This forms a gelatinous floc which coats the upper layers of sand grains and aids materially in filtering out sediment and bacteria. The pot type of chemical-feeding apparatus is used in most small installations. One can be seen in the plan view of Fig. 12-2, and details are shown in Fig. 12-4. It is charged with the chemical in lump, briquette, or crystal form. The flow of water through the pot is caused by the pressure difference on each side of an orifice or venturi tube. Since the pressure difference depends upon the rate of flow through the orifice or tube, the amount of water and hence the amount of chemical dissolved by the water flowing through the feeder are automatically proportioned to the amount of water passing through the filters. The desired dosage is set by the regulating valve. Either potash alum (potassium aluminum sulfate) or ammonia alum (ammonium aluminum sulfate) is the coagulant used, and sal soda or soda ash (sodium carbonate) is the akaline agent.

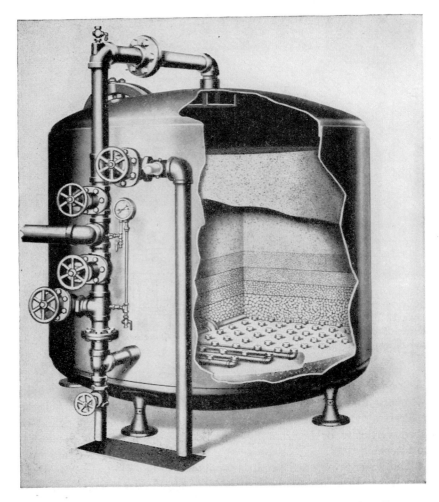

FIGURE 12-3 Sectional view of vertical pressure filter. (*Courtesy of Infilco Inc., Tucson, Ariz., and Public Works Magazine.*)

Ammonia alum has the disadvantage of adding ammonia to the water, which tends to form chloramines with chlorine, reducing the efficiency of disinfection. The quantity fed is usually about 2 oz per sq ft of filter area over a period of 6 to 8 hr, starting immediately after the filter is backwashed.

Many operators dislike the pots and consider them inefficient. Feed can be controlled better by open tanks, which are obtainable commercially, and feeding is done into a surge tank (if there is one), into the suction side of the recirculation pump, or by use of a small pump. These tanks allow use of the cheaper filter alum (aluminum sulfate) and

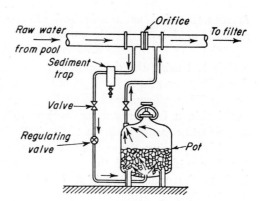

FIGURE 12-4 Flow diagram of pot-type feeder for crystal alum or sodium carbonate.

powdered sodium carbonate. The water must be sufficiently alkaline in reaction to produce a proper floc. Even though the original water carries the requisite alkalinity, which is not always the case, it will be used up in the recirculation process and generally must be replaced by the addition of sodium carbonate or some other chemical. Alkalinity is measured by titration, with a methyl-orange indicator; the procedure is given in "Standard Methods for the Examination of Water and Wastewater" [12]. This is not to be confused with pH, the latter being only indirectly related to alkalinity. The alkalinity test measures the concentration of the alkaline anions, the bicarbonates, carbonates, and hydroxides, which tend to buffer the pH above 7.0. When these are removed from solution or changed by chemical reaction through the addition of acidic compounds, such as the coagulants and chlorine gas, the pH drops very rapidly. Consequently, as a factor of safety, an alkalinity of at least 50 mg/l should be maintained. A rule of thumb is to add 0.5 mg/l of alkalinity for each milligram per liter of alum and 1.2 mg/l of alkalinity for each milligram per liter of elemental chlorine dosage.

Authorities differ on the correct pH range. Those specified in state standards vary from "above 7.0" to "8.0 to 8.9." The reason for this is that there are advantages and disadvantages to each side of the pH scale, and the relative importance of each must be weighed in recommending an optimum range. Assuming that sufficient alkalinity is present, the optimum pH for alum coagulation is 7.2 to 7.6; that for efficient disinfection by chlorine is 4.0 to 8.5; that for efficient algae control is above 8.1; and that for avoidance of eye irritation is 7.0 to 8.4. Generally, a range of 7.5 to 8.0 will be a satisfactory balance of these factors. When high free chlorine residuals are maintained (Arts. 12-3 and 12-9), a range of 8.0 to 8.9 is considered acceptable.

Chlorine gas and alum tend to lower the pH, and hypochlorites tend to increase it. If it is necessary to lower the pH, sodium bisulfate is recommended as a safe and effective compound to use, though muriatic acid is frequently employed.

The test for pH as used by swimming-pool operators is a colorimetric test using the dye indicators bromothymol blue and phenol red, depending on range. Both are bleached by chlorine concentrations as low as 0.2 mg/l and will affect the pH reading by as much as 0.5. To avoid this, a few crystals of sodium thiosulfate may be added to the sample prior to the addition of the indicator.

After passing through the filter, where all the floc and sediment together with most of the bacteria are removed, the water is forced back to the pool, being heated on the way if temperature conditions require it. The disinfectant may be added to the water before it is filtered, as shown in Fig. 12-2, or just before it enters the pool.

The filters are cleaned by the process of reversing the flow through the filter. This is accomplished by manipulating the various valves shown in Fig. 12-3. The wash water, carrying with it the floc, sediment, and bacteria which have accumulated in the filter, is wasted into the sewer. If the installation is a large one and consists of a battery of filters, one is washed at a time, and filtered water from the others is used. In a one-filter layout it is necessary to wash with water from the original source of supply. Pool water may also be used, but this, of course, is undesirable unless the first water filtered after washing is wasted. Where less than four pressure filters are used, a special wash-water pump may be a desirable provision to ensure an adequate backwash rate. Rate controllers, devices that keep the filtration rate constant between washings, are highly desirable but are not usually installed in small filtering systems because of their cost. For large pools, those holding 100,000 gal or more, such equipment should be used. Rate-of-flow gages can be provided in most instances as an aid to control. Filters should be equipped with pressure gages on influent and effluent lines.

Recirculation systems have a hair catcher in the return line through which the water passes before it reaches the pump. This is a metal strainer which catches hair, lint, and other solids which may clog the pump and form masses in the filter. It is arranged so that removing a plug allows the accumulated material to flow out.

In general, swimming-pool filters are operated at 2 to 3 gal/sq ft of filter area per min and are backwashed at 15 gal/(sq ft)(min).

12-7. Maintenance of the Pressure Sand and Gravel Filters. Some operating difficulties may appear in recirculating systems. The sand grains of the filters may cement together, or mud balls may form to the extent that filtration is ineffective. These effects may be due to back-washing with an insufficient amount of water or overdosing with alum. Filters should be inspected once each season. This is done by back-washing the filter, draining the water well below the top of the sand,

and removing the manhole cover from the filter. The sand should be level, with no pools of water standing on it and no cracks or pulling away from the filter shell. A hole or trench should be dug in the sand at least 1 ft deep, and the sand taken from the various levels should be carefully examined. The situation may require a redesign of the washing system in order to obtain more water. If there are four or more filters, the recirculation pump should be able to backwash properly; otherwise a special pump will be required, or pulverized anthracite coal may be substituted for the sand. It is lighter than sand and can be washed with only half as much water as sand. The standard washing rate is a 24-in. rise of the water per minute through the sand.

If backwashing a filter does not remedy the clogging, organic matter may be removed by using lye or sodium hydroxide. This is done as follows: Draw the water level by means of the drain valve down to within 2 in. of the sand, and add 1 lb of the chemical for each square foot of the filter. Allow this to act on the bed for several hours. Then draw the water down partway through the bed, and repeat the process. Follow this with a thorough backwashing. Care must be taken in handling the lye and also the wash water containing it, or burns may result. The above treatment will not clear clogged nozzles or perforations in the underdrain system. When these occur, the manufacturer of the filter should be consulted. Certain acids or sodium bisulfate can be used to clear the openings. About 2 lb of sodium bisulfate per sq ft of filter surface is added, followed by the soaking procedure described above.

Some operators wash filters only after they note a reduction in the rate of filtration. It is better, however, to wash when the pressure difference reaches a certain amount, such as 5 psi or about 10 ft, as shown by the pressure gages.

12-8. Diatomaceous Earth Filters. During World War II, the Army adapted filtering systems previously in use in the petroleum and chemical industries for treatment of water for drinking purposes in the field. This filter, which involves the application of a filter aid, has since become widely used at swimming pools. It is well adapted to this field in that, generally speaking, relatively nonturbid water is applied to the filter.

The filter design takes many forms, but as generally used in swimming pools, it consists of a steel shell containing porous elements (tubes, leaves, disks, or trays), referred to as septa, of metal, stone, or plastic. The septa may be wire-wound or covered with cloth, such as Dacron, to produce the required even porosity, with openings generally less than 0.005 in. It is equipped with a "precoat feeder," which places the filter aid in suspension and feeds it into the water flowing into the filter shell. The filter aid deposits on the outside of the septa, forming a coating which remains as long as the pressure is maintained. Turbidity,

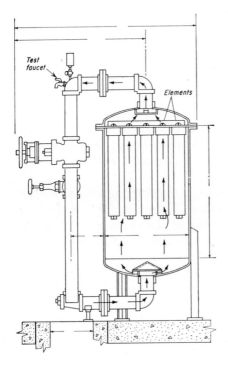

Test
faucet

Elements

some bacteria, and even amoeba cysts become enmeshed in the coating and are thus removed from the system.

The filter aid is usually diatomaceous earth (microscopic fossils of marine plants), but other materials may be used, such as asbestos fiber or expanded perlite. Both diatomaceous earth and perlite are found in extensive deposits in this country.

The usual charge of diatomaceous earth in the precoat is about 0.125 lb/sq ft of septa. During the precoating, water is recirculated through the filter or wasted. Afterward the filter is placed "on line" and kept in continuous operation while more filter aid is fed by means of a "body feeder" in the makeup line. The rate of filtration is the same as for sand and gravel filters, 2 to 3 gpm per sq ft of septum surface.

When the differential pressure between the influent and effluent attains 25 to 50 psi, the filter is taken out of service, and the filter-aid coating is removed and wasted. This is done by various methods, depending on the make of filter, and may consist of backwashing by reversal of flow, by applying air pressure, or by manual shaking (spinning the elements by turning an external crank). In some small installations, the filter shell is opened, and the elements are cleaned by hosing.

Some diatomaceous earth filters operate by means of a vacuum applied to the interior of the septa. In these, the septa are submerged

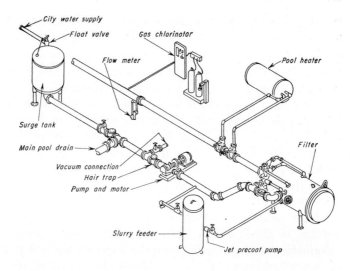

City water supply

Float valve

Gas chlorinator

Flow meter

Pool heater

Surge tank

Main pool drain

Vacuum connection

Hair trap

Pump and motor

Filter

Slurry feeder

Jet precoat pump

FIGURE 12-6 Isometric drawing of typical equipment room: diatomite filter, precoat pump, heater, chlorinator, surge tank, and piping. (*Courtesy of Kinetrol Company, Dallas, Tex.*)

in open tanks containing the recirculated water. The vacuum filters are cleaned when the vacuum reaches 10 to 15 in. of mercury.

As long as the diatomaceous earth filters are operated properly and the septa are kept in repair, they are highly effective. It is obvious, however, that if the coating does not cover the septa fully, little or no filtration occurs.

12-9. Disinfection of Pool Water. While filtration of the pool water removes all ordinary suspended matter, it does not remove all bacteria. Hence some means of disinfection must be applied. Disinfection processes are much more effective in clear water than in turbid water carrying much organic matter.

The hypochlorites, of either calcium or sodium, have been extensively used to disinfect pool water. Solutions of hypochlorites can be pumped or injected into the recirculation system of a pool by the use of appropriate commercial apparatus. For fill-and-draw pools, intermittent dosage is accomplished by sprinkling a solution of the chemical over the surface of the water or by dragging a cloth bag containing the proper amount through the water. However, this has to be done with care to assure a uniform and effective dosage.

Liquid chlorine (a liquid under pressure in the containers, but a gas as fed to water) is generally used in large pools. Several manufacturers furnish apparatus which feed controlled amounts of chlorine gas wherever desired. If water is recirculated, the chlorine is added to the water just before it reenters the pool or before it goes to the filter.

Feeding just ahead of the filter requires more chlorine, but it tends to keep the filter sand in better condition by destroying organic growths, such as fungi. The advantages of chlorine gas over hypochlorites are that it does not lose strength in storage as the latter do and that it is generally more economical for large installations (Art. 2-18).

The most satisfactory method of controlling disinfection is by retaining a slight excess of chlorine (a residual) over and above that required to satisfy the demand of the organic matter in the water. The excess can be determined by the use of the orthotolidine test, described in Art. 2-19. The standards mentioned above recommend a residual of 0.4 to 1.0 mg/l. The dosage necessary to retain this must be learned by experiment. Methods of calculating dosages are the same as those used for treating drinking water, given in Art. 2-20. In recirculation systems, residuals can be maintained by means of proper setting of the chlorinator which is feeding into the recirculating water. During periods of heavy patronage, the water should be tested at frequent intervals throughout the day for residuals, the samples being taken from both the shallow and deep ends of the pool.

The addition of chlorine so that available chlorine residuals are obtained provides a distinct advantage as far as disinfection is concerned, and the pool operator should strive to maintain free chlorine residuals to the exclusion of combined available chlorine residuals, which contain the less effective chloramines. Experience in maintaining high chlorine residuals (equal to, or greater than, 1 mg/l) indicates that a greater margin of safety is produced than through the use of residuals on the order of 0.4 to 0.6 mg/l. High free-residual chlorination of swimming-pool water is claimed to reduce eye irritation, as compared with combined residuals. It also improves algae control by permitting higher pH values, 8.0 to 8.9.

Free available residuals may be obtained by adding enough chlorine to destroy the ammonia present; usually a dosage of about ten times the ammonia content is required. The ammonia is converted to nitrogen and hydrochloric acid if the pH is confined to a range of 7.5 to 8.5. This is the "break-point" chlorination process, described in Art. 2-22.

Hypochlorites of calcium, sodium, and lithium are also used for disinfection of swimming-pool water. Calcium and lithium hypochlorites are solids and most often are used in the granular form. Sodium hypochlorite is always in solution form. The strength of these compounds is expressed in terms of "available" chlorine (Art. 2-18) and is 70 per cent for calcium hypochlorite, 35 per cent for lithium hypochlorite, and 5 per cent for sodium hypochlorite solution. They are generally fed as a solution diluted to 1 per cent or 10,000 mg/l available chlorine (Art. 2-20) by a small diaphragm or reciprocating pump or siphon feeder. Other methods of feeding calcium hypochlorite include using submerged baskets or dissolving cylinders, in which case the chemical is used in tablet form and is placed in the feeder.

Bromine has been used for disinfecting swimming-pool water since World War II. It is growing in popularity, having been recognized by the standards of several but not all states. It is a liquid at room temperature and may be fed into recirculation systems with a relatively simple injection apparatus in which water simultaneously dilutes the chemical and conveys it into the system. The recommended residual is 1.0 mg/l or above, which does not cause skin or eye irritation. The residuals may be determined by means of orthotolidine. Since bromine is a severe skin irritant, burning on contact, it must be handled with caution and stored in recessed floor or wall-hung units to avoid accidental spillage.

Iodine is also employed as a swimming-pool disinfectant. It is a highly efficient bactericide and is claimed to effect disinfection without eye irritation. Sodium or potassium iodide, from which free iodine can be released by chlorine or another oxidizing agent, is the form generally employed. Residuals of 0.4 mg/l have been found to be effective.

The chlorinated cyanurates (chloramides), in powder form, are also employed as disinfectants. In these compounds chlorine is combined with nitrogen and remains stable as long as the material is kept dry and free of organic matter. When they are dissolved in water, chlorine is released which responds to tests for free chlorine. Among the advantages of their use is the minimal change in pH.

Public health authorities prefer the halogens (chlorine, bromine, and iodine) and compounds of them for disinfection of pool water because residuals can be maintained which provide a factor of safety in the disinfecting procedure. Other chemicals and methods have been used but have been found less satisfactory. They include ultraviolet ray, ozone, and ionized silver.

12-10. Natural Bathing Places. In artificial pools the most important consideration with respect to the water is that it not be contaminated after it enters the pool. At the natural bathing places, which may be beaches, lakes, or slightly improved pools in streams, the original condition of the water must also be considered. Here bacteriological tests of the water do not tell the full story, for the total count and tests for coliforms do not differentiate between the members of the coliform family, which originate with animals and cultivated fields, and the dangerous contamination caused by sewage from dwellings, hotels, factories, municipal sewage works, and the bathers themselves. The tests must therefore be supplemented by a sanitary survey covering sources and possibilities of dangerous contamination. Little has been accomplished with regard to water standards for natural bathing places.

One state has rated ocean bathing places at various depths and tide levels on the basis of analyses as follows:

Average coliforms
per 100 ml

Class A	0–50
Class B	51–500
Class C	501–1,000
Class D	Over 1,000

At the same time, a sanitary survey was made of the same areas, covering such matters as sewer outlets and shore currents which would spread pollution, and a similar letter rating was adopted on this basis. A close correlation was found between the survey and the analysis rating. The letter ratings may be interpreted as good, doubtful, poor, and very poor.

The bacterial limits for natural bathing waters recommended by West Virginia, Great Lakes and Upper Mississippi River Boards, TVA, and New York State are indicated in Table 12-1.

Combined sewer overflows in the beachfront metropolitan areas of the United States are cause for concern. During a storm, regulators will allow the excess flow to be discharged directly into a watercourse. The initial discharge from a combined sewer overflow contains highly concentrated raw sewage which has been stored in the sewers. In some cases this problem has been minimized by passing the overflow into storage basins and chlorinating it. The eventual answer, however, appears to be complete separation of the storm and sanitary systems.

Table 12-1. BACTERIAL LIMITS FOR NATURAL BATHING WATERS AS RECOMMENDED BY FOUR AGENCIES

Water classification	Coliform density per 100 ml			
	West Virginia	Great Lakes and Upper Mississippi River Boards	Tennessee Valley Authority	New York State
Satisfactory for bathing . . .	0–1,000	100–500	0–50	0–1,000
Satisfactory with reservations .	....	501–1,000	51–500	1,000–2,400
Use doubtful; not recommended	......	1,001–10,000	501–1,000	50 per cent of samples, over 2,400
Do not use.	......	10,001–100,000	Over 1,000	Evidence of infection from area

SOURCE: Eugene L. Lehr and Charles C. Johnson, Jr., Water Quality of Swimming Places, *Public Health Rept.*, vol. 69, no. 8, 1954.

Leptospirosis is a problem of natural bathing places. The natural reservoirs of the causative organism are rats and domestic animals. These organisms are excreted in urine and remain viable in water for several weeks. A number of epidemics have been traced to swimming in contaminated water.

Another factor making natural bathing places less satisfactory than artificial pools is the problem of providing supervision and lifeguards. Unless definitely limited areas are roped off, adequate supervision is virtually impossible. Even then, the deep water boundaries can be patrolled only with difficulty.

12-11. Disinfection and Bathing Loads for Natural Bathing Places. Whether or not disinfection is employed, efforts should be made to eliminate sources of sewage pollution of small ponds or streams used for bathing, and sanitary surveys of watersheds are recommended. Chlorine can be applied to the inlet water continuously, or several applications may be made over the area during bathing periods, with the same residuals as recommended for artificial pools.

Disinfection of large bodies of water by feeding liquid chlorine from a "chloroboat" has been successful in a few cases. Bathing areas several acres in extent have been chlorinated by use of pipe systems laid on the bottom through which chlorine solution or chlorinated water is applied and the water is to some extent recirculated since the solution water is withdrawn from the pool. Whether disinfection should be applied to natural bathing areas will depend not only upon the safety of the water but also upon the amount of water available and its dilution by action of tides and currents.

In small natural pools it is possible to correlate the amount of water with the bathing load. It should probably never be less than 500 gal per bather without disinfection. The Becker formula can be used in relating the load to the volume of diluting water. This formula is $Q = 6.25\ T^2$, where Q is the quantity of water per bather in gallons, and T is the replacement period in hours. For example, if the flow is such as to replace the pool volume in 8 hr, then Q will be 400 gal, and the number of bathers permitted in 8 hr would be the capacity of the pool divided by 400.

12-12. Pool Construction. In sizing public pools, consideration can be given to providing a capacity in proportion to the tributary population. It has been found that between 5 and 10 per cent of the population of cities with 30,000 inhabitants or less will provide the maximum attendance at a public pool. This decreases with the size of the city. Average daily attendance is about 2 or 3 per cent of the population. For motels, a rule of thumb used is to allow one person per unit up to 50, and thereafter one person per two units.

The loading capacity of a pool can be determined as follows:

diving area, 12 persons maximum within 10 ft of the diving board or platform; swimming area (that part deeper than 5 ft, not counting the diving area), one person per 24 sq ft; and nonswimming area, 70 to 80 per cent of the entire pool area, one person per 10 sq ft. These figures assume that a large proportion of pool users are not in the water at all times.

Pools are of various shapes and dimensions. Outdoor pools are frequently oval, with the shallow water at the edges and the deep water in the middle. The usual swimming pool, however, is rectangular, shallow at one end and deep at the other. Pools which are to be used for athletic contests must have a minimum length of 60 ft; otherwise the minimum should be 40 ft for public and semipublic pools. For racing it is also necessary that each contestant have a free lane 5 ft wide. For these reasons, the smaller swimming pools are quite commonly 60 ft in length with the width a multiple of 5 ft, the most popular size for indoor pools being 30 by 60 ft.

The depth of a pool should receive careful consideration during design, particularly the proportion of the shallow and deep parts. As the pools considered become smaller, the proportion of shallow area will become smaller, for the space for diving will remain constant. Deep water for diving should extend a distance of 10 to 15 ft beyond the end of the springboard to minimize the chance of accidents. Usually the minimum depth of water is 3 ft, and maximum depth 9 ft. Depths should be clearly marked by tile inlays, by figures painted at the pool edges, or by conspicuous signs.

The bottom slopes of pools should be gradual enough to prevent slipping. A fall of 1 ft in 20 ft will be safe in the shallow area. Where the water is over 5.5 ft deep, steeper slopes are permissible. In pools less than 42 ft in length, a maximum slope of 1 ft in 8 ft is advisable. There should, of course, never be sudden drops.

Pools are usually constructed of reinforced concrete, sometimes with a tile surface. They should be impervious, smooth of surface, and easy to clean. Concrete polished with carborundum bricks immediately after removal of the forms makes an excellent surface. The rounding of corners and the avoidance of recesses also facilitate cleaning. A light-colored finish, when accompanied by clear water, makes a more attractive pool and also allows lifeguards or attendants to discover submerged bodies easily.

If concrete curbing and runways are used, they should be given a wood-float surface that will prevent slipping. The walks or runways around the pool should slope gently away, about ¼ in./ft, or be otherwise arranged so that no drainage will enter the pool from them.

Runways should be not less than 4 ft wide. It is not advisable to have grass or sand plots within the pool enclosure, as grass and sand will be carried into the pool on the feet of bathers and result in unsightly water. Entrance to the pool should be at the shallow end.

Scum gutters are recesses in the pool wall extending completely around the water edge at the water level. They receive overflow, scum, and floating matter and act as expectoration troughs. There is no objection to their being arranged to receive drainage from runways, in which case the latter are sloped slightly to the pool. The gutters may drain to the pump in the case of recirculation pools or directly to the sewer. They should have drainage outlets at not more than 15-ft intervals and should slope to the outlets. They are sometimes molded to form the life rail, in which case they should be deep enough so that the hand will not touch bottom, about 2 or 3 in. It has become quite common practice to utilize the scum gutters as part of the recirculation system. In others words, a percentage of the swimming-pool water is returned via the scum gutters to the purification equipment. Advantages of this method are that it (1) maintains the water level constantly at the overflow point, (2) improves circulation efficiency by increasing the number of withdrawal points, and (3) provides for purification of the most highly contaminated portion of the water.

There is a growing tendency to utilize mechanical skimmers to replace the more expensive scum-gutter construction, particularly in small pools. The skimmers may be of the floating type, or they may be recessed at various points in the walls. These are generally connected with the pump suction. At least one should be provided for every 800 sq ft. It is required that the devices be adjustable up to at least 50 per cent of the capacity of the swimming-pool filter system. Other features specified are automatic adjustment to variations in the water level over a range of 2 in., provision of a device to prevent air lock in the suction line, and provision of a removable and cleanable basket or screen.

The "water-level deck type" of swimming pool has been installed in a number of cases in recent years. Here the water level is maintained with the peripheral overflow, and there are no scum gutters as such. Water is flushed over the walls onto a floor which is sloped to deck drains, spaced at about the same distance as scum-gutter outlets would have been. This type of construction also requires the use of a balancing tank to maintain the pool level.

Diving boards should be covered with corrugated sheet rubber or some other rough material to prevent slipping, but in the interest of athlete's-foot prevention they should not have fabric or wood surfaces. In indoor pools, 13 ft of headroom is required above a springboard. No diving tower greater than 10 ft in height should be used in public pools. The minimum safe depth of water is 8 ft. If diving platforms are more than 5 ft and up to 7 ft above the water, the minimum depth should be increased to 11 ft; for a height up to 10 ft, a depth of 12 ft is needed.

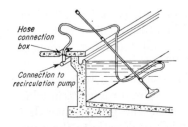

FIGURE 12-7 Suction arrangement for cleaning bottom and sides of pool.

Lifeguards should be instructed to prevent congestion of swimmers in the water near the boards in order to minimize the chance of accident.

The inlets and outlets of continuous-flow pools must be carefully placed to ensure a complete change of water and the absence of stagnant portions. It is recommended that inlets be installed, at least in the shallow portion of the pool, so that each serves 15 lin ft. The main drains are usually placed at the deepest point of the pool and vary in number according to the width. In general, the drains should not be placed farther than 10 ft from a sidewall.

If steps are used rather than ladders, they should be recessed and not allowed to extend into the pool. Indoor pools require adequate ventilation but should be so arranged that no drafts will strike the bathers. Infrared heating has been applied with success in indoor pools.

12-13. Cleaning Pools. Cleaning of pools is necessitated by heavy sediment or by algae growths on the bottom walls and sidewalls. Cleaning can be accomplished by draining the pool and scrubbing the sides and bottom. This causes considerable expense in labor, loss of water, and operating time. Suction cleaners, specially designed for cleaning pools, may be used for removing sediment without draining the pool. The apparatus consists of a suction tube with a stiff brush within the suction nozzle. It is connected to the suction side of the recirculation pump, which is arranged to bypass the mingled foreign matter and water to the sewer or to conduct it to the filter. Special inlet connections for the suction hose must be placed at intervals around the pool. About 6 in. of water is removed from the pool during the operation of cleaning.

Algae growths, though harmless, except for making surfaces slippery, are unsightly and are likely to discolor the water, give it an unpleasant odor, and increase chlorine demand. Their development can be prevented by dosing with copper sulfate at the rate of 10 to 20 lb per million gal. The chemical can be applied either by dragging it through the water in bags or by adding it continuously to recirculated water. Chlorination also tends to prevent algae growths and will do so if a proper residual is constantly maintained. A very important factor in algae control is the maintenance of pH at a proper level (Art. 12-6).

Quaternary ammonium compounds when used in the presence of a disinfectant increase the effectiveness of the disinfectant in attacking

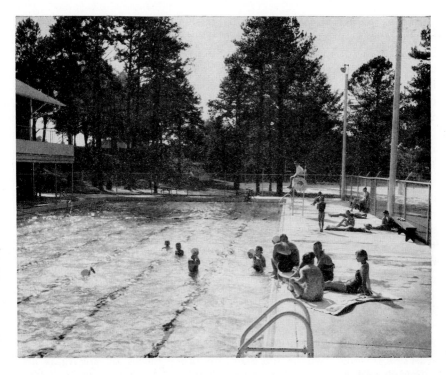

FIGURE 12-8 City pool at Greenwood, S.C. Note fenced enclosure, lifeguard, guard rope, and scum gutter. (*Courtesy of Inertol Company.*)

algae because of the consequent lowered surface tension. The dosage recommended is 1 gal per 50,000 gal of water initially, followed by 1 qt. per 50,000 gal every 6 days. Certain highly toxic algicides have been marketed, some even containing mercury, which should not be used because of specific sensitivity of some of the pool patrons. No algicide should be used in a public pool unless the label shows the active ingredient, the ingredient is known to be safe for use, and instructions for use are clearly given.

Once pool walls have become discolored and slimy with algae, chemical treatment may have but little effect in their removal, particularly if the walls are rough. Emptying and scrubbing will then be necessary. Scrubbing with 5 per cent hypochlorite slurry or solution has been found effective in completely removing the slime. Where algae troubles are expected, continuous but light treatments, about 0.5 mg/l, with copper sulfate are commonly applied as a preventive measure. This is especially likely to be necessary in outdoor pools because exposure of the water to sunlight promotes heavy growth of algae; indoor pools may also have trouble at times. Rubber-base waterproof enamels resist algae intrusion.

12-14. Safety Provisions. Attendants should be stationed at all pools for lifesaving purposes. They should be expert swimmers and should be skilled in lifesaving and resuscitation. A certificate in lifesaving, as awarded by the Red Cross, is a logical requirement. If the pool is large, it is of advantage to place the guard on an elevated platform where he can easily survey the whole pool. One chair should be provided for each 2,000 sq ft of pool surface.

A first-aid kit should be on hand at each pool. The safety equipment required will depend to some extent on the size of the pool. If the minimum horizontal dimension is less than 30 ft, the following should be provided: (1) one or more poles, each longer than one-half of the width of the pool and capable of being extended to all parts of the pool bottom, constructed preferably of bamboo, and having a shepherd's crook at the end with an opening of at least 18 in. between the tip of the hook and the tip of the pole; (2) one or more throwing ring buoys, each having a maximum diameter of at least 15 in. and with a $\frac{3}{16}$-in. line at least as long as the maximum width of the pool; and (3) one or more "flutter boards," each approximately 1 ft by 3 ft by 2 in. and capable of supporting a weight of at least 20 lb in the water.

At pools with a minimum width of more than 30 ft, the above requirements are modified to the effect that the hooked poles must be at least 15 ft long, two or more of the other pieces of apparatus are required, and the ring buoys must be attached to at least 60 ft of line. In addition, blankets should be available and a telephone installed.

Fewer injuries will occur if the pool is not overcrowded. A minimum of 24 sq ft per person is considered necessary, except within a radius of 10 ft of a diving board, which may be considered to serve only 12 persons, including those waiting to dive. Not more than two or three persons should be allowed in the diving area at one time while diving is in progress.

While deaths from electric shock in swimming pools are rare, every means should be taken to prevent them. The water in the pool will carry electric current, and current leakages may occur from faulty fixtures. Most of the accidents have resulted from flooded underwater lights. Investigation has shown that moisture can enter through the connecting cord normally employed if it is present in a deck box. A method of "potting" the terminal areas of both the lights and deck boxes can be used to prevent this from occurring and also to insulate the terminals effectively and permanently. Essentially it involves filling the terminal cavities with electrical epoxy resins. Kits with instructions for making this modification on existing installations are available.

The 1962 revision of the National Electrical Code includes for the first time a special section on swimming-pool wiring Its principal feature is that all lighting fixtures, niches, deck boxes, diving stands, ladders, piping systems, reinforcing steel, pumps, filters, feeders, and metallic objects within 5 ft of the pool must be grounded by 14-gage or larger wire run back to the power panel. The code contains a recommendation that if a circuit voltage greater than 30 volts is employed, a fail-safe current-leakage detector be installed.

12-15. Control of Bathers. Of great importance is supervision of the bathers. The entrance into the pool of persons with communicable diseases or with open wounds or bandages should be prohibited. This is necessary, not only to prevent contamination of the water, but also to protect the bathers themselves. Serious sinus trouble has been attributed to infectious material being forced by the water into the interior cavities of the head when bathers are suffering from ear discharges, colds, or respiratory infections. This prohibition, with the other instructions mentioned below, should be made plain by means of placards displayed at the entrance to the dressing rooms and inside them.

The need for requiring swimmers to take shower baths before entering the pool is recognized but not always enforced. The quality of the pool water reflects, to a very great extent, the degree to which this requirement is complied with. The showers, to be effective, must be taken before the bathing suit is put on; soap should be used, and the water should be warm. Inspection is necessary to enforce the rule. A set of personal regulations should be posted.

Eating and smoking in the pool enclosure are also prohibited in order that foreign material will not be thrown into the water. In general, it is good practice to segregate spectators in street clothes in such a manner that they do not have access to the pool enclosure.

12-16. Suits and Towels. Swimming suits, unless properly treated, are likely to harbor many bacteria. Although at most pools it is the practice to allow patrons to bring their own suits, it would probably be better to require that all use suits furnished by the pool management so that they may be washed and sterilized after each use. Cleaning and practical sterilization of suits and towels are accomplished by thorough washing with hot water and soap, followed by complete drying. Cold-water washing and air drying should be prohibited. A chemical treatment may be applied, consisting of soaking the suits for 5 min in a 1,000-mg/l solution of a quaternary ammonium compound. A further valuable requirement is that the stock of suits and towels be large enough to allow storage of the clean supply for 24 hr, thus reducing the danger of the patron being issued a dirty suit at rush times.

Clean suits and towels should never be allowed to come in contact with unwashed stock or be stored on shelves or in baskets which have held it. The issuing of clean suits and towels at the same counters where dirty suits and towels are turned in is dangerous.

12-17. The Bathhouse. Of the bathhouse equipment, the toilets and showers are the most important. The usual minimum requirements are based on maximum pool loading and are one shower for each 40 swimmers, one toilet for each 40 women, and one toilet and one urinal for each 60 men. One lavatory with hot and cold water should be available for each 60 patrons. Drinking fountains should be provided.

The shower-bath heads should preferably be of the shoulder-high slanting-jet type. This will allow use without wetting the hair, which is desirable if rubber bathing caps are worn. Precautions should be taken with showers, by means of check valves and other apparatus, to prevent hot water from entering the cold-water pipes and to ensure proper mixing of the hot and cold water.

The locker room must be well ventilated and, if possible, separated from the shower rooms in order to prevent excessive moisture from entering. The lockers themselves are usually ventilated by means of doors of expanded metal or doors having slots or perforations. While ventilation of the lockers is much needed, the possibility of stealing from the stored clothing by means of wire hooks should be considered.

12-18. Small Pools. Particularly in the Southern states, the construction of small pools of a private and semipublic nature is growing in popularity. Motels and hotels, for example, frequently provide them for use by their customers. They are also being constructed to serve apartment houses and real estate subdivisions and residences. Quite often their size invites departure from accepted standards which were written primarily for the municipal type of pool. Examples of such departure are failure to provide the floor slopes recommended in Art. 12-12 in the nonswimming section, nonobservance of recommended recirculation rates, utilization of skimming devices rather than scum gutters, and utilization of substitutes for the generally accepted masonry construction. These bear watching on the part of health departments, not only because of substandard features, but also because trained and qualified operation is as important in these installations as in the larger community pools.

To assure that public health principles are observed in the design and operation of all pools, ordinances should be adopted incorporating public health standards, and the installation of pools should be controlled by a permit system in which the health department has a voice. The provisions of such an ordinance should also cover location, nuisance features (from the standpoint of neighborhood annoyance), fencing, materials of construction, quality of water supply, plumbing, and disposal of waste wash water and pool contents. In one state it is recommended that a pool with a capacity greater than 750 gal be equipped with a complete recirculation system including filters and disinfection equipment.

Bibliography

1. "Recommended Practice for Design, Equipment and Operation of Swimming Pools and Other Public Bathing Places," American Public Health Association, New York, 1957.
2. Swimming Pools: Disease Control through Proper Design and Operation, CDC Training Manual, *Public Health Service Pub.* 665, 1959.
3. Mollohon, Cecil S., and Mary S. Romer: Public Health Significance of Swimming Pool Granuloma, *Am. J. Public Health*, vol. 51, no. 6, June, 1961.
4. Mallmann, W. L.: Cocci Test for Detecting Mouth and Nose Pollution of Swimming Pool Water, *Am. J. Public Health*, vol. 52, no. 12, December, 1962.
5. Laubusch, Edmund J.: Disinfection of Public Swimming Pools, *Public Works*, vol. 89, no. 6, June, 1958.
6. Griffin, Attmore E.: H_2O: The Operator as Water Chemist, *Swimming Pool Age*, vol. 37, no. 1, January, 1963.
7. Byrd, Oliver E., *et al.*: Safety of Iodine as a Disinfectant in Swimming Pools, *Public Health Rept.*, vol. 78, no. 5, May, 1963.
8. Typhoid Traced to Bathing at a Polluted Beach, *Public Works*, vol. 91, no. 5, May, 1961.
9. Frances, Saul: How Good Is Your Present Algaecide? *Swimming Pool Age*, vol. 36, no. 11, November, 1962.
10. Doughty, Donald: Progress in Electrical Safety, *Swimming Pool Age*, vol. 37, no. 1, January, 1963.
11. Timm, E. E.: The Role of Electrical Epoxy Resin in Pool Safety, *Swimming Pool Age*, vol. 37, no. 7, July, 1963.
12. "Standard Methods for the Examination of Water and Wastewater," 11th ed., American Public Health Association, New York, 1960.

13

LIGHT

13-1. Light and health are related in several ways. The bactericidal effect of light has been mentioned elsewhere. Light appears to have a stimulating effect upon the blood, particularly that portion of the blood supply which is in the outer parts of the body, and this stimulation apparently helps the body to overcome tuberculosis infection. Sunlight has been found to be a specific in the treatment of rickets. The ultraviolet rays here appear to be the active agents. On the other hand, excessive exposure to sunlight is known to cause skin cancer.

Inside illumination is receiving ever-increasing attention from physicians, engineers, educators, and employers. This interest in illumination has resulted in a recognition of the effect of insufficient lighting upon

438

the eyes, the comfort, and the production of workers and upon the efficiency of schoolchildren. The importance of good lighting in reducing accidents and the need for street lighting that can cope with modern high-speed traffic have also been emphasized.

Measurement of Light

13-2. The *intensity of light source* is measured by the *standard candle*. This is the light given by a candle which has been internationally agreed upon so that it is approximately uniform.

The *intensity of illumination* is measured by the *foot-candle*. This is the illumination given by a source of one candle to an area 1 ft away from the source (see Fig. 13-1).

The *luminous flux* is the amount or quantity of light, and its unit is the *lumen*. In Fig. 13-1, the area *A* is 1 sq ft, and since it is 1 ft away from the candle, it is illuminated to an intensity of 1 ft-c. Strictly speaking, the surface should be curved so that each point is equidistant from the candle. The total amount of light passing through the area *A*, if it is considered to be transparent, is 1 lumen. Therefore, the lumen is the quantity of light required to illuminate 1 sq ft to the intensity of 1 ft-c. The lumen is useful in specifying the amount of light which a light source, or luminaire, must supply. For example, if 100 sq ft must be illuminated to an intensity of 10 ft-c, 1,000 lumens will be required.

The *brightness* of a surface which is emitting or reflecting light is expressed in *candles per square inch* or in *lumens per unit of area*. A surface that is emitting or reflecting light in a given direction at the rate of 1 candle/sq in. of projected area has a brightness in that direction of 1 candle/sq in. Or, a surface which has a brightness equal to the uniform brightness of a perfectly diffusing surface emitting or reflecting 1 lumen/sq ft has a brightness of 1 ft-L. (foot lambert). The *foot-lambert* is also the average brightness of any surface emitting or reflecting light at the rate of 1 lumen/sq ft. The *lambert* is the brightness of a surface emitting or reflecting 1 lumen/sq cm. Since it is brightness which affects the seeing process, the foot-lambert rather than the foot-candle is the primary factor in the consideration of eye comfort and efficiency of seeing.

13-3. The Inverse Square Law. In Fig. 13-1 it will be seen that if the surface is removed, the light which has illuminated it also illuminates

FIGURE 13-1 Illumination at *A* is 1 ft-c. The illumination on surfaces varies inversely as the square of the distance from the source to the surface.

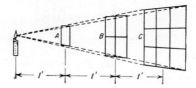

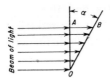

FIGURE 13-2   The cosine law.

B, but B is larger in area than A and therefore is less intensely illuminated. Since the two areas are bases of pyramids, their areas are proportional to the squares of their distances from the candle which is at the vertex, and if their respective distances are 1 ft and 2 ft, the area of B is four times the area of A, and its intensity of illumination is only one-fourth as much. Similarly, the area of C is nine times that of A, and its illumination is $\frac{1}{9}$ ft-c. Hence the rule may be stated that the intensity of the illumination on a surface varies inversely as the square of its distance from the light source.

13-4. Cosine Law. In Fig. 13-2 the surface OA is perpendicular to the path of the light ray from the source of light, the source being considered so far away that light rays are practically parallel. The surface OB is at an angle α to the ray. The illumination on the two surfaces is inversely proportional to their areas; hence

$$\frac{\text{Illumination of } OB}{\text{Illumination of } OA} = \frac{OA}{OB}$$

But OA/OB is the cosine of the angle α.

The rule then may be stated that illumination on a surface not perpendicular to the path of the rays is proportional to the cosine of the angle between the surface and the perpendicular surface.

13-5. Photometry. This is the measuring of the intensity of a luminous source or the brightness of an illuminated surface. Photometers are devised for determining the luminous intensity of an unknown source. They involve the principle of comparison of a known source with one of unknown intensity and make use of the inverse square law [2].

A simple photometer, which illustrates the principle of photometry, is the bar type (Fig. 13-3). It consists of a paper or cloth screen with a waxed or greased spot. Two mirrors are arranged so that both sides of the screen can be viewed simultaneously. The screen is arranged so that it can be moved between two sources of light, one of known intensity,

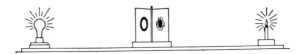

FIGURE 13-3   Bar photometer showing use of oblique mirrors (photometer not balanced).

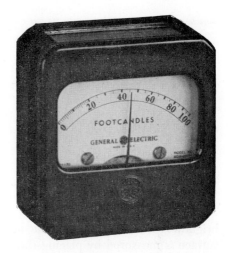

FIGURE 13-4   Foot-candle light meter.
(*Photograph courtesy of General Electric Company, Cleveland, Ohio.*)

such as 1 or more candles. The greased spot transmits more light through it than the plain section of the screen. It reflects less light, however, than the surrounding paper. Hence, if the paper is illuminated to the same intensity on both sides, the spot becomes indistinguishable from the surrounding paper. The distances are measured, and the inverse square rule is then applied.

For checking illumination, the foot-candle meter is very useful. It has the further advantages of being small, portable, and inexpensive. It can be used by inspectors in determining and measuring illumination at the factory worker's bench or at the schoolroom desk (see Fig. 13-4). Two sources of error in an inexpensive light meter are that it does not react to colored light as the eye does, and that it requires a correction for light which reaches it at an angle. In order to correct for the latter, the meter should be held perpendicular to the light direction and the reading multiplied by the cosine of the angle through which the meter was rotated to the vertical. Meters are obtainable that are corrected for this factor and for color.

Measurement of intensity of illumination is important, but it must be recognized that it is only one factor in the matter of obtaining eye comfort and efficient seeing. The brightness of objects, which is related to the reflection of the light cast upon them, and the contrast between the brightness of various surfaces in the field of view are equally important. Brightness is measured by brightness meters. Rough approximations of brightness can be obtained with some types of foot-candle meters. For reflecting material, the cell is placed against the test surface and then drawn away slowly until a constant reading is obtained (a distance of 2 to 6 in.). The meter reading at that point multiplied by 1.25 to allow for light striking the cell at oblique angles is the approximate

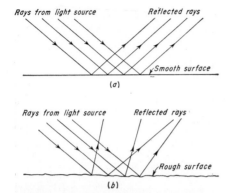

FIGURE 13-5   Types of reflection. (*a*) Regular or specular reflection; (*b*) diffused reflection.

brightness in foot-lamberts. The foot-lambert brightness of an emitting surface is measured by placing the cell against the surface and multiplying the reading by 1.25.

13-6. Reflection. Whenever light strikes a surface, the light is absorbed or reflected. If the surface is rough and black, practically all is absorbed. If the surface is light-colored, a large proportion will be reflected. The law of reflection is that the angle of incidence equals the angle of reflection. This means that the angle which a ray of light makes with a surface it strikes is the same as the angle which the reflected ray makes with the same surface. As shown in Fig. 13-5, if the reflecting surface is very smooth or polished, the parallel or approximately parallel rays of incident light are reflected in parallel or nearly parallel lines. The eye, therefore, sees on the surface the image of the source of light. This type of reflection is known as regular or specular reflection. If the reflecting surface is rough, it is, in effect, made up of many small planes arranged at various angles, with the result that the incident light is reflected in lines that are not parallel. This is known as diffused reflection, and the eye which intercepts the rays can perceive no image of the source.

Most surfaces have a combination of specular and diffuse reflection characteristics. A newly varnished desk top, for example, would have mostly specular and little diffused reflection. Certain types of paper will combine diffused with specular reflection to the extent that there will be reduced contrast and visibility. This is called a veiling reflection or reflected glare.

Reflection resulting from wall and ceiling surfaces is very important in the illumination of rooms, particularly in daylight lighting and the indirect and semidirect systems of artificial lighting. Of the light which strikes walls or ceiling, part is absorbed, and the balance is reflected to strike other surfaces, where more is absorbed and the balance reflected, and so on until it is all absorbed. Each reflection contributes to illumination over that of the source alone. Therefore ceilings, walls, and floors

Table 13-1.   REFLECTION FACTORS OF
PAINTS OF VARIOUS TINTS

Classification	Reflection coefficient, per cent
White plaster	90–92
Flat mill white (mat)	75–90
Light cream	74
Light pink	67
Light yellow	65
Light blue	61
Light buff	58
Light gray	49
Light green	47
Medium blue	36
Medium gray	30
Red	13

of low absorbing and high reflecting powers aid materially in illumination. The lighter colors reflect more light than the darker ones, black being completely absorbent unless the surface is highly glazed or polished, in which case there is some specular reflection. Table 13-1 gives reflection factors for paints of various colors.

13-7. Contrast. Visibility is obtained by bringing lumens from the lamp or lamps to produce foot-candles of illumination on the work or any object in which the observer is interested. Merely bringing lumens is not sufficient; for visibility, some of the light must be reflected, and the surface must thus have a brightness. For example, if the object or work receives 30 ft-c and 60 per cent is reflected, the brightness of the work is 18 ft-L, while 40 per cent of the light is absorbed. If this surface is close to another one that reflects little or no light, the contrast makes for visibility. As an example, the black ink of printing reflects little or no light, while the paper on which the letters are printed reflects nearly all the light. Hence there is a high contrast, visibility on the task is good, and reading is easy. Conversely, printing with a medium blue ink on pale blue paper would be much lower in visibility because of lack of contrast. At the extreme, sewing with black thread on black cloth is exceedingly difficult because of the almost complete lack of contrast. It can be said that good visibility depends upon a high *brightness contrast* of the critical detail to its background.[1]

---

[1] This is also called "per cent contrast," which is the ratio of the brightness difference between an object and its background to the brightness of its background. In the case of the blue printing on light blue paper (see Table 13-1), it would be $\frac{61 - 36}{61} \times 100 = 41$ per cent. In the case of black printing on white paper, assuming that the printing absorbs all the light and that the white paper reflects all the light, the contrast would be $\frac{100 - 0}{100} \times 100 = 100$ per cent.

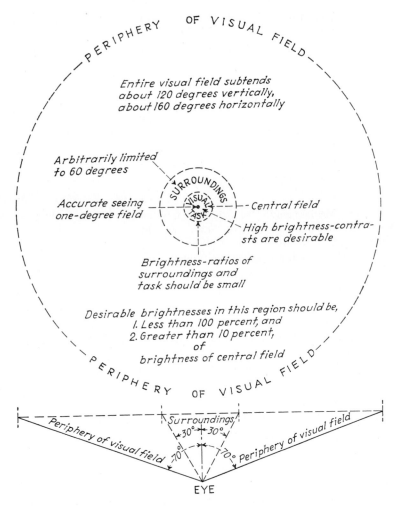

FIGURE 13-6 A diagrammatic analysis of the entire visual field, indicating the importance of brightness, brightness-contrast ratios in its various parts, and suggested limitations. (*Reproduced by permission from M. Luckiesh, "Light, Vision and Seeing," D. Van Nostrand Company, Inc., Princeton, N.J.*)

The term *brightness ratio* is used to apply to the brightness of any two surfaces. It may be the ratio of the average brightness of the visual task to that of some surface in the surroundings. It is necessary to recognize three fields of vision in connection with brightness ratios and their effects upon vision (see Fig. 13-6). The visual task, whether it is reading a book or filing a casting, is called the *central field*. In the center of the central field is an area of 1 deg where very accurate seeing is required. The surrounding field extends approximately 30 deg on each side of the line of sight. Thus its total area is 60 deg in the center of the total visual field. The peripheral field is outside the surrounding field and includes an area of about 120 deg vertically and 160 deg horizontally centering on the line of sight.

As already indicated, high brightness ratios are desirable in the visual task to avoid excessive eyestrain. In the recommended standard practice for the lighting of schools, it is required that the brightness ratio between the visual task and nearby surfaces in the surroundings—a desk top, for example—be 1 to $\frac{1}{3}$. In other words, the desk top or other immediate surroundings of the task should not be less than one-third as bright as the visual task and no brighter than the task. We may say in general that in the surroundings the brightness ratio between the task and those surroundings should be small. In the entire field of vision of the eye, control is also necessary. Brightness ratios in this region should be less than 100 per cent and greater than 10 per cent of the brightness of the task; in other words, the ratio should be between 1 and $\frac{1}{10}$.

Glare occurs when there are high brightness ratios anywhere in the field of vision. It may be *direct glare,* which is due to bright light sources or areas inside or outside the room. The sources or areas may be quite small and very bright, or relatively large and with lower brightness. *Reflected glare* may be due to the image of some bright light source reflected in glass table tops, polished furniture, glazed paper, etc.

Glare causes discomfort and directly influences the ability and the continued urge to see. It tends to be cumulative in its effects. A minor glare, which might be negligible when exposure is short, may become of serious importance after long exposure. Conditions which do not appear glaring while persons are performing tasks requiring only casual seeing may become uncomfortable when a critical task is to be performed, such as recognition of small but important details. This is because reflected glare reduces the brightness contrast on the task. A reduction of visual acuity and strain and nervousness may soon develop. Careful brightness surveys, made with instruments, will frequently indicate conditions that should be corrected. Corrections, including prevention of veiling reflections, are made by using proper types of luminaires, eliminating polished surfaces and surfaces with very high reflecting power from the field of view, and brightening the surrounding areas against which the source of the glare is seen. Figure 13-7 shows how light sources in the 0- to 45-deg zone will cause loss of contrast on the task by reflected glare.

13-8. Shadows. If the light falling upon an object comes from one direction only, a sharp and dense shadow results. If the intensity of illumination is high, glare results on some surfaces. Also, it is difficult

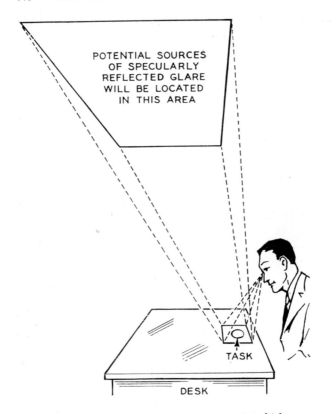

POTENTIAL SOURCES
OF SPECULARLY
REFLECTED GLARE
WILL BE LOCATED
IN THIS AREA

TASK

DESK

FIGURE 13-7   Method for determining zone in which potential glare sources may be located. (*Reproduced by permission from "Illuminating Engineering Society Lighting Handbook, 3d ed., Illuminating Engineering Society, New York,
1959.*)

to distinguish completely between the object and its shadow, and thus
there is a distortion of objects. Complete absence of shadows is possible
only when the intensity of illumination is the same from all directions.
This would be undesirable because its monotony would be tiresome to
the eye, and the shape and contour of objects would be difficult to dis-
cern. The shadows should, therefore, be of the proper quality, *i.e.*, soft
and luminous, so that an object is clearly distinguishable from its shadow
and without harsh contrast in intensity of illumination. A rough test is
to hold a pencil horizontally several inches above a white surface. If
the shadow is blurred and not sharply outlined, light diffusion has been
attained. The required uniformity of illumination is obtained by a proper
ratio of the spacing distance of light sources to their height of mounting. A rough rule is that the spacing distance should be equal to the
height.

Table 13-2. RECOMMENDED MINIMUM LEVELS OF ILLUMINATION
FOR OFFICES

Tasks	Foot-candles on tasks
Cartography, designing, detailed drafting	200
Accounting, tabulating, bookkeeping, business-machine operation, reading poor reproductions	150
Regular office work, reading good reproductions, reading or transcribing handwriting in hard pencil or on poor paper, active filing, mail sorting	100
Reading or transcribing handwriting in ink or medium pencil on good-quality paper, intermittent filing	70
Reading high-contrast or well-printed material, tasks not involving critical or prolonged seeing, such as conferring, or in areas such as inactive files and washrooms	30
Tasks in corridors, in elevators, on escalators, and on stairways. . .	20

SOURCE: "Illuminating Engineering Society Lighting Handbook," 3d ed., Illuminating Engineering Society, New York, 1959.

13-9. Standards of Illumination Practice. The Illuminating Engineering Society has prepared standards or codes of practice for application to schools, industrial plants, and offices [1]. Lighting of schools and industrial plants is discussed in Chaps. 15 and 16. Recommended intensities of illumination for office lighting are given in Table 13-2. The intensities given are commensurate with the difficulty of the various seeing tasks and the current cost of lighting. These values should be obtained by proper design and then maintained by proper cleaning and replacement of deteriorated or failed lamps. Initial values should be increased by some percentage to offset depreciation of lamps and dirt accumulation, which may reach 30 to 50 per cent depending upon character of maintenance, dust conditions, and design of luminaires with respect to the gathering of dust.

Recommended brightness ratios are as follows: between tasks and surroundings, 3:1; between tasks and remote surfaces, 10:1; between luminaires (or windows) and adjacent surfaces, 20:1; and anywhere within normal field of view, 40:1. These are the recommended maximums; reductions are desirable.

Room finishes, especially of ceilings, are important in determining brightness ratios between lighting equipment and its surroundings. Color and reflectance of surfaces have much effect upon utilization of light, as indicated in Art. 13-6. The following reflection factors are recommended: ceilings, 75 to 85 per cent; walls, 50 to 60 per cent; desk tops, 35 per cent; furniture, 30 to 35 per cent; and floors, 30 per cent. Dull finishes (mat) are recommended for all painted and other surfaces.

13-10. Natural Lighting. In spite of the great strides which artificial lighting has made in late years and the difficulties sometimes encountered

Table 13-3.   REPRESENTATIVE LEVELS OF
ILLUMINATION

	Foot-candles
Starlight	0.0002
Moonlight	0.02
Street lighting	0.6–1.2
Daylight:	
At north window	50–200
In shade (outdoors).	100–1,000
Direct sunlight	5,000–10,000
Office lighting	30–50

in obtaining effective natural light, the latter is the standby for homes, schools, offices, and even industrial establishments where possible.

The recommended window-glass area of a workroom is usually 15 to 20 per cent of the floor area. Windows on only one side of the room usually give satisfactory illumination if the width of the room is less than twice the height from the floor to the top of the windows. Large rooms, such as auditoriums, may require windows on both sides. For best working conditions in rooms lighted by windows, the distance of any working space from the windows should be no more than twice the height of the top of the windows.

The amount of light furnished by windows to a point is largely dependent upon the sky area visible at that point. Windows facing blank walls get and transmit only reflected light. The lighting values of such windows, therefore, in addition to the amount of any sky visible depends upon their brightness and the reflection factors of the outside surfaces. Satisfactory lighting can usually be obtained when the visible sky subtends an angle of at least 5 deg at any working point in the room. It is recommended that the sky exposure be at least 50 sq deg, preferably 5 deg vertically and 10 deg horizontally. Without special precautions window lighting results in larger proportions of light and perhaps glare from sunlight at points near the window. The closer windows are to the ceiling, the greater is the angle of the entering light to the line of vision, and thus danger of glare is reduced. Shades are used to give protection from glare, but the ordinary shade may cut off too much light. Shades of light yellow, light buff, or tan cause diffusion of light and prevent glare without absorption of too much light. For schools double shades are advisable, both operating from the middle of the window. Venetian blinds are valuable in deflecting light toward the ceiling. Where the sky is obstructed by buildings, prismatic glass in the windows greatly improves the natural lighting by distributing the light rays to the inner parts of the room. Basement lighting can also be effectively done with prismatic glass.

Skylights are used to supplement windows and should be used to a

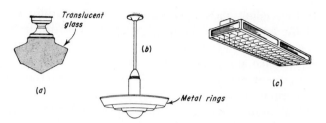

FIGURE 13-8   Luminaires. (a) Direct-indirect, or diffused; (b) indirect; (c) fluorescent, direct-indirect with egg-crate louvers to shield eyes from glare.

greater extent than at present. The saw-tooth roof for industrial plants lends itself to effective lighting. The glass side of the saw tooth should be toward the north rather than the south in order that the glass may transmit diffused daylight rather than direct sunlight.

13-11. Artificial Light. There are five systems of artificial lighting: direct, direct-indirect, semidirect, semi-indirect, and indirect.

In *direct lighting* 90 to 100 per cent of the light of the luminaires is directed in angles below the horizontal directly toward the usual working area. Direct lighting may be local or general. Since local lighting involves droplights close to the work, considerable glare may result unless shades are provided. When direct lighting is used, the luminaires should be placed high, preferably not less than 20 ft, unless enclosed in diffusing glassware to prevent glare. Glare is reduced if the ceiling is illuminated by good reflection from surfaces. Direct lighting has the advantage of being highly efficient, as little or no light is absorbed before striking the work. It causes harsh shadows, and glare results from reflection on smooth or glazed surfaces. Deep reflectors may be used, however, to hide the filaments and prevent direct glare, but they have no effect upon reflected glare.

In *direct-indirect* or *general diffuse lighting* the light is distributed equally in all directions, although strictly direct-indirect luminaires produce very little light in angles near the horizontal, and accordingly they are more desirable. In general the predominant lighting is from the downward component since it is not reflected. With these systems direct and reflected glare may be noticeable.

In *semidirect lighting* 60 to 90 per cent of the light output is directed downward to the work. The small upward component illuminates the ceiling and thus reduces the brightness ratio between the luminaire and the ceiling. The luminaires have reflecting surfaces above the light sources to deflect most of the light downward. Glass or plastic enclosures or louvered bottoms provide diffusion and shielding.

In *semi-indirect lighting* 60 to 90 per cent of the light is directed to the ceiling and upper walls, while dense diffusing glass allows some of the light to pass through directly downward. If the diffusing glass of the reflector is good, all glare and high brightness are avoided. The ceiling surface and upper walls must be highly reflecting. As the downward component increases toward 40 per cent, direct and reflected glare may require attention.

In *indirect lighting* 90 to 100 per cent of the light is directed toward the ceiling and upper sidewalls, from which it is reflected to all parts of the room. As the ceiling thus becomes the light source, care must be taken that it is not a source of glare. Careful attention must be paid to room finishes. They must be as light in color as possible and kept in good condition. Luminaires have opaque inverted reflectors and are frequently set in recesses at the ceiling or in architectural coves.

No one system can be recommended to the exclusion of the others. Direct lighting gives high utilization and therefore lower cost, but good lighting on the task is attained only by close spacing of luminaires or the use of large-area–low-brightness equipment. Indirect lighting provides good light on the work, but utilization is low. The intermediate systems combine the characteristics of both these in varying degrees.

Much of the advantage of lighting systems, particularly in industrial plants, is lost through the accumulations of dust and dirt on bulbs and reflectors. This is particularly important in the indirect and semi-indirect systems. In some plants regular inspections of the lights are made by a responsible employee for the purpose of replacing burned-out bulbs and cleaning bulbs and reflectors.

13-12. Fluorescent Lighting. Although the gas-filled tungsten filament incandescent lamp is still the most widely used illuminant, the fluorescent lamp is increasingly popular. It consists of a glass tube filled with mercury vapor and having an electrode sealed in each end. When the electric current is turned on, an arc is formed by current flowing through the mercury vapor. The arc generates some light but much more invisible ultraviolet energy, which excites fluorescent chemicals which coat the inside of the tube. Various fluorescent substances are used to obtain different colors. So-called daylight tubes are obtainable, but in practice they have been found to be objectionable, except where very accurate color discrimination is required. They tend to blur the visibility of objects and are unflattering to the human complexion. A slight yellowish tint to the light, which is obtainable in the "standard" daylight tubes and which occurs naturally in incandescent bulbs, is satisfactory.

An advantage is that the equipment which uses fluorescent lamps is much lower in brightness in the direct and reflected glare zones and provides a larger and more uniformly illuminated area. Shadows are also much softer. It is possible, however, to have brightness in such lamps so high that high brightness ratios occur, with detriment to eye comfort and efficiency. Complaints that there is too much light or that the light from the fluorescent lamps is hurting the eyes are usually caused by direct glare. Although shielding the light source so that the worker cannot see the lamp usually eliminates the complaint, care should be taken that no other unfavorable circumstances are also present

Fluorescent lighting is economical in use of electrical current. For example, a 60-watt coil tungsten filament lamp emits 13.9 lumens/watt, while a 40-watt white fluorescent lamp emits 58 lumens/watt. These figures are for lamps which have been in use for 100 hr. New lamps give off more light. In general, fluorescent lamps produce 40 to 65 lumens/watt. The smaller use of current also reduces the heat generated by the lamp.

13-13. Good Lighting and Production. Good lighting safeguards eyesight and reduces accident hazards. It also saves the worker's time and cuts down the amount of spoiled work and is, therefore, economically profitable to the employer. This is an argument which should never be neglected by the sanitarian.

A report by the Illuminating Engineering Society indicates that the whole cost of good lighting is usually equal to the cost of about 3 min of the worker's time each day. Hence, if it saves 3 min daily it pays for itself regardless of the cost of poor lighting. Tests made in shops as to the effect of light upon production indicated that increase of the average illumination from 0.2 to 4.8 ft-c increased production in varying amounts from 6 to 100 per cent, with an average of 35 per cent. Increased illumination from 4.6 to 12.7 ft-c gave increases varying from 8 to 27 per cent and averaging 15 per cent.

It should be pointed out that a good lighting system is not an accident but the product of careful planning that considers the type of work to be done, the size of the room, and the reflecting factors of the walls and ceiling. Manufacturers of luminaires can give the characteristics of the various types, and these combined with the room dimensions, candle power of the bulbs installed, reflection factors of the walls and ceilings, and spacing and mounting of the luminaires allow accurate design of illumination.

Bibliography

1. "Illuminating Engineering Society Lighting Handbook," 3d ed., Illuminating Engineering Society, New York, 1959.
2. Staley, K. A.: "Fundamentals of Light and Lighting," Bulletin LD-2, Large Lamp Department, General Electric Co., Cleveland, Ohio, 1960.
3. Phelps, E. B.: "Public Health Engineering," vol. 1, John Wiley & Sons, Inc., New York, 1948.
4. Boast, W. B.: "Illumination Engineering," 2d ed., McGraw-Hill Book Company, New York, 1953.

5. Croft, T.: "American Electrician's Handbook," 7th ed., rev. by Clifford C. Carr, McGraw-Hill Book Company, New York, 1953.
6. Luckiesh, M., and F. K. Moss: "The Science of Seeing," D. Van Nostrand Company, Inc., Princeton, N.J., 1944.
7. "Recommended Practice for Office Lighting," Illuminating Engineering Society, New York, 1960.
8. "American Standard Guide for School Lighting," Illuminating Engineering Society, New York, 1960.
9. "School Lighting Application Data," Illuminating Engineering Society, New York, 1960.

14

HOUSING .

14-1. Poor housing is a contributor to low physical and mental efficiency, and its relation to prevalence of disease is easy to recognize. Certainly if we consider public health work to be aimed at obtaining optimum conditions for physical and mental well-being, in addition to preventing disease, we must include improvement of housing in the program. Since poor housing is related to poverty, public opinion has tended to consider it an unavoidable evil, and up to two decades ago what little had been done was confined to a few laws or city ordinances directed at landlords and tenants to prevent some of the worst abuses. The growing strength of the public health movement and the development of a more active community conscience have led to comprehensive studies as to what constitutes good housing and how the economic and legal hurdles which have intervened can be traversed or removed [1, 2].

The American Public Health Association through well-qualified committees has formulated housing requirements and has grouped them under four headings: the satisfaction of fundamental physiological needs; the satisfaction of fundamental psychological needs; protection against communicable disease; and protection against accidents [3]. The discussion of housing needs as presented in this chapter follows these principles.

Housing which does not comply with the more important requirements as to sanitation or which is in urgent need of repairs is known as "substandard" housing. An area in which substandard housing predominates, frequently accompanied by overcrowding, is known as a "slum." The Committee on the Hygiene of Housing of the American Public Health Association in its appraisal method [4] of measuring the quality of housing considers that each of the following conditions represents a basic deficiency and that any dwelling having four or more such deficiencies is an extreme slum: (1) contaminated water supply; (2) water supply outside living unit or structure; (3) toilet shared or outside the structure; (4) bath shared or outside the structure; (5) more than 1.5 persons per habitable room; (6) overcrowding of sleeping rooms; (7) less than 40 sq ft of sleeping area per person; (8) lack of dual egress; (9) installed heating lacking in three-quarters of rooms; (10) lack of installed electricity; (11) rooms lacking a window; and (12) serious deterioration.

The term "blighted area" is applied by city planners to those sections of a city which are undesirable for residential purposes and which are not in demand for commercial or industrial purposes. They frequently are adjacent to high-value business districts, and many property owners will not maintain properly the buildings in them in the hope that business will soon move in. Similar districts also tend to develop in or near industrial areas. Because of the traffic and noise, the more prosperous people do not care to live in them, and the consequence is that buildings are converted to cheap rooming houses and tenements with high probability of their developing into slums. City planning which eliminates or prevents blighted areas is a means of slum prevention, but slum clearance, while also related to good city planning, is more closely connected with housing improvement.

14-2. Heating and Ventilation. As already discussed, the factors controlling heat loss from the human body are air temperature, relative humidity of the air, air movement, and temperature of such surrounding surfaces as walls, floors, ceilings, windows, and radiators, since the body radiates to them or receives radiant heat from them, according to which has the higher temperature. In the usual home in winter, air movement and humidity are not likely to be of importance. Air temperature and mean radiant or wall temperature when combined are called "operative temperature," and ordinarily it is the mean between the air temperature and the wall temperature. For normal persons who are wearing the usual type of clothing and are at rest, this should be 65°F at knee height, 18 in., in order to prevent chilling of the legs and feet. Air temperatures may be increased or decreased to compensate for deviations in the mean radiant temperature. In rooms occupied by old people or young children, the operative temperature may have to be 70°F at knee height. With ideal heating, temperatures at ankle height and at 5 ft would be almost identical. Unfortunately it is not uncommon for ankle-height temperature to be 65°F, the 5-ft temperature 70°F, and the ceiling temperature 80°F—a total differential of 15°F. In poorly constructed dwellings, where proper temperatures may be difficult to achieve and heating facilities may be inadequate, the total differential may conceivably be as much as 30°F or more.

Climate is a factor in design of heating facilities as well as housing, but it should be possible to attain the above requirements under ordinary winter conditions. Heating engineers have adopted, as a basis for design, an outside temperature 15°F above the lowest recorded temperature for a 10-year period.

Insulation, which is also useful in reducing heating costs, is an important item in reducing temperature differentials from floor to ceiling. Flooring materials of high heat-conducting potential, such as concrete or tile, should be avoided, particularly where children may play on the floor. Windows can be insulated by curtains.

For low-rent housing in one- or two-story dwellings, the free-standing circulator type of stove is lowest in cost but is inferior for comfort to the circulating heater enclosed in a central distribution chamber and discharging warm air to adjacent rooms through grilles. Central heating is preferable for apartments and perhaps for large groups of one- and two-family houses using either steam or hot water. Indirect heating with hot air may also be used.

Ventilation of homes is also concerned with adequate heat loss from the body. The factors involved are air temperature, mean radiant temperature, relative humidity, and air movement. In cold weather, operative temperature will be the determining factor and should not exceed 75°F in the zone of occupancy, or discomfort will result. Overheating in the winter season is common, and prevention should be possible by control of heating sources without resort to opening windows. Here steam heating and hot forced air provide flexibility in control.

In summer, air cooling and dehumidification are desirable but uneconomical for the low-rent house. The attic fan is practical as a means of drawing cool night air into a house to encourage sleep. Cross ventilation should be provided in each house by the proper placing of windows. They should also extend to within 6 in. of the ceiling so that hot upper air can escape. Windows of the casement type which swing either horizontally or vertically may be preferable to the ordinary double-sash type. They may also be used to deflect air currents in desired directions. Another factor of importance in summer is exposure to prevailing winds so that maximum air movement is obtained. Summer sunshine, particularly in the late afternoon, is undesirable in rooms principally occupied in the daytime. This must be considered, however, in relation to the amount of direct sunshine desired in winter.

A third requirement in ventilation is a sufficient air interchange, particularly in the heating period, to prevent accumulation of odors from human bodies, cooking, or various heat sources. The rate of air interchange required to prevent the accumulation of odors is variable, depending upon the total space involved, the number of persons present, and the degree of activity.

Such an air change is obtained automatically in cold weather by normal leakage of air through ceilings and walls of usual porosity and around normally constructed doors and windows. The modern trend is to use a minimum floor area and ceiling height requirement in preference to the cubic-foot determination. Section 8 of the APHA "Proposed Housing Ordinance" [6] states, in part: "Every dwelling unit shall contain at least 150 square feet of floor space for the first occupant thereof, and at least 100 additional square feet of floor space for every additional occupant thereof, the floor space to be calculated on the basis of total habitable room area."

Fumes, odors, soot, and grime may enter by windows from industrial and other neighborhood sources, and they are not always subject to effective control under antinuisance regulations. Such possibilities, together with the direction of prevailing winds, are factors which should be considered in the choice of housing sites.

14-3. Lighting. Lighting of houses must be planned for both natural and artificial light. Definitions of the lighting terms used here are found in Chap. 13.

NATURAL LIGHTING. The minimum intensity of illumination in any occupied space should be 6 ft-c on a horizontal plane 30 in. above the floor. With unobstructed exposure to the sky, this illumination will be attained in clear weather in the latitude of Washington, D.C., 39°, with a window-glass area of 15 per cent of the floor area, provided also that walls and ceilings are light in color. Since the average brightness of the sky varies both with latitude and with different regions of the country, corrections must be made. The average daylight illumination is 25 per cent higher in the states between the Mississippi and the Rocky Mountains and about 46 per cent higher in the states between the Rockies and the Sierra Nevada and Cascade Mountains than in the Eastern states. It is possible, therefore, that in the Plains and Plateau states, window percentages may be lower and thus housing costs can be reduced. Correction for latitude can be made at the rate of 2 per cent increase of the percentage for each degree of latitude north of 39° North, and the same rate of decrease for each degree south. Thus at 45° North latitude the window area would be increased by 12 per cent of 15 per cent, or to 17 per cent of the floor area.

The percentages given are for practically unobstructed sky. If there are trees or buildings which obstruct the sky, increased window area is required. The 15 per cent figure applies to sky angles[1] from 90 to 86 deg; from 86 to 82 deg to 16 per cent; from 82 to 78 deg to 17 per cent; etc. Since windows should extend almost to the ceiling for both ventilation and lighting, an increase in area required by local conditions should be obtained by increasing their width.

Placing windows as high as possible gives the greatest sky angle in all parts of the room and thus secures the greatest lighting effectiveness. Windows extending to less than 30 in. from the floor tend to cause glare and obstruct furniture placement without increasing illumination to any extent. Inside walls should have reflection factors of at least 50 per cent, and ceilings, 70 per cent. A mat-finish (dull) paint should be used because glossy paints produce glare. Venetian blinds and window shades are useful to prevent glare, the former being especially valuable in allowing reflection to inner parts of the room.

Direct sunlight is desirable, for at least part of the day, for all dwellings, especially in winter. Sunlight, particularly its ultraviolet rays, is recognized as being of value to the body. The amount which enters a dwelling depends upon the sky angles of the windows and the orientation of the buildings. For dwellings in rows a desirable orientation is to face 20 to 30° east or west of south. This allows sunshine to penetrate the yard on both sides of the structure. Casements which open substantially throughout their area are more desirable than double-hung windows for admitting ultraviolet rays of sunlight. Ordinary window glass eliminates most of the ultraviolet rays.

ARTIFICIAL ILLUMINATION. Sufficient illumination should be arranged so that all areas in the room may be covered by adequate light without glare, with at least three convenient electrical outlets in the living room and two in other rooms. For accurate illumination with regard to foot-candle requirements, it is suggested that the Illuminating Engineering

[1] The sky angle is the angle between the vertical and a line from the lowest window sill to the lower edge of the visible sky.

Society standards be followed. For the control of glare, all bulbs should be shielded from view by suitable reflectors, globes, and shades to prevent excessive brightness against the background of the luminaire. Ceiling fixtures of the semi-indirect type and floor lamps of the direct-indirect type go well together for local and general illumination. Shades of table and floor lamps should be of such thickness and color that their surfaces are not a source of glare.

14.4 Protection against Excessive Noise. Effects of excessive noise are given in Art. 16-11. Noises should be excluded from dwellings to the extent that the noise level does not exceed 50 db (decibels) (Art. 16-11); 30 db should be the upper limit in sleeping rooms. Housing sites should be chosen away from such sources of noise as factories, highways, railways, and athletic fields. Automobile horns and radios should be controlled. Small enclosed courts should be avoided in housing developments since noise may be reflected from the building walls.

Noises which are transmitted by the air in a multifamily dwelling can be reduced about 50 db by party walls equivalent to an 8-in. brick wall. Apartment doors opening into public passageways should be fitted to exclude noise.

Noises which are transmitted by the structure, such as footsteps or furniture moving, can be reduced about 15 db by proper construction. Airborne noise can also be reduced [7]. Two thicknesses of wood flooring on standard joists with a lath and plaster ceiling effect a reduction of 10 to 15 db. If the laths or ceiling boards are fastened to the joists with spring clips and the floor is laid so as to allow some "play" between the subfloor and the joists, a reduction of well above 15 db may be obtained. Concrete floors are effective against airborne but not against structure-borne noise. All plumbing, steam pipes, and valves should be correctly designed so that steam "hammer" and "singing" in valves do not occur. Refrigerating and heating equipment, pumps, and blowers should be so installed that vibrations are not transmitted to the structure. Plumbing stacks and water riser pipes should preferably not be located in living-room or bedroom walls.

14-5. Provision of Adequate Exercise and Play Space for Children. Playground and recreation space is considered to be essential to the physical and mental well-being of children and adults. It should be considered by all who are concerned with the construction of homes. This is primarily a problem of neighborhood and city planning and must be considered from the standpoints of the types of recreation to be provided (including indoor recreation), the amount and location of existing recreation facilities, the availability of trained recreation leaders, etc. In any case play spaces for very young children should be provided within each large group or block of buildings. Athletic fields within ½ mile are desirable for adolescents.

14-6. Water Supply. The source of water for a single dwelling or a housing project should, wherever possible, be a city supply which is controlled as to quality by health authorities. If a well or some other individual supply must be used, methods of construction and protection should be as described in Chap. 2. Within the building the water supply should be protected from contamination by cross-connections or fixtures which have inlets at insufficient distances above the highest possible water level in the fixture. Where defects are found to exist, corrections should be made. Routine inspections of large projects should include checking on alterations which may be made from time to time.

14-7. Excreta Disposal. Water-carried sewerage should be available for all dwellings as the best means of preventing the spread of disease by flies or in other ways. A separate toilet should be available for each family, and it should be located high enough above the sewer to avoid danger of flooding. Compartments in which toilets are located should have floors and walls of material as nearly impervious as possible. The room should be well lighted, preferably by a window in daytime. The house-drainage system should be tight. Possible backing up of sewage or storm water into basements should be considered when the site of the dwelling is chosen. If back flooding of basements is feared, the hazard may be minimized by installing a check valve and gate valve in the branch serving the basement fixtures, or the outlets of the basement fixtures may be discharged into a sump from which an electrically operated pump can raise the sewage to discharge it into the sewer. Such pumps should be of the centrifugal type with a float-controlled automatic start when the sump is full and a stop when it is empty.

Isolated dwellings may have water-carried sewerage with a disposal system or some type of privy, both as described in Chap. 4.

14-8. Prevention of Vermin. Accumulations of organic refuse breed flies, and piles of lumber and similar refuse provide harborage for rats and should not be permitted. Ratproofing as described in Art. 9-54 should be applied. Pools of standing water should be eliminated. If they are ornamental, frequent inspections should be made to determine the presence of mosquito larvae. If found, fish or larvicides may be used (Chap. 9). Screening of windows and doors is a necessity for excluding flies and mosquitoes.

Where the population to be housed is likely to be infested with lice or bedbugs, treatment of clothing, bedding, and furniture may be desirable. Bedbugs and roaches which have invaded dwellings can also be eliminated. Methods are described in Arts. 9-37 to 9-39.

14-9. Food Storage. The observance of low temperatures for food storage is economical, but it is also a sanitary measure. As discussed in Chap 7, certain pathogenic bacteria propagate in some foods, so that food poisoning or infection may result through ingestion of improperly preserved food. Every home should have facilities for storing food at 50°F or less. The amount of refrigerated space required for an urban home depends upon the marketing habits and size of the family.

14-10. Provision of Sufficient Space in Sleeping Rooms. Experience in institutions and army barracks has shown that if the center-to-center distance between cots is less than 6 ft or the floor area per cot is less than 50 sq ft, the spread of communicable disease by mouth spray is likely to occur. Satisfactory spacing of cots would provide 3 ft of clear space between them. That is the essential point.

Protection against Accidents

14-11. Materials and Construction. Building codes specify materials and methods of construction, and if they are followed no danger should exist. Termite infestation sometimes causes accidents by weakening joists or stairways. Hence, in zones of serious infestation, wood members should be avoided in foundations, and the clearance between the ground and woodwork should be at least 6 in. outside and 18 in. inside the foundation. The underspace should be cleared of wood scraps and ventilated with screened openings. Termite shields of metal of proper design are necessary between foundation wall or columns and woodwork.

14-12. Fire Protection. This calls for construction methods and materials which do not result in fire hazards and which provide adequate facilities for escape in case of fire. Elimination of fire hazards calls for more details than can be given here, but some important requirements should be pointed out. Electrical wiring should follow local codes. Stoves and heaters should be mounted clear of combustible floors and walls, but if they are near walls, there should be adequate air space and fireproof mats or screens. Flues carrying hot gases also should be insulated from walls by thimbles and should be properly supported. Chimneys should be supported by foundations on the ground, and all wood joints or partition members should be at least 2 in. away from them with the intervening space properly insulated with mortar or other material. Chimneys should be lined with fire-clay tile, and the joints should not coincide with the masonry joints.

In multiple buildings, stairways should be enclosed in fire-resistant materials. In buildings over two stories high, fire-resistant materials should be used in exterior walls, roofs, and first-tier beams, particularly between apartments and between stair halls and apartments and all shafts. Dwellings over four stories should have noncombustible floors and floor joists; those over six stories should be noncombustible throughout.

When framing with combustible members leaves hollow walls, fire stops, preferably of noncombustible materials, should be placed. On roofs, wooden shingles are undesirable because of possible ignition by sparks blowing from burning buildings. Most noncombustible types of roofs have sufficient insulating value to prevent ignition of the supporting boards. Protection offered by metal roofing can be increased by placing asbestos felt between the roofing and the boards.

Exits in case of fire should be carefully considered. Multiple dwellings should have at least two exits from each living unit, and the doors of these exits should open outward. An exception to two exits in multiple dwellings may be made if the stairways are in separate fire-resisting enclosures having self-closing doors at each floor.

14-13. Accident Prevention. Accidents occurring in the house include electric shocks and burns, gas poisoning, and falls [8]. Danger of electric shock can be reduced by placing live conductors so that they are not exposed to contact and by grounding metal enclosures of electrical appliances so that failure of insulation cannot cause shocks. All portable appliances and pendant fixtures should be so placed that no person can come simultaneously in contact with the fixture and plumbing or gas pipes, or the fixture and other grounded metal. In no case should a wall switch be placed so the occupant of a bathtub can reach it. If because of lack of room the switches or convenience outlets must be placed within reach of plumbing fixtures, the cover plate must be nonmetallic. In laundries and kitchens, or wherever hands may be wet, electric lights should be controlled by wall switches or pull chains which have an insulating link in them.

Protection against gas poisoning should be obtained by the precautions described in Art. 10-21.

Falls may be caused by a wide variety of conditions which are difficult to foresee, but it is clearly essential to use safeguards on bathtubs, stairs, windows, balconies, and roofs. Bathtubs, particularly those of the built-in type surrounded by tile, should have handholds available. Steep stairs should be avoided; the angle of slope should be between 30 and 36 deg, and the sum of the width of the tread and twice the riser height should be 24 to 25 in. Satisfactory values are 10 in. for the tread width and 7 to 7½ in. for the riser. Steps, of course, should be uniform in dimensions. Stairs should have handrails, particularly outdoor stairs. Winding stairways too narrow for a foothold at the rail side are especially dangerous.

Window sills that are less than 30 in. from the floor should be avoided, especially at stairway landings. If such sills are unavoidable, one or more crossbars should be installed to prevent children from falling out; built-in screens are desirable from this standpoint. Casement windows, if designed with enough clearance at the hinges to permit washing from the inside, minimize the dangers in window cleaning. Rails or parapets are essential around porches, balconies, and accessible roofs, even if the fall is only 2 or 3 ft. In the North all sloping roofs which may have a pitch of perhaps 15 to 55 deg and which terminate over steps or walks should be equipped with snow guards to protect passersby. Good lighting is a necessity for all walks and stairs.

Protection against traffic accidents is not a detail of housing proper, but location of housing projects should be considered with traffic conditions in mind. Traffic hazards are greatly reduced if residential streets are planned so as to discourage through traffic. In some new housing communities this is done by using dead-end streets. Usual pedestrian routes should be planned so that it is unnecessary to cross a major traffic way except by overpasses or underpasses. Blind corners should be avoided by the proper placing of buildings and shrubbery. In planning the location and other aspects of playgrounds, special precautions are required in order to isolate them from traffic.

Satisfaction of Fundamental Psychological Needs

14-14. Privacy. Privacy, to some degree and during some periods, is a necessity to most people. The ideal would be a room of one's own for everybody. This is not always possible, but at least a bedroom should have to be shared with only one other person and one of the same sex, except in the case of married couples and young children. Separate bedrooms for the sexes are required at the age of ten years by English law (and by the city of Toronto, Canada), although some American authorities think they should be required at the age of eight. Sleeping rooms of children over two years of age, according to psychiatric opinion, should be separate from those of parents. Bathrooms, toilets, and bedrooms should be accessible from halls or living rooms, not through other bedrooms.

Regulations against overcrowding also promote privacy. English legislation requires that not more than two persons occupy a bedroom. Two rooms are required for three persons, three rooms for five persons, four rooms for seven and one-half persons, and so on. Bathrooms are not counted as rooms. Infants under one year of age are not counted as persons, and children between one and ten are counted as half persons. In dwellings, the practices of taking in boarders and subrenting rooms must be controlled. As families increase in size, some provision must be made for obtaining appropriate living units.

One of the most vexatious problems facing cities is the control of the conversion of old houses into "hot-plate" apartments and rooming and boarding houses. From the public health standpoint, conversion of single-family residences into multifamily or rooming houses is not necessarily undesirable as long as such conversion is done according to minimum standards of occupancy and facilities. This problem, of course, ties in with the discussion in Art. 14-19, "Zoning and Housing." Most zoning ordinances assume that a land-use pattern, once established, remains relatively unchanged. This, of course, is not the case, for neighborhoods mature, and certain changes are unavoidable. Zoning laws should therefore be written with these changes in mind in order to encourage honorable maturity within minimum standards for conversion.

14-15. Provision for Normal Family and Community Life. This could be called provision for sociability. Opportunities must be given for adolescent boys and girls to meet under wholesome conditions. This requires a living room of adequate size which can be used by all members of the family, plus reasonable space for withdrawal elsewhere during periods of entertainment. In housing projects where space has been kept to a minimum in order to attain low rents, community meeting rooms for special entertaining are available. In some cases, accommodations for overnight guests have been included.

A normal community life for dwellers in a housing project is something of a compromise. They should not be cut off from the rest of the city, and there should be easy communication with the city's centers of culture and business. Other community facilities which should be easily accessible are schools, churches, entertainment, shopping, libraries, and medical service. If they are not available, at least some should be supplied as a neighborhood facility, if not for the project alone. This is a phase of city planning as applied to the particular area.

Another factor allied to the above, which may be mentioned as a reason for good housing rather than as a factor in planning, is the better morale of persons who live in decent home surroundings. Persons who live in substandard houses, particularly children, may develop a feeling of inferiority which can lead to serious social consequences.

14-16. Provision for Cleanliness and Convenience. Obviously an ample supply of safe water is a necessity for personal and home cleanliness. Clean hands have a part in preventing the spread of disease, but cleanliness is also a factor in promoting good morale. Where water must be carried into a house, it is obvious that insufficient amounts are used. Hence every dwelling, for the protection of health and maintenance convenience, should have facilities within the building to assure adequate quantities of safe-quality water. About 20 gal per person per day is the minimum for household use. The minimum facilities should include a washbasin, kitchen sink, and bathtub or shower. Hot water should also be provided.

To facilitate household cleaning, interior surfaces should be nearly impervious, with all joints as tight as practicable. Surfaces should be readily washable, and design should avoid, as far as possible, dust-catching angles and pockets.

In large housing projects, suitable chutes which discharge garbage and rubbish to incinerators have been used. Outdoor receptacles are discussed in Art. 5-21.

Housing and Government

14-17. Housing Regulation. It is recognized that housing improvement, with its accompaniment of lessening slums, reduces crime, fire, and disease. Recognition of these facts has opened the way to invoking the police power of government to prevent dangerous housing, to require remedies, and to punish violators. Since police power in intrastate matters is vested in the states, the control may be applied by state laws or, in cities, by means of city ordinances. City ordinances cannot contravene in any particular the laws of the state in which they are located, but they may be more detailed. Four methods of legal control of housing have developed, and these are briefly described below [9]:

1. General housing laws, as passed by Michigan and Iowa, are based upon the excellent model-housing law written by Lawrence Veiller in 1920. These laws deal with construction and upkeep of single-family and multifamily dwellings and also with sanitary facilities, required space, lighting, etc. In some states they provide for a housing enforcement official. Other states have enacted housing statutes of the old-line tenement-control type, which, of course, apply only to multifamily dwellings. Usually state housing laws apply only in cities over a certain size.

2. Some cities have adopted comprehensive local housing codes as ordinances. These incorporate the essential features indicated under (1).

3. Special laws or ordinances are passed defining unsafe or substandard

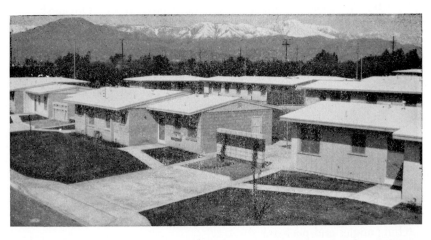

FIGURE 14-1   Redlands Homes, a 75-unit low-rent housing project in Redlands, Calif. (*Photograph courtesy of Public Housing Administration, Washington, D.C.*)

dwellings and providing for remedial action by demolition, repair, abatement, or closure. These were usually passed to control flagrant conditions, but they are not sufficiently comprehensive.

4. Enabling acts may be passed by a state legislature or city council. These define the problems and the ends to be gained but leave to the proper department or official the authority to set the standard which will remedy matters. These standards are written in a code of administrative regulations, have the force of law, and can be enforced by the officer designated by the enabling law. For example, the enabling act includes a clause which, in the interest of health and morals, gives to a particular official the power to prescribe minimum standards of space per family or per person. In order to apply this provision, the responsible official formulates such requirements as may be needed and attends to their enforcement.

The establishment of administrative regulations has some advantages over the codes established in detail by law or ordinance. The latter can be amended only by a new law or ordinance, and obtaining this may be slow and difficult. The administrative code, on the other hand, can be made as detailed as necessary, and, what is more important, details can be easily changed if found to be impractical or in order to meet new conditions or advances in knowledge. Housing officials prefer this type. An example of such a housing code is that of Baltimore. The effect of its application in a portion of the city, using the American Public Health Appraisal method, is reported by Johnson and McCaldin [10].

14-18. Enforcement of Housing Regulations. Housing regulations, in addition to health matters, involve fire protection, structural condition, plumbing, and electrical wiring. This presents complications for enforcement which would involve at least three departments—fire, health, and building—considering that electrical, plumbing, and building inspection are all in the building department. To meet this situation in Hartford, Conn., it was proposed that nine inspecting items be assigned to a combined inspectorate of the building and fire departments, that eight be the responsibility of the health department, and that two (ventilation and heating) be handled jointly. In Cincinnati, which operates under a modern building code with comprehensive housing regulations for new and old dwellings, the building department has a force of special housing inspectors under a special supervisor, which inspects annually every dwelling in the major substandard areas, issues orders, and makes follow-up inspections to see that orders have been complied with. Fire hazards are inspected by the fire department.

It is apparent that the Cincinnati system is far better coordinated than the Hartford plan. Duplication of inspections is kept to a minimum, record keeping is simplified, and enforcement is easier. In general, therefore, it may be said that a single housing authority in a city is to be

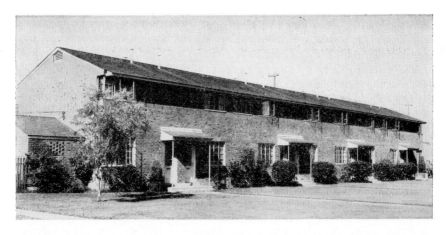

FIGURE 14-2 New Helvetia, a 310-unit low-rent public housing project in Sacramento, Calif. (*Photograph courtesy of Sacramento, Calif., Housing Authority.*)

preferred, although compromises as to a division of the inspector's duties are possible if the local situation makes them necessary. However, a central housing office and official are necessary for the keeping of housing records (including the inspection reports), the issuing of orders for vacating unfit housing, the demolition of unsafe buildings, and the remedying of other violations, together with the follow-up of such orders.

14-19. Zoning and Housing. City planning is becoming more and more important in urban affairs. Two of its important features are control of zoning and subdivision of land. Control of land subdivision requires landowners to conform to certain regulations when they develop the land for residential or business purposes. The regulations cover minimum lot sizes and dimensions and width of streets, and in the case of large developments, the subdividers are encouraged to dedicate a portion of the land for parks and playgrounds. This type of regulation controls the density of population per acre and also assures a street width that suits neighborhood requirements. Minimum lot sizes can be varied in different districts to suit different income groups. Also, by proper attention to street widths and their relation to traffic movement, it is possible to discourage through traffic and thereby reduce accidents, particularly to children. Such planning also permits a reduction in the total street area, which, in turn, lowers first cost and maintenance cost of streets and thus reduces housing costs by lowering selling values of lots and taxes.

Zoning regulates the bulk of buildings, *i.e.*, the proportion of the lot that may be occupied by the building, and the uses to which the building may be put. The city is divided into districts: industrial, of which there may be several subdivisions, such as heavy and light; commercial, with several subdivisions; and residential, subdivided into apartment, high-value, and low-value, the latter having smaller lots for the smaller houses built for low-income families. Forming districts according to uses prevents industries and commercial firms from building high structures or establishing offensive or dangerous industries in residential areas. The zoning ordinances are very explicit as to space around residences to ensure sufficient light and air, and the heights of the buildings are also restricted. This is done by specifying the minimum allowable width of side yard, length of rear yard, and setback from the front line of the building lot. If row houses are permitted, minimum allowable widths of courts between the houses are specified. Required open space differs somewhat in the different residential districts, being somewhat smaller in the low-value districts. Similar restrictions are also placed upon apartment-house districts and commercial districts, although these are much more liberal. In a commercial district, for example, the allowable building height at the front lot line may be one and one-half times the street width from lot line to lot line. If the owner wishes to build higher, he must set the next stories back a required distance. By another setback he may go still higher. This procedure allows the construction of skyscrapers without excessive interference with sunlight to other buildings.

It will be apparent that zoning and housing are allied. A city that is logically zoned has aided housing in several ways. It has ensured better living conditions in newly constructed dwellings. The encroachments of industry and business into residential districts has been curbed, and this helps to prevent the formation of blighted districts, undesirable for residential purposes, which soon develop into slum areas.

14-20. Municipal Housing Programs. The difficulty of obtaining suitable houses in sufficient number for the low-income families has led to many housing schemes. Some industrial plants have built their own towns, including not only the streets, sewers, waterworks, and other utilities but also the homes. These developments have not all been satisfactory from the standpoint of housing or other considerations. In some projects the homes are sold to employees on easy payments, while in others they are rented at a rate sufficient to allow a moderate or only a nominal return on the capital invested. The advantage to the worker is the avoidance of paying for large construction profit and the costs of the involved financing which accompanies present-day building.

Strictly municipal housing involves construction, maintenance, and rental at moderate rates of modern homes by the cities. It has been tried by European cities with success. Municipal tenements in London have apparently been profitable, although there is a question whether profits would have been shown if the usual accounting methods of business had been used. As a rule such municipal schemes have resulted in financial loss. There are other important considerations. To result in any appreciable betterment to the large populations concerned, municipal housing requires enormous sums of money. Furthermore, to avoid disaster, these sums must be expended with much more business acumen than is usually displayed by a city council or commission. Finally, experience abroad has shown that the demolition of a slum preliminary to the erection of model tenements or dwellings usually results in the original dwellers' scattering into, and actually increasing the congestion of, other slums, while the new model tenements, when completed, are occupied by an entirely different class of persons. The plan suggested in Art. 14-21 would overcome some of the difficulties mentioned.

14-21. Federal Government and Housing. The Federal government, by the Housing Act of 1937 and its frequent amendments, is showing increasing interest in the improvement of housing. The first prerequisite for federally aided low-rent public housing is a state enabling law permitting localities to establish housing authorities and to accept Federal aid to build and operate low-rent housing. Most of the states have such legislation. Generally the enabling law authorizes municipalities and/or counties having acute housing problems to establish a local housing authority. This enabling legislation permits local housing authorities to negotiate with, and receive aid from, the Federal Housing Authority (FHA). After an ordinance or resolution is adopted by the local governing body, the housing authority commission (usually composed of five members) is appointed by the head of the local government. The commission generally serves as an independent body. The actual administrative duties are performed by a salaried staff headed by an executive director. In Arizona, Michigan, and New Mexico, housing authorities are branches of the local government.

The Housing Act of 1954 places much emphasis on the prevention of slums and blight and provides tools with which to attack problems of community deterioration. It generally involves redevelopment, rehabilitation, or conservation of properties or some combination of these three types of activity [11]. Redevelopment consists in the acquisition by the local housing agency of all or part of a project area, the clearance of the site, the installation of utilities and facilities necessary to prepare the land for re-use, and the sale of the land for redevelopment in accordance with a predetermined plan. Rehabilitation preserves as many buildings in the area as possible and requires their improvement and the upgrading of the area to eliminate existing substandard conditions and to prevent future deterioration. Conservation applies remedial measures in areas where deterioration is threatening even though blight has not developed far enough to require redevelopment or rehabilitation. Under this Act local communities are required, as a condition of receiving Federal assistance in the form of grants and long-term FHA mortgage insurance, to develop and put into operation a *workable program,* using all resources available, to eliminate and prevent slums and blight.

Section 220 of the Housing Act provides special mortgage-insurance assistance in urban-renewal areas. It may be used for the rehabilitation and conservation of existing salvable houses through the refinancing of an existing mortgage plus paying the cost of home improvements. It may also be used to assist in financing new sales or rental housing for single-family or multifamily structures. Section 221 authorizes the FHA to insure mortgages on new or rehabilitated housing for sale or rent to families displaced from urban-renewal areas or by other governmental action causing displacement, such as the construction of schools, highways, and other public improvements. Mortgage insurance is available for new homes and for the purchase and repair of existing homes. Section 221(d)(3) of the Housing Act of 1961 establishes a below-market rental housing program for displaced families and other low- and moderate-income families. The mortgage financing for a new or rehabilitated rental housing project can bear an interest rate below the market rate, and the FHA can insure the mortgage with reduced insurance premiums or no premiums. These mortgages are available in communities having a workable program certified by the Housing and Home Finance Agency (HHFA) and may be obtained by nonprofit corporations or associations, limited dividend corporations, and cooperatives. Section 207 of the 1961 Act authorizes grants to public or private bodies to develop and demonstrate new or improved means of providing houses for low-income families. Section 213 provides financing for management-type cooperative housing. Section 203K provides home-improvement loans in amounts from $2,500 to $10,000 per dwelling unit for the improvement of homes outside urban-renewal-project areas. These loans may be for terms of up to 20 years or three-fourths of the remaining economic life of the property, whichever is less, and do not require the refinancing of existing mortgages on property. Housing for the elderly can be provided under several programs administered by the HHFA. They include direct loans through the Community Facilities Administration, public housing, and FHA-insured mortgages. The Federal National Mortgage Association is rechartered under the Act, so that private investments are gradually being substituted for Federal investments, and private rather than Federal funds are being used for the purchase of mortgages.

The *workable program* as interpreted by the HHFA should include the following basic elements to be approved:

1. Sound local housing and health codes
2. A general "master" plan for the community's development
3. An appraisal of the neighborhoods and kind of treatment needed

4. An effective administrative organization to supervise the program

5. Financial capacity to carry out the program

6. Arrangements for the rehousing of displaced families in satisfactory facilities, a difficult problem for low-income families [12]

7. Community-wide citizens' participation and support

Such a program is good for a community to undertake if it is ready to help itself with or without Federal aid. To summarize, under the *workable program*, the Federal government can provide:

1. Loans and grants—up to two-thirds of the net cost, three-fourths for cities of under 50,000 population—for clearing areas or replanting blighted areas for rehabilitation

2. Special FHA mortgage insurance to share the risk of private investment in the rebuilding and rehabilitation of these replanned urban-renewal areas

3. Special FHA mortgage insurance for low-cost private housing, new or rehabilitated, for displaced families

Other aids that can be used for urban-renewal purposes are:

1. Preliminary loans and annual subsidies for low-rent public housing for low-income families where wanted and needed

2. Special assistance for general planning and experimental approaches for urban renewal and technical and professional help on the community's particular urban-renewal problems

Most of the states have passed laws to promote slum clearance. Under these laws, cities may condemn and purchase land for slum clearance and re-use for such public purposes as parks; or the city may sell part or all of the land to private interests for redevelopment for housing purposes, or it may use the land itself for housing projects.

Another promising development has been the interest of large business concerns in housing as an investment, rather than as a speculation. The Metropolitan Life Insurance Company has constructed large-scale housing projects which not only return a reasonable profit but also allow reasonable rentals. This is an indication of the possible results of a combination which has hitherto been conspicuously absent from the housing industry in the United States: careful planning, economical methods of financing, large-scale production with its economies, absence of the motive of speculation or sale at a profit, and careful management.

Bibliography

1. Housing and Health, *Public Health Service Pub.* 718, 1959.

2. "Report of Expert Committee on the Public Health Aspects of Housing," World Health Organization, Columbia University Press, International Documents Service, New York, 1961.

3. "Basic Principles of Healthful Housing," 2d ed., American Public Health Association, New York, 1950.
4. "An Appraisal Method for Measuring the Quality of Housing," pt. I, "Nature and Uses of the Method," 1945; pt. II, "Appraisal of Dwelling Conditions: Vol. A—Directors Manual, Vol. B—Field Procedures, Vol. C —Office Procedures," 1946; pt. III, "Appraisal of Neighborhood Environment," 1950, American Public Health Association, New York.
5. "Principles for Healthful Rural Housing," American Public Health Association, New York, 1957.
6. "Proposed Housing Ordinance," American Public Health Association, New York, 1952.
7. "Impact Noise Control in Multifamily Dwellings," Federal Housing Authority, 1963.
8. Velz, C. J., and F. M. Hemphill: "Home Injuries," School of Public Health, University of Michigan, Ann Arbor, Mich., 1962.
9. "A Primer on Rehabilitation under Local Law Enforcement," National Association of Real Estate Boards, Committee on Rehabilitation, Washington, D.C., 1960.
10. Johnson, R. J., and R. O. McCaldin: Housing Rehabilitation and Enforcement of Housing Laws, *Public Health Service Pub. 451*, 1955.
11. "Program for Community Improvement (Workable Program)," Housing and Home Finance Agency, Washington, D.C., 1960.
12. Banks, J. G.: The Social Implication of Urban Renewal, *Am. J. Public Health*, vol. 53, no. 1, January, 1963.

15

INSTITUTIONAL SANITATION

15-1. The provision and maintenance of an environment conducive to health at institutions of all types—including general hospitals, chronic-disease hospitals, convalescent homes, maternity hospitals, geriatric facilities, schools, jails, and prisons—encompass all the features of a well-rounded community public health program. To some extent the needs of the various institutions vary, depending on their uses. Although the fundamentals of water supply, plumbing, sewage disposal, heating, ventilation, and vermin control are much the same at all types of institutions, standards for lighting, recreational space, and special service facilities entail a close study of the type of institution, its uses, and the individuals involved.

Institutional sanitation is a recognized activity of health departments at both the local and state levels. It is a function of the state to establish standards and to promulgate rules and regulations which permit the local representatives to supervise effectively the construction, maintenance, and operation of the institutions. The state should offer consultation services which may be utilized by the institution operators and designers as well as by local health departments. Another very important function of the state health department is the review of plans and specifications for new institutions. Close liaison between the state health department and such other state agencies as prison boards, hospital boards, and education departments is most helpful in carrying out this program.

Schools

15-2. The school health and sanitation program depends upon the size of the school, whether it is a rural or city school, the age group to be served, and the availability of health services from official and volunteer agencies other than those provided directly by the school administration. The rural school is required to provide many services that are furnished by the community in urban areas, and the absence of local health departments and volunteer health agencies increases the school's responsibilities. Standards for school health and sanitation are the responsibility of the state health department, and the local health agencies cooperate with the educational authorities in applying these standards. The state health department is also responsible for consultative services which are essential in implementing the more complicated phases of the program.

The complexity of school sanitation problems, along with the high degree of susceptibility of school children to communicable diseases, makes the role of the sanitarian one of great importance.

15-3. School Health Program. A school health program should include service in the following seven areas [1]:

1. *Control of communicable disease.* This includes daily observation by the teacher, who should be instructed to note the signs and symptoms of illness. Although no attempt should be made to diagnose the specific disease or to treat the illness, the teacher should be alert to such evident signs as flushed face, rash, difficult breathing, abnormal cough, and pallor and should also ascertain the presence of such symptoms as chills, fever, and headache. The child who exhibits these abnormalities should be excluded from the classroom and sent to the office of the school nurse or principal, where the teacher's findings can be verified. The child is then sent home with a note of suggestion that the family doctor be called in for specific diagnosis and treatment. The note

should also inform the parents that if the illness is a communicable disease, the child should not be returned to school until he has a readmission certificate from the local health officer.

2. *Minimizing noncommunicable defects.* This includes observations by the teacher as well as by specially trained individuals to detect any evidence of defective vision, hearing, speech, posture, and teeth in the children. When defects are noted, the parents should be informed, with a recommendation that remedial care be given. It is advisable that follow-up visits by staff members be made. If financial difficulties prevent the parents from taking prompt, effective action, the community services and facilities should be utilized.

3. *Provision of health essentials in the school environment.* This is school sanitation, which is discussed in detail later in this chapter.

4. *Provision of health essentials through nutrition.* Many children are poorly fed because of poverty and ignorance. The provision of lunches in the school helps the poorly nourished child and inculcates good eating habits. The policy governing the school lunch program is a local matter and thus differs materially from place to place; however, most schools offer the lunch at cost or less to ensure that it is well received. The Federal government through the Department of Agriculture makes many food items available to the school lunch programs and provides a small cash subsidy for each child served. This permits the school to offer free lunches to underprivileged children without creating

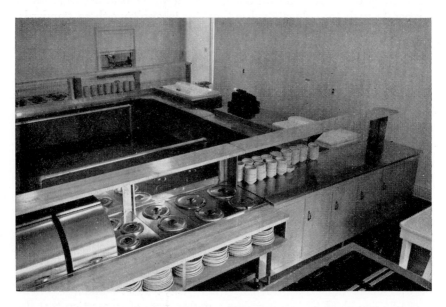

FIGURE 15-1 Serving tables of a school lunchroom. Note protective glass screen. (*Pharr–San Juan, Tex., Independent School District.*)

a serious drain on the local funds. The lunches should be prepared under the direction of a nutritionist, or at least with the consultation and periodic supervision of one.

The furnishing of lunches requires a kitchen, serving room, and dining room and involves all the usual sanitary problems connected with food handling. The methods used should comply with the standards set forth in Chap. 7 with due consideration given the laws of the state in which the school is located. Some special considerations for school installations include the rounding of all table corners and the provision of at least 16 in. and preferably 18 in. of level space per child at tables where food is consumed.

5. *Provision of adequate physical activity for the children to promote their development of basic physical skills.* This includes provision for play and sports—both supervised and unsupervised, indoor and outdoor. The related facilities of playground space, equipment, gymnasium, and dressing rooms all require consideration in this connection.

6. *Health education.* The school curriculum should include sufficient material on health education to enable the child to form proper habits in regard to diet; care of teeth; sleep; protection of eyes, ears, and other sensory organs; posture; safety; and cleanliness. Teaching should include the relationship of the individual, the school, and the community to the various aspects of the spread of communicable diseases and the role of sanitation in their control.

7. *Integration of school and community health programs.* It is essential that the school health program provide continuity with the preschool phase of the community program. It should also be correlated with the work of the local health department. This is especially true in the control of communicable disease and the solution of sanitary problems.

15-4. Location. The health and safety program of the school starts with the selection of the site and its development. The size of the school campus and the external social, industrial, and commercial environmental factors play important roles in the success or failure of a school health program. In rural areas the selection of a site is usually easier than in the case of urban schools; however, the considerations are similar. Minimum site areas should consist of 5 acres plus 1 acre for each 100 pupils to be served at elementary schools, and 10 acres plus 1 acre for each 100 pupils at secondary schools. The site should be well drained and free from certain hazards such as ravines, bluffs, etc. Health and safety features of the adjoining properties should be thoroughly studied in the selection of a site, since disease, insects, rodents, and vermin are no respecters of property lines.

Noise, bad odors, and traffic congestion connected with industrial and commercial centers are to be avoided, and such traffic arteries as main streets and highways, as well as railroad lines, are both noisy and hazardous. If possible, however, access to the school should be such that pupils are permitted the opportunity to utilize the community facilities. The distance of travel required of both the walking and the bus-carried pupils should also be a factor in location. For elementary-school children, ¾ mile is considered the maximum for walking and a 30-min bus ride one way the maximum for motor transport. For secondary schools the maximum walking distance should not exceed 2 miles, and the one-way bus ride should not exceed 1 hr. In some sparsely settled areas, these factors must be balanced with other considerations and a compromise reached which is advantageous to the pupils served.

Another matter which should not be neglected in school locations is the opportunity to establish surroundings which are pleasing to the eye, thus helping to instill a feeling of pride, contentment, and happiness in the pupils. Accessibility of utilities such as water, electricity, gas, and sewer, if possible, as well as of fire protection, should be considered in the selection. In addition, the educational administrator must give thought to other factors, such as population growth, consolidation, annexation, and type of education plan projected.

15-5. Building. The program of education and the age level served are reflected in the building and particularly in the grouping of the various services, as well as in the educational departments. Provision should be made for expansion as to both total pupil load and program coverage. Some consideration is usually given to the flexibility of the building to permit revision of the educational program conveniently.

The service facilities, along with the administrative units, form the core or hub of the school plant and should be located in such a manner as to permit good operation and supervision as well as easy access for the delivery of supplies and equipment. Noisy activities such as shops, music departments, and indoor physical education facilities should be separated from the academic departments. In elementary schools, the primary grades are usually grouped together at such a location that the children may have access to the nearer playground areas, and the older students can then utilize larger playground areas at a greater distance from the building.

The entrances are located to permit sheltered dismounting from buses and cars. It is also advisable to plan the school layout to permit community use of the auditorium, cafeteria, and general-purpose rooms with a minimum of interference with the classroom areas. Many local community and climatic conditions must be considered in the planning of a school building, and none is of greater importance than the natural lighting, heating, and ventilation arrangements, upon which the use and comfort of the school are dependent. In the South, where heat loss is relatively unimportant but cross ventilation is essential, the practice of using a sprawling finger design with orientation of the rooms to expose window walls to the prevailing breeze is frequently adopted. Open single-loaded covered corridors are popular in dry, warm areas, whereas in damp or cold climates closed halls are necessary to afford protection from the elements to students when moving from one area to another. Under certain industrial or climatic conditions where fog, cloud cover, or smoke interferes with the reliability of natural light, it is an economical practice to disregard sky light in the building design since artificial light must be provided in such quantity as to meet the total need.

15-6. Interior Finish. Experience gained from using existing buildings provides valuable insight for the school administrator as to the materials and finishes which are readily adaptable to the local school and community needs. Serious thought should be given to the serviceability of various materials, since an initial capital investment saving may result in such a serious sacrifice in service that maintenance burdens are excessive.

For floors, the softwoods are undesirable because they have a comparatively short life, whereas hardwoods give good service if properly installed. Even after prolonged neglect, hardwood floors can be sanded and refinished to recover the qualities of a new floor. Asphalt-tile floors have been widely used in schools. They are cheap, easy to replace, light-colored, and easy on the feet. The disadvantages of asphalt tile are that it is subject to indentation, scarring, and deterioration from grease, oils, spirit-solvent waxes, kerosene, gasoline, and turpentine [2]. Rubber or vinyl flooring is similar to asphalt tile except that it is more expensive, and the colors are brighter. Cork flooring has a limited use, particularly where acoustical qualities are indicated. It requires rather extensive maintenance, such as lacquer or varnish seal and protection against alcohol. Concrete floors are useful in corridors, auditoriums, and similar places; however, special consideration for their hardness is essential, or they tend to become dusty. Terrazzo floors are attractive if properly sealed and serviced; however, they are expensive and may be slippery unless nonskid chips are used in the surfacing. Acids, abrasives, or strong alkaline cleaners should not be used on terrazzo. Ceramic-tile floors are satisfactory. They are cleaned with neutral soaps or mild detergents with damp mopping followed by a clean-water rinse. Slate and marble are too soft for heavy use and tend to crack and chip. Quarry tile is useful in laboratories, kitchens, and similar places. Plastic tile, linoleum, and grease-resistant rubber tile have been found useful in kitchens and lunchrooms, where ease of cleaning is essential.

For interior walls the recent trend has been toward the use of exposed brick and cinder block. They are cheaper than plaster walls and present a pleasing appearance when painted. For partition walls, sheetrock, plywood, and other light materials are popular, because they permit economical remodeling. Chalkboards are found in nearly all class rooms and usually become part of the wall surface. Slate boards are los ing favor since their light absorption is very high. Glass, composition, and plastic boards, usually green in color and with a light reflectivity of 20 to 25 per cent, are now commonly used. With most composition boards, care must be taken not to allow moisture to be absorbed, or they will deteriorate rapidly.

In schools with a heavy dependence on natural light, the prismatic glass block has been used extensively with clear-glass vision strips below the glass-block area. The vision strip is usually placed in windows of the awning or pivot type to permit ventilation.

Wall surfaces in classrooms should usually have a light-colored smooth mat finish. For kitchens, dining rooms, and similar areas the finish should be smooth and washable.

Ceiling surfaces receive attention for acoustical treatment, and fiber-glass board and vegetable fiberboard as well as sheetrock are extensively used. A flat white finish is essential for good light reflectivity.

15-7. Light and Color. The importance of good lighting and some of the various factors which enter into providing an acceptable visual environment have been mentioned in Chaps. 13 and 14. Modern educational methods are dependent upon a well-lighted environment for much of their effectiveness, and more research and development have gone into this aspect of school plants than into any other one phase. It has been said that what is learned by the child is learned by the whole child and that what is seen by the child is seen by the whole child—not just the eye. The whole body is involved in seeing; nerves, muscles, and circulation all play a part.

To see with ease and comfort results in a minimum use of energy, and fatigue does not occur as readily. The handicaps to seeing, such as glare, dim lights, and poor balance of illumination, all tend to create muscular and nervous tension, which prematurely brings on fatigue. The function of school lighting is to produce conditions which permit the performance of visual tasks efficiently with a minimum of strain and effort. Children's energies should be used for growth of sturdy bodies and the development of sound mental and emotional processes, not for combating the visual difficulties which result from poor lighting.

Until recent years, the intensity of light was considered the only criterion worthy of consideration, but now the quality of the light is also considered important for proper eye comfort and visual efficiency. Quality includes, in addition to quantity or intensity, such things as location of source, color, brightness, and the reflective characteristics of floor, ceiling, walls, and furnishings. All these factors make up the brightness balance not only of the visual task but of the entire visual field. It is desirable to have no area in the entire visual field brighter than the task, nor should any area be less than one-third as bright as the task. These conditions, along with a general high level of illumination, are the goals which should be sought [3, 4].

Light sources which are in the visual field, such as windows and light bulbs, must be toned to diffuse and distribute the light over a wider area. This is accomplished by using some type of shielding which diffuses and distributes the light. For windows, such equipment as translucent diffusers and deflectors are practical, as are blinds and light shades. Drapes and other dark or opaque materials reduce the available light without accomplishing the desired distribution. For light bulbs the indirect-light fixture directs the light rays to reflecting surfaces, where further diffusion is accomplished. All these procedures tend to reduce the local or spot brightness; thus, a step toward smaller brightness ratios in the visual field is accomplished.

The Illuminating Engineering Society has suggested that school lighting for various types of visual tasks be sufficient to maintain levels on the task area corresponding to the values given in Table 15-1.

The most common source of light used in schools until recent years has been natural light, and it is still used very extensively in most schools. The variables of natural light, such as orientation of light openings, sun rotation, cloud cover, and seasonal conditions, make the effective use of natural light a complex matter and can be coordinated for efficient use only part of the time. Formerly, it was considered advisable to have windows on one side of the room and to arrange the seating so that the light came to the child from the left side. Now the considerations of brightness, contrasts, limitations, glare control, shadow reduction, and other quality factors and the efforts being made to obtain a high over-all illumination level have opened the lighting design to the use of multilevel lighting. Bilateral window arrangements, entire upper wall areas of prismatic light-directional glass blocks, improved elementary roof design, and skylights have been used effectively. The trend toward single-story construction and the use of open and single-loaded corridors

Table 15-1. MINIMUM RECOMMENDED LEVELS OF ILLUMINATION IN SCHOOLS

Tasks	Foot-candles on tasks
Reading printed material	30
Reading pencil writing	70
Reading spirit-duplicated material:	
Good	30
Poor	100
Drafting, benchwork	100
Reading chalkboards, sewing, lipreading	150

SOURCE: "Illuminating Engineering Society Lighting Handbook," Illuminating Engineering Society, New York, 1958.

have freed the designer of many of the handicaps to light utilization which previously existed. Multiple light sources make it mandatory that glare be eliminated and that light diffusion and direction be applied with a minimum of light loss.

In orienting the classrooms of the South and particularly the Southwest, direct sunrays should be kept out of the major light openings, and shielding, direction, and diffusing should be practiced if any direct sunlight is used. In the northern part of the country, direct sunlight is considered psychologically desirable, and glare, as well as high brightness contrast, results. To offset these handicaps more attention is given to seating arrangements, and for extremely difficult cases some internal shielding is applied.

Sky light represents sunrays that have been diffused and thus rendered more usable. Every effort should be made to utilize sky light and to inhibit the entrance of direct sunlight. Such external shields as canopies, overhanging roofs, louvered overhangs for windows, and external horizontal or vertical venetian blinds have been used successfully, so that in the warmer climates the heat control effected is of considerable value. Shielding and diffusing by interior equipment are accomplished by using venetian blinds, center-hung double shades, diffusers, and louvers.

In order to prevent glare (Art. 13-7) there must not be too much contrast between the brightnesses of the tasks and the various surfaces in the schoolroom. Table 15-2 gives the minimum ratios necessary for comfortable visual conditions in the schoolroom.

In planning for a balance of brightness, it is necessary to consider artificial light either to supplement the natural light or to provide all light if the facilities are to be used in the evenings. Frequently the artificial lighting is placed in both roles. To utilize one set of lighting fixtures for all purposes, it is suggested that the various fixtures be placed on separate switch circuits which permit using only selected fixtures in the supplementing role and all fixtures when natural light is eliminated. Light fixtures may be divided into five classes: direct, semidirect, general-diffusing, semi-indirect, and indirect. As indicated by the names, the percentage of light directed downward and the percentage of light

Table 15-2.   MINIMUM BRIGHTNESS RATIOS FOR
SCHOOL LIGHTING

Area	Brightness ratio
Tasks to immediate surroundings	3:1
Minimum for chalkboards to surroundings	1:3
Tasks to surroundings more remote	10:1
Tasks to large remote bright areas	1:10
Luminaires or windows to surroundings	20:1

directed toward a reflecting surface are different in the five categories, varying from 100 to 90 per cent of the light directed down in the first class to 100 to 90 per cent directed to reflecting surfaces in the fifth class. See Art. 13-11. The direct-type fixture is not considered satisfactory except for very limited use—for example, local lighting for tasks such as operating machines, reading dictionaries, etc. The semidirect fixture has limited school use in corridors, locker rooms, and storerooms. The general-diffusing fixture produces glare and shadow, which are undesirable features for classroom lighting. In spite of these defects, this type of equipment has been extensively used in the past. The semi-indirect fixture utilizes the ceiling as a primary reflecting source with a small percentage of light directed down and a limited amount of glare. This type of fixture can be successfully used in most classrooms. The indirect fixture usually is equipped with an opaque or only slightly translucent surface on the bottom and sides, with the light being reflected against the ceiling for further redirecting and diffusing. This type of fixture produces light with the most desirable qualities, but it does have a lower efficiency of light production per energy-unit input than the other types.

Since the advent of fluorescent-light fixtures, there have been many discussions on the relative advantages of the two types of artificial light-

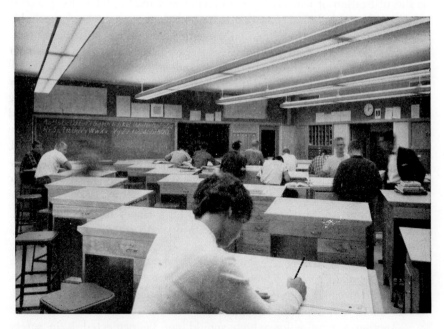

FIGURE 15-2 A well-lighted classroom. Note luminaires that minimize reflected glare and troublesome shadows. (*Courtesy of General Electric Company.*)

ing. In general, it is usually possible to provide satisfactory lighting utilizing either incandescent- or fluorescent-light fixtures if proper consideration is given to wattage, glare, location, and the reflective values of the various room surroundings. Local conditions usually control the relative advantages of one or the other, and thus some of the major points to be investigated are outlined below.

Incandescent fixtures and bulbs are cheaper in first cost than fluorescent fixtures; however, the incandescent light requires a higher wattage to produce a given brightness and, thus, is more expensive to operate. Incandescent lights produce large quantities of heat, whereas fluorescent lights are relatively cool. Fluorescent lights may be advantageous if the local building wiring is overloaded, since the current requirements are lower. Both types of light bulbs have been improved to give longer-lasting service, and, likewise, new light fixtures of both types are designed for easy maintenance and cleaning and high efficiency. Formerly, the phosphorus used in fluorescent light bulbs was a toxic material, and the danger from broken tubes was rather extensive; however, the present-day material is relatively inert, and broken tubes are no more hazardous than any other cutting object.

The use of color in schools is of great significance since it plays a very important part in establishing the brightness ratios which are essential for visual ease and comfort. Another consideration in choice of color is the utilization of various light sources. Color may differ in its qualities under different light sources, depending on the components of the light. Color exerts an important influence on the alertness of the room occupants and may tend to soothe the user or, if clashing colors or sharp hues are used, to produce nervousness and fidgeting on the part of the teachers and children. From the standpoint of lighting, the reflective factors of the various colored surfaces are of such importance in imparting the proper light brightness for visual tasks that precedence should be given to these factors in selecting colors.

The recommended reflective factors for classroom surfaces are shown in Fig. 15-3. The wall surface has the same factor as the ceiling for 18 to 20 in. below it. The factors given preclude the use of slate boards, oiled floors, or dark-finish tile.

A nongloss finish should be used on all surfaces to eliminate glare. Colors have usually been associated with warmth or coolness—blue and green indicating coolness, and yellow, orange, and red suggesting warmth. Usually the cool colors are used in sunny rooms and warm colors in sunless rooms. Likewise, color plays a part in making rooms seem large or small. The light colors seem to enlarge the room, and dark colors make the room appear smaller.

Another use of color which should not be neglected is in safety work. The standardizing of colors for moving parts on machinery as

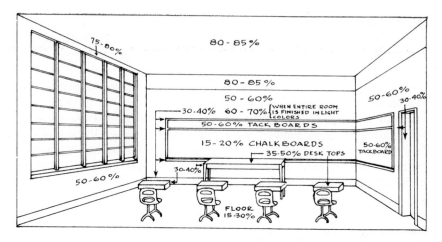

FIGURE 15-3   Recommended classroom reflective values.

well as fire-fighting equipment is a practical procedure that should be considered in school plants.

15-8. Heating and Ventilation. The atmosphere of the various parts of the school must be healthful and comfortable for the particular activities for which the room is used. It thus becomes necessary for the heating and ventilation systems to accomplish the following:

1. Supplying of clean air in sufficient quantities to dilute the room air below the threshold of body-odor detection and to remove dust, fumes, obnoxious gases, and humidity. (A system that accomplishes these goals also supplies sufficient oxygen for the occupants.)

2. Maintenance of a uniform room temperature without rapid fluctuations.

3. Supplying of heat for balancing losses from the human body.

4. Supplying of makeup heat for room and building losses.

5. Removal of excess heat caused by body radiation, conduction, evaporation, or external conditions.

6. Diffusion of the atmospheric temperature without pronounced drafts or stratification.

As may be noted, some problems require constant attention, while others occur alternately, such as the provision of makeup heat under certain conditions and the removal of excess heat under other conditions.

In some climates, the provision of proper heating of the schools takes precedence over ventilating, while in areas where a mild climate exists, the ventilating and cooling must receive major attention. There are numerous methods of heating; however, all depend on radiation, conduction, convection, or a combination of them to distribute the heat uniformly from the source to the room generally. It is usually better to have a central heating plant than room-fired heaters, which multiply the maintenance and operation duties of the custodial staff. Simple systems usually offer advantages in that the school staff is able to service and maintain the equipment, while the more complex types require skilled specialists. The fuel chosen depends on the locality; however, oil and gas fuels usually permit more nearly automatic operation and eliminate the problem of ash removal and disposal. Also, recent experiences in prolonged interruption of coal deliveries suggest the necessity of installing a large bunker space to store coal. Special consideration for student safety must be included in the planning, particularly if gaseous fuels are used. Explosions may result in mass injuries and death as well as a rapid spread of fire over a wide area.

For many years, the most common heating system used in schools consisted of a low-pressure steam boiler with steam radiators located in the various rooms. The systems have been modified to the extent that hot-water boilers have been added, and the distribution of the heat may be accomplished by means of hot-water radiators, forced warm-air systems, or radiant-heating panels. The forced-air system offers certain advantages in that it may be designed for cooling as well as heating, and it permits control of fresh air, which may be filtered and tempered.

While central heating is usually more desirable than room-fired heaters, there are numerous installations which lend themselves to individual control for convenience and economy. Room heaters which are equipped with circulating fans permit good distribution of heat.

The effectiveness, safety, and economy of any heating system are dependent upon the controls. The fuel controls, pressure relief valves, and makeup water valves should be the best available, since the safety of the facility and of the occupants is dependent upon their prompt operation. Automatic controls produce more efficient operation, and the economies in fuel and man-hours more than offset the initial investment. Thermostats and humidostats, if humidity-control equipment is utilized, provide much more sensitive control of these atmospheric qualities than manual adjustment using thermometers and psychrometers for indicating instruments. Locked controls which prevent tampering by unauthorized persons should be used in all public locations, such as classrooms, corridors, etc.

Ventilation standards are much more flexible than heating standards since the socioeconomic status of occupants, the activity for which the room is used, and general climatic conditions all have valid effects on the design criteria. Studies have been made to determine the minimum amount of fresh air per person needed to keep body odor below an objectionable level on the basis of cubic space per person, as affected by the age and socioeconomic status of the occupants. For example, a study by the Harvard School of Public Health, in which grade-school children were used as subjects, shows that with 200 cu ft of space per person of average economic background there is a need for 21 cu ft of fresh air per person per min but that occupants of a lower-than-average socioeconomic status require 38 cu ft of fresh air per person per min. Likewise, greater supplies of air are necessary if vigorous rather than sedentary activity is taking place.

Except in the case of exceedingly warm conditions, the ventilation requirements are based on body-odor control. For dissipating heat, the quantity of air supplied, the temperature of the incoming air, the water-vapor content of the air, and the air movement are all factors which affect the comfort of the room occupants. Drafts may be uncomfortable if velocities of over 25 fpm are obtained when the air is appreciably cooler than the body; however, during warm weather, velocities of up to 100 fpm may be tolerated very well. See Art. 10-15 for a discussion of outlet velocities.

The dissipation of body heat is dependent upon the surrounding atmosphere's taking up the heat in one form or another. Most of the heat disposal in warm weather is accomplished by vaporization of perspiration from the body surfaces. The vapor content of the air thus materially influences the effectiveness of this process. Dehumidification of incoming air could effect a material benefit even if the air was not cooled in the process. It is obvious that the conductive effect of room air in cooling is dependent upon the temperature differential between the body to be cooled and the air. The heat-absorption capacity of dry air is very low, and thus the quantity of air which is needed to remove excess heat by the process of raising the air temperature is large.

The use of air conditioning in schools has not gained favor to any great extent because the cost of operation is rather high and the initial investment is likewise considerable. Another factor in the slow application of air conditioning is the relatively light use of school buildings during the warmest months of the year. Many of the newer schools have provided limited air conditioning for audio-visual rooms, auditoriums, cafeterias, and other similar special service rooms. Most of these air conditioners provide dehumidification, cooling, and filtration of the air, with a comparatively high percentage of air being recirculated.

In arid parts of the country, the conditioning is accomplished by air filtration and vaporization of water with little or no recirculation. This desert-type equipment is much more economical in initial cost, as well as in operation, than the mechanical refrigeration type, but it has a limited effectiveness in that it is useful only if the incoming air has a low vapor content. Central air-conditioning equipment can be used most economically with hot-air heating systems which permit the use of the air-filtration equipment and the distribution ducts and grilles for all-year heating and cooling.

In the southern part of the United States, various types of fans have been used to increase the air movement and circulation. The most satis-factory installations are of the exhaust type which permit gravity re-placement of exhausted air. The primary advantages are that these sys-tems permit lower fan speeds with less noise, fewer drafts, and a high rate of air change. Blower-type fans which are located to have an air intake from the outside permit an increased air change. With these, how-ever, drafts are common, and high-speed operation, with its concomitant of increased noise, is frequently required. General circulating fans, such as ceiling fans, floor fans, and stand fans, are not recommended. One of the primary objections to their use is the increased opportunity for disease transmission as a result of the spread of droplet-borne infectious organisms as well as dust- and lint-carried organisms.

Natural ventilation, depending on windows, doors, transoms, and louvers, is widely used and can be rather effective if properly designed, installed, and utilized. One of the most serious deficiencies noted in natural ventilation systems is the lack of an adequate opening for the exit of stale air. In general, there is no static-pressure differential, and the velocity force is sufficient to function effectively only if the exit-air area is equal to the entrance area and is located to permit cross-ventila-tion movement without short-circuiting. Since used air which is to be exhausted is usually warmer than incoming air, the exhaust opening should be near the ceiling, where the warm air accumulates. Fresh air that enters the room at a low height, at least 18 in. above the floor to avoid excess pickup of dust and lint, contacts the occupant's body and breathing zone. After this contact and use, the air is warmed and rises out of the occupied area of the room. If natural ventilation is used during the heating portion of the year, some tempering of the intake air should be accomplished by passage over heated surfaces before it con-tacts the occupants.

In this country, the comfort temperature is between 68 and 72°F for most people; however, older persons may find that temperatures nearer 75°F are desirable. Likewise, if vigorous activity is being per-formed by the occupants, lower temperatures may be desirable. If humidity control is being practiced, the range from 30 to 50 per cent is most comfortable for normal individuals, although 45 per cent is recom-mended as a minimum by some authorities [1].

15-9. Noise Control. School buildings should be so designed that noise will not be an annoyance. Excessive noise causes irritation, mental and emotional strain, and distraction and inefficiency of children, teachers, and employees. The acceptable noise levels in decibels (see Art. 16-11) are given in Table 15-3. It will be noted that the acceptable outdoor noise level at school sites is less than 70 db. Higher levels would require difficult and costly treatment of walls and corridors to reduce them to 30 to 35 db in the classrooms.

Table 15-3.   ACCEPTABLE NOISE LEVELS
IN SCHOOL AREAS

Type of room	Acceptable noise levels, db
Classrooms	35–40
Cafeterias	50–55
School sites (outdoor noise levels)	Less than 70
Health rooms	Less than 45
Hearing-test rooms	Less than 40
Music rooms	Less than 40

In the design of buildings, internal noise-making equipment should be so planned that sound will be absorbed. Special areas such as auditoriums should be acoustically designed. Sound surveys made with sound-level meters will indicate areas of undesirable noise levels, and corrective measures may then be applied. These include placing of acoustic tile on walls and ceilings and use of special acoustic plaster or fabrics containing lead. Noise from outside sources can be reduced by brick barrier walls or by screen planting. A cypress hedge about 2 ft in thickness will reduce noise to the extent of 4 db [2].

15-10. Furnishings. School furniture which is not designed for the particular use to which it is put can create hardships that interfere with the educational programs of the users and promote the development of physical deformities, even to the extent of permanently accentuating abnormalities. Properly designed desks, tables, and chairs are particularly important since the students use this equipment for prolonged periods. Size and shape should be considered in the light of the ages, stages of physical development, and functional requirements of the potential users. Adjustable furniture is available, and while the initial cost is higher than that of some other types, it may prove more economical in the long run if the cost of education and of treatment for physical deformities is considered.

The furnishings should also be selected to harmonize with the lighting and to suit climatic conditions and educational requirements. Furniture should be light and sturdy to permit movement as needed. In primary grades the extensive use of paints, clays, and other handiwork objects requires that the finish be durable and resistant to cleaning materials as well as to the supplies provided students for school use. Special finishes may be required in certain educational rooms, involving such factors as heat resistance in rooms where cooking, pottery making, and certain physical sciences are taught. In warm or humid climates such furniture as desks and chairs should fit the users in a manner which permits them to wear loose clothing and which allows intimate ventilation of the body surfaces. In all instances the coloring of the furnishings should blend with other interior finishes, particularly as to depth of color. This may be explained as a method of obtaining uniformity of brightness, regardless of the light intensity.

15-11. Plumbing. School plumbing fixtures include water closets, urinals, lavatories, and drinking fountains in all buildings. Under some conditions such special fixtures as sinks, showers, and hydrotherapeutic vessels may also be utilized. To avoid repetition, only the basic fixtures are discussed in this chapter; information on special fixtures is given in Chap. 11, which deals with their general uses.

Fundamentally, all plumbing fixtures used in schools should be smooth, attractive, and corrosion-resistant. They should be designed without sharp edges, corners, and crevices. White or bright finishes permit easy visibility of dirt, and this promotes better cleaning. Toilets and lavatories should be installed in well-lighted and well-ventilated rooms. Dry, clean restrooms and plumbing fixtures can be maintained free from fecal and urine odors. School management which practices good restroom cleanliness, good ventilation, and normal maintenance finds that chemical deodorants are unnecessary.

The water closets used in the primary grades should be small in size, 11 or 12 in. high. Preschool age groups may find the 10-in. height useful. The regular-sized water closets, 14 in. high, should prove satisfactory for all older school groups. Some manufacturers build a 13-in. water closet for intermediate grades, but the majority of administrators do not feel that this special size is needed. All water closets should be equipped with a U-shaped seat of impervious material that is not subject to checking or cracking.

If the water pressure is at least 18 psi, the flushometer-valve type of flushing device is the most acceptable. The advantages of this type of valve are that a more vigorous flushing action is obtained, less water is used, and no delay between flushing cycles exists. The maintenance problems are reported as less frequent with the flushometer-valve unit than with the holding tank. Where low water pressure exists, the flush-tank water closet is required. In both types a siphon breaker or anti-backflow device is required to prevent possible pollution. These devices should be inspected at least once a year to determine whether they are still in good condition, since infrequent use permits corrosion and deterioration to occur without noticeable effect on the operation of the flushing device.

The same consideration regarding height of the fixture should apply to urinals. The urinal should be wall-hung rather than floor-mounted. The latter is difficult to clean, easily soiled, and frequently subject to clogging.

Lavatories should be mounted at various heights from 24 to 30 in. from the floor, depending on the age of the children to be served. The 24-, 26-, and 30-in. fixtures have been found most useful. To promote proper hand washing, all lavatories should be equipped with hot and cold water discharged through a mixing faucet. The discharge should be located above the overflow, and the valves should not be spring-loaded. Flush-valve types are very beneficial if the water is not of a scale-forming quality. They do serve to save water and to avoid water-hammer problems and overflows, but for many waters the positive-action manually operated valves prove most sensible. Training in the school, as in the home, can effectively eliminate the objection commonly raised to the use of this type of valve. Schools are in existence to teach conservation of manpower and resources, and water is one of America's critical resources.

School lavatories should not be equipped with drain stoppers as all hand and face washing should be accomplished with running water that has not been contaminated from water in the lavatory bowl left by a previous user.

Drinking fountains should never be located in close proximity to other plumbing fixtures, particularly waste disposal fixtures. The drinking fountain should be mounted 30 to 40 in. above the floor with the 30-, 36-, and 40-in. fixtures being the most popular. Measurement of height on these units is the vertical distance from floor to fountain orifice, while on other fixtures the measurement is from floor to overflow rim. The fountainhead should be of the angle-jet mouth-guard type with an antisquirt device. The valve should be either hand- or foot-operated, and a pressure-control regulator should be an integral part of the valve. The jet from the orifice should be regulated to rise not more than 4 in. vertically above the orifice, and the arc should not extend more than 10 in. horizontally from the orifice. The discharge orifice should be not less than ¾ in. above the overflow rim of the water basin.

In warm climates, there is a trend toward installing refrigerated drinking fountains, and while this practice is common and readily accepted, special precautions should be taken to prevent school pupils from drinking cold water while they are overheated. This may be accomplished by providing two supplies of different temperature or by connecting only tap water to fountains in places where students congregate following strenuous exercise.

The number of plumbing fixtures needed per student is a widely debated subject, and there are many standards. Table 11-1 lists minimum facilities recommended by the Coordinating Committee for a National Plumbing Code [5]. Recommendations for institutions other than schools are included.

15-12. Water Supply and Sewage Disposal. The water supply should be obtained from a public supply, and sewage disposal should be conducted via a public sanitary sewer if practicable. In the absence of public service, the principles as set out in this book for individual water systems and private sewage systems should be used as a guide (see Chaps. 2 and 4).

Water use for domestic purposes at day schools is usually less than 20 gal per person per day even in schools that have gymnasiums and cafeterias. Many elementary schools use 5 gal per person per day or less for domestic purposes. In the more arid regions, the extensive use of water for maintenance of lawns, athletic fields, and playgrounds greatly exceeds the domestic water use. The design of the school water-service lines should take this into consideration.

Usually a design figure of 15 gal of sewage per person per day is adequate. For individual-system design the sewage should be classed as weak with less than 0.07 lb of biochemical oxygen demand per capita per day with the suspended-solids content also low. Rarely does grease present a problem.

In choosing a type of sewage disposal system it should be remembered that the school is closed for a long period of each year and that it is advisable to avoid plant processes that require close supervision or highly technical operation since operation will be in the hands of school personnel who are not sanitation specialists.

15-13. Cleaning and Maintenance. The cleaning and maintenance program of a school plays an important part in the health and education of the building users. Of importance to the tax-paying public is the improved serviceability of a plant which is preserved through an effective maintenance program. A schedule which includes the various tasks—both daily and weekly duties and those that must be performed only at infrequent intervals—pays dividends through the avoidance of neglect of critical matters.

Cleaning is usually considered a separate function from maintenance; yet one of the primary records of a complete cleaning program is the reduction of deterioration due to excess wear, corrosion, and grit. Many large and well-organized school systems have training programs for their custodial staffs which are designed to stress proper cleaning procedures and maintenance practices. Many expensive repairs can be avoided if the custodial staff is alert to the care of the equipment it services.

The various surfaces to be cleaned require different kinds of cleaners and different types of brooms, brushes, or mops. Some surfaces may be cleaned with detergents in water, while other surfaces may be seriously damaged by the water or the ionization of the detergent. See Art. 15-6. Some surfaces require vigorous buffing, while others are scratched and permanently damaged by stiff bristles. Most suppliers of cleaning supplies have developed charts which specify the type of agent and the applicator needed for various surfaces. Many of these charts refer to a specific kind of material which is handled by the cleaning supply house, but this is a handicap in preparing specifications for open bidding by the purchasing agent. Most manufacturers and trade associations have prepared instructions for the installation and care of their products. By the use of these informative guides, the school may develop its own charts based on ingredients and results without reference to brands.

The properly equipped, alert, and trained custodian can and will perform preventive maintenance in the course of his routine duties. Examples of such actions are replacing washers and gaskets in plumbing fixtures; adjusting pressure controls; replacing pull cords, tapes, or other frayed or broken items; tightening bolts or screws; oiling moving parts; and noting for early repair defects that will require future attention. The tasks in this last category might include touching up disfiguring marks, filling cracks, removing small spots of corrosion, and replacing cracked or broken window glass, etc. For the proper procedure for accomplishing this type of care, the manufacturer's instructions are the most reliable.

In addition to the routine preventive maintenance, some major and highly specialized jobs occur. Only in very large school systems is it practical to have specialized personnel on the staff. Other schools find it economical to hire the service required in the open market. Quite frequently, permitting the handyman type of employee to do technical and delicate work results in permanent damage to expensive equipment.

The most effective cleaning and maintenance program is found where the administration not only furnishes good equipment and high-quality supplies but also hires alert and progressive personnel and provides them with basic training and frequent refresher courses.

Hospitals

15-14. The basic concepts of sanitation in a hospital are no different from those related to hotels, schools, and eating establishments since certain areas of the hospital render the same basic services. The major difference is in the greater degree to which cleanliness and sterilization are practiced; for the patient in the hospital, perhaps a simple medical, surgical, or obstetrical case, may develop some communicable disease after admission, or the patient may be admitted because of a communicable disease.

15-15. Physical Structure and Maintenance. The basic physical structure of a hospital is the same as that of any fireproof hotel. Special precautions are taken in the way of exits, fireproofing, wiring, etc., to reduce the possibility of fire and to make it easy to remove bedfast patients. Schools and hotels are designed to be cleaned regularly, but in a hospital the cleaning is much more frequent and important. Halls and other public areas should be mopped and washed every day. Floors are particularly important since dust and bacteria tend to settle on them. Wet pickup vacuum cleaners are preferred. The floor is first moistened with a detergent and bactericide; the machine then scrubs the floor and picks up the liquid, which is discharged into a tank [6]. The patients' rooms must be thoroughly scrubbed after each patient leaves. Because of the frequent washing and the strong bactericides which are often used, the wall and floor surfaces must be designed to take this punishment as well as the abuse of being struck by carts and stretchers and being maltreated by the public. For this reason, some form of glazed tile or a vinyl plastic sheeting is frequently used. All paint is usually a high-quality enamel.

The outbreaks of antibiotic-resistant staphylococcus infections sometimes occurring in hospitals must depend for prevention upon good sanitation in the hospital. Airborne staphylococci have been implicated in operating-room and nursery infections. Ventilation systems may provide transportation throughout the hospital. In general the air-pressure gradient should be from clean to dirty areas, but open doorways may cause trouble [6]. Cleaning and disinfection practices should keep airborne bacteria to a minimum.

In general, the food-handling and dish-sterilization rules followed are the same as those observed in a good modern restaurant; however, extra care must be taken in dish and eating-utensil sanitizing. The smallest of hospitals should have a dishwashing and dish-sanitizing machine.

15-16. Central Supply and Sterilizing Areas. The typical hospital has several features that are not found in any other type of building. The central supply and sterilizing area is responsible for the sterile and sanitary condition of nearly all items used by the patients that are not supplied by the kitchen. Autoclaves using saturated steam under pressure are used to sterilize surgical supplies and equipment, syringes, textiles, enamelware, and rubber goods. Dry heat is preferred for sterilizing needles and sharp cutting instruments. Gaseous sterilization, using ethylene dioxide, is coming into increasing use. Laundry is washed for 25 min at 165°F or over and is then rinsed and ironed. Clean linen must be kept separate from soiled articles. Laundry chutes are difficult to keep clean and should be avoided.

15-17. Hospital Plumbing. The plumbing fixtures differ to some extent from normal units [5]. All bedrooms and examining rooms should have hand-washing facilities, but the faucets should be of the gooseneck type, and the handles should have wrist or elbow blades. Some units, particularly those in operating rooms, have foot- or knee-operated controls. Many toilets are equipped to wash bedpans and thus save the nurse time. Many sinks used in surgery and delivery areas are equipped

with flushing rims or special traps to catch plaster and instruments overlooked in the linen.

No under-rim plumbing fixtures of any kind should be permitted
(Art. 11-22). The danger of back siphonage from a bedpan washer, for
example, is readily apparent.

15-18. Operating and Delivery Rooms and Nurseries. The operating
rooms and delivery rooms present many sanitation problems. Safety from
explosive mixtures of anesthetic gases and oxygen must be ensured by
using conductive floors and explosion-proof electrical outlets. The areas
must be particularly easy to clean and must be scrubbed and disinfected
before each use. Year-round air conditioning with humidity control is
almost a necessity in these sections of the hospital. The maintenance of
a relative humidity of 50 to 60 per cent helps reduce the static electricity
and the possibility of explosions. The air-conditioning-system filters
should remove at least 90 per cent of the particulates of 1 to 5 μ in size.
A minimum ventilation rate of 12 room volumes of outdoor air with no
recirculation is necessary to keep airborne contaminants low [8]. Air of
operating rooms may be recirculated when the room is not in use.
Blankets and linen from the patient's room should not be transferred
with the patient to the operating room, and this restriction also applies
to beds and to stretchers when they transport persons to the operating
room.

The delivery room and nursery also require a high degree of sanitation control. Here also, the washing of the room and bassinets is almost
continuous. No more than 12 bassinets should be housed in each room,
and a limit of eight is recommended. There should be not less than 24
sq ft of floor space per bassinet, and 30 sq ft is recommended. Cubicles
for bassinets are also recommended [8]. The air is usually conditioned
the year around to control temperature and humidity. The air-conditioning machine must supply the same type of air, and without recirculation,
as is provided for the operating and delivery rooms, but from an independent source.

15-19. Isolation Areas. The handling of contagious diseases in a
hospital requires, in some cases, the reservation of special sections for
diseased patients in which there is no recirculated air from or to other
parts of the hospital (all air is supplied from the outside and is exhausted
to the outside). No equipment leaves the area. Even the dishes are
washed and sterilized in a special workroom set up for this purpose.
If provision for complete segregation in this manner is not made, the
isolation must be accomplished through the technique of the personnel.

15-20. Refuse Disposal. There is always a considerable amount of
refuse from a hospital presenting unusual problems. The normal rubbish,
such as paper, boxes, etc., may be handled in the conventional manner.

The edible garbage must be stored in closed containers and in a screened area. It should not be fed to hogs, for the possibility of the garbage being contaminated by infectious agents is always present. Hot water or steam should be provided for cleaning the cans.

One form of rubbish that is always present is a wet, contaminated group of items that come from surgery and delivery rooms. The infective or bloody bandages and human wastes that cannot be permitted to enter a sanitary sewer require special consideration. Usually a gas-fired incinerator is supplied that can accommodate material containing 80 to 90 per cent moisture.

Nursing Homes and Related Institutions

15-21. Nursing Homes. These are homes designed to care for the aged and infirm. They should be planned from the standpoint of the safety, health, and convenience of the patient or guest residing in the home. It is recommended that such homes be single-story buildings constructed of the most fire-resistive materials and that the building be located on adequate grounds with access to public transportation, churches, shopping centers, and hospitals.

Special features of the building and general equipment should include slip-resistant floors and corridors not less than 8 ft in width equipped with handrails on each side. All patient rooms should be outside rooms opening onto the corridor. It is recommended that ceilings in corridors, recreation rooms, detention rooms, nurses' stations, and utility rooms be acoustically treated. Wherever possible, ramps should be installed in lieu of steps; however, if steps are required they should be easy-tread and equipped with handrails. Handrails or safety grips are also needed in bathrooms, adjacent to the bathtub, shower, water closet, and lavatory. Drinking fountains and lavatories should be projected from the wall in order that they may be easily approached at the front by wheelchair patients.

Doors to bathrooms and toilets should be 3 ft wide with metal kick plates on both sides and should swing out. An inswinging door could be blocked if the patient should meet with some accident and fall against the door. Toilet stalls should be equipped with curtains instead of doors. Bathtubs should be set on the floor, and it is recommended that the tub be accessible from both sides and one end. It is important that hot water at all fixtures used by patients be thermostatically controlled to provide a temperature of not more than 110°F. Emergency call buttons should be installed in all toilets and bathrooms as well as in the individual patient quarters.

More liberal allowance should be made for storage space in nursing homes and other related facilities than in most public institutions. A room for medicine preparation and storage should be directly connected to the nurses' station. A utility room large enough to contain a small electric pressure sterilizer; a nonpressure utensil sterilizer with booster; and a clinical sink with drainboards, counter, and storage cabinets is needed. Provision should also be made for the storage of stretchers and wheel chairs as well as for linen-supply and general-equipment storage. In addition to the closet space provided in bedrooms for the personal possessions of patients, a unit should be provided for the storage of such bulky items as trunks, luggage, and seasonal changes of clothing.

Special consideration should be given to designing a heating system that maintains constant uniform temperatures, avoids drafts, and controls odors.

Jails

15-22. Physical Structure. Buildings which are used for jails should be structurally sound, secure, and fire-resistive and properly heated, ventilated, and lighted. The elimination of exposed wiring, wood partitions, and other combustible material is essential.

15-23. Cleanliness and Maintenance. Proper cleanliness and sanitation are absolute essentials in jail operation to maintain the health and morale of the inmates as well as to provide protection for the community against the spread of disease which might originate with the inmates. The jail authorities are obligated to maintain high standards of maintenance and repair practices through the allocation of funds in sufficient quantity to meet the needs. There is no excuse for lack of cleanliness, since a liberal supply of labor is readily available as long as the jail is occupied. This, along with soap, hot water, brushes, and mops, permits the administration to enforce the provision of a clean and sanitary building at all times. The official in charge should establish routine rules and regulations, as well as a policy, which ensure proper cleanliness, and he should then supervise the strict application of these instructions. A daily routine of work should be instituted with provision for incorporation of weekly and other periodic duties into various daily schedules. Allocation of specific tasks to prisoners, supervision of their progress, and inspection of the results should be the responsibility of paid employees rather than of trusties or other prisoners.

15-24. Examination of Inmates and Inspections. The local health officer or medical officer should examine all inmates upon admission or as soon thereafter as possible. He should also promulgate rules for care of sick prisoners and prescribe standards for isolation of all patients suspected or known to have communicable diseases. The health officer or his representative should make frequent inspections of the premises for insanitary or unsafe conditions. Likewise, the fire marshal should be called upon to assist the jail administration in maintaining proper fire safety facilities and services.

15-25. Lighting and Ventilation. The building should be well lighted, ventilated, and heated to promote a healthful and clean environment. All cells should receive some natural light, and the artificial lighting should be sufficient throughout the building to permit easy visibility at all times. Cells, dormitories, dayrooms, and work areas should have sufficient artificial light to permit reading without eyestrain.

The interior of the jail should be of a durable finish which permits effective cleaning. The surfaces should be light in color to reflect light effectively. The pastel colors also tend to make the environment more pleasant and materially assist in promoting cleanliness.

Natural ventilation is not always sufficient to keep the air fresh and free from disagreeable odors, especially during periods of inclement weather. The use of a forced-air ventilation system has many advantages, since it can be designed to operate effectively in all types of weather. The heating system should be so installed that a uniform temperature can be maintained throughout the building. It is preferable to have a day temperature of 68 to 72°F and a night temperature of 60°F in the cells and dormitories, offices, guardrooms, and similar areas.

15-26. Water Supply and Sewerage. The water-supply and sewage disposal systems are usually a part of the community system, so that other local authorities are responsible for the provision of the necessary safeguards. The installation of sanitary drinking fountains throughout the jail is essential, and if the water is tepid to warm, it may be advisable to provide coolers. In those rare instances where the jail must maintain its own water-supply or sewage disposal systems, the standards for individual systems explained in Chaps. 2 and 4, respectively, should be applied. Under these circumstances it is also advisable to request the local health authorities to make inspections and tests at regular intervals.

15-27. Pest Control. Vermin, insect, and rodent control is an essential administrative responsibility. The building should be ratproof, and every effort to eliminate rat feeding or harborage in the immediate vicinity should be applied. Likewise, all exterior windows and doors should be effectively screened, and insect breeding on or near the jail premises should be eliminated. Head and body lice, bedbugs, and roaches can be effectively controlled by thorough inspection of the new prisoners and their garments; enforcement of high standards of personal hygiene, including frequent bathing and laundering of clothes, bed linen, bath towels, and other washable items; and maintenance of clean premises, particularly the kitchen, dining room, and prisoners' living quarters. Personal cleanliness should include required bathing for all prisoners at least twice a week and daily bathing for food handlers, cleaning personnel, and prisoners who do heavy labor. If possible, any prisoner should be permitted to bathe daily if he so desires. In the event of an infestation of vermin, insects, or rodents, the services of a competent exterminator should be engaged.

A well-secured enclosure which is clean, free from sharp or dangerous objects, and well drained should be provided for outdoor exercise of all prisoners. If an outdoor area is not available, a well-ventilated enclosure which admits sunlight should be provided.

15-28. Food Service. The food for prisoners should be procured, prepared, and served in accordance with the provisions cited in Chap. 7. Since prisoner labor is available, every effort should be made to operate a food service within the jail rather than to obtain food from an outside source, except in extremely small jails. Three meals should be served daily; however, if only two meals can be provided, the quantity of food supplied should be the same. The serving periods should be spaced to avoid any unduly long period without food. Prisoners are interested in the quantity, taste appeal, and variety of food rather than in its nutritional value. Good and attractive food proves valuable in maintaining discipline, high morale, and reasonable health, whereas monotonous or unpalatable food is a source of illness and resentment and may even provoke violence or an attempted jailbreak.

While the prisoner helpers in the food service should be inspected for communicable disease and closely supervised for cleanliness, it is essential that a well-qualified employee-cook, capable of planning menus and preparing and serving food in an appetizing manner, be in charge of the kitchen and dining room.

15-29. Cell Furnishings. Each cell or dormitory room should be equipped with a metal bed and a clean mattress, mattress cover, pillow, pillowcase, sheets, and blankets for each inmate. There should also be a cabinet or locker for each inmate's personal belongings, a stool or chair, and a table. Each room or cell should have a trash container and a unit for the disposition of cigarettes. The cells should have a washbowl and a water closet, and community facilities may be used in dormitory rooms. There should be one shower for each 15 inmates and one water closet and one lavatory for each eight prisoners where community facilities are used. The cell should be designed to provide 50 sq ft of floor space for each prisoner, and in the case of dormitory rooms additional space is highly desirable.

Bibliography

1. School Health Program: An Outline, *Public Health Service Bull.* 834, 1960.
2. Environmental Engineering for the School, *Public Health Service Bull.* 856, 1960.

3. "School Lighting," Large Lamp Department, General Electric Co., Cleveland, Ohio.
4. "American Standard Guide for School Lighting," Illuminating Engineering Society, New York, 1962.
5. "Report of the Coordinating Committee for a National Plumbing Code," U.S. Department of Commerce, Domestic Commerce Series, no. 28, 1962.
6. "Cleaning, Disinfection and Sterilization: A Guide for Hospitals and Related Facilities," California Department of Public Health, Berkeley, Calif., 1962.
7. Hospital Sanitation, *Sanitarian*, vol. 23, September–October, 1960.
8. Haldeman, J. C.: Design Features Affecting Asepsis in the Hospital, *Public Health Service Pub.* 930-D-9, 1963.
9. "Illuminating Engineering Society Lighting Handbook," Illuminating Engineering Society, New York, 1958.

16

OCCUPATIONAL HEALTH

16-1. Occupational health work, frequently called industrial hygiene, is concerned with conservation of the health of the worker. Insofar as it accomplishes this end it affects not only his well-being but also the prosperity of his family and the community. It also influences favorably his employer's production, labor turnover, and profits. The fact that science can eliminate work hazards and improve the worker's health has so proved itself to industrialists that the cost of such work in many of the more progressive industries is now charged off to production. This cost averages about $20 per year per employee, although it varies considerably in the various industries, but it pays returns, not only in the ways already mentioned but also in reduced absenteeism and improved employee morale.

The newer concept of occupational health embraces nonoccupational as well as occupational influences on the worker's health. It is also being extended to all the gainfully employed, not only to industrial workers; *i.e.*, the occupational hazards of the nonmanufacturing group are being studied, and protection is being applied to workers in various services, such as transportation and the utilities. The more progressive states are also becoming concerned with the 9,600,000 agricultural workers who may be exposed to various insect poisons, herbicides, fungicides, and fertilizers under conditions approximating those of manufacture. The migratory farm workers present an additional and special problem. They are particularly exposed to nonoccupational diseases by reason of their poverty, nomadic life, and lack of sanitary facilities in their usual environment.

16-2. Health Work in Industry. Authorities consider that an effective occupational health program in an industrial plant should include three types of service: medical, engineering, and safety. These services will be discussed in detail.

1. *Medical service*. This work is carried on by physicians, dentists, and nurses. It can be further subdivided as follows:

a. Physical examinations. These are given to new employees in order to eliminate those unfit for work, or those who have some latent condition which could be aggravated by a new exposure, and also to guide in assigning applicants to suitable work. Current practice tends to "preplacement" examinations since it is now recognized that certain operations can be satisfactorily performed by persons with limited disabilities. The examinations in many cases, and preferably so, are as searching as those given for life insurance. They also have a value for the workman in that they uncover both major and minor defects that he or the plant physician may take steps to remedy. Included under this activity may also be the instruction of new employees as to the occupational hazards they will encounter in the plant. Periodical physical examinations are important since they have the advantage of revealing previously unsuspected working hazards. The physician then is responsible not only for seeing that proper treatment is given but also for notifying the employer and the governmental authority having jurisdiction so that corrective measures can be taken to prevent injury to other workers. Workers known to be exposed to poisons or other hazards should be examined frequently. Periodical routine examinations are also useful in the discovery of nonoccupational defects which can be remedied before irreparable harm is done. In this phase of the examination the usual confidential relationship between doctor and patient should be preserved in order to overcome the employee's possible objections and to obtain his cooperation in the examination program.

b. Supervision over working conditions. The physician is the health officer of the plant. In this capacity he should acquaint himself with the toxic materials and harmful processes that exist there and their effects upon the workers. He should analyze sickness records as an aid to discovering hazards and be able to recommend or outline the necessary preventive measures. He should be able to interpret the engineers' reports on health hazards and apply them effectively.

c. *Health preservation in the plant.* This includes dental and optical services and treatment of injuries and illnesses. Under this heading may also be placed provision for rest and recreation and supervision or inspection of food-handling establishments. Health education should be stressed in the industrial plant. This may be the function of the nurse who treats injuries. Furthermore, the prevention of health hazards requires not only the installation of preventive measures but also their intelligent use. Hence the employee should be fully informed as to what has been done and the reasons therefor. Through educational measures he can be given an accurate evaluation of the conditions under which he works so that he will be neither unnecessarily alarmed nor unduly careless at his work. These and other aspects of health education may be discussed by the same employee groups who meet periodically to discuss the safety problems of their plant. In other words, reduction or elimination of health hazards is a product of teamwork between management and the employee.

d. *Home and community problems.* While too much work in this direction may result in the accusation of paternalism, which, by that name at least, is distasteful to many Americans, undoubtedly much can be done by visiting nurses and by industrial physicians toward bettering home conditions. At this point it may be well to point out that a few employers now realize, as in all likelihood many more will later, that the stimulation of municipalities to obtain good water and milk supplies and the application of health measures in general pay dividends to industry. Since the large industries are heavy taxpayers, their influence may do much in this respect.

2. *Engineering and safety services.* The application of engineering to industrial hygiene requires basic engineering training in addition to knowledge of ventilation; chemistry of dusts, fumes, gases, and vapors; radiation; noise; physiology; toxicology; industrial sanitation; and the broad field of public health. Many industrial plants have no engineers on their staffs, and very few have their own industrial hygiene specialists. These plants may utilize the services of the governmental industrial hygiene bureaus, Federal, state, or local, to obtain impartial surveys and expert consultation. If this is done, the plant management should assign some responsible person, preferably an engineer, to work with the industrial hygiene consultant—this, of course, in addition to the necessary cooperation with the plant physician.

The safety engineering service is more likely to be organized by the plant. It may be headed by a safety engineer or by a man who is acquainted with the processes and who is required to familiarize him-self with accident hazards and methods of prevention.

a. Engineering in occupational health. The engineer is expected to recognize potential hazards and to design or recommend suitable con-trols before they develop—preferably in the design stage of a process. If hazardous conditions or processes already exist, engineering methods leading to remedies should be applied. These are (1) the determination of the plant conditions that are causing the hazard; (2) the use of precise quantitative measurements or statistics to establish the exposure or other factors that result in injury or disease; and (3) the devising of methods of controlling or minimizing the dangerous conditions and study of their effectiveness.

b. Safety. The safety engineer has the necessary training or knowl-edge to recognize conditions or practices that might result in accidental injuries to workers. His work might well be correlated with the physical examinations mentioned above. All industrial operations must be de-signed so that they can be done safely. Moving parts likely to injure workers must be guarded. In certain operations, workmen are required to wear safety shoes, goggles, hard hats, special gloves, and other protective clothing. Women workers should wear hairnets and practical work clothes, of designs made by the U.S. Women's Bureau. Stairways and pits must have adequate hand- and guardrails. Daily inspections of all operations should be made by the safety engineer. Safety committees, made up of workmen—one for each shop and operating under a central plant committee—have been found useful in investigating accidents, formulating safety rules, making recommendations, and seeing that rules are complied with. The plant physician and safety engineer should be members of the central safety committee. Each plant should have at least one first-aid or stretcher crew composed of interested employees who have had some special training.

16-3. Programs for Small Plants. Small industrial plants cannot, of course, afford a staff of specialists in occupational health fields. In many plants, however, the employees are exposed to hazards and should receive protective services. Such services can be established, employing a part-time physician and a nurse [15]. Preferably the physician should have a knowledge of industrial hazards. He should also understand the type of program the management desires and needs. His duties will include:

1. Maintenance of a healthful environment. Since specialists will be lacking, he should recognize when they are needed and persuade the manage-ment to hire them.
2. Making diagnoses and giving treatments for illnesses.
3. Giving health examinations.
4. Keeping medical records.

5. Applying immunization procedures when they are applicable to the hazards.

6. Providing health education and counseling.

It is recommended [15] that 2 physician-hr per week be provided for the first 100 employees and 1 additional hr per week for each 100 additional employees.

16-4. Govermental Control. While some large industries are able to provide all the health services mentioned in the previous articles, the many workers in small industries must depend for health protection upon the state and local health departments, which, in turn, must be supported by adequate laws. The national laws affecting the health of workers are concerned with hours of employment of Federal employees, safety devices for railroads, and also protection of workers employed by Federal government contractors against physical and chemical occupational hazards. The states have many and varied laws governing factories and mines. Some of the earliest were concerned with inspection of steam boilers, dust removal, regulation of working hours of minors and women, and provision for fire exits. These were later followed by requirements concerning the reporting of occupational disease, the installation of safety devices, the provision of proper ventilation and lighting, and the sanitation of workrooms and toilet rooms. To enforce these requirements most states have corps of factory inspectors. In addition, all states have workmen's compensation laws applying to accidental injuries but covering some occupational diseases also.

Laws that are more specific and comprehensive are required. Preferably such laws, or city ordinances, should be enabling in their nature. This would allow health officials to make and enforce regulations and would have the advantage of flexibility to meet changing conditions.

16-5. Organization for Occupational Health. The real and potential progress in the field of industrial hygiene is indicated by the fact that over forty states have industrial hygiene services in actual operation on the state level. In addition to this, many of the larger municipalities, such as Detroit, Houston, and Los Angeles, have full-time industrial hygiene programs, while over 254 other city health departments are prepared to offer some type of related service in this field. However, most of these cities provide more extensive services of a technical nature in cooperation with the state occupational health organization. In most states, the work is in a separate division or bureau of the health department, where it is also identified occasionally as the industrial hygiene division or the industrial health division. In a few states, it is a function of the labor department. The Navy, Army, Air Force, and Atomic Energy Commission have well-organized industrial health units which conduct programs and surveys of their major installations. The

Navy has an industrial hygienist at most of its shore stations. The Army and Air Force have traveling teams to cover the United States and some overseas installations.

A separate occupational health unit of a state or city has a director who may be a physician, an engineer, or a chemist. The work is divided between a medical section and an engineering section. The physician handles medical and clinical investigations of occupational diseases and serves as a connecting link between industry and the various preventive medical services offered by the state health department. Such contact will also include consultation and cooperation with the health services provided by the larger industries of the state.

The engineer handles all problems concerned with environmental control of industrial hazards, makes investigations in industrial plants, and collects samples as needed. He is the connecting link between industry and the environmental-control services offered by the state health department.

The laboratory is separate from other state laboratories and is available for such medical, chemical, and biological tests as may be required. Administratively it is responsible to the director, but the physician and engineer work directly with it, the former for medical laboratory work and the latter for engineering investigations.

Nursing consultation is carried on under the direction of the physician with as much coordination as may be necessary on the part of the engineer.

Many variations are noted from the above type of organization, whether in the state or municipal service. If the unit is in the bureau of sanitary engineering, the medical services are obtained as needed from some other bureau, probably that for control of communicable diseases, which may have a specialist in industrial medicine. Or all the technicians, physicians, engineers, and nurses may work together in the same office as a functional unit; however, each type of personnel will be administratively responsible to some bureau, for example, the physicians to the bureau of communicable disease and the engineers to the bureau of sanitary engineering. The general health department laboratory may perform the laboratory services needed.

The Public Health Service has a Division of Occupational Health in Washington, D.C., a Research and Training Facility in Cincinnati, and an Occupational Health Field Station in Salt Lake City. It works closely with the other four environmental health divisions of the Bureau of State Services of the Public Health Service. This organization carries on extensive research work in the field of occupational health hazards, offers related laboratory services, and assists in organizing state work and training its personnel. Results of research and major field studies are published in bulletins and technical publications. It also provides a directory, which is revised periodically, of all local, state, and Federal government industrial hygiene personnel.

16-6. Occupational Hazards. Most processes and operations of industry involve one or more potential threats to the health and safety of the worker. These are called occupational hazards, and most of them may be eliminated, or much reduced, by the application of engineering methods. Lists of these hazards are available from various sources [1, 2]. Very broad classifications of the most important hazards are given below:

1. Excessive air temperatures and humidities, radiant heat, and cold
2. Compressed air
3. Dust, fumes, and gases
4. Poisons
5. Excessive noise
6. Poor illumination, glare, and extreme light
7. Repeated motion, pressure, or shock
8. Infections
9. Radiation hazards
10. Accidents
11. Poor plant sanitation

16-7. Industrial Poisons. In many industries, poisonous materials are produced or used or appear as impurities in otherwise safe substances. Some occur as gases, fumes, mists, vapors, or dusts which are breathed with the air; others are liquids or solids which may be absorbed through the skin. Some which are solids or liquids may form fumes or gases and thus be absorbed in several ways. Note that the poisons mentioned are not ingested and that, generally speaking, industrial poisons are not taken through the mouth, although it is possible for a workman to handle food while he has poison on his hands. Inspired poisons are far more important. As an example, a person can safely ingest twenty times the lead concentration which, if inhaled, would show systemic toxic effects.

Poisons absorbed through the skin may cause dermatitis, or skin inflammation, which is a common industrial ailment. In some cases it may occur as an individual sensitivity to a substance, or allergy, when other workers have no difficulty. One of the common industrial poisonings is due to lead, either from breathing fumes, dust, or droplets or from contact. Particularly hazardous is spray painting with lead paints or molten lead. Brush painting is less dangerous. The manufacture of storage batteries and leaded gasolines and the pouring of leaded steel and iron are hazardous. Lead poisoning also occurs during the smelting of lead and the glazing of china and earthenware and in the printing trades. The preparation of arsenic and the making of commercial poisons have also been found to be dangerous. In the zinc, brass, and copper trades the fumes of the metals themselves and their impurities are deleterious. Carbon monoxide, a product of incomplete combustion, has caused deaths through the agency of blast furnaces and in mine explosions and from being inhaled in various exhausts. Mercury poisoning was formerly found among hatters and in trades where amalgams of mercury are used. Benzol and other coal-tar products, petroleum products, and many new organic solvents used as spray-paint thinners and degreasing agents represent other occupational hazards. The cleaning agent carbon tetrachloride has figured in many poisoning cases. Mention should also be made of beryllium, which is widely used in the atomic energy program; toluene diisocyanate and other diisocyanates used in polyurethane foams, which cause response at very low levels; the epoxy resins, which cause severe dermatitis; and toxic fuels and oxidizers used in rocketry, such as unsymmetrical dimethyl hydrazine, liquid fluorine, and nitrogen trioxide. A list of poisons and threshold limits is given in Appendix B.

The prevention of sickness and death from these causes requires recognition of the hazard and the application of expert medical and engineering knowledge. These measures cannot be discussed in detail here, although some general rules for the protection of workers may be mentioned:

1. Construction of buildings so that the dangerous processes are isolated.

2. Use of apparatus that is adapted to its special purpose, kept in good order, and constructed, as far as possible, to prevent escape of dangerous materials.

3. Use of exhaust fans and ducts, placed as close to the source as possible, so that poisonous airborne materials are removed quickly. These require careful design, with due consideration to the character of the dust, fumes, or gases and the allowable concentration of the deleterious material in the air [3].

4. Avoidance, as far as possible, of direct contact between the workmen and dangerous substances.

5. Replacement of particularly dangerous production methods with less dangerous methods and substitution of less dangerous chemicals or agents for the more dangerous ones, even though greater production expense results thereby. This is often not feasible.

6. Instruction of workmen as to the hazards of the process they are working in, with frequent repetition of such instructions. The workmen should be instructed in the signs of the poisoning or other injury that may be expected and in the importance of consulting with the plant physician when suspicious signs appear. They should also be taught the precautions that should be taken to avoid poisoning or other injury. Warning placards should be used to supplement other instructions.

7. Supervision of dangerous operations by responsible and well-informed persons.

8. Employment of all personal means appropriate to the hazards encoun-

tered, such as suitable clothing, gloves, goggles, and respirators. These devices should not, however, replace the better alternative of attacking the basic causes of the hazards. Furthermore, such safety devices are not always used and may get out of order or otherwise lose their efficiency without being suspected. The only respiratory equipment that should be used is that which has the approval of the U.S. Bureau of Mines and the U.S. Department of Agriculture [5, 6].

9. Periodical medical examinations with provision for transferring workmen who show signs of poisoning to other occupations.

10. Requiring of body cleanliness on the part of workers. This includes bathing and changing of clothing at the end of the working day. Work clothing must be frequently cleaned in nonhazardous ways. This requirement places upon the industry the responsibility of furnishing suitable clothing lockers, washrooms, and shower baths.

11. Lunches should not be eaten in the workrooms. This requires the industry to furnish lunchroom facilities.

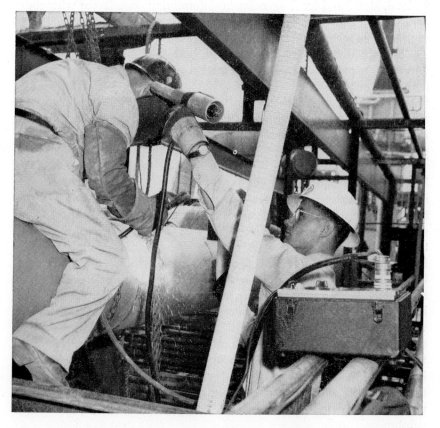

FIGURE 16-1 Portable equipment used to collect welding fumes. (*Photograph courtesy of J. W. Hammond, Humble Oil and Refining Company.*)

Many of the industrial poisons are airborne, such as fumes, gases, dusts, and vapors, and are difficult to collect and determine. The impinger or the electrostatic precipitator may be used if it is known that the poisonous material is a dust. Impingers are also useful for most toxic gases. Sampling methods have been developed for many atmospheric contaminants, and concentrations which may be tolerated by workmen have been established for some [4, 8].

16-8. Threshold-limit Values. As a result of many observations and much experience, much has been learned of the effects of certain substances upon workers, and this knowledge has been translated into allowable concentrations. The knowledge is by no means complete, and especially where the experience is limited, there are differences of opinion as to threshold limits. Each year the Threshold Limits Committee of the American Conference of Governmental Industrial Hygienists reviews the list of threshold-limit values published the preceding year. The 1963 list appears in Appendix B. These values serve as a guide for Federal, state, and local agencies in determining compliance with codes or safe practices and are helpful to industry as bases for the design of protective measures.

Threshold limits are based on the best available information from industrial experience, from experimental studies, and, when possible, from a combination of the two. These values are based on various criteria of toxic effects or on marked discomfort; thus, they should not be used as a common denominator of toxicity, nor should they be considered the sole criterion in proving or disproving diagnosis of suspected occupational disease.

Threshold-limit values should be used as guides in the control of health hazards and should not be regarded as fine lines between safe and dangerous concentrations. They represent conditions under which it is believed that nearly all workers may be repeatedly exposed, day after day, without adverse effect. The values listed in Appendix B refer to time-weighted average concentrations for a normal workday of 8 hr for persons in average health. The amount by which these figures may be exceeded for short periods without injury to health depends upon a number of factors such as the nature of the contaminant, whether very high concentrations even for short periods produce acute poisoning, whether the effects are cumulative, the frequency with which high concentrations occur, and the duration of such periods. All must be taken into consideration in arriving at a decision as to whether a hazardous situation exists. Special consideration should be given to the application of these values in assessing the health hazards which may be associated with exposure to combinations of two or more substances.

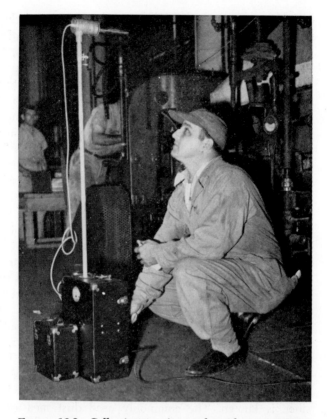

FIGURE 16-2 Collecting an air sample with a precipitator to determine the lead content near a soldering machine used in can making. (*Courtesy of Texas State Department of Health.*)

16-9. **The Dust Hazard.** Workers in many industries are exposed to a serious health hazard as a result of dust inhalation. The injurious effects of inhalation of a harmful dust are proportional to the amount of dust breathed, which, in turn, is related to the amount of dust in the atmosphere and the length of time it is breathed.

Dusts may be classified as inert, irritating, or toxic. The inert ones do not poison the body, although they may cause undesirable effects. Irritating dusts have an immediate and local effect. They include lime and other caustics, picric acid, soap powder, and some cereal dusts. Toxic dusts are differentiated from irritating dusts in that they result in remote or systemic poisoning rather than immediate local effects.

The inert dusts include those of vegetable and animal origin, such as are encountered in woolen and carpet manufacturing, spinning and weaving, and jute and paper manufacturing, and they are less harmful than other types, although a considerable amount of respiratory disease is attributed to them. Metallic and mineral dusts, to which grinders, polishers, printers, and file and tool workers are exposed, are considered more dangerous in predisposing persons to respiratory disease.

Dusts containing silica, which are incident to stonecutting, sandblasting, rock drilling, and certain processes in coal mining, are especially dangerous. Silica enters into a chemical reaction in the lungs to form fibrous tissue, the resulting injury being known as "silicosis," which in turn sets up conditions favorable for a fatal pulmonary tuberculosis. Asbestos dust has the same effect as silica, the resulting disease being known as "asbestosis," with pulmonary tuberculosis as the aftermath. Preventive measures include mechanical removal of the dusts by exhaust systems, which should be properly designed and then tested to make sure that they are reducing the atmospheric dust content below the danger point; enclosure of the work, such as the barrel method of sandblasting; the use of wet processes to diminish dust production; and the requirement that workmen wear respirators or helmets (either plain or, in especially dangerous processes, with special air supplies pumped under pressure to the helmets) over the nose and mouth.

Threshold limits of atmospheric dust contents, as given in Appendix B, are expressed in millions of particles per cubic foot as measured by various types of apparatus. Also given is a formula for determining the allowable number of particles of siliceous dusts when the per cent of silica is known. The commonly used dust measurer is known as the "Greenburg-Smith impinger." It consists of a pump which draws the air to be sampled through a glass tube and impinges it at high velocity against a glass plate which is submerged in water, or other suitable liquid, in a flask. The dust is arrested, wetted by the liquid, and trapped. After sufficient air has been sampled, a portion of the liquid is removed to a suitable counting chamber or cell for a microscopic count of the particles. Another type is the electrostatic precipitator, which can be used for the collection of dusts, fumes, and mists for chemical analyses.

16-10. Radiation Hazards. The general subject of radiation hazards and protections is discussed in Chap. 17. The industrial use of radioactive compounds, such as luminous paints, has long been recognized as a serious industrial health hazard. In textile and paper mills radioactive static eliminators which are improperly shielded or stored have been reported. Radioactivity is much used in industry for density and thickness gages, oil-well logging, element tracing, and nondestructive inspection of welding. In the future, as nuclear energy is adapted for industrial purposes and as betatrons, radioactive isotopes, and atomic power piles become commonplace, the accompanying hazards from both dangerous radiation and radioactive salts and gases will increase the demands for

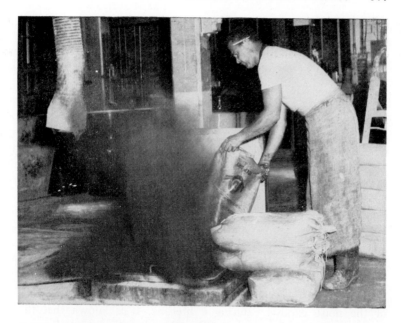

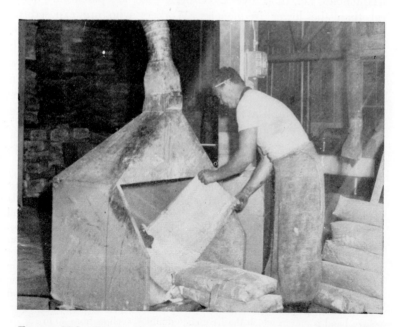

FIGURE 16-3 Upper, emptying paint pigment sacks without a hood; lower, the same process under a hood. (*Photographs courtesy of J. W. Hammond, Humble Oil and Refining Company.*)

industrial hygiene services. Uranium mining is now presenting a hazard to workers, as shown by an excess of deaths from lung cancer.

16-11. Industrial Noise. Noise, which is defined as unwanted sound, is a problem of municipal and industrial environments. A discussion of noise as a municipal problem will be found in Arts. 18-10 and 18-11. Probably most important is the undesirable hearing change resulting from long exposures to noises at high pressure levels. This has become legally significant since the courts may award compensation to workers who have suffered hearing losses resulting from industrial exposure.

Sound levels or pressures are expressed in decibels,[1] and frequencies in cycles per second. Different frequency levels are not perceived equally by all persons, and also high-frequency sounds are perceived to be louder or noisier than low-frequency sounds of the same sound-pressure level. Therefore, loudness of a sound will not be the same to all persons, and two sounds of the same pressure level will not be equally loud.

The effects of noise exposure on hearing will depend upon (1) the pressure level of the noise, (2) the frequency of the noise, (3) the distribution of the exposure during a workday, and (4) the total duration of the noise exposure during a lifetime. It is known that the higher frequencies, *i.e.*, those over 2,000 cycles/sec, are potentially more harmful than the lower frequencies. Workers who are exposed to noise levels that exceed 85 db in frequencies of 600 to 4,800 cycles/sec will notice a slight change of hearing, or temporary threshold of hearing shift, at the end of the day. This has some relation to a permanent threshold shift. There are indications that this may lead to a permanent threshold shift after an exposure of 5 to 10 years, although much research is required to establish this relationship. Obviously, if audiometer tests of temporary threshold shifts would permit the prediction of future permanent hearing impairment of workers, preventive measures would

[1] Strictly speaking, the decibel rating of a sound is a ratio, and as generally used it is the ratio of the level of the sound in question to the smallest sound distinguishable to the human ear. For example, if the levels of two sounds are as 10:1, the sounds differ by 10 db; if they are as 100:1 (or 10^2:1), the sounds differ by 20 db; if they are as 1,000:1 (or 10^3:1), they differ by 30 db. Stated mathematically, the common logarithm of the sound-level ratio multiplied by 10 expresses the ratio in decibels. The bel is the basic unit, but the decibel, which is 0.1 bel, is more convenient for practical use. Noise-measuring instruments show sound levels in decibels as compared with the smallest sound distinguishable to the human ear.

The frequency of a sound in cycles per second is also important. Sound levels, therefore, are frequently measured and reported in octave bands of frequency. An octave band is one in which the frequency doubles, such as from 20 to 75; 75 to 150; 150 to 300; 300 to 600; 600 to 1,200; 1,200 to 2,400; and 2,400 to 4,800, all in cycles per second. Some sound-level meters have scales and filter networks that provide a single measure of sound level that weights the middle and high frequencies and thus correlates better with the loudness level than the over-all sound-pressure level does.

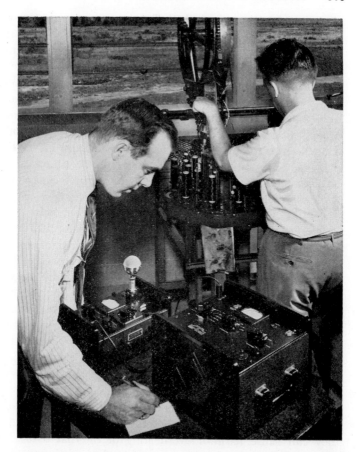

FIGURE 16-4   Noise-evaluation study being made with a sound-level meter and frequency analyzer in an industrial shop. (*Photograph courtesy of General Radio Corporation, Cambridge, Mass.*)

be more readily applied and accepted. A great deal of research is required, however, concerning exposures at various levels and frequencies before a valid method of making predictions can be formulated. The matter is further complicated by the fact that the ears of some persons are more easily injured by noise than the ears of others. The average worker will not be aware of hearing impairment until it affects the speech range, *i.e.*, 500 to 2,000 cycles/sec. Noise apparently has no other health effect than hearing impairment. Nervousness, stress, and other effects reported from exposure to loud noises are overcome by adaptation.

   In most industries where injuriously loud noises exist, the noise volume cannot be reduced to a safe level by the use of sound-absorbing walls or sound-conditioning of machinery. Injury can be prevented only by reducing the noise level of the sound reaching the inner ear. Cotton in the ears does not provide sufficient protection, but properly worn ear protectors will reduce most noises to a safe level [12, 13, 14].

16-12. Light as a Hazard. Ultraviolet light and infrared light, which are given off by glowing metals, are hazards to furnacemen, glassworkers, and electro-welders. Ultraviolet light causes conjunctivitis, skin burn, and skin cancer. Welding with the inert-gas metal arc emits ten to twenty times as much ultraviolet light as the common metal-arc process using heavily coated electrodes and is, therefore, much more dangerous. Infrared light, which is also emitted in welding, causes eye damage, and long exposure may result in cataracts. Protection for welders is obtained by wearing reflective helmets and clothing. For other workers, safety glasses may be sufficient.

16-13. Heat. The effects of excessive heat may be noted among stokers, smelters, blast furnacemen, glassworkers, kiln and pottery men, etc. The effects of heat will progress through the comfort zone to discomfort—where personnel problems, error increase, and possibly reduction of output may be expected—and will finally cause physiological strain. The physiological effects are colic and cramps, heat exhaustion, and heat stroke. For persons at rest, effective temperatures (see Art. 10-8) should not exceed 90°F; for sedentary workers, not over 85°F; and for men engaged in heavy work, not over 80°F. Protection against heat may be attained by insulating and enclosing heat sources, by shielding workers from radiant heat, and by using local exhaust ventilation and general building ventilation [17, 18].

Microwaves, which are used in connection with radar equipment, may be considered a hazard. At frequencies of less than 1,000 megacycles, they can cause harmful overheating of internal tissues. The hazard is minimized by restriction of persons from hazardous areas.

16-14. Compressed Air. Divers and workmen in caissons who work in air at greater than atmospheric pressure are exposed to a disease known as the bends. The increased pressure causes air to be dissolved in the blood, a condition which is not dangerous unless the air pressure is suddenly greatly reduced. Bubbles of nitrogen then form in the veins and arteries and interfere with circulation, collapse and death being very likely to occur. The danger is overcome by reducing the air pressure gradually. Deep-sea divers are raised to the surface in successive stages. After leaving work, caisson workers are held in a special air lock or chamber for several hours while the pressure is slowly reduced. This permits the dissolved nitrogen to leave the blood without bubble formation.

16-15. Repeated Motion, Vibration, Pressure, and Shock. Using the same muscles in the same motion for many hours in the day may affect them so that the worker loses the ability to continue the operation, although the muscles respond to his will in all other respects. This condition is called an "occupational neurosis." The well-known writer's cramp is an example, but trap drummers, cigar rollers, milkers, engravers, dancers, letter sorters, and followers of many other occupations are sometimes affected. The use of vibratory tools in industry, especially in automobile and aircraft factories, is increasing. No one knows very much about the effects of vibration at the present; however, the Occupational Health Program of the Public Health Service is currently studying this particular type of exposure. Rest and medical attention are required by the victims of this condition.

16-16. Infections. Certain occupations present hazards from infections. Anthrax has occurred among tanners, hide handlers, and workers in leather and hair. As far as possible, hides and hair should be disinfected. Workers with open cuts should not handle unsterilized hides or hair; gloves should be worn; and washing facilities are necessary. Dust can be reduced by ventilation but should be removed by downward ventilation to carry the dangerous material away from the faces of the workers. Dairymen, butchers, and slaughterhouse employees are exposed to brucellosis, or undulant fever. Millers, dishwashers, and cigar makers are liable to fungus diseases.

Metalworkers use oily or soapy liquids to cool the metal while it is being cut. Such cutting compounds are used and returned many times. Frequently they become vehicles for large numbers of pus-forming bacteria and are responsible for spreading wound infections and furunculosis (boils). The remedy is sterilization of the compound by heat in a central reservoir before it is recirculated. Some of the newer disinfectants are now being investigated and may prove satisfactory to add to cutting compounds.

Plant Sanitation

16-17. The sanitation of industrial plants is directed toward obtaining proper conditions for conserving health and improving the efficiency of the worker. This includes proper ventilation, heating, and lighting; the furnishing of pure drinking water; adequate toilet facilities; adequate and clean lunchrooms; and good housekeeping of the plant in general. A highly important provision is the delegation of responsibility for sanitary conditions to some qualified person. In factories having organized medical or health services, the necessary inspections should be made by some member of the health organization. Leaving this important matter to the individual foremen of various departments is unsatisfactory. Even in the smaller plants, where more dependence must be placed upon state or city factory inspectors, instructions, responsibility, and the necessary authority should be given to some permanent member of the working force. It has been suggested that the personnel manager be charged with this responsibility because of his advantageous relationship with labor and management.

16-18. Ventilation. The ventilation of industrial plants should be based upon the comfort standard discussed in Chap. 10, considering the activity required of the worker by his occupation. This may change the usual relationships of temperature, humidity, and air movement to bring the atmospheric conditions into the comfort zone. Natural or artificial means may be employed to get this result. An additional requirement is that at least 20 sq ft of floor space and 200 cu ft of air space be provided for each workman.

In addition to what may be called normal ventilation, the problem of removing injurious dusts, fumes, vapors, and gases must be solved. This requires exhaust systems that should be designed by experienced engineers to remove the undesirable substances at their source. Of equal importance is the fact that such systems should be operated at all times when protection is needed and that they should be properly maintained.

Ventilation systems, particularly in the Northern states, sometimes include recirculation of air in order to conserve heat. Recirculation of air containing toxic dusts is not permitted by some states, even after cleaning. Cleaning and recirculating of exhaust air containing odorous, irritating, or toxic gases and vapors is generally not practical.

16-19. Illumination. Many states have adopted lighting codes to ensure sufficient lighting to reduce unnecessary eyestrain and to prevent accidents. Table 16-1 gives standards for some representative industrial operations. The illumination should be measured by a foot-candle meter at the place of work with due attention to proper brightness ratios and prevention of glare. Supplementary lighting is sometimes necessary to give proper illumination for special types of work. Here also care should be taken to avoid high brightness ratios in the field of vision. A ratio of 10:1 should not be exceeded, and 5:1 is a preferable limit.

16-20. Water Supply. The supply should, of course, be pure, satisfying the standards of the Public Health Service. If the water is derived from a private source, precautions outlined in Chap. 2 should be applied to prevent contamination, and tests should be made periodically. Not less than 20 gal per capita per working day is required for drinking, washing, and other purposes. The consumption of drinking water alone varies from 2 qt to 2 gal, depending on the type of work and the temperature.

A possible danger is the use of unsafe supplies for fire-protection or industrial purposes. Too often the auxiliary water is accessible for drinking by careless or uninformed workmen, or if the two supplies are cross-connected, the supposedly safe supply may become polluted. Cross-connections are so dangerous that they should not be permitted.

Table 16-1.   RECOMMENDED MINIMUM LEVELS OF ILLUMINATION
FOR CERTAIN INDUSTRIAL PLANTS

Foot-candles on tasks

Automobile manufacturing:	
Frame assembly	50
Chassis assembly line	100
Final assembly and inspection line	200*
Body manufacturing:	
Parts	70
Assembly	100
Finishing and inspecting	200*
Meat packing:	
Slaughtering	30
Cleaning, cutting, cooking, grinding, canning, packing	100
Jewelry and watch manufacturing	500*
Shoe manufacturing, leather:	
Cutting and stitching	300*
Making and finishing	200
Materials handling:	
Wrapping, packing, labeling	50
Picking stock, classifying	30
Loading, trucking	20
Inside truck bodies and freight cars	10
Cloth products industries:	
Cloth inspection	2000*
Cutting	300*
Sewing	500*
All plants, toilets and washrooms	30

* Obtained with a combination of general lighting plus specialized supplementary lighting. Care should be taken to keep within recommended brightness ratios.

SOURCE: "Illuminating Engineering Society Lighting Handbook," Illuminating Engineering Society, New York, 1958.

Exposed piping should be distinctively colored or lettered, and taps or faucets on unsafe supplies should be placarded or removed.

The common drinking cup should be prohibited in favor of drinking fountains, readily accessible and preferably furnishing water at not under 46°F. The number of fountains required varies from one for 50 men to one for 200 men, depending upon the plant arrangement. See Table 11-1.

16-21. Toilet Facilities. Observation of many plants indicates that the workmen may be protected against plant hazards but not against those of the toilet room and washroom. In all toilet rooms the floor and sidewalls should be impervious to moisture to a height of 6 in., including the angle formed by the floor and sidewalls. Floors, sidewalls, and ceilings should have an easily cleaned finish. Toilet rooms and washrooms should have window openings to the outside air or should be provided with ventilation systems which provide at least six air changes per hour. The glass window surface should not be less than 10 per cent of the floor area. If insufficient natural illumination is available, artificial light should be provided at the level of 30 ft-c.

Water closets, lavatories, and sinks should be of porcelain or vitreous china. The most sanitary water-closet seats are of impervious material and are either U-shaped or split type (open front and back). Water-closet bowls should be set free from all enclosing walls and should be so installed that space around them can be easily cleaned. If the washroom is not combined with the toilet room, one or more washing faucets should be placed in the toilet room. For the number of water closets, urinals, lavatories, and showers required in manufacturing establishments, see Table 11-1.

The recommended type of urinal is the vitreous-china individual stall with the waste pipe in the floor. They may be located at convenient points in the plant, but there should always be urinals in the toilet room.

Washing faucets are more desirable than the individual washbasin or lavatory because they are less likely to spread infections among the users. Hot and cold water should run from the same faucet, and it is desirable that there be automatic regulation of the hot water to not more than 125°F. Circular wash fountains with treadle-operated water valves and soap dispensers have been found satisfactory. Liquid soap in dispensing containers, rather than cake soap, should be furnished, and no common towels should be used.

Showers should discharge at an angle from the wall rather than from overhead. Hoods may be advisable to carry off vapors. As much privacy as possible should be provided in baths and dressing rooms, particularly where women are employed.

The floors and ceilings of locker rooms should conform to the requirements for toilet rooms and washrooms. In fact, locker rooms and washrooms are frequently combined. A well-ventilated locker should be furnished to every employee. The room itself also requires good ventilation, or the odors from used clothing will be noticeable. An alternative to lockers is the ceiling hook, an arrangement which allows complete drying and airing of clothing. Each workman is allotted a combination of two hooks and a wire basket for shoes, etc., all of which are attached to a chain which runs over a pulley suspended close to the ceiling. After the clothing is raised to the ceiling, the chain is locked to a device below. This system has been widely used at steel plants, mines, and chemical works.

Where 10 or more women are employed at any one time, at least one retiring room should be provided for their exclusive use. The space provided should be at least 60 sq ft of floor area, with an increase of 2 sq ft for each additional woman employee above 10. At least one couch or bed should be provided where 10 women are employed. The recommended minimum number of beds is one for 100 women or less; two beds for 100 to 250; and one additional for each additional 250 women employed.

It is of great importance that janitors be made responsible for the condition of toilet rooms, washrooms, and locker rooms and for the placement of soap, towels, and paper. But this is not sufficient. There should be frequent inspections of the rooms by responsible executives of the plant staff.

Where employees are permitted to eat their lunches at their place of employment, a space should be provided for this purpose that will be adequate for as many workers as may wish to use it at one time. A covered receptacle is supplied for waste food, paper, etc., and employees should be required to use it for the disposal of all such wastes. No employee should be permitted to eat any food where there are poisonous materials or other substances injurious to health.

Bibliography

1. Occupational Hazards and Diagnostic Signs, *U.S. Dep. Labor Bull.* 582.
2. Hunter, D.: "The Diseases of Occupations," Little, Brown and Company, Boston, 1955.
3. Brandt, A.: "Industrial Health Engineering," John Wiley & Sons, Inc., New York, 1947.
4. Jacobs, M. D.: "The Analytical Chemistry of Industrial Poisons, Hazards and Solvents," 2d ed., Interscience Publishers, Inc., New York, 1949.
5. "Information Circular No. 785," U.S. Bureau of Mines, Washington, D.C.
6. Respiratory Devices against Certain Insecticides, *U.S. Dep. Agr. ARS* 33-76, Supplement 1, April, 1963.
7. The Industrial Environment: Its Evaluation and Control, *Public Health Service Pub.* 614.
8. "Air Sampling Instruments," American Conference of Governmental Industrial Hygienists, Cincinnati, Ohio, 1960.
9. Drinker, P., and T. Hatch: "Industrial Dust," 2d ed., McGraw-Hill Book Company, New York, 1954.
10. Patty, F. A. (ed.): "Industrial Hygiene and Toxicology," 2d ed., vols. I and II, Interscience Publishers, Inc., New York, 1958.
11. "Industrial Ventilation: A Manual of Recommended Practice," 7th ed., Conference of Industrial Hygienists, Committee on Industrial Ventilation, Cincinnati, Ohio, 1962.
12. Glorig, A.: The Problem of Noise in Industry, *Am. J. Public Health,* vol. 51, no. 9, September, 1961.
13. Clark, W. E., and A. C. Pietrasanta: Community and Industrial Noise, *Am. J. Public Health,* vol. 51, no. 9, September, 1961.
14. Yaffe, C. C., and H. H. Jones: Noise and Hearing, *Public Health Service Pub.* 850, 1961.
15. Guide to Small Plant Occupational Health Program, Committee on Public

and Professional Affairs of the Council on Occupational Health, *Arch. Environ. Health,* vol. 5, no. 4, October, 1962.

16. "Illuminating Engineering Society Lighting Handbook," Illuminating Engineering Society, New York, 1958.
17. "Industrial Ventilation: Manual of Recommended Practice," Committee on Industrial Ventilation, American Conference of Governmental Hygienists, Lansing, Mich.
18. Lee, D. H. K.: "Heat and Cold Effects and Their Control," Course Manual, Public Health Service.

17

RADIOLOGICAL SANITATION

17-1. Radiological health, which is the public health aspect of the use of ionizing radiation, is becoming increasingly important as nuclear energy is used to an ever-increasing extent in medicine and industry. Radiological sanitation is necessary to prevent human injury since it is the environmental factors, such as air, water, food, and industrial operations, which bring radioactive material into the human body or into dangerous proximity to it. The use of radioactivity in medical work requires environmental safeguards to prevent injury to using personnel and office workers. The specialist in radiological health and safety is found in major hospitals where radioactive materials are used, where reactors are operated, and on the staffs of state health departments and

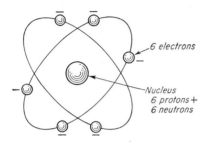

6 electrons

Nucleus
6 protons+
6 neutrons

FIGURE 17-1   The atom of carbon 12. It
is stable and occurs in nature.

the larger local health departments. The sanitary engineer and sanitarian, under present conditions, should have some knowledge of radiological hazards to health and protection therefrom.

17-2. Atomic Structure. All matter is made up of atoms.[1] The atom consists of a nucleus surrounded by a group of electrons moving orbitally about it. The nucleus is made up of particles called protons and neutrons. The proton has a positive electric charge. It is very small, but its mass is some two thousand times that of the electron. The neutron is neutral in charge and has about the same mass as a proton and an electron combined. A free neutron will spontaneously split into a proton and an electron. The electron has a very small mass and a negative electric charge. Normally the atom is electrically neutral, having equal numbers of positively charged protons in the nucleus and negatively charged electrons in orbit.

The number of protons or electrons present in a chemical element is called the atomic number, and each element has an atomic number according to the number of its protons or electrons. For example, one isotope of hydrogen, the simplest element, has only one proton and one electron, and thus its atomic number is 1. A stable isotope of lithium has three protons and three electrons, and its number is 3. The atomic number for chlorine is 17; for iron, 26; and for lead, 82. The atomic number of an element should be distinguished from its mass number, which is based upon the mass or quantity of matter in its nucleus. It is the mass number which is used in making chemical calculations in which mass is involved, and it is the sum of the protons and neutrons.

An atom of the same element may have differing numbers of neutrons in its nucleus. Chemically it remains the same, but its mass is slightly different. These slightly varying atoms of the same element are known as isotopes. Every element has three or more known isotopes; for example, hydrogen, as mentioned above, has one proton and one electron in its atom, with an atomic number 1 and mass number 1. But there are other isotopes of hydrogen. One has a single neutron in its nucleus in addition to its single proton. The atomic number remains the

[1] A glossary of radiological terms is provided in Appendix C; they are not defined in this chapter except where some explanation is considered necessary.

same, but the mass number is 2. Another hydrogen isotope has two neutrons in the nucleus, and its mass number is 3. These three isotopes are known as hydrogen 1, hydrogen 2, and hydrogen 3. They are also called protium, deuterium, and tritium, respectively. In so-called "heavy water," the hydrogen component is deuterium. It is used in reactors to slow down neutrons. Carbon has at least five isotopes, carbon 10, 11, 12, 13, and 14, the figures indicating the mass numbers, but the atomic number remaining the same.

In the nuclei of most atoms the forces holding the nuclear particles together are balanced, and the balance is hard to upset. Nuclei of this sort are called stable. In other nuclei there is spontaneous rearrangement with ejection of charged particles and final attainment of more stable combinations of protons and neutrons. These unstable isotopes are called radionuclides, radioactive isotopes, or radioisotopes. They are characterized by a relatively high number of neutrons in the nucleus as compared with the number of protons.

Each element has at least one radioisotope. Some occur in nature, such as those of radium, thorium, and uranium, while others can be made artificially by means of the nuclear reactor or otherwise. Figure 17-2 shows radioisotope formation by means of a neutron stream. In both natural and artificial types, radioactive decay takes place, and simpler nuclei are formed, with other combinations of protons and neutrons; if the number of protons is changed, transformation to a different element results.

17-3. Radioactivity. Radioactivity is the process whereby unstable nuclei undergo spontaneous atomic disintegration with liberation of energy. The process, also known as decay, is characterized by the emission of one or more types of radiation, such as alpha particles, beta particles, and gamma radiation [1].

ALPHA RADIATION. The heavier elements have very large nuclei, and this is considered to be a cause of their instability. The nuclei become smaller through the ejection of protons and neutrons in groups of two of each. These are known as alpha particles. They have two positive electric charges and constitute the nucleus of the element helium. Since the number of protons in the original nucleus has been reduced by two, an atom undergoing such decay becomes a new element. Thus emission of an alpha particle changes uranium to thorium, and radium to radon. Alpha particles are emitted at high velocity but quickly dissipate their energy and can penetrate matter for only a short distance. They are usually a health hazard only when the radioisotopes have been ingested or otherwise absorbed in the body and radiate internally. In that case they are a very important internal hazard.

BETA RADIATION. Unstable isotopes have a high proportion of neutrons to protons in their nuclei. In their progress toward stability, they

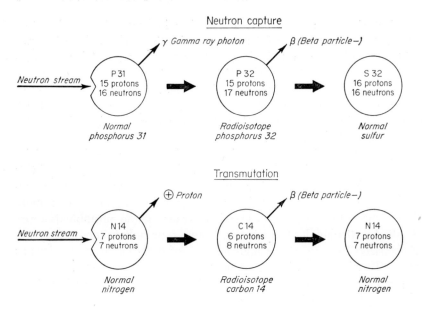

FIGURE 17-2 The processes by which radioisotopes are formed by bombardment of nuclei with neutrons, and the resulting decay products.

emit electrons; these are known as beta particles. Such a splitting may occur spontaneously, but it can be brought about by adding an extra neutron to the nucleus, as shown in Fig. 17-2. Such splitting is called fission, and it is the process (neutron bombardment) which is used in nuclear reactors. The smaller atoms produced by fission have an excess of neutrons as compared with stable isotopes of the same elements. As previously stated, a neutron has approximately the same mass as a proton and an electron, and if a free electron is left alone it will change into a proton and an electron. Therefore, if an atom is able to expel electrons, each such expulsion will result in one of the neutrons of its nucleus being converted to a proton. Each such conversion will bring the atom nearer to a stable proton-neutron ratio. This emission of electrons is known as beta radiation. Beta particles generally have high velocities. They are only moderately penetrative and dissipate their energies relatively quickly, but they can be a health hazard as either internal or external radiation.

PRODUCTS OF DECAY. Obviously the emission of alpha and beta particles changes the number of protons and neutrons within the nucleus and thus changes the atom, the result being a new isotope of the original element or a new element. These products of decay are known as daughters, and the original element is the parent. The daughters may be unstable also and decay still further until finally a stable atom is reached. Uranium 238, for example, decays to thorium, protactinium, radium, radon, polonium, and bismuth, until it becomes stable lead 206. Yttrium 90 is a daughter of strontium 90, the mass weight remaining nearly the same. In this case the loss of a negative beta particle from a neutron leaves a positive charge, or proton. The process has reduced the neutrons by one and increased the protons by one, and the sum is the same. The changed number of protons, however, has changed the chemical nature of the atom. Figure 17-2 shows this in the decay of carbon 14 to nitrogen 14.

GAMMA RADIATION AND X RAYS. When alpha and beta particles are emitted, they leave in the nucleus excess energy which may be discharged as gamma rays. Since they are energy and not particles, they do not change the characteristics of the radioisotope. Gamma rays are high-energy "photons," rays similar to light and radio waves but much shorter in wavelength and of much higher frequency. They resemble X rays, and actually the longer gamma rays are identical with the shorter X rays, so that the radiations are indistinguishable. The term "gamma ray," however, is applied to radiations of short wavelength having their origin in atomic nuclei.

X rays are produced by subjecting a metal or other dense target to bombardment with a stream of high-speed electrons. The electrons are formed by passing a high-voltage current through a vacuum from a cathode to an anode. The atoms of the target anode are surrounded by intense electric fields; when the electrons strike these fields, a part of their energy is converted into continuous X rays, which emerge in all directions from the target. The vacuum tube is enclosed by a shield of lead or other dense material with a small opening through which the useful beam can pass. The higher the voltage used to form the electron stream, the more penetrating the resulting X rays are. The voltage used may be from 50,000 to more than 10 million. Gamma rays and X rays are especially dangerous because of their long range and high penetrative ability.

OTHER TYPES OF RADIOACTIVITY. Nuclear reactors and accelerators, such as betatrons and cyclotrons, produce other types of radioactivity in the form of neutrons, protons, and conversion electrons.

Background radioactivity is the radiation produced by cosmic rays and the trace amounts of radioactive isotopes which are naturally present in the environment or which have been disseminated as a result of man's use of nuclear energy. Cosmic rays are high-energy particulate and electromagnetic radiations which originate outside of the earth's atmosphere.

ENERGY. The amount of energy released in nuclear reactions is of importance because of the effects it may have upon persons or matter exposed to the various rays. One method of calculating energy is of interest. It utilizes the fact that the forces in atomic nuclei manifest themselves in their respective nuclear masses. According to Einstein's equation, the relationship can be expressed as

$$E = mc^2$$

where E is the energy equivalent of the mass m, and c is the velocity of light. If m is expressed in grams and c is taken as 3×10^{10} cm/sec, then E will be in ergs; that is,

$$E = 3^2 \times 10^{20} \, m$$

To change ergs to calories, divide by 4.2×10^7. The energy change in any nuclear reaction can be obtained by inserting for m in the equation the difference in mass resulting from the nuclear reaction.

Measurement of the energy actually generated, however, is made by other means, and the energy is expressed in units related to the means of measurement. A special unit, the electron volt (ev), is used to express molecular and nuclear energy. One electron volt is the energy given to a single electron as it moves across an electrical potential difference of 1 volt. The volt is the same unit employed to measure electrical potential in its ordinary use. One electron volt is 1.7×10^{-12} erg. One million electron volts (Mev) is enough energy to lift a milligram one-millionth of a centimeter. The energy of the bonds holding molecules of chemical compounds ranges from fractions of electron volts to 10 or 12 ev. The nuclear binding energy holding protons and neutrons together in the nucleus of an atom is of the order of millions of electron volts.

17-4. Half-life of Radioisotopes. Decay of a radioactive isotope is caused by the disintegration of the individual atoms of which it is composed, with the release of energy in the forms of alpha and beta particles and gamma rays. There is no known means of speeding or slowing the rate of decay. Among the identical radioactive atoms, disintegrations occur at random, and no prediction can be made as to when a particular nucleus will decay. It is possible, however, to estimate with accuracy the number that will disintegrate in any given length of time. Since very large numbers disintegrate, the number doing so in any one time interval follows the laws of probability. The number decaying in any given interval of time is proportional to the number originally present and can be estimated with sufficient accuracy. If the interval chosen is that in which 50 per cent of the atoms disintegrate, then in each successive interval of the same length 50 per cent of the remaining radioactive atoms will decay. Such a time interval is known as the radioactive half-life. After seven half-lives the radioactivity of a radioisotope will have been reduced to about 1 per cent.

The half-lives of the known radioisotopes range from fractions of seconds to billions of years. Nitrogen 12[1] has a half-life of 13/1,000 sec; iodine 131, of 8.05 days; carbon 14, of 5,760 years; and radium 226, of 1,622 years. Half-lives are expressed exponentially. For example, uranium 238 has a half-life of 4.49×10^9 years, or 4,490 million years.

17-5. Ionization. Ionizing radiations—whether they are the alpha, beta, gamma, or other rays produced by radioactive decay, by radiation-producing machines, or by cosmic sources—all react upon any matter which absorbs them by forming pairs of electrically charged fragments called "ions." Gamma rays do not, however, produce ions directly. They knock electrons from atoms and impart some of their energy to the electrons, and these form ions. Ionization can occur in any kind of matter, and when it takes place in living tissue, animal or plant, changes occur that may affect health. The extent of the ionization and damage depends upon the length of exposure, the amount and energy level of the radiation received, and the importance of the organ or part of the body affected [2].

The fact that charged particles or photons ionize gases is made use of to measure radioactivity. If an electrical potential is maintained across a gas, a small charge flows through the gas chamber each time a charged particle traverses it; this is the result of positive ions and negative electrons collecting on the cathode and anode, respectively. The Geiger counter makes use of this method and is used principally for the measurement of beta and gamma rays.

17-6. Units of Radiation and Radioactivity. Radiological health workers commonly make use of several units of rate of radioactive disintegration. The curie is a unit of rate of radioactive disintegration. It is the quantity of any radioactive material in which the number of disintegrations per second is 3.700×10^{10}. This is a large amount of radioactivity. Practically speaking, a gram of pure radium in equilibrium with its decay products is 1 curie of radium.

The units that are in general use, together with their symbols, are as follows:

Curie—C = 3.7×10^{10} disintegrations per second
Millicurie—Mc = 10^{-3} curie = 3.7×10^7 disintegrations per second
Microcurie—μC = 10^{-6} curie = 3.7×10^4 disintegrations per second
Micromicrocurie—$\mu\mu$C = 10^{-12} curie = 3.7×10^{-2} disintegrations per second; also known as the picocurie

Some instruments are calibrated to give results in curies. Others give merely the number of disintegrations per unit of time, and these are known as counters.

---

[1] Nitrogen 12 means that the mass number of this particular isotope is 12, whereas the commonly stated mass number for the more abundant nitrogen is 14.

17-7. Radiation Dosage. The radiation delivered to a specified area or volume or to the whole body is known as the dose. In the glossary will be found definitions of various terms applied to dosage.

The units recommended [3] for use in connection with dosage are as follows: the curie, for activity (see Art. 17-6); the roentgen, for exposure; the rad, for absorbed dose; and the rem, for absorbed dose modified by its biological effect.

The *roentgen* is the quantity of X or gamma rays that will produce in air ions carrying one electrostatic unit of electricity of either sign per cubic centimeter at standard temperature and pressure.

The *rad* is defined as 100 ergs of absorbed energy per g of absorbing material. One rad is approximately equal to the absorbed dose delivered when soft tissue is exposed to 1 r (roentgen) of medium-voltage X radiation. Thus in many situations of interest in medical radiology, but not in all, the numbers of roentgens of exposure and rads of absorption associated with a particular medical or biological effect are approximately equal.

The absorbed dose in *rems* is related to the *relative biological effectiveness* (RBE) of the particular nuclear radiation. The RBE of a given radiation is defined as the ratio of the absorbed dose in rads of gamma or X radiation (of a specified energy) to the absorbed dose in rads of the given radiation having the same biological effect. The value of the RBE for a particular type of nuclear radiation depends upon the dose rate, the energy of the radiation, the kind and degree of the biological damage, and the nature of the organism or tissue under radiation. The unit which takes these effects into account is the rem (roentgen equivalent man). It can be expressed as

$$\text{Dose in rems} = \text{RBE} \times \text{dose in rads}$$

All radiations capable of producing ionization (or excitation)—*i.e.*, alpha and beta particles, X rays, gamma rays, and neutrons—cause injury of the same general type. The various radiations, however, differ in the depths to which they penetrate the body and in the degree of injury from a specified amount of energy absorption. The difference, as indicated above, is expressed by the RBE. The RBE for gamma rays and X rays is approximately unity, although it varies somewhat with the energy of the radiation, as stated above. For beta particles, the RBE is also close to unity; for alpha particles, it has been variously reported as 10 to 20; for thermal neutrons, 2.8; and for fast neutrons (1 to 10 Mev), 10.

The *internal dose* is radiation from radionuclides which have been inhaled or ingested or which have otherwise entered the body. Such dosage is especially dangerous since it subjects the body tissues to highly effective bombardment. Even alpha particles are highly injurious inside the body. Dosage to the skin or the internal body burden can be estimated from the known radioactivity of air that is breathed or of water or foods that are ingested.

The *biological half-life* is the time necessary for half the radionuclide to be eliminated from the body or some organ. The *effective half-life* is the resultant of the biological half-life and the radioactive half-life of the radionuclide. It will depend upon its distribution in the body and whether its chemical characteristics are such that it is cumulative or is slowly or rapidly eliminated. Strontium 90, for example, being chemically similar to calcium, accumulates in the bones and delivers its principal dose there.

17-8. Instruments Used for Detection and Measurement of Radiation. There are three principal types of radiation detectors: (1) Ion collectors, which have charged electrodes that collect the ions in a gaseous medium by the radioactive energy applied. These include the electroscopes, ionization chambers, Geiger counters, and proportional counters. (2) Scintillators, in which alpha or beta particles or gamma rays produce flashes of light when they strike certain substances. (3) Chemical dosimeters, in which permanent chemical changes are observed. This is the effect used in photographic film dosimetry.

Another method of classification of the above instruments is as follows: (1) Pulse counters, which indicate and record the passage of individual alpha or beta particles or gamma quanta.[1] The count rate of the sample will be the number of counts per unit of time divided by the instrument efficiency, and this gives a measure of the activity of the sample. (2) Integrating instruments, which give a reading dependent upon the number and ionizing density of particles or quanta passing through the detector over a period of time. Electroscopes and film badges are in this class. (3) Instruments which measure the flux of particles or rays through the detector. They indicate dose rate and are used to measure the radiation level in the vicinity of intense beta-gamma sources for accurate assay of high-activity beta-gamma samples.

Much used by engineers and sanitarians in area surveying and monitoring for radioactivity are the portable survey meters which are pictured in Fig. 17-3. These are rate meters and give readings in milliroentgens per hour. Background activity is first obtained before a counter is used to determine the activity of a radioactive material.

For monitoring of air doses to workers exposed to radiation, two types of dosimeters are used. A pocket electroscope, which resembles a fountain pen in size and shape, is used, and also a film badge, which contains X-ray film. These are attached to the clothing during working

[1] Quanta are "packages" of radiant energy (not particles) which, according to the quantum theory of physics, characterize light, gamma rays, X rays, and radio waves.

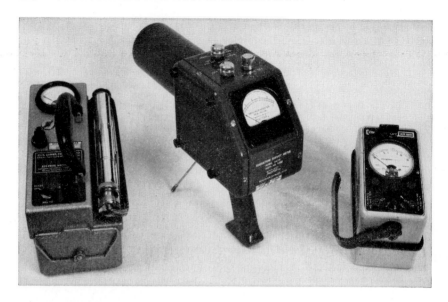

FIGURE 17-3 Three types of radiation instruments (rate meters) used for area monitoring. (*Courtesy of Texas State Health Department.*)

hours and are examined and renewed when necessary; they provide a record of total exposure.

17-9. Maximum Permissible Radiation Exposures. There has been much investigation of permissible radiation dosages, and it is still in progress. Recommended figures, therefore, are subject to change as knowledge is increased. Handbook 69 of the National Bureau of Standards [4] gives the following basic rules, which were formulated by the National Committee on Radiation Protection:[1]

BASIC RULES

Accumulated Dose (Radiation Workers)

A. *External exposure to critical organs. Whole body, head and trunk, active blood forming organs, eyes or gonads:* The Maximum Permissible Dose (MPD) to the most critical organs, accumulated at any age, shall not exceed 5 rems multiplied by the number of years beyond age 18, and the dose in any 13 consecutive weeks shall not exceed 3 rems.

Thus the accumulated MPD $= (N - 18) \times 5$ rems where N is the age in years and is greater than 18.

Comment: This applies to radiation of sufficient penetrating power to affect a significant fraction of the critical tissue.

B. *External exposure to other organs. Skin of whole body:* MPD =

---

[1] The rules are given here without the accompanying discussion. It is recommended that the Handbook be obtained by those interested in further study.

1($(N - 18)$ rems, and the dose in any 13 consecutive weeks shall not exceed 6 rems.

Comment: This rule applies to radiation of low penetrating power.

Hands and forearms, feet and ankles: MPD = 75 rems/year and the dose in any 13 consecutive weeks shall not exceed 25 rems.

C. *Internal exposures.* The permissible levels from internal emitters will be consistent as far as possible with the age-proration and dose principles above. Control of the internal dose will be achieved by limiting the body burden of radioisotopes. This will generally be accomplished by control of the average concentration of radioactive materials in the air, water or food taken into the body. Since it would be impractical to set different MPC values for air, water and food for radiation workers as a function of age, the MPC values are selected in such a manner that they conform to the above stated limits when applied to the most restrictive case, *viz.,* they are set to be applicable to radiation workers of age 18. Thus, the values are conservative and are applicable to radiation workers of any age (assuming there is no occupational exposure to radiation permitted at age less than 18).

The maximum permissible average concentrations of radionuclides in air and water are determined from biological data whenever such data are available, or are calculated on the basis of an average annual dose of 15 rems for most individual organs of the body, 30 rems when the critical organ is the thyroid or the skin, and 5 rems when the gonads or the whole body is the critical organ. For bone seekers the maximum permissible limit is based on the distribution of the deposit, the RBE, and a comparison of the energy release in the bone with the energy release delivered by a maximum permissible body burden of 0.1 microgram of radium 226 plus daughters.

Emergency Dose (Radiation Workers)

An accidental or emergency dose of 25 rems to the whole body or a major portion thereof, occurring only once in the lifetime of a person, need not be included in the determination of the radiation exposure status of that person.

Medical Dose (Radiation Workers)

Radiation exposures resulting from necessary medical and dental procedures need not be included in the determination of the radiation exposure of the person concerned.

Dose to Persons in the Neighborhood of Controlled Areas

The radiation or radioactive material outside a controlled area, attributable to the normal operations within the controlled area, shall be such that it is improbable that any individual will receive a dose of 0.5 rem in any 1 year from external radiation.

The maximum permissible body burden of radionuclides in persons outside the controlled area and attributable to the operations within the controlled area shall not exceed one-tenth of that for radiation workers.

This will generally entail control of the average concentrations in air or water at the point of intake, or at the rate of intake to the body in foodstuffs, to levels not exceeding one-tenth of the maximum permissible concentrations allowed in air, water, and foodstuffs for continuous occupational exposure. The body burden and concentrations of radionuclides may be averaged over periods up to 1 year.

The maximum permissible dose and the maximum permissible concentrations of radionuclides as recommended above are primarily for the purpose of keeping the average dose to the whole population as low as reasonably possible, and not because of the likelihood of specific injury to the individual.

The MPC levels mentioned above under internal exposures for air and water are given for various radionuclides in microcuries in Handbook 69. They are given for 40-hr exposures per week and 168-hr exposures per week. The maximum permissible body burden is also given in microcuries, and the type of radiation of the radionuclide is given, i.e., alpha, gamma, beta, or electrons. Procedures are also given when radiation is derived from a mixture of radionuclides or if they are unknown.

Radiation dosages to exposed workers are checked by means of dosimeters which are worn attached to the clothing (Art. 17-8).

17-10. Harmful Effects of Radiation. Existing knowledge of the harmful effects of radiation has been derived from observations of persons who were exposed to explosions of atomic bombs or who worked with X rays and radium before the need for protection was recognized and from animal experimentation. Much is yet to be learned as to the dosage levels above which harmful results can be expected. The dosages given in Art. 17-9 are considered to be reasonably safe for persons who are employed where radioactive materials are produced or used [2, 5].

Massive doses of radioactivity will result from atomic bombs (fission) or hydrogen bombs (fusion) or from accidents at nuclear reactors. The median lethal dose is 400 to 600 r. This means that about 50 per cent of the persons exposed will probably die in 1 month. The survivors will require 6 months for recovery. At a dose of 750 r, there will be few or no survivors.

For smaller doses the time period of exposure will have much influence upon over-all effects. For example, total body irradiation in a short period of time, such as occurred in Japanese bomb casualties and a few accidental exposures in nuclear energy plants, caused injury to the blood-forming tissues and the intestinal tract as well as leukemia and other delayed effects in various organs. With exposures at a lower level over a period of years, such effects as skin cancer and leukemia may appear. Shortening of life-span is noted in experimental animals, but there is some doubt whether this applies to man. No bad effects have been noted where present permissible dose levels have been adhered to [2].

The lethal or injurious dose for partial body irradiation in general far exceeds that for the whole body. A small volume of tissue may receive thousands of roentgens without causing death. This permits X-ray and radium therapy. Injudicious or careless exposures may result in damage, particularly to workers with the radioactive materials that are used therapeutically. Studies of such exposures indicate such results as anemia, leukemia, cancer, skin damage, and cataracts. The threshold dose for cataract production is 600 to 1,000 r from X rays (200 kv) to the eyes. For equal energy absorbed from neutrons, the RBE is 5 to 10.

Much attention has been given to possible genetic effects of radioactivity, but less is known with certainty than about other harmful effects. It is supposed that undesirable mutations may occur in the offspring of individuals who have been exposed to irradiation, particularly of the gonads. What little is definitely known has been determined from animal experiments using relatively large doses. What effect, if any, will result from increases in low-level doses to the general population is not known. The doses given in Art. 17-9 for populations near controlled areas are considered to be below those that will have important genetic effects. The significant doses for this hazard are those received prior to the end of the reproductive period.

It should be pointed out that persons who have received internal doses of radioactive materials are not dangerous to other persons. Also, exposure to radioactivity, except in massive doses, has no effect upon fertility.

17-11. Radiological Sanitation. This is essentially the protection of the general public and workers exposed to radioactivity from excessive exposures; it is accomplished through environmental-control measures. The protective measures required will depend upon the conditions under which the radioactivity is generated or used.

URANIUM MINING. The principal hazards in this process are the gases radon and thoron, particularly the former. Both are daughters of radium which themselves decay into radioactive daughters. In underground mines good ventilation is necessary to prevent injurious concentrations. This is of importance to workers in occupational health.

FUEL PROCESSING. This includes concentration and refining. The process separates uranium from its daughters, which are wasted to the environment, particularly to waste water. Stream pollution, therefore, is a hazard. In the handling, storage, and fabrication of enriched fuels hazardous amounts of radioactive materials may escape as the result of criticality accidents.

REACTORS. The engineering of reactors is a complicated matter which is concerned with the use of materials in their construction that will provide the maximum safety against accidents and contamination of coolants. Monitoring of the environment around the reactors and of the personnel as to dosages received is necessary. At air-cooled reactors, argon 41 may be produced and discharged into the atmosphere, but it has a half-life of only 1.8 hr. Radioactive dusts may also be emitted, but this is avoided by filtration of the air supply to remove dust that would be made radioactive and also of the exhaust to remove radioactive particles which have flaked from surfaces. Dilution into the atmosphere is accomplished by high stacks. Continuous measurements of air conditions are carried on, and if undesirably high concentrations result, the power of the reactor is reduced.

In single-pass water-cooled reactors, the water is first treated to remove suspended solids and dissolved impurities. Traces remain, however, and more may be added by contact with the aluminum surrounding the fuel elements, or small leaks may develop. Many of the radionuclides so produced are short-lived. At Hanford the coolant is held 1 to 3 hr before it is discharged into the Columbia River. After 35 miles of travel the activity has decayed to less than 10 per cent of its original value.

At other water-cooled reactors, the coolant water is treated by filtration to remove suspended impurities and is then passed through ion-exchange resins to remove dissolved impurities. During use there may be some leakage by corrosion or otherwise, and radioisotopes will get into the cooling water. Other waters will become contaminated with water used for decontaminating parts removed for repair, laundering workers' clothes, and laboratory washings. These waters are also treated as above and are stripped of gas by passing them over plates exposed to a countercurrent of steam.

X-RAY MACHINES. The hazards inherent in the use of X-ray machines are excessive exposures of persons exposed for diagnostic purposes or for treatment and excessive exposures of persons using the machines or working in the vicinity of the machines. The avoidance of excessive doses of radioactivity to persons receiving treatments or examinations is primarily a matter of medical concern. Safety measures include use of filters to absorb soft radiation that adds to exposure but serves no useful purpose; use of faster films to reduce doses needed for diagnosis; use of cones to restrict the area of body part being irradiated; and shielding of the room, including doors, in which the machine is located [15].

The use of X-ray fluoroscopes for shoe fitting is forbidden as being a source of unnecessary irradiation to persons being fitted and a possible danger to operators. Competent orthopedists have stated that no benefit is derived from their use.

USE OF RADIOACTIVE MATERIALS. There are many uses for radiation in medical diagnosis, therapy, and research; in agricultural and other research; and in industry [17]. They constitute an important problem because of their number and the aggregate of workers and patients involved. The necessary precautions will be briefly mentioned.

Licenses[1] are required for the acquisition, possession, or use of certain sources of ionizing radiation. These are granted by the Atomic Energy Commission or by the state in which the applicant is located. The Commission and the licensing states have regulations for protection against ionizing radiation [17, 19]. These set forth maximum exposures for workers and require the use of dosimeters, the keeping of dosage records, and the instruction of workers. Cautionary labels and signs are required on containers and in radiation areas. Surveys or evaluations of radiation hazards that may exist incident to production, presence, use, or disposal of radioactive materials are also required. Disposal methods are stipulated in the regulations, and use of other methods requires special approval.

RADIOACTIVITY IN THE ENVIRONMENT. Accidents at reactors, though rare, may occur that release radioactive material to the environment. Coolants—air and liquid—are discharged into the atmosphere and streams. Testing of nuclear weapons results in fallout which contaminates soil, water, and foliage.

17-12. Monitoring of Air, Milk and Other Foods, and Water. The Federal Radiation Council [6] in 1962 formulated daily intake levels of certain radionuclides, with 12-month totals, as acceptable health risks for large general population groups, compatible with the orderly development of the nuclear industry in the United States:

Iodine 131—100 micromicrocuries per day, or a total of 36,500 micromicrocuries per year[2]

Strontium 90—200 micromicrocuries per day, or a total of 73,000 micromicrocuries per year

Strontium 89—2,000 micromicrocuries per day, or a total of 730,000 micromicrocuries per year

Radium 226—20 micromicrocuries per day, or a total of 7,300 micromicrocuries per year

The above figures might be called significant levels and do not represent the difference between safety and danger. Exposures even many times above the stated levels would not result in detectable incidence of disease. As applied to fallout, the guides can be taken as indications that detailed evaluation of possible exposure risks might be needed.

[1] There are numerous exemptions as to license requirements. The reader should obtain state requirements and those of the Atomic Energy Commission.

[2] The guide for iodine 131 is set for the most susceptible group—infants and small children. For adults the iodine 131 guide could be tenfold larger, or 365,000 micromicrocuries per year.

AIR. The Public Health Service conducts surveillance of airborne radioactivity by means of 72 stations at which continuous sampling of dustfalls is done. The radioactivity of particulates is found, and also the gross beta activity. This measures the effects of fallout of fission products from nuclear weapons tests [6].

MILK. Fallout of fission products to vegetation which is consumed in pastures by cows is soon indicated by radioactivity of the milk. A slower uptake would be through soluble radionuclides being absorbed by roots from rainwater. The Public Health Service conducts a national program, with state and local health agencies cooperating, in sampling pasteurized milk, which is tested in the Service laboratories for strontium 89, strontium 90, and iodine 131. It should be pointed out that determination of the identity of radionuclides requires elaborate laboratory facilities and procedures [6].

WATER. Some ground waters contain radioactive materials derived from soluble radionuclides in the ground. Surveillance of radioactivity due to fallout is confined to surface waters. The Public Health Service tests waters sampled at 119 stations for plankton population; organic chemicals; chemical, biological, and physical quality; and radioactivity. The radioactivity of the dissolved solids will show the quality of the treated water, since nearly all suspended solids are removed by treatment. Gross alpha and beta determinations are made on both suspended and dissolved solids, and strontium 90 determinations on total solids only. It was found that nuclear installations may contribute additional alpha or beta activity, whereas fallout contributes primarily to additional beta activity [6].

Some states, including Texas, have conducted statewide sampling and testing programs to determine the present radioactivity of their surface waters [7]. The data so obtained will be valuable in the future to determine the increase above natural radioactivity resulting from fallout, the development of nuclear industries, and the disposal of radioactive wastes into streams.

The Public Health Service Drinking Water Standards adopted in 1962 assert that approval of water supplies containing radioactive materials shall be based upon the judgment that the radioactivity intake, when added to that from all other sources, is not likely to result in an intake greater than the radiation protection guidance recommended by the Federal Radiation Council. See Art. 2-9.

17-13. Environmental Protection from Nuclear Power Reactors. Nuclear power reactors will soon be a feature of industry in the United States, and their effects upon the nearby environment will be the concern of health authorities. Procedures followed by the New York State Health Department [8] prior to the construction of a 535,000-kw nuclear power plant are of interest. This plant is to be a pressurized water reactor with an oil-fired superheater. A comprehensive radiological monitoring plan was developed for the environment within a 20-mile radius of the plant.

The possibility exists that a reactor system might fail and permit release of radioactive materials into the containment vessel and that leakage therefrom might give the public a dosage in excess of normal annual tolerance. Such accidents would be rare, and as a further precaution the power company surrounded the steel containment vessel with a second concrete structure. The other hazards would be low-level liquid wastes, which would be discharged into the Hudson River, and radioactive gases, also low-level.

The first procedure was to establish the background radioactivity before the plant was built so that comparison would be possible after its construction. Accordingly samples of water, fish, plankton, bottom mud, soil, vegetation, and rabbit thyroid were routinely collected and analyzed. Fallout stations were maintained. A background gamma survey of the atmosphere was made by helicopter. A sampling program was then agreed upon with the power company, the local health departments, and the New York State Health Department cooperating. The monitoring program covered (1) a continuing radiological sampling program and (2) emergency planning in case of accidental over-releases. After the agreement the company received a permit to construct the plant.

The continuous sampling program includes the following: (1) Weekly samples of the water intake and condenser discharge for gross beta radioactivity of dissolved and suspended contents. If a quarterly composite indicates that more than 5 curies have been released during that quarter, isotopic analyses are made. (2) Quarterly—as permitted by the weather—samples of plankton, fish, shellfish, and mud would be given gamma spectrometric analyses and radiochemistry analyses as the spectrometric findings dictate. (3) The discharge of radioactive gases will be limited to such a rate that iodine 131 concentration is less than 3×10^{-10} microcuries/cu cm, which is the off-site limit of the National Committee on Radiation Protection. The entire environment around the reactor will be sampled if total releases of this radionuclide exceed 55 millicuries per month. Sampling for iodine 131 will also include vegetation and milk from the area dairies. This is considered important because of the radiosensitivity of the thyroid gland in children. In order to keep within the prescribed limit, the company will collect and retain waste gases in holding tanks for 90 to 120 days before releasing them to the atmosphere. This will permit decay of the short-lived nuclides, of which iodine 131 is one, having a half-life of 8.05 days.

It is unlikely that large quantities of radioactive materials could escape from the plant. The worst accident would be rupture of the reactor core, but the containing sphere would allow only a slow leakage of radioactive materials, and no great direct radiation exposure would result to persons outside. A more important hazard from this and lesser accidents would be deposition of radioactive materials on crop and pasture lands and their appearance in water, milk, and other foods. A study indicated that allowable limits would not be exceeded. Of course, surveillance would be increased, and emergency measures could be applied if required.

17-14. Disposal of Radioactive Wastes. Wastes may be solid, liquid, or in a form that will contaminate the atmosphere. Low-level liquid wastes are those resulting from ore processing, decontamination work including laundering, use of reactor coolant, laboratory research, and medical diagnostic and therapeutic work. The isotope concentration will range from trace amounts to several millicuries per liter [10].

High-level liquid wastes are produced in the processing of spent fuel elements to recover fissionable material. Normally these wastes are permitted to cool for several days to permit short-lived isotopes to decay.

Low-level liquid wastes may be stored in tanks or in open pits where evaporation will take place, or they may be allowed to seep into the soil near the surface from covered trenches, discharged into deep formations, or discharged into streams and oceans [10]. Chemical precipitation will remove significant proportions of suspended radionuclides from water. A special hazard resulting from disposal of wastes to surface waters is that algae and other plankton will take up and concentrate radioactivity. Fish will eat the plankton, and these in turn may be eaten by humans [18].

High-level liquid wastes have been buried or placed in containers and sunk in carefully chosen areas of the oceans. Experiments have been conducted regarding disposal of such wastes in those geological formations known as salt domes and salt beds and into beds of impervious clay.

Solid wastes result from mining and processing of radioactive ores, from many laboratory and shop operations, and from those chemical operations producing sludges. Their levels of activity may vary from a few multiples of the background to 2 to 150 r/hr at the container surface. Disposal is by burial, by incineration if combustible, or by remelting if metallic. Incineration will reduce bulk and concentrate the radioactivity in less volume for burial. Consideration should be given to the possibility of air contamination and radioactive fallout.

Radioactive atmospheric contaminants are gases and particulates, either solid or liquid. They are produced in mining and ore processing which results in uranium- or radium-bearing dust. Radon gas will be associated with its parent radium. Uranium and thorium particulates may be created by the production and processing of uranium metal and thorium metal. Air-cooled reactors, where the cooling air contains dust and is exposed to neutron flux near fuel elements or shielding, will produce induced radioactivity. Active rare gases such as argon 41 may result. The use of spray cooling water which contains minerals will produce active aerosols. Certain radioactive gases in effluent cooling air will decay to radioactive particulates less than 0.2 μ in size [5].

The ventilation methods used in industrial hygiene include use of hoods or enclosures over dust- or fume-producing operations which discharge into ventilating systems. The methods of dust removal described in Art. 3-14 may then be applied. Solids and liquids so obtained may be disposed of as indicated above for solid and liquid wastes. Filters, etc., will become contaminated and may require decontamination. Gases or air still containing radioactive particles may be dispersed to the atmosphere by means of stacks.

The disposal of radioactive wastes is controlled by the Public Health Service, state health authorities, and local health officials.

17-15. Health Departments and Radiological Health. Control of sources of ionizing radiation for protection of the public and employed persons against the hazards of radiation exposure is a government function for which official health departments should be given major legal responsibility [14]. The Public Health Service, the Bureau of Standards, and the Atomic Energy Commission have made investigations that have related doses to health. The Public Health Service conducts short courses in the various aspects of radiological health for health workers. The Office of Civil Defense disseminates information regarding nuclear disasters. Most states have adopted legislation regarding radiation sources, the requirement of registration and licensing of isotope users, waste disposal permits, and radiation protection regulations and have established advisory groups on atomic energy development and control [15].

Local health departments should exercise control over uses of X-ray equipment [14, 15, 16, 17] and nuclear energy sources used in industry.

If the air and water in an area contain radioactive materials, it is possible that significant contamination will appear in the milk and foodstuffs produced in the area. Monitoring will then be desirable. It is important, however, that the public health officials be competent to evaluate such radiation with the total radiation in the community.

Bibliography

1. O'Kelley, G. D.: "Detection and Measurement of Nuclear Radiation," National Academy of Sciences, Office of Technical Services, U.S. Department of Commerce, 1962.
2. "The Biological Effects of Atomic Radiation," National Academy of Sciences, Washington, D.C., 1960.

3. Radiation Quantities and Units, International Commission on Radiological Units and Measurements, *Natl. Bur. Std. U.S. Handbook* 84, 1962.
4. Maximum Permissible Body Burdens and Maximum Permissible Concentrations of Radionuclides in Air and Water for Occupational Exposure, *Natl. Bur. Std. U.S. Handbook* 69, 1962.
5. "Public Exposure to Ionizing Radiations," American Public Health Association, New York, 1958.
6. *Radiological Health Data*, vol. III, no. 12, December, 1962.
7. Drynan, W. C., and E. F. Gloyna: "Radioactivity in Texas Surface Waters," Sanitary Engineering Research Laboratory, Civil Engineering Department, University of Texas, Austin, Tex., 1960.
8. Davies, S., and M. H. Thompson: Protecting the Environment around a Nuclear Power Reactor, *Am. J. Public Health*, vol. 52, no. 12, December, 1962.
9. "Radiological Health Handbook," Public Health Service, Robert A. Taft Sanitary Engineering Center, Cincinnati, Ohio, 1961.
10. Blatz, H. (ed.): "Radiation Hygiene Handbook," McGraw-Hill Book Company, New York, 1959.
11. "Disposal of Low Level Radioactive Wastes into Pacific Coastal Waters," National Academy of Sciences, Washington, D.C., 1962.
12. "Nuclear Attack and Industrial Survival," McGraw-Hill Publications, New York, 1962.
13. "Effects of Nuclear Weapons," Atomic Energy Commission, 1962.
14. Environmental Health Planning Guide, *Public Health Service Pub.* 82, rev. 1962.
15. X-ray Protection Design, *Natl. Bur. Std. U.S. Handbook* 50, 1952.
16. Medical X-ray Protection up to Three Million Volts, *Natl. Bur. Std. U.S. Handbook* 75, 1961.
17. "Radioisotopes in Science and Industry," Report of the United States Atomic Energy Commission, 1960.
18. Eisenbud, M.: "Environmental Radioactivity," McGraw-Hill Book Company, New York, 1963.
19. "Radiation Control in Texas: Policies and Procedures," Texas State Department of Health, Austin, Tex., 1962.

18

MISCELLANEOUS ENVIRONMENTAL PROBLEMS

18-1. Control of the environment to prevent accidental injuries and deaths comes within the definition of sanitation (page 2). Safety programs to reduce the toll of accidents have been conducted for many years, and the effects can be seen in the downward trend shown in Fig. 18-1. There is still, however, much to be accomplished.

Accidents have been variously defined. One given by Arbous [1] has been accepted by some writers: "In a chain of events, each of which is planned or controlled, there occurs an unplanned event, which, being the result of some nonadjustive act on the part of the individual (variously caused) may, or may not result in injury. This is an accident." Accidents do not just happen; the "nonadjustive act" may result from

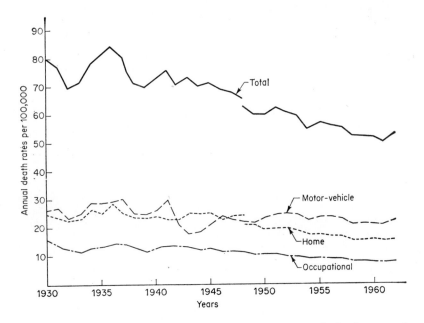

Figure 18-1 Annual death rates from accidents—motor-vehicle, home, and occupational. The gap in the curves for total and home accidents is caused by a change in nomenclature in the International Causes of Death. (*Figures from the National Safety Council.*)

ignorance, carelessness, or inattention in the operations of daily life or in the design or construction of machinery or buildings.

18-2. Magnitude of the Problem. Figure 18-1 gives the annual death rates from all accidents and also for three categories of accidents. These figures are significant to the student, but more striking are the figures of actual deaths, all accidents, and various types of accidents for the years 1958 to 1962 as shown in Tables 18-1 and 18-2.[1] These figures do not, however, depict the whole accident toll. The National Safety Council estimates [3] that there were 9,900,000 disabling injuries from accidents[2] in 1962. These were divided as follows: work, 2,000,000; motor-vehicle, 1,500,000; public, 2,100,000; and home, 4,300,000. These figures and those in the tables indicate that for deaths and injuries the home is a hazardous place.

Accidental deaths ranked according to age groups are highly significant. Between the ages of one and thirty-four, accidents are the lead-

---

[1] The accident category "public—non-motor-vehicle" applies to accidents occurring in streets and public buildings and during recreative activities.

[2] This means disabling beyond the day of the accident. Figures are based upon studies of ratios of disabling injuries to accidental deaths, except for work injuries, which have a broad representative reporting.

Table 18-1. PRINCIPAL CLASSES OF ACCIDENTAL DEATHS, 1958–1962

Year	Total*		Motor-vehicle		Public—non-motor-vehicle		Home		Work	
	Deaths	Rate†	Deaths	Rate†	Deaths	Rate†	Deaths	Rate†	Deaths	Rate†
1958	90,604	52.3	36,981	21.3	16,500	9.5	26,500	15.3	13,300	7.7
1959‡	92,082	52.2	37,910	21.5	16,500	9.3	27,000	15.3	13,800	7.8
1960	93,806	52.1	38,137	21.2	17,000	9.4	28,000	15.6	13,800	7.7
1961	92,249	50.4	38,091	20.8	16,500	9.0	28,000	15.6	13,500	7.4
1962	97,000	52.2	40,900	22.0	17,000	9.1	28,500	15.3	13,700	7.4

* Duplications between motor-vehicle, work, and home accidents are eliminated in the total column.

† Rates are deaths per 100,000 population.

‡ 1959 includes Alaska; 1960 and later years include Alaska and Hawaii.

SOURCE: Figures are estimates by the National Safety Council and are based on data from the National Vital Statistics Division, state and city health departments, and other sources.

Table 18-2. PRINCIPAL TYPES OF ACCIDENTAL DEATHS, 1958–1962

Year	Motor-vehicle	Falls	Fires, burns	Drownings*	Railroad	Firearms	Poison gases	Poisons (except gas)
1958	36,981	18,248	7,291	6,582	2,480	2,172	1,187	1,429
1959	37,910	18,774	6,898	6,434	2,291	2,258	1,141	1,661
1960	38,137	19,023	7,645	6,529	2,391	2,324	1,253	1,679
1961	38,091	18,691	7,102	6,525	2,246	2,204	1,192	1,804
1962	40,900	19,800	7,500	6,400	2,200	2,000	1,400	1,700

* Includes drownings in water-transport accidents.

SOURCE: National Safety Council.

ing cause of death. They are the second most common cause between thirty-five and forty-four; the fourth, between forty-five and sixty-four; and the fifth at age sixty-five and over.

18-3. Epidemiology of Accidents. McFarland and Moore [2] advocate the epidemiological approach. Epidemiology has already been defined (Art. 1-1). It is being applied to other diseases, and it is applicable to accident prevention. The method can be described as making determinations of *who, when, where,* and *how.*

An epidemiological study of home accidents would include the following: the persons involved—ages, sex, and possibly other status, such as housewife; time of accidents during the day; location of accidents, such as kitchen, bathroom, stairs, or yard; and details as to type of accidents, which may be falls, poisonings, cuts, burns, etc. There may also be contributing factors, such as economic status of the family; location of the home—whether in a slum area or not; and habits or customs of the persons involved. When the basic data are known, the remedies will be apparent or will become so after further study.

The epidemiological method is employed in the prevention of traffic accidents. For example, study of types, frequencies, and sites of accidents points out needs for traffic lights or improvements at street or highway intersections; the age grouping of drivers in accidents has resulted in courses for drivers in the high schools; and knowledge of types of common injuries has caused automobile designers to change details of steering wheels and to install seat belts. Safety engineers and safety committees in industry have followed similar methods.

18-4. Accident Prevention. Accident-prevention activities in the occupational field have been carried out by the larger industries, not only as a humanitarian measure, but also because of the economic advantages in reduction of time lost from work and reduction of compensation insurance costs. Responsibility for safety is assigned to some person, who may be called the safety director or safety engineer; in smaller plants it may be one of the executives. Training in safety procedures is given to supervisors and workers, accident records are kept, medical and first-aid services are available, and periodic physical examinations are given.

Traffic safety has been a concern of the police, particularly of the traffic squads. Many cities now have traffic engineers, among whose duties is the study of traffic accidents and the application of such remedial measures as may be applicable to the streets. Mention has already been made of courses for drivers in the high schools. Education of the public through newspaper items, posters, etc., is widely used.

Figures given in Art. 18-2 indicate that the school years are among those during which accidents are the chief cause of death. Safety education and school safety measures are therefore important. It is recommended [2] that each school system have a safety coordinator or specialist whose duties are indicative of the school safety program. They include development of the safety curriculum; improvement of safety education; provision of safety education in cocurricular activities; establishment of procedures for the maintenance of a safe school plant and other facilities; coordination of various community agencies in the promotion of the school safety program; and promotion and maintenance of continuous evaluation of the school safety program. The safety curriculum is usually integrated with other courses. Such instruction should be adapted to the age of the children. Automobile driver education is given separately. The attainment of a safe school environment includes proper maintenance of buildings, equipment, and grounds; provision

of fire-fighting equipment and holding of fire drills; use of safety practices in special rooms and areas, such as school shops and gymnasiums;
and safety on streets around the school area and in school bus transportation. School safety patrols are used on the school grounds, in school
buses, and at street crossings near the schools. School physicians, nurses,
and teachers should all cooperate in the safety program.

Public accidental deaths are due in large part to recreative activities.
By causes, they are as follows: drowning, including boating accidents,
43 per cent; firearms, 8 per cent; falls, 7 per cent; air transport, 10 per
cent; and all others, 32 per cent. These figures indicate the need for
educational and regulatory measures to prevent drowning and boating
accidents and also for education in the handling of firearms. Safety
features of swimming pools are discussed in Chap. 12. It should be
pointed out that playgrounds reduce traffic accidents among children
who would otherwise be playing in the streets or in other unsafe places.

Home accidents are responsible for more than one-fourth of all
accidental deaths; for nearly two-thirds of those among children under
five years of age; and for almost half of those among people sixty-five
years old and over. They also are responsible for more nonfatal injuries
than any other category. Table 18-3 gives types of fatal accidents as
they occurred in various age groups. The importance of prevention of
home accidents is apparent, but influencing the householder is difficult.
The approach has been largely educational and along the following lines:
(1) Measures directed to protect the small child, such as storage of
medicines, detergents and cleaning agents, and insecticides and other
poisonous materials so that small children do not have access to them;
avoidance of potentially dangerous toys; avoidance of thin plastic films

Table 18-3. DEATHS IN HOME ACCIDENTS, 1961

Types of accidents	Age groups, years						
	0–4	5–14	15–24	25–44	45–64	65–74	75 and over
All types	5,800	1,300	800	2,200	3,400	3,200	9,800
Falls.	500	80	20	200	900	2,000	8,100
Fires, burns	1,200	650	200	850	1,200	600	900
Suffocation, ingested objects . .	1,300	30	20	80	100	70	100
Suffocation, mechanical . . .	1,300	30	10	20	20	10	10
Poisons, solid or liquid . . .	400	30	120	400	400	100	50
Firearms	70	300	170	250	300	60	50
Poison gases	30	40	90	170	250	70	50
Other home accidents. . . .	1,000	140	170	230	230	290	540

SOURCE: "Accident Facts," National Safety Council, Chicago, 1962.

used as bed covers; permitting of no open fires to which the child can come into contact and safe storage of matches; and removal of dangerous rubbish from yards. (2) Some general precautions are making firearms inaccessible to children and keeping them unloaded; labeling all poisons; enforcing proper smoking habits, *e.g.*, no smoking in bed; proper venting of room and water heaters; protecting heaters so that clothing of girls and women cannot come in contact with flames; taking precautions in the use of flammable cleaning fluids or using only nonflammable agents; and removing flammable rubbish from basements, closets, and attics. (3) It will be noted that falls are important in the accident figures for all ages and particularly for persons sixty-five years of age and older. Prevention includes the following: Necessary climbing should be done only on ladders of good design; stairways should be properly designed and provided with handrails; windows should be guarded against children falling out; and bathtubs and showers should be provided with convenient hand holds. Also see Art. 14-13 and [3].

Educational measures are much used in preventing home accidents. These include use of leaflets and pamphlets, newspaper items, and talks. Schools have been enlisted in the fight; they give instruction to school-children, and some have provided their students with home-inspection forms so that they can check conditions and discuss them with their parents. Housing inspectors and visiting nurses may also make valuable suggestions.

18-5. Organization for Accident Prevention. Governmental agencies have been slow to support accident-prevention work, although this outlook is now changing. Industry was quick to see the value of adopting safety measures. Private agencies have concerned themselves with safety, and through their efforts health departments are manifesting more interest.

The National Safety Council is a clearinghouse for accident statistics. It furnishes leadership and information to local safety organizations and provides services for government departments, industry, insurance companies, schools, etc. It publishes much information on many phases of safety, and these are available as leaflets and pamphlets at small cost to any organization.

The Public Health Service has a Division of Accident Prevention, which conducts a program aimed at encouraging and assisting state and local health and other agencies in the development, operation, and improvement of local accident-prevention programs. It provides technical services to state and local authorities, plans and conducts research, and aids in the administration of a grant program to aid in the development of research at universities and elsewhere. It also provides interchange of information for poison-control centers throughout the country.

Some state health departments have accident-prevention divisions.

Their activities include encouraging and assisting local and private agencies in development, operation, and improvement of local programs and providing technical services to local agencies.

The local activities will be carried out by the local health department [4], police and traffic-control agencies, and the fire marshal's organization for fire-prevention inspections; all these agencies will perhaps be assisted by a local safety council made up of interested persons. The health department's activities will, of course, depend upon the interest manifested by its director and also upon the funds he has available.

If a division of accident prevention is established, its functions should include:

1. Coordination of accident-prevention work carried on by other agencies and cooperation with such agencies.

2. Encouragement of effective enforcements of all codes, such as housing, electrical, building, etc., which are related to accidents.

3. Training of nurses and inspectors of the health department so that in their visits to homes, premises, and places of business they will be alert for accident hazards and take the appropriate measures. Training may also be given to recreation supervisors and schoolteachers.

4. Study of local accident statistics so that accident-prevention work can be directed where most needed.

5. Carrying on of a continuous educational campaign.

There are over four hundred poison-control centers located throughout the country. They have information which is furnished by manufacturers of the poisonous ingredients of many commonly used cleaning agents, polishes, insecticides, etc., which are used in households. A physician who must treat a child who has swallowed furniture polish, for example, can telephone the poison-control center, give the brand name of the product, learn its composition, and thereby be aided in giving the proper treatment.

Sanitation of Public Conveyances

18-6. Railways. The Bureau of State Services of the Public Health Service has jurisdiction over the sanitation of interstate carriers, and details as to sanitary requirements and procedures are obtainable from that agency. The term "interstate carrier" as applied to railways is very broad and includes, by court decision, railways which are entirely within a state but which connect with a line that crosses the state boundary. Hence practically all railways are under Federal supervision in regard to sanitation as well as other matters. The sanitary problems of railways are concerned with dining cars, water supply, and excreta disposal. The first-named presents the usual problems of food handling and is not discussed here. Only an outline of the requirements for the latter two can be given; for more details the reader is referred to the "Handbooks on Sanitation" of the Public Health Service [6, 7, 8].

WATER SUPPLY. The water supplies of the railways are carefully supervised. The standards of quality mentioned in Art. 2-9 were formulated by the Public Health Service to apply to interstate carriers, but they have been widely adopted by the states and cities. Actual inspections of the sources of supply, usually municipal systems, are made by sanitary engineers of the state health departments, who also take samples for testing in the state laboratory. The results of the survey and tests are sent to the Public Health Service, together with a recommendation by the inspecting engineer. If findings are favorable, a certificate of approval is issued. If minor deficiencies are found, a provisional certificate is issued pending the making of improvements. If they are not made or if major deficiencies are found at the first inspection, the supply is disapproved and cannot be used.

The water-supply problem, therefore, is largely a matter of safety in production, treatment, and distribution of municipal supplies. However, safety must also be attained at the points where the water tanks of the cars are filled, which frequently are the railway yards. The filling is done by hose from faucets, which must not be flush with the ground surface, lest contaminated water accumulate around them, and which must be placed or guarded in such fashion that they are not exposed to spattering from car toilets. Guards are placed over the ends of hoses so that they cannot come into contact with the ground. If buckets are used, they must have covers and must be used for this purpose only. Water tanks must be kept clean, and since ice may be contaminated by handling, it is placed in a separate compartment from the water. The ice must, however, be handled in a sanitary manner.

EXCRETA DISPOSAL. In yards and terminals, toilets are kept closed, and tanks are attached during cleaning and flushing. These tanks are emptied and cleaned in such fashion that the water supply is not endangered. Railway-car toilets discharge wastes and flushing water directly to the tracks, and the only sanitary restriction has been the locking of toilets while cars are in stations or the placing of signs in the toilets requesting that no flushing be done while the train is in, or passing through, a station. Sanitary authorities have been concerned with possible danger to water supplies near railways and to track workmen by discharge to the tracks, but an inquiry by Maxcy [9] indicated no definite proof that the practice had caused waterborne epidemics or had any effect upon the death rate for typhoid fever among track and yard employees of railroads.

The practice of scattering fecal matter along tracks is disagreeable to contemplate. Studies have been made [10] to determine the amount and character of the discharges, and further investigations are in progress to develop some device to reduce the wastes to a finely divided condition so that they will not be conspicuous and then to disinfect them by means of heat before they are scattered to the track.

18-7. Vessels. The sanitary problems of passenger and other vessels include food handling, water supply, and rat control [11, 12]. The water-supply problem for interstate vessels is handled in the same manner as for railways, with the same precautions as to quality and distribution at the docks. Careful attention must be given to the ship's plumbing to prevent cross-connections of the drinking-water system to polluted supplies. This is particularly necessary on vessels plying the Great Lakes. Rats must be controlled by fumigation or otherwise. Vessels which make international voyages and which come from known plague-infested ports are fumigated to kill rats under the supervision of the Public Health Service. Other vessels may also make use of the same service from time to time. The Service also gives consultation service to ship designers and builders to the end that rat harborages may be reduced.

18-8. Airplanes. Planes engaged in interstate service present the same problems regarding food and water as railways [13]. Excreta are caught in tanks and disposed of at the airport. The principal sanitary problem concerns planes on international flights, which may convey infected mosquitoes for long distances in a few hours. Jungle yellow fever is endemic in large areas of Africa and South and Central America, and epidemics of urban yellow fever may arise in the cities. Obviously, unless precautions are taken, an infected mosquito may enter a plane and be carried to another country, and an epidemic may result. Obviously too, precautions should be taken whether there is a known epidemic in an airport city or not. Another danger is the introduction of a new vector of mosquito-borne disease to an area. An instance of this was the appearance in eastern Brazil of *Anopheles gambiae,* apparently introduced by a fast boat from Africa. This mosquito is a very efficient malaria vector, and, as it found conditions in that portion of Brazil very favorable, it caused a severe epidemic of malaria. The Rockefeller Foundation in cooperation with the Brazilian government was able to exterminate the species in Brazil by careful work adapted to its breeding habits.

Mosquitoes in airplanes are killed by aerosols containing pyrethrins and other insecticides. The aerosol should be released before passengers enter the plane at the beginning of a trip. Since mosquitoes may enter with passengers, another release should be made just before the next stop. This is not always done, but certainly there should be a final release just before landing at the last airport of the trip.

18-9. Buses. The principal sanitary problem which may arise in connection with buses or motor coaches is the motor exhaust. The exhaust gases include dangerous carbon monoxide and should not be allowed to enter the conveyance. Some cities, therefore, have ordinances requiring that exhaust pipes be free from leaks and that the discharge point be located so that there is a minimum of danger of exhaust gases entering the coach.

Community Noise Abatement

18-10. Sources of Noise. Noise in industry has been discussed in Art. 16-11. Here community noise will be treated. The principal sources of community noise are (1) automobile or truck traffic; (2) railway trains and other rail transit systems; (3) aircraft on the ground or in flight near terminal areas; (4) building equipment, such as air-conditioning blowers, compressors, etc.; (5) construction and maintenance equipment; (6) electrical distribution transformers; and (7) factories from which noises escape to the surrounding area. The last four sources are likely to be of importance only in certain localities. They may be of public concern where schools, apartment houses, or office buildings are located near airports or in hotel rooms that have openings toward rooftop mechanical equipment of a nearby building.

Noise that does not impair hearing is primarily a nuisance and causes no health hazard, although claims have been made that work output in offices has been improved by reducing the noise level. Adaption to noises is usually accomplished. Noise levels are measured by decibels (Art. 16-11), and surveys have indicated that street traffic din may range from 60 to 80 db. The noise of a subway train will reach 94 db, and a steamship whistle 93 db. In city residences the average noise has been found to be 31 db, with variations from 22 to 45 db. In offices the noise may vary from 72 to 32 db, with an average of 51 db.

18-11. Noise Prevention. Overcoming the community noise nuisance requires (1) education of the public; (2) cooperation of industrial firms, utility companies, truck owners, businessmen, and city authorities; (3) a reasonable and enforceable antinoise ordinance; and (4) a coordinating agency or commission.

The public must be informed as to the desirability of reducing unnecessary noise, particularly with regard to blowing of automobile horns, loud radios, etc.

Utility companies may cooperate by reducing noises of streetcars, elevated railways, and subways. Subways and elevated railways can be so constructed in the future that noise is much decreased, although remedying existing conditions is impracticable. Trucks and taxis can be kept in repair, and drivers can be instructed to avoid unnecessary noise. Steel buildings may be constructed by welding rather than riveting. Automobile horns can be used that are free from shrill and inharmonic overtones.

Soundproofing of homes and office buildings should not be overlooked. Materials are available that reduce transmission of sound through walls and damp it after it has entered. Fans, compressors, and other noisy equipment items can be enclosed. In offices noisy processes, such as typewriting, can be segregated in small rooms rather than placed all in one large room, where the resultant noise is the sum of all. Such precautions make it possible to keep the noise of homes and offices below 30 and 35 db, respectively; in any case, the noise level in homes should not exceed 50 db.

An ordinance[1] is required to define unnecessary noises and provide for punishment of infractions. Heavy penalties defeat the purpose of the ordinance. Small fines, up to $5, should be levied for violations, and enforcement is easier and more efficient if violators who admit their guilt can pay their fines to the tax receiver without having to appear in court. Of course, provision must also be made for trial of the accused who claims that he is not guilty. Policemen should have the responsibility of enforcing the ordinance.

Some agency should be established to coordinate antinoise activities and keep the matter before the public. If this is not done, enforcement soon becomes perfunctory and then ceases altogether. The commission should be made up of interested persons and city officials, with a sanitary engineer from the health department as technical consultant.

Motels, Trailer Parks, Camps, and Migratory Labor Camps

18-12. Motels and Tourist Courts. These facilities for the traveler present no sanitary problems if located where they will receive city services. If not located in a city, they must provide their own water supplies and disposal methods for sewage and refuse. Water supplies will usually be wells, which should be located, constructed, and equipped so that the water will be adequate in amount and safe (Art. 2-39). The supply should be checked by the local health authorities; if there is no active local authority, the approval of the state health department should be obtained. Table 18-4 gives the amounts of water required for motels and courts and for other services, such as restaurants, service stations, swimming pools, picnic grounds, etc., which are frequently provided by motels.

The amounts of sewage may be assumed to be the same as the water-supply requirements given in Table 18-4. The disposal method

---

[1] A model noise ordinance is obtainable from Public Administration Service, Chicago.

Table 18-4. GUIDE FOR WATER USE

Type of establishment	*Gallons per day*
Bathhouses (per bather)	10
Camps:	
Construction, semipermanent (per worker)	50
Day, with no meals served (per camper)	15
Luxury (per camper)	100–150
Resorts, day and night, with limited plumbing (per camper)	50
Tourist, with central bath and toilet facilities (per person)	35
Courts, tourist, with individual bath units (per person)	50
Clubs:	
Country (per resident member)	100
Country (per nonresident member present)	25
Motels:	
With bath, toilet, and kitchen facilities (per bed space)	50
With bed and toilet only (per bed space)	40
Parks:	
Overnight, with flush toilets (per camper)	25
Trailers with individual bath units (per camper)	50
Picnic areas:	
With bathhouses, showers, and flush toilets (per picnicker)	20
With toilet facilities only (per picnicker)	10
Restaurants:	
With toilet facilities (per patron)	7–10
Without toilet facilities (per patron)	2½–3
With bars and cocktail lounge (additional quantity per patron)	2
Service stations (per vehicle)	10
Swimming pools (per swimmer)	10
Workers, day (per person per shift)	15

SOURCE: Manual of Individual Water Supply Systems, *Public Health Service Pub.* 24, rev. 1962.

used should meet the approval of local and state health authorities. It should not endanger the water supply. Methods suggested for trailer parks of various sizes in Art. 11-23 are applicable to motels. Discussions of the methods will be found in Chap. 4.

Covered garbage cans should be supplied for each living unit. For disposal of refuse a simple type of incinerator may be used. It will reduce the bulk of the refuse, but garbage will not be completely consumed, and therefore ashes and other residue may be buried to prevent odors and fly breeding. A sanitary landfill may be used for residue or for the total refuse. Care should be taken that buried material will not pollute the water supply.

Sanitary inspection of motels and tourist courts should cover the following: water supply, sewage disposal, and plumbing; refuse collection and disposal; proper lighting of dwelling units and grounds; ventilation of dwelling units, including proper venting of gas heating and cooking facilities; screening of dwelling units and kitchens; control of rats, mice, cockroaches, and other vermin; and cleanliness of living units, including floors, rugs, mattresses, and linens and whether linens are changed after each use. If a restaurant is operated and a swimming pool is among the attractions, the requirements of Chaps. 7 and 12 should be applied.

18-13. Summer Camps. It is estimated that over five million children go to summer camps each year; many adults also visit them. Many states require permits for such camps. These are not granted until preliminary inspections indicate that health hazards will not exist, and the permits may be revoked if considered necessary. State regulations require that each camp have at least one person who is familiar with the state requirements as to sanitation and who is responsible for the operation and maintenance of the hot- and cold-water systems, the sewage and refuse disposal systems, the swimming pool, the food handling, the refrigeration, and the cleanliness of all buildings and the grounds.

Table 18-4 gives the amount of water that is required per person in camps. The source of supply should meet the approval of local and state health authorities and should satisfy the requirements as to safety indicated in Chap. 2. Table 18-5 gives required number of baths, showers, etc. Toilets must be within convenient distances from sleeping quarters, in general not over 150 ft. Sewage disposal methods must also meet local and state health department approval. Applicable methods are given in Chap. 4 and Art. 11-23. Refuse should be placed in covered cans and disposed of as indicated in Art. 18-12. Swimming-pool operation should comply with the recommendations of Chap. 12.

Buildings should be structurally safe and should be screened. They should have easily cleanable floors, provide adequate ventilation, and have fire extinguishers (Art. 18-14).

Food handlers should have toilets near the kitchen. Hand-washing facilities with hot and cold water and paper towels should be made available to them. Food storage, handling, and washing and sanitization of dishes and other utensils should apply methods given in Chap. 7. Kitchen and dining room should be screened against flies, and rodents

Table 18-5. NUMBER OF FIXTURES RECOMMENDED
FOR SUMMER CAMPS

Type of fixture	Number of persons per fixture	
	Male	Female
Water closets	12–15	10–15
Urinals.	15–20	. . . .
Showers	12–15	12–15
Lavatories	10–15	10–15

and other vermin should be controlled. Refuse should be stored in covered metal cans placed on racks about 12 in. from the ground and should be emptied at least once a week. For disposal methods and for applicable sanitary inspections, see Art. 18-12.

18-14. Migratory Labor Camps. Migratory farm laborers, in many cases accompanied by their families, follow harvests to work some weeks or less at one location and then move to another. Between four and five hundred thousand people take part in this migration [17]. Living accommodations are provided by the farmers for whom they work. In some cases the living facilities have been so primitive as to present serious health hazards. State health departments are assisting local health departments to remedy conditions, although the obstacles are numerous. The farm proprietor wishes to spend as little as possible for accommodations which are used only a short period of each year. His water supply may be meager, and he assumes that the workers will not appreciate showers, water closets, or commodious living quarters. Education and pressure are necessary to bring about improvements. State regulations may include the following requirements.

Water required will be 35 gal per person per day. Its quality must meet the standards of the state health department, and it should be available at all times in all habitable buildings. Hot and cold water should be available for bathing, dishwashing, and laundering. For the required number of fixtures, Table 18-5 will apply. One laundry tray, washtub, or other laundry facility should also be furnished for each 25 persons or fraction thereof.

Separate washrooms, bathrooms, and toilet rooms should be provided for each sex, and they should be plainly marked. If located in the same building, they should be separated by solid walls or partitions extending from the floor to the roof. Adequate dressing space should be furnished adjacent to bathing facilities.

A toilet facility should be located not further than 200 ft from the door of each sleeping room. For common toilet facilities, toilet paper should be furnished. All toilet, wash, bath, and laundry buildings should have impermeable floors sloped to drain and should be adequately lighted and ventilated.

In camps where separate family living units are provided and where they include bath and toilet facilities, these should be placed in a separate room that is reached without passing through a bedroom. If a kitchen is provided, it should include a sink and water supply.

Sewage disposal, if no city sewers are available, will ordinarily be by septic tank and tile disposal field. If a non-water-carried system is used, it should be of a type approved by the state health department. In that case no privy should be located within 50 ft of a kitchen.

Garbage and other refuse should be deposited and stored in covered metal cans of not over 32 gal capacity. For disposal methods see Art. 18-12.

Dormitories, living units, and common kitchens should be screened. Mosquitoes, flies, rodents, and other vermin should be controlled. If sleeping facilities, such as cots or bunks with mattresses, are furnished, they should be filled with clean straw or other suitable material free from dust and vermin. Mattresses and ticks should be laundered or otherwise sanitized between assignments to different employees. Beds or bunks should be at least 12 in. above the floor. Triple-deck facilities should be prohibited, and in quarters other than for family groups, double beds should be prohibited. Single beds should be spaced not closer than 36 in. laterally or end to end. Double-deck beds should be spaced not closer than 48 in. laterally and 36 in. end to end, with a clear height from mattress to ceiling of at least 36 in. The clear space above the lower mattress of a double-deck bed should be at least 27 in. to the bottom of the upper bed.

Safety provisions include the furnishing and maintenance of first-aid facilities and fire extinguishers. Units of fire-extinguishing equipment should be provided for each 1,000 sq ft of floor space, and it should not be necessary to travel more than 100 ft to reach the nearest unit. A unit consists of (1) soda and acid—one 2½-gal or two 1½-gal containers; (2) foam—one 2½-gal or two 1½-gal containers; (3) vaporizing liquid (carbon tetrachloride)—two containers, any size from 1 qt to 1 gal; and (4) water—one 2½-gal (stored pressure) or two 5-gal (pump type) containers.

The camp site should be well drained and free from water-holding depressions. Standing water within 200 ft of the edge of the camp should be drained or treated with a mosquito larvicide during the mosquito breeding season. No camp structure should be located less than 200 ft from a food-processing plant or from barns, pens, or similar quarters for livestock or poultry. Some recreation space should be provided that is appropriate to the size and occupancy of the camp.

The Federal government made funds available in 1962 as grants to the state and local tax-supported agencies and to private nonprofit organizations to finance programs that will benefit the migratory worker and his family. Programs have included family health service clinics, camp construction, sanitation services, and health education projects. The Public Health Service administers the grants.

18-15. Mobile-home Parks. There are over two million trailer coaches being used as temporary or permanent homes in the United States, and the number is increasing. Plumbing, heating, and wiring systems of the homes have been standardized to make them more habitable [14]. City ordinances and state regulations have been found necessary to control the grounds where the trailers park for short or long periods. City ordinances may prohibit parking for residential purposes except at designated parks [15].

The site should be well drained with no breeding places for insects and rodents and should be free from smoke, odor, and noise. If possible, city water and sewer service should be available.

Each mobile-home space should be clearly marked. Space provided should allow at least 15 ft of side-to-side spacing between homes, 10 ft of end-to-end spacing, 10 ft to any adjoining property line, 25 ft from the sideline of any public street or highway, and 15 ft from any building or structure [16]. Some regulations require a minimum of 1,000 sq ft (40 by 25 ft) per mobile home and also require that provision be made for a few homes up to 50 ft long.

Table 18-4 gives 50 gpcpd as the probable water consumption. The New Jersey regulations specify 125 gal per day per mobile home. The water and sewer connections required are described briefly in Art. 11-23.

Trailer parks should be equipped with electric power, and all systems and equipment installed should be in accordance with local ordinances or the current National Electrical Code. A properly grounded waterproof electrical receptacle should be provided for each home space, and each home should be suitably grounded. A properly sized over-current device should be installed as an integral part of each outlet.

Fire protection is obtained by requiring that a fire hydrant be located within 400 ft of all the mobile homes or park buildings, if water is supplied by a public system. If otherwise supplied, a riser pipe 2 in. in size located not over 300 ft from all the homes is required. Sufficient 1½-in. fire hose to reach the homes is also required. A fire-extinguishing unit (Art. 18-14) is also required to be available for each home, or approved pump tanks, water barrels, and buckets must be provided. A fire alarm is also required.

Refuse containers should be covered, flytight, and rodentproof. They should provide at least 6 gal/day per mobile home space and should be located not more than 150 ft from any home space. They should be emptied at least once per week. Containers should be located on racks or in holders to minimize spillage. The racks or holders should have 12 in. of clear space beneath them. Containers should be emptied at least weekly. If collections are not made by city forces, disposal should be by methods indicated in Art. 18-12.

Parks which accommodate trailers not equipped with toilets and baths must provide a service building equipped to furnish hot and cold water. This should provide for 10 units or less: one water closet for males and two for females; one urinal; two lavatories each for males and females; and one shower each for males and females. For each

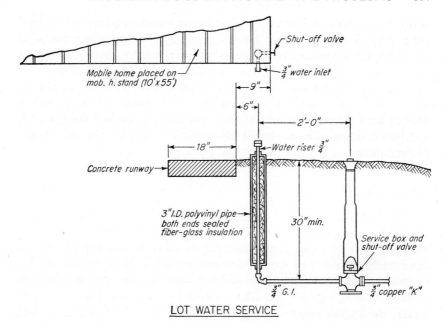

LOT WATER SERVICE

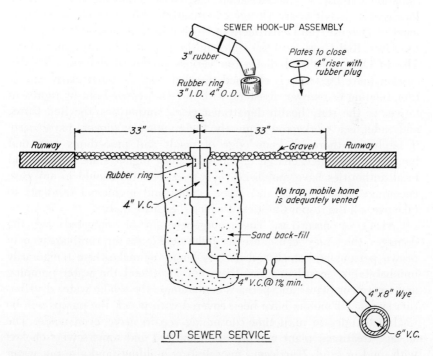

LOT SEWER SERVICE

FIGURE 18-2 Water and sewer connections for mobile homes. (*Recommended by the Mobile Homes Manufacturers Association.*)

additional 10 units or less, one of each fixture mentioned should be added for male and female, except for the urinals, which may be substituted for the male water closets to the extent of not more than one-third of the total closet requirements. One slop sink should also be provided.

The service building should be separated for male and female. It should be well ventilated and screened and should have a window area at least 12 per cent of the floor area and an interior finish that is moisture-resistant. Floors should be of impervious material and sloped to floor drains.

Disaster Sanitation

18-16. Public health is often endangered when disasters occur and should be considered in preparedness measures. Congress created the Federal Civil Defense Administration to cushion the impact and to function in the relief of natural disasters as well as those which are due to bombing or other military action. A system of radar stations has been established and warning procedures developed. To cope with an enemy attack, the FCDA provides training in rescue work, evacuation, gas and radiation defense, decontamination, and construction of bomb shelters. Its disaster activities are closely coordinated with those of the Department of Defense, the Department of Health, Education, and Welfare, the American Red Cross, and the state and local civil defense organizations. The FCDA publishes bulletins on various phases of defense. The discussion here, however, is confined to relief matters, particularly sanitation, relating to nonwar disasters, with the work carried out by representatives of the state health department, local authorities, the Red Cross, and volunteer workers. Frequently the sanitary engineer, particularly if he has a thorough knowledge of needs and procedures may find himself in complete charge of all work until higher state officials and local authorities have mobilized their resources. He should in any case encourage local officials and other county and municipal residents to take over all the responsibilities of which they are capable.

TYPES OF DISASTERS. The emergencies to be expected and the damages they may cause are as follows: *Floods* in rural areas may drown persons and stock and destroy homes or make them temporarily uninhabitable; in urban areas they may also flood the water pumping and treatment plants and perhaps contaminate the whole water distribution system. If motors have been covered with water, the pumps will be unable to operate until time-consuming repairs have been made. The sewage treatment plant may also be damaged and some sewers choked with mud or sand. *Hurricanes* may destroy buildings and also put water pumping and treatment plants out of operation. Collapse of buildings means extensive plumbing damages and heavy leakage of water. All city services, including light, power, and telephone, may be disrupted. *Fires* and *explosions,* if extensive, may have all the effects of hurricanes. *Earthquakes,* which are sometimes accompanied by fires, may result in much breakage of water mains and sewers, in addition to causing the other damages cited.

PREPARATION. The state health department which has prepared itself has designated a sanitary engineer in each district to function in case of disasters. He should have available for instant use a mobile water filter and chlorinator with a stock of chlorine or hypochlorite, depending upon the type of apparatus. The representatives of chlorinator manufacturers sometimes have portable units which they are willing to place at the disposal of an engineer in emergencies, and he should be ready to call for this assistance when needed. He should also know where gasoline- or motor-driven pumps can be obtained for emergency water service. Fire department pumpers have sometimes been used for this purpose. For information as to such emergency shelter as tents, he should make contact with Army, including National Guard, and Navy authorities in his district. If there are local committees for relief work, the engineer should confer with them, explain his plans, and learn theirs. The same applies to the representatives of the Red Cross. If there are regional waterworks associations, he should encourage them to form emergency sanitation committees that will obtain the following lists: names of trained waterworks and sewage works operators in the area; equipment that can be obtained for use during an emergency, such as tank trucks, repair equipment, insect sprayers, and refuse collection equipment; major plumbing concerns; and local utility concerns. If waterworks associations are not available, he must use other methods to obtain such information. He should also have on hand a list of equipment and supplies that can be obtained from the state and local health departments.

RELIEF WORK. The primary human needs in an area which has been struck by disaster are medical services, safe water, food, and shelter. If the weather is severe, fuel and warm clothing are also essential.

Medical services, which may include immunization against typhoid fever, are furnished by state, local, or Red Cross authorities, which also furnish the supplies.

If a refugee camp is set up, an emergency water supply may be established by means of a mobile water treatment plant and chlorinator; if tank trucks are available, they may be used to convey water from some safe supply. The food, including milk, should come from safe sources and be properly handled in the camp. If warehouses or similar buildings are not available for emergency housing, it may be necessary to obtain tents, which must be properly placed on a suitable, well-drained site. Refuse must be collected and removed. If no city service is available, it may be possible to obtain trucks and drivers from the state highway department. If sewerage is not available, some type of emergency latrines may have to be established to be replaced with pit privies as quickly as possible. Tools and materials should be available, and able-bodied male refugees should be put to work, under skilled supervision, digging pits for privies and refuse disposal and constructing privy buildings, tent floors, rough tables, benches, and other necessities. If the camp is located in an undamaged urban area, it may be possible to have electric lines and gas pipes run for lighting and cooking at a central kitchen.

Dead bodies must be collected and placed in temporary morgues for identification and later burial. Carcasses of animals may be removed by meat-packing plants, which usually have trucks and hoists. Insecticides should be used freely around garbage storage and disposal areas, toilets, barracks, and food-handling points. Airplane application of DDT may be advisable to control flies and to prevent malaria in areas which have been flooded. Observations should be made as to the need for rodent control.

In cities it may be necessary to chlorinate the water distribution system throughout if it has been contaminated by unsafe water. Emergency pumps may have to be set up. If important damage has been done to the waterworks, pipe, fittings, and other equipment may be needed. Reference to the lists mentioned above will enable the engineer or local waterworks man to obtain them quickly. If he needs skilled assistance, he can call upon men listed as available. If many plumbing systems have been damaged, it may be necessary to plug broken lines so that adequate water pressure can be built up. Thereafter permanent repairs may be made. If sewers are clogged, rods and other cleaning apparatus will be needed for rapid cleaning.

Bibliography

1. Arbous, A. G.: Accident Statistics and the Concept of Accident Proneness, *Biometrics*, vol. 7, p. 340, 1951.
2. Halsey, M. N. (ed.): "Accident Prevention," McGraw-Hill Book Company, New York, 1961.
3. "Accident Facts," National Safety Council, Chicago, 1962.
4. Suggested Home Accident Prevention Activities for Health Departments, *Am. J. Public Health*, vol. 46, no. 5, May, 1956.
5. Velz, C. J., and F. M. Hemphill: "Home Injuries," School of Public Health, University of Michigan, Ann Arbor, Mich., 1962.
6. Handbook on Sanitation of Railroad Passenger Car Construction, *Public Health Service Pub.* 95.
7. Handbook on Sanitation of Railroad Servicing Areas, *Public Health Service Pub.* 66.

8. Handbook on Sanitation of Dining Cars in Operation, *Public Health Service Pub.* 83.
9. Maxcy, K. F.: "An Inquiry into the Public Health Hazard of Sewage Disposal from Railway Conveyances," Association of American Railroads, 1946.
10. Wolman, A., and L. K. Clark: Human Waste Disposal from Railroad Passenger Cars, *Am. J. Public Health*, vol. 38, no. 5, May, 1948.
11. Handbook on Sanitation of Vessel Construction, *Public Health Service Pub.* 393.
12. Handbook on Sanitation of Vessels in Operation, *Public Health Service Pub.* 68.
13. Handbook on Sanitation of Airlines, *Public Health Service Pub.* 308.
14. "Plumbing, Heating and Electrical Systems in Mobile Homes," American Standards Association, New York, 1963.
15. "Mobile Home Park Sanitation with Suggested Ordinance," prepared by Public Health Service, Mobile Homes Manufacturers Association, Chicago.
16. "Mobile Home Parks," New Jersey State Sanitary Code, Trenton, N.J., 1963.
17. "Housing for Migrant Agricultural Workers," *U.S. Dep. Labor, Bull.* 235, 1961.

19

VITAL STATISTICS

19-1. While the sanitarian cannot ordinarily be a statistician, he should be sufficiently acquainted with vital statistics and their uses to be able to apply them to his work. Morbidity statistics, which are the statistics of disease, and mortality statistics, which are concerned with death and the causes of death, indicate more or less clearly the healthfulness of a community and the success or failure of health work. What is even more important, they may give valuable clues as to the character of work that is required. Birthrates are of somewhat less importance to the sanitarian but are useful in other lines of health activities. The prediction of future population is essential in connection with the planning of such sanitary improvements as water treatment plants, sewage disposal works, and sewer extensions. Complete studies of vital statistics include many other items, such as marriage and divorce rates and characteristics of the population of the country as to age, race, etc.

19-2. Sources of Vital Statistics. Vital statistics are obtained from several different agencies. Population and its characteristics are obtained from the official enumeration made by the Bureau of the Census. Birth and death statistics are obtained from certificates that are required by state laws from attending physicians or midwives. Physicians are also required by law to report cases of certain diseases, known as notifiable diseases, to the local health officers, who transmit the reports to the state health officers. The state health officers in turn report to the Communicable Disease Center of the Public Health Service. The National Center for Health Statistics collects and compiles health statistics of a more general nature and publishes them. These sources of vital statistics are discussed in detail in the following articles.

19-3. Census. The United States census is taken every 10 years by the Bureau of the Census, which is a part of the Department of Commerce. A staff of enumerators works simultaneously in all parts of the country and of the outlying possessions, completing the collection of data in about 30 days. The information is obtained through questions which may be classified under the following headings: place of abode, tenure of home, personal description, citizenship, nativity, and occupation. The census reports give the population by various civil divisions. The population is divided into states; the states into counties; the counties into boroughs and towns; and the cities into wards. The population of the rural regions and villages is also indicated. Data are also given for about two hundred standard metropolitan statistical areas, which are whole counties or groups of counties (Art. 21-2). The study of the vital statistics of any section of the country must be based upon its total population and the characteristics, age grouping, sex distribution, etc., of that population. The importance of the census reports which give this fundamental information therefore cannot be overestimated.

19-4. Death Certificates. Death certificates are required by the laws of the various states. They include information as to name, usual residence, age, race, nativity, conjugal condition, occupation, and date of death of the deceased. These questions may be filled in by any competent person, usually the funeral director. Place and date of burial or removal must be given by the funeral director. The cause or causes of death and circumstances surrounding it must be given by the physician in attendance. If no physician has been in attendance, the required burial-transit permit is not issued until the case has been referred to the local health officer or coroner. In suspicious cases an investigation must be made by the coroner, justice of the peace, or other proper official before burial is permitted. In case of accident, suicide, or homicide, in-

CERTIFICATE OF DEATH

BIRTH No.	STATE OF		STATE FILE No.	

1. PLACE OF DEATH
a. COUNTY

2. USUAL RESIDENCE (*Where deceased lived. If institution: Residence before admission*)
a. STATE   b. COUNTY

b. CITY, TOWN, OR LOCATION   c. LENGTH OF STAY IN 1b   c. CITY, TOWN, OR LOCATION

d. NAME OF HOSPITAL OR INSTITUTION (*If not in hospital, give street address*)   d. STREET ADDRESS

e. IS PLACE OF DEATH INSIDE CITY LIMITS?   YES ☐ NO ☐   e. IS RESIDENCE INSIDE CITY LIMITS?   YES ☐ NO ☐   f. IS RESIDENCE ON A FARM?   YES ☐ NO ☐

3. NAME OF DECEASED (*Type or print*)   First   Middle   Last   **4. DATE OF DEATH**   Month   Day   Year

5. SEX   **6. COLOR OR RACE**   **7** MARRIED ☐ NEVER MARRIED ☐ WIDOWED ☐ DIVORCED ☐   **8. DATE OF BIRTH**   **9. AGE** (*In years last birthday*)   IF UNDER 1 YEAR | Months | Days   IF UNDER 24 HRS. | Hours | Min.

10a. USUAL OCCUPATION (*Give kind of work done during most of working life, even if retired*)   **10b. KIND OF BUSINESS OR INDUSTRY**   **11. BIRTHPLACE** (*State or foreign country*)   **12. CITIZEN OF WHAT COUNTRY?**

13. FATHER'S NAME   **14. MOTHER'S MAIDEN NAME**

15. WAS DECEASED EVER IN U. S. ARMED FORCES? (*Yes, no, or unknown*) (*If yes, give war or dates of service*)   **16. SOCIAL SECURITY NO.**   **17. INFORMANT**   Address

MEDICAL CERTIFICATION

18. CAUSE OF DEATH   [*Enter only one cause per line for (a), (b), and (c).*]   INTERVAL BETWEEN ONSET AND DEATH

PART I. DEATH WAS CAUSED BY:
IMMEDIATE CAUSE (a) _____

Conditions, if any, which gave rise to above cause (a), stating the underlying cause last.   DUE TO (b) _____
DUE TO (c) _____

PART II. OTHER SIGNIFICANT CONDITIONS CONTRIBUTING TO DEATH BUT NOT RELATED TO THE TERMINAL DISEASE CONDITION GIVEN IN PART I(a)   **19. WAS AUTOPSY PERFORMED?**   YES ☐ NO ☐

20a. ACCIDENT ☐   SUICIDE ☐   HOMICIDE ☐   **20b.** DESCRIBE HOW INJURY OCCURRED. (*Enter nature of injury in Part I or Part II of item 18.*)

20c. TIME OF INJURY   Hour a. m. p. m.   Month, Day, Year

20d. INJURY OCCURRED   WHILE AT WORK ☐ NOT WHILE AT WORK ☐   **20e.** PLACE OF INJURY (*e. g., in or about home, farm, factory, street, office bldg., etc.*)   **20f.** CITY, TOWN, OR LOCATION   COUNTY   STATE

21. I attended the deceased from _____ , to _____ and last saw her/him alive on _____

Death occurred at _____ m on the date stated above; and to the best of my knowledge, from the causes stated.

22a. SIGNATURE   (*Degree or title*)   **22b. ADDRESS**   **22c. DATE SIGNED**

23a. BURIAL, CREMATION, REMOVAL (*Specify*)   **23b. DATE**   **23c. NAME OF CEMETERY OR CREMATORY**   **23d. LOCATION** (*City, town, or county*)   (*State*)

24. FUNERAL DIRECTOR   ADDRESS   **25. DATE RECD. BY LOCAL REG.**   **26. REGISTRAR'S SIGNATURE**

FIGURE 19-1   The standard death certificate. (*Public Health Service, 1956.*)

formation is obtained as to the nature of the injury and the time and place it occurred. The death certificate, after being made out and signed by the physician and the undertaker, must be filed by the latter with the local registrar, and a burial-transit permit is issued. Copies of death certificates and burial permits are kept by the local registrar, who transmits the original death records to the state registrar for permanent filing in the state bureau of vital statistics. Copies of vital records may be filed locally by the county or city clerks and/or by the county or city health departments.

Death registration assists in the prevention and detection of crime. It is valuable in the settlement of property, inheritance, and life insurance cases. The fact that causes of death are recorded has resulted in statistics which have played a large part in the control of disease.

```
                          CERTIFICATE OF LIVE BIRTH
STATE OF                                              BIRTH NO.
```

STATE OF	CERTIFICATE OF LIVE BIRTH BIRTH NO.	

1. PLACE OF BIRTH
   a. COUNTY | 2. USUAL RESIDENCE OF MOTHER (*Where does mother live?*)
   a. STATE | b. COUNTY

b. CITY, TOWN, OR LOCATION | c. CITY, TOWN, OR LOCATION

c. NAME OF (*If not in hospital, give street address*) HOSPITAL OR INSTITUTION | d. STREET ADDRESS

d. IS PLACE OF BIRTH INSIDE CITY LIMITS? YES ☐ NO ☐ | e. IS RESIDENCE INSIDE CITY LIMITS? YES ☐ NO ☐ | f. IS RESIDENCE ON A FARM? YES ☐ NO ☐

CHILD
3. NAME (*Type or print*) First   Middle   Last

4. SEX | 5a. THIS BIRTH SINGLE ☐ TWIN ☐ TRIPLET ☐ | 5b. IF TWIN OR TRIPLET, WAS CHILD BORN 1ST ☐ 2D ☐ 3D ☐ | 6. DATE OF BIRTH Month Day Year

FATHER
7. NAME First   Middle   Last | 8. COLOR OR RACE

9. AGE (*At time of this birth*) YEARS | 10. BIRTHPLACE (*State or foreign country*) | 11a. USUAL OCCUPATION | 11b. KIND OF BUSINESS OR INDUSTRY

MOTHER
12. MAIDEN NAME First   Middle   Last | 13. COLOR OR RACE

14. AGE (*At time of this birth*) YEARS | 15. BIRTHPLACE (*State or foreign country*) | 16. PREVIOUS DELIVERIES TO MOTHER (*Do NOT include this birth*)
a. *How many OTHER children are now living?* | b. *How many OTHER children were born alive but are now dead?* | c. *How many fetal deaths (fetuses born dead at ANY time after conception)?*

17. INFORMANT

18. MOTHER'S MAILING ADDRESS

I hereby certify that this child was born alive on the date stated above. | 18a. SIGNATURE | 18b. ATTENDANT AT BIRTH M. D. ☐ D. O. ☐ MIDWIFE ☐ OTHER (*Specify*)
| | 18c. ADDRESS | 18d. DATE SIGNED

19. DATE RECD. BY LOCAL REG. | 20. REGISTRAR'S SIGNATURE | 21. DATE ON WHICH GIVEN NAME ADDED BY (*Registrar*)

FOR MEDICAL AND HEALTH USE ONLY
(*This section MUST be filled out*)

22a. LENGTH OF PREGNANCY COMPLETED WEEKS | 22b. WEIGHT AT BIRTH LB.   OZ. | 23. LEGITIMATE YES ☐ NO ☐

(SPACE FOR ADDITION OF MEDICAL AND HEALTH ITEMS BY INDIVIDUAL STATES)

FIGURE 19-2   The standard birth certificate. (*Public Health Service*, 1956.)

The records also have a local value in the detection and suppression of epidemics of communicable disease.

19-5. Birth Certificates. Birth registration is invariably required by the states. Registration is carried out by means of birth certificates, which are made out by the physician or midwife who attended the birth or, if the birth was nonattended, by the parents. The certificate contains the date and place of birth; the name and sex of the child; the name, age, race, birthplace, and residence of the parents; and the occupation of the father. As in the case of death certificates, birth certificates are filed with the local registrar, who may keep a permanent record of them and transmit them to the state registrar, in whose department they are permanently filed.

As registration of birth is of great importance not only to the community but to the individual, parents should insist that the physician file a birth certificate without delay. The local health officer should know how many infants there are in his community and what proportion of the total have died. From birth certificates, he can plan his infant and child hygiene work to safeguard the health of the newborn child and the mother. In cities where health work is well organized, public health nurses visit every home in which a birth has been registered. Some of the more frequent uses of birth records are for obtaining passports, marriage licenses, drivers' licenses, and pension benefits. They are also used for entering military service, obtaining employment, and receiving retirement benefits. To summarize, a birth certificate is important to the individual as the best means of proving age, parentage, and citizenship.

19-6. Morbidity Reports. State laws require that all cases of certain diseases be reported to the state health department by the attending physician immediately after the diagnosis is made. If there is an active local health department, the reports pass through the office of the local health officer or epidemiologist, who is thereby kept informed of the incidence of disease and the existence of actual or threatened epidemics. He may then take the necessary control measures, or in the absence of local action, the state authorities may function. Good cooperation by local physicians in disease reporting is important.

The diseases required to be reported are known as notifiable diseases. The list varies in different states, but usually it will include the communicable diseases and some others that are of particular interest such as pellagra and cancer. A city may by ordinance require reporting of diseases which are not on the state list.

The national morbidity reporting system covers all the states, the District of Columbia, and Puerto Rico, and it is administered by the Communicable Disease Center of the Public Health Service. Data so obtained are published weekly and annually and provide the information necessary for the detection of epidemics and the determination of trends in disease incidence. The data are available to all health departments, news media, and other interested agencies and individuals. Procedures in reporting to the Communicable Disease Center are given in the "Manual of Procedures for National Morbidity Reporting" [1]. Some diseases are required to be reported by state health offices by telephone or telegraph to the Center as soon as a case is diagnosed or suspected or a death is attributed to them. They are then reported, as required by International Sanitary Regulations, to the epidemiological intelligence system of the World Health Organization, which in turn publishes them or may broadcast them if the situation justifies it. The diseases in this category are cholera, plague, plague in rodents, relapsing fever (louse-borne), smallpox, epidemic typhus fever (louse-borne), and yellow fever.

Reports of other cases of notifiable communicable diseases are telegraphed weekly by state health officers to be consolidated in the Morbidity and Mortality Weekly Report. The notifiable diseases are anthrax, aseptic meningitis, botulism, brucellosis, diphtheria, encephalitis (infectious), hepatitis (infectious and serum), malaria, measles, meningococcal infections, poliomyelitis, psittacosis-ornithosis, rabies in man, tetanus, tularemia, typhoid fever, typhus fever (flea-borne and murine), typhus fever (tick-borne), Rocky Mountain spotted fever, rabies in animals, and streptococcal sore throat, including scarlet fever.

Epidemics which occur are also reported by the states by mail. These are also placed in the Weekly Report. Certain diseases are under special surveillance, and these are reported by mail by state epidemiologists. These diseases are poliomyelitis, diphtheria, hepatitis in adults, malaria, smallpox, and influenza. All these, except influenza, are also among the notifiable diseases to be reported. Mail reports are also submitted of cases of tuberculosis, venereal diseases, and diseases transmissible from animals to man. The Center also receives weekly mortality reports from the city health officer or registrar of vital statistics of the city. These are given in the Morbidity and Mortality Weekly Report mentioned above.

The local health officer keeps a record of the diseases reported. The importance to the local health officer of the prompt reporting of diseases by the attending physician cannot be overestimated. It enables him promptly to apply quarantine, isolation, and other measures and thereby prevent an epidemic. His knowledge of the occurrence of a few cases of such a disease as typhoid fever may allow him to apply measures which will stop an incipient typhoid outbreak. In tuberculosis control, prompt registration of the cases ensures the valuable preventive and educational work of the nursing service. A comparison of current morbidity reports with those of former years gives some indication of the value and efficiency of public health work. Morbidity reports are, of course, dependent upon the cooperation of the physician and his compliance with the law. The health officer is frequently called upon to take a firm stand in the enforcement of the state laws requiring such reports. Enforcement of such requirements is as much a part of the public health work as the study of epidemics or milk sanitation.

19-7. Registration Area. The states were not equally progressive in passing adequate laws requiring the registration of births and deaths, and in some cases enforcement of the law was neglected. The result of this condition was that the statistics of some states were not complete and were far from reliable. The Bureau of the Census recognized the birth and death records of a state or any subdivision if, after a careful check, it became convinced that at least 90 per cent of births and deaths were registered, and such recognition placed the state, city, or county in the registration area. A relaxation of diligence in collection and registration might cause it to be dropped from the area. At present all the states are included in the birth- and death-registration areas.

19-8. Population. The vital statistics of any particular subdivision are based upon its population, and this information may be obtained from the census reports. However, the census gives the population only at 10-year intervals. The calculation of a death rate based upon the population given in the census report of 5 or 6 years previous may be far from accurate. It becomes necessary, therefore, to make some approximation of the population for the year in question. This may be done in several ways. The simplest method is by arithmetical progression. The increase per year during the preceding census period is found by dividing the total increase for that period by 10. It is then assumed that the yearly increase for the following census period will be the same. For example, a city of 100,000 population in 1960 gained 20,000 from 1950 to 1960, or an average annual increase of 2,000. The arithmetical method assumes that the annual gain will continue to be 2,000 and will have reached 6,000 by 1963; therefore the population of the city will be 106,000 in 1963. This method has the merit of simplicity and has been widely used. It cannot be extended too far into the future. Local conditions which tend to modify population growth and local information such as number of voters, number of names in the directory, and the school attendance should also be considered in population estimates.

Populations sometimes increase by geometrical progression, *i.e.*, in the same manner as money increases by compound interest. Therefore, applying this method to population increase is sometimes more correct than the arithmetical method. It can be applied easily by means of a formula identical with that used in compound interest computations. It is

$$P_n = P_c(1 + r)^n$$

where P_c is the population at the last census, r is the annual rate of increase expressed as a decimal, n is the number of years after the census, and P_n is the population at n years after the census. To use this formula for the city mentioned above, the average rate of increase for the preceding 10 years must be obtained by substituting 100,000 and 80,000 for P_n and P_c, respectively, and 10 for n, and solving for r. The value of r is found to be 0.0226. To find the population in 1963, 100,000 is substituted for P_c, 0.226 for r, and 3 for n, and P_n (the answer) is found to be 106,993.

In areas undergoing rapid population changes, neither the arithmetic nor the geometric progression method is likely to be adequate. In many states an agency of the state government, *e.g.*, the state health department, makes annual estimates for counties and cities. Such an agency frequently uses methods utilizing the current birthrates and death rates and estimates the loss or gain by migration.

The prediction of population of cities over long periods, 15 years or more, is more complicated and subject to large errors. The possibility of annexations is an important factor. It should also be recognized that there is a tendency toward decreased rates of growth as cities become larger. One method of making forecasts, briefly outlined, is as follows:

1. Plot a population curve over the past census reports.
2. Extend this curve, following the general direction of the known points.
3. Plot the curves of older and larger cities.
4. Other curves showing the arithmetical, geometrical, and 1 per cent rates of growth may also be plotted as guidelines.
5. After carefully considering the possible decreased rate of growth, the possible annexations, the industrial and commercial situation, etc., as well as the previously plotted curves, draw a curve to show the expected increase. In some states assistance in making population predictions can be obtained from state agencies such as planning commissions.

19-9. Death Rates. These are expressed as so many per year per 1,000 of the population. The crude death rate is expressed as the number of deaths in one year occurring per 1,000 of the whole population and may be found from the following formula:

$$\text{Death rate per 1,000} = \frac{\text{number of deaths}}{\text{total population}} \times 1,000$$

The crude death rates of various localities are sometimes compared for the purpose of arriving at the relative healthfulness of the areas. A little consideration demonstrates that crude death rates are not always indicative of the health of a community. Death rates are high among very young children and among the aged. Therefore the locality containing a large percentage of either of these two classes will have a higher crude death rate than another community having a high percentage of young adults, irrespective of health conditions. Comparisons can be made by means of specific death rates, *i.e.*, by finding the death rate among the population of a certain class. For instance, the annual specific death rate for children between five and nine years of age is as follows:

$$\text{Specific death rate} = \frac{\begin{array}{c}\text{number of deaths of children} \\ \text{5 to 9 years of age}\end{array}}{\begin{array}{c}\text{total number of children 5 to} \\ \text{9 years of age}\end{array}} \times 1,000$$

In this formula the number of deaths of children between the ages of five and nine is obtained for the year in question and is then divided by the total number of children of that age in the community in that year.

The specific death rate may be similarly found for other ages, for the sexes, and for the locality of dwelling, *i.e.*, urban or rural. The specific death rates which may be computed are, of course, dependent upon the tabulations as to age, etc., given by the census reports for various localities. Dr. Raymond Pearl [2] points out the value of specific death rates covering such other factors as race, including color and country of birth of person and parents, and occupation.

Since the death rates vary for different ages, it is apparent that the variation in age distribution of populations makes it impossible to compare death rates unless they are standardized or adjusted. The standardized, or adjusted, death rate (indirect method) is obtained by applying the specific death rates for the various age groups (sex groupings may also be used) of some standard population, say, the registration area, to the corresponding age groups of the living population of the particular locality. This gives the number of deaths that would have occurred in the locality if the specific death rates of the standard population had prevailed there, and dividing the number of deaths so obtained by the total living population of the locality gives the expected death rate. The formula

$$\frac{\text{Death rate in standard population} \times \text{death rate of locality}}{\text{Expected death rate of locality}}$$

gives the ratio or corrective factor by which the crude death rate of the locality differs from the death rate of the standard population as a result of the differences between the age distributions of the two populations.

The standardized, or adjusted, death rate (direct method) of a locality is the reverse of the rate described above. The formula is

$$\frac{\text{Sum of (age-specific death rates of locality} \times \text{corresponding}}{\text{populations by age in standard population)}}{\text{Total standard population}}$$

As the formula indicates, the standardized rate is obtained by applying the specific death rates observed in the locality to the corresponding groups in the standard population and dividing the sum of these deaths by the total standard population.

19-10. Causes of Death. Since the causes of death as reported on the death certificates are of great value in studies of vital statistics, it is important that there be uniformity in the medical terms used to describe them. To bring about such uniformity, international commissions have met from time to time to adopt standard classifications of causes of death. The latest, or seventh, classification was made in Paris in 1955 by the International Conference for the Decennial Revision of the International Lists of Diseases and Causes of Death. This list is used by the states in compiling vital statistics. The International List is divided into 17 groups as follows:

Section	Numbers
1. Infective and parasitic diseases	001–138
2. Neoplasms	140–239
3. Allergic, endocrine system, metabolic, and nutritional diseases	240–289
4. Diseases of the blood and blood-forming organs	290–299
5. Mental, psychoneurotic, and personality disorders	300–326
6. Diseases of the nervous system and the sense organs	330–398
7. Diseases of the circulatory system	400–468
8. Diseases of the respiratory system	470–527
9. Diseases of the digestive system	530–587
10. Diseases of the genitourinary system	590–637
11. Deliveries and complications of pregnancy, childbirth, and the puerperium	640–689
12. Diseases of the skin and cellular tissue	690–716
13. Diseases of the bones and organs of movement	720–749
14. Congenital malformations	750–759
15. Certain diseases of early infancy	760–776
16. Symptoms, senility, and ill-defined conditions	780–795
17. Accidents, poisonings, and violence	800–999

Death rates by cause are expressed as the number from the specified cause per 100,000 population.

19-11. Some Factors Affecting Death Rates. In addition to the age groupings, which have already been mentioned as affecting death rates, there are other factors concerned. There may be a large number of non-resident deaths in an area because of the presence of hospitals which attract patients from other communities, thereby unfavorably affecting the local death rate. Therefore, the rate by place of residence should usually be used in studies of mortality. The occupational, social-class, or ethnic composition of the population also significantly affects the death rate.

19-12. Birthrates. These are usually expressed as so many per year per 1,000 population. The birthrate based on the whole population is termed the crude birthrate, which can be found by using the following formula:

$$\text{Birthrate per 1,000} = \frac{\text{number of births in 1 year}}{\text{total population}} \times 1,000$$

While the crude birthrate is the one generally used, it is apparent that the birthrates for various localities cannot be properly compared in many cases. Obviously, the number of births depends to a considerable extent upon the age distribution of the population, the sex distribution, and, particularly, the number of the female population who are of child-bearing age (ordinarily considered to be from fifteen to forty-four years). The birthrate based upon the number of females of child-bearing age may be about five times as great as the crude birthrate.

In some 2 to 3 per cent of all reported deliveries, the child is born dead. This is termed a fetal death and is not considered either a birth or a death in the computation of birthrates, death rates, or infant-mortality rates. The standard certificate of fetal death (stillbirth) is used in registering these events.

If birthrates for local areas are to be compared, it is necessary that such rates be computed on the number of births for the area by place of residence of the mother rather than by place of occurrence.

19-13. Infant Mortality. One of the most important aspects of vital statistics is infant mortality. The infant-mortality rate is suggestive of several things. It reflects very closely the social welfare of a community and also serves as one of the most sensitive indexes of its sanitary condition. This is due to the close connection between the health of infants and the quality of the milk supply, the presence of flies, the condition of housing, and, to some extent, the availability and purity of the water. Therefore the alert health officer scrutinizes very closely the infant-mortality figures. These figures are expressed as the number of deaths of infants under one year of age per every 1,000 births occurring in the same year, and they are expressed as the following formula:

$$\text{Infant mortality} = \frac{\text{infant deaths in 1 year}}{\text{births in same year}} \times 1,000$$

It is almost impossible to determine in midyear the total number of infants under one year of age, but with good registration of births and with a fairly stable population the number of births registered for any one year is practically equal to the number of infants under one year of age. Infant mortality varies greatly in different cities and even in the different sections of a city. In general, there has been a decline in infant-mortality rates during the last quarter century. For instance, in the registration area of the United States, the infant mortality was 99.9 in 1915, 47.0 in 1940, 29.2 in 1950, and 26.0 in 1960. It must be remembered that the infant-mortality rate for a local area may be adversely affected if the percentage of completeness of birth registration is considerably below that of death registration. Infant deaths, however, are also under-registered in some areas.

19-14. Morbidity Rates. These are expressed as the number of cases of a specific disease occurring in one year per midyear population expressed in thousands or, more frequently, in hundred thousands. Morbidity rates are usually based upon the entire population but may be computed for certain age groups or classes. Incompleteness due to poor reporting of disease is the weak point of morbidity rates. To a great extent, morbidity rates depend upon the environmental conditions which directly or indirectly cause disease or lowering of resistance. The study of the morbidity rates of diseases which are specifically connected with some particular condition, such as industrial diseases and typhoid fever, is of great value to the health officer and sanitarian.

The fatality of a disease is the ratio between the number of deaths due to the disease and the number of cases of it and is usually expressed as a percentage. The determination of the fatality rate of a disease is complicated by incompleteness of morbidity reports. For instance, typhoid fever was for many years considered to have a fatality rate of 10 per cent. On the basis of case and death reports, it may appear even higher. Careful investigations in connection with typhoid epidemics have established the fact that the fatality rate is considerably less than 10 per cent under usual conditions.

19-15. Statistics. Environmental health engineers and sanitarians will sometimes find it useful to apply statistical methods to data they are using in order to determine their significance. For example, if certain health measures are carried out and a change in morbidity or mortality figures is then reported, it can be determined whether the change is probably due to chance or whether it can be ascribed to the work accomplished. A method of arriving at statistical significance will be described.[1] A few definitions will be needed.

Frequency distribution is an arrangement of numerical data according to size or magnitude.

The *arithmetic mean* of a number of items is obtained by adding all the items together and dividing the total by the number of items. It is frequently called the average. It is greatly affected by extreme values.

The *quadratic mean* is the square root of the mean square of the items (root-mean-square). Its formula is

$$\text{Quadratic mean} = \sqrt{\frac{\Sigma(x^2)}{N}}$$

where $\Sigma(x^2)$ is the sum of the squares of the items, and N is the number of items.

The standard deviation of a series of data is a form of average deviation from the mean. It is computed by taking the quadratic mean of the deviations from the arithmetic mean.

It is assumed that an investigator takes 10 coins and makes a large number of throws, recording the number of heads turned up at each throw. If he then makes a frequency distribution of the number of heads turned up at the individual throws and plots these frequencies vertically against the number of heads on the horizontal axis, he will have a curve of the shape shown in Fig. 19-3. This is known as the "normal frequency curve," and the plotting in the same manner of any data dependent upon

---

[1] Mathematical proof of the method is not given here. For such proof and other applications of statistical methods, the reader is referred to the works on statistics given in the bibliography of this chapter.

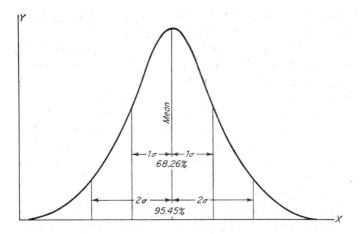

Figure 19-3 **A normal frequency curve.**

chance will have the same general shape, although the peak may be higher or lower relative to the other points on the curve. Normal frequency curves can be drawn, if sufficient data are available, for annual rainfall data and for cases of disease or causes of death in definite populations. The curve of collected data may, however, be "skewed"; *i.e.*, it may not be symmetrical about the peak.

To return to coin tossing, if it is resumed and in a series of throws a frequency of heads appears that is far to the right or left of the area under the curve, there would be basis for belief that some factor other than chance was affecting the appearance of heads. If the standard deviation is obtained from the data used in making the curve, it will have a value along the x axis. It is expressed as σ and is shown in Fig. 19-3. Its value is such that the area between the two vertical lines each distant 1σ from the mean is 68.26 per cent of the total area under the curve. A horizontal line that is 2σ in length on each side of the mean, or twice the standard deviation, when verticals are drawn will enclose 95.45 per cent of the total area. This means that if an item in new data is twice the standard deviation on either side of the mean, there is less than a 5 per cent chance, or less than 1 in 20, that the difference was caused by chance. A value at 3σ on either side of the mean will enclose an area of 99.73 per cent of the total, indicating that there is only a 0.27 per cent probability that the difference is due to chance. It is usually considered that when the difference between an item of data is less than or exceeds the arithmetic mean by 2σ or more, the figure is statistically significant. Use of this concept will be illustrated.

A medium-sized city had a relatively large area and was inhabited by persons of low economic status, and there were no sewers and numerous insanitary privies. Many homes had shallow wells of poor construction, and others had outside faucets; in some cases one faucet served a number of houses. Garbage and other refuse were stored in open containers, and collections were inefficient and were made at weekly intervals. In 1958 and 1959 an improvement campaign was instituted which resulted in installation of sewer connections, abolishment of unsafe water supplies and outside faucets, requirement of covered refuse containers, and semiweekly collecting by the city. The deaths from dysentery and diarrhea among children four years of age and under reported for the years 1941 to 1958 are given in Table 19-1; the reported

Table 19-1. COMPUTATION OF STANDARD DEVIATION

Year	Number of deaths (D)	Deviation from mean (mean $-$ D) $= x$	x^2
1941	38	-3	9
1942	45	$+4$	16
1943	43	$+1$	1
1944	37	-4	16
1945	36	-5	25
1946	32	-9	81
1947	39	-2	4
1948	51	$+10$	100
1949	49	$+8$	64
1950	47	$+6$	36
1951	43	$+2$	4
1952	37	-4	16
1953	34	-7	49
1954	41	0	0
1955	43	$+2$	4
1956	46	$+5$	25
1957	41	0	0
1958	37	-4	16
Total . .	739	0	466
Mean . .	41		25.9

$$\sigma = \sqrt{\frac{\Sigma(x)^2}{N}} = \sqrt{\frac{466}{18}} = \sqrt{25.9} = 5.09$$

Year	Number of deaths (D)
1959	30
1960	21
1961	19
1962	17
Total	87
Mean	21.75

$$\frac{41 - 21.75}{5.09} = 3.78$$

deaths for the years 1959 to 1962 are also given. It is desired to determine whether the later death figures, after the improvements were made, are statistically significant or due merely to chance.

In Table 19-1 the mean number of deaths[1] per year is first computed as 41. The values of x are then found. For example, for 1941 x is the difference between 38 and 41, or 3. For the whole series the algebraic sum should be zero. Should the mean prove to have a decimal portion, such as 41.31, the algebraic sum may not be zero. In this case the difference can be prorated among the x items or ignored. The x^2 values are found and added without regard to plus or minus signs. The standard σ, it will be remembered, is the quadratic mean of the deviations from the arithmetic mean. The computation is shown in Table 19-1.

The number of deaths in 1959 was 30, or 11 less than the arithmetic mean of the original series, which was 41. Then $11 \div 5.09 = 2.16$. This is statistically significant since it is more than twice the standard deviation. The mean of the years 1959 to 1962 is obtained as 21.75. The computation shown in the table indicates that the difference between the new mean and the old is 3.78σ, which is so great that there is only a very remote possibility that the reported reduction in deaths is due to chance.

Should data be obtained which, when plotted, give a skewed curve, the procedures here given are still applicable since the mathematical difference in results is negligible.

Bibliography

1. "Manual of Procedures for National Morbidity Reporting," Public Health Service, Communicable Disease Center, January, 1962.
2. Pearl, Raymond: "Introduction to Medical Biometry and Statistics," W. B. Saunders Company, Philadelphia, 1940.
3. Linder, F. E., and R. D. Grove: "Vital Statistics Rates in the United States," chaps. II–IV, Government Printing Office, Washington D.C., 1943.
4. Swaroop, Satya: "Introduction to Health Statistics," E. & S. Livingston, Ltd., Edinburgh and London, 1960.
5. Hill, A. B.: Principles of Medical Statistics, *Lancet*, London, 1955.
6. Croxton, F. E.: "Elementary Statistics with Applications in Medicine," Prentice-Hall, Inc., Englewood Cliffs, N.J., 1953.
7. Kenney, J. F., and E. S. Keeping: "Mathematics of Statistics," 3d ed., D. Van Nostrand Company, Inc., Princeton, N.J., 1954.

[1] It is assumed here that the total population of children under four years of age is unchanged during the period. This may not be the case. Specific death rates for this age and cause could be used in the same manner as deaths, with the population of that age determined from birthrates and death rates and with an estimate, if considered necessary, for the effects of migration.

20

PUBLIC HEALTH ORGANIZATIONS

20-1. The protection of the health of the citizen is a function of government. The needs, however, vary according to the governmental agency involved. The principal health agency of the national government, the Public Health Service, is organized to meet specific emergencies and to carry out particular routine duties. The health departments of the various states, in general, resemble each other in organization and functions. There is resemblance also between the organizations of the state departments and the local agencies, those of the cities and counties. But the detailed functions of the various departmental divisions of the local departments are necessarily different from those of the states. For instance, the bureau of communicable disease control in a state department, though having the same object as a similarly named division or bureau of a city health department, has a different field to cover and directs its activities accordingly.

In addition to government health organizations, there are a number of private health agencies, supported by endowments, contributions, or public subscription, which cover certain fields of health work either independently or in cooperation with the governmental agencies.

20-2. Health Activities. The activities of health departments vary somewhat not only according to the governmental agency involved but also according to the size of the community served and, to some degree, the local conditions. In some cities, by custom, health departments have retained certain functions which, it is felt, should be undertaken by other agencies—for instance, garbage collection and disposal. However, health authorities are agreed that certain activities should be duties of public health services, and these are listed below. Of course, many of them are not included by certain departments, possibly because funds or interest is lacking or perhaps because the particular problem is absent.

A. Vital statistics
  1. Registration
  2. Classification
  3. Verification
  4. Interpretation
B. Communicable disease control
  1. Reporting
  2. Record keeping
  3. Verification of diagnoses
  4. Laboratory control
  5. Control practices
  6. Investigation of sources of infection and epidemics
  7. Isolation, quarantine, release, and disinfection
C. Maternal and child health
  1. Prenatal service
  2. Infant hygiene
  3. Care of the preschool child
  4. Health of the schoolchild
    a. Physical examinations
    b. Correction of defects
    c. Sanitation of school buildings
    d. Health education
    e. Recreation
D. Chronic diseases
  1. Reporting on registration
  2. Screening and detection
  3. Statistical studies
  4. Follow-up
E. Environmental health

    1. Control of atmospheric pollution
    2. Water supply
    3. Waste disposal
       a. Excreta and sewage
       b. Refuse
    4. Food sanitation
       a. Milk sanitation
       b. Meat inspection
       c. Sanitation of food-handling establishments
    5. Housing
    6. Insect and rodent control
    7. Occupational health
    8. Radiological health
    9. Swimming-pool and bathing-place sanitation
   10. Accident prevention
   11. Nuisance inspections
F. Laboratory
    1. Bacteriological and virological examinations
    2. Chemical examinations
    3. Research
G. Public health education
    1. Bulletins, circulars, and periodicals
    2. Newspaper articles, radio programs, and telecasts
    3. Exhibits
    4. Lectures and motion pictures

In addition to the above activities, some cities also conduct clinics for mental hygiene, drug addiction, and various other special purposes. Clinics for infants and children and for tuberculosis and venereal diseases are usual. Dental clinics for schoolchildren are now common. Some departments also have nutritionists on their staffs. A newcomer in the public health field is geriatrics, which is concerned with diseases and health conditions of old age. The greater proportion of the population in the older age group is focusing attention on the need for planning an acceptable and realistic program and guide for the older age group. Its work is placed in the division of chronic disease control.

Other activities of some health departments are administration of medical care programs, rehabilitation, and administration of hospitals. These, however, are sometimes placed in welfare departments.

20-3. Vital Statistics. This work, as discussed in Chap. 19, includes the registration of births, marriages, and deaths. It also includes tabulation and analysis at monthly intervals of the data obtained. The reports of the reportable diseases sent in to the division or bureau of communicable diseases should also be tabulated.

Although a register is kept by active city and county health departments, the state organization is the final repository for the death and birth certificates. The National Center for Health Statistics in the Public Health Service at Washington collects tabulated reports of births, morbidity, deaths, and causes of death from the states and some municipalities. It analyzes such reports and publishes statistics.

The Metropolitan Life Insurance Company of New York also keeps vital statistics of a group of 17 million insured persons. Various bulletins and studies based upon its records are issued by the company from time to time and are of great value.

20-4. Communicable Disease Control. As this has been discussed to some extent elsewhere, it is touched upon but briefly here. The epidemiological work of this division includes a system of reporting of all the ordinary communicable diseases with systematic investigation of each reported case. In the more serious diseases, such as diphtheria, smallpox, bubonic plague, and poliomyelitis, verification should be made by a medical officer. Specimens are taken for laboratory diagnosis or release, or both, in diphtheria, typhoid fever, syphilis, and epidemic cerebrospinal meningitis. Cases are hospitalized if proper precautions cannot be taken at home. Many health departments furnish biologics for prevention of infectious diseases. Public health education pays dividends in stimulating and securing adequate community immunization levels of such diseases as smallpox, diphtheria, whooping cough, tetanus, typhoid fever, and poliomyelitis. In some areas of other continents, bubonic plague and cholera are important. From the public health standpoint, health departments are primarily interested in securing immunization levels of a community to prevent a major outbreak of the disease. Should an epidemic of a communicable disease occur, this division institutes measures to determine the natural history of the disease and, utilizing this knowledge, plans a strategy of control and decides where and how control measures may be applied.

Tuberculosis control, through the use of mass case-finding techniques, antimicrobial drugs, and major chest surgery, has brought about a marked decline in the mortality rate. However, in certain states and larger cities where tuberculosis is still a major problem, separate divisions are maintained. In some areas, however, certain parts of this work, such as that of outpatient clinics and visiting nurses, are supported or furnished by voluntary health agencies. The control methods used include effective reporting of cases; consultation services; screening techniques, such as mass chest X-ray surveys and tuberculin testing, ascertaining that each case receives proper nursing and medical care in adequately staffed hospitals or at home; and provision for adequate follow-up and vocational rehabilitation for arrested cases.

Much progress has also been made in venereal disease control. With the advancement of modern therapy, the treatment of gonorrhea is as trifling as that of the common cold, and more certain. Today complications of the disease are rarely encountered, but because of its reinfectious nature, the morbidity of gonorrhea, despite modern treatment, remains high, and control is therefore very difficult. Modern therapy has also brought about a remarkable decline in the morbidity of syphilis, bringing us close to the reservoirs of infection, and it is now timely to consider eradication rather than mere control. If syphilis is to be numbered, as it should be, with smallpox, yellow fever, malaria, typhoid fever, and diphtheria, among the extinct or nearly extinct diseases in the United States, we shall need to revise our epidemiological approach to it. The decline in syphilis has been followed by an increase, indicating that more vigorous measures will be required if the disease is to be eradicated. In the control program of today, emphasis must be placed upon reporting of all cases to the local health authorities (reporting is required by all the states), contact investigation, and prophylactic use of penicillin. There should be precise legislation providing for the examination of the presumably infected and their compulsory treatment when indicated.

20-5. Maternal and Child Health. This very important branch of health work may be divided into two major classifications: complete maternity care and a program for child health.

Maternity care includes premarital education and counseling, preconceptive advice and instruction, prenatal care, delivery care, and postnatal care. In planning these services, consideration is given not only to the physical factors involved but also to the mental, emotional, social, and economic situations.

A health program for children must take into consideration the physical factors in the child's life situation and, here again, also the emotional, social, mental, and economic aspects. This program can be subdivided into the care of the newborn, or neonatal care; infant care; care of the preschool child; and a health program for the school-age child. A comprehensive program varies according to the age levels and includes health appraisal; counseling; mental health; communicable disease control; nutrition instructions; dental health; health education, including special activities for the handicapped child; and the control of environmental conditions which affect the child's growth and development.

20-6. Chronic Diseases. In state or other health departments chronic diseases may be cared for by a bureau of adult health or geriatrics. The treatment of chronic diseases is a function of the private physician; however, health authorities have recognized that through community effort, early detection of disease can be stimulated, early treatment started, disease arrested, and the burden of aftercare of indigent patients reduced.

Heart disease and cancer are leading causes of death. Diabetes is a major chronic degenerative disease affecting over 2 per cent of our population. Tuberculosis is communicable but chronic in character. Arthritis is the chief cause of morbidity and disability. These diseases are often silent in their early stages.

The activities of the local health authorities in regard to chronic diseases include:

1. Detection or case finding from the reports of physicians, hospitals, and clinics and through mass screening. This procedure permits early treatment.
2. Programming measures to arrest the disease.
3. Advising on nursing homes and aftercare for indigent patients.

20-7. Environmental Health. Control of environment has been discussed in detail elsewhere and needs no further elaboration here. All such work, however, is not included in the work of the health department, although practice varies in this regard. In general only those activities which are directly concerned with health are placed in the city health department. Refuse collection and disposal, for instance, are often excluded and are handled by some other department. Research along such lines has, however, been carried on by the state health agencies and by the Public Health Service. In cities the care of small water supplies, from the standpoint of safety, is invariably entrusted to the health department, but purification of the public supply is supervised by the water department. Excreta disposal in unsewered areas is a recognized activity of health departments, but maintenance and operation of city sewers and sewage treatment plants are likely to be functions of some other city agency. Plumbing inspection may or may not be included in the health department, but in most cases the city sanitary engineer or some other health official is placed on the examination board which licenses plumbers. Nuisance inspection is invariably conducted by the health department inspectors of cities and counties, but of late its removal elsewhere has been urged.

The theory of such elimination of activities from the health department is good. There are other practical considerations, however, which, for some time to come at least, may necessitate a departure from theory. To the average person many of these functions, particularly nuisance inspection, belong in the health department, and it will be blamed for poor performance even though not responsible. On the other hand, such work is conspicuous and if well done may gain financial support for the less spectacular, though more important, activities.

In all environmental health problems, however, the health department may be called upon to give advice; hence it is important for health officials to have a thorough understanding of all branches of sanitation. Also, since all the allied sanitary matters are strictly of an engineering nature, it is of value for the health department to have a sanitary engineer who can represent the health department and at the same time meet the engineers of other city departments on common ground.

Good administration indicates that safety and sanitation features be incorporated in the design, construction, and maintenance of streets, utilities, public buildings, industrial plants, recreational areas, and housing projects and in city and regional planning in general. Good communication with most governmental and some private agencies is highly desirable.

20-8. Laboratory. The laboratory of a health department makes chemical and bacteriological examinations of milk, water from public and private supplies, bottled waters, and possibly sewage or sewage-polluted waters; chemical, bacteriological, and microscopical examinations of foods and drugs; and bacteriological and microscopical examinations for diagnosis and release in diphtheria, tuberculosis, typhoid fever, malaria, syphilis, gonorrhea, pneumonia, and—in the South—hookworm and other intestinal parasitic diseases. Research should also be carried on along the lines of bacteriology, virology, and chemistry as they pertain to public health.

20-9. Public Health Education. Health education not only teaches healthful living to children and adults but also instructs in the principles of community hygiene. It therefore is doubly valuable in that it helps the individual directly and also brings about recognition of the value of public health work, resulting in better cooperation between the citizen and the health department. The recognized methods of health education as accomplished by health departments are as follows: preparation of an annual report showing clearly the work done, results accomplished, costs, and future needs; publishing and distribution of weekly or monthly bulletins to physicians, nurses, teachers, social workers, and prominent persons so that they may be informed about current health problems; preparation of radio scripts, television recordings, and newspaper stories and articles on timely subjects; holding exhibits illustrating and demonstrating health work; operating a lecture service for various organizations; and stimulation of health instruction in the schools by arousing the interest of the school authorities and teachers and cooperating in instruction. Departments of education of many of the larger cities have health education specialists on their staffs.

20-10. Public Health Law. Public health activities are controlled by legislative bodies in two ways: by the passage of laws and by the appropriation of funds for health work. Much of the work of health departments is educational in nature, but those activities which affect the actions of persons or use of their property must be authorized by laws or by recognized legal principles, such as the police power of government [1, 2].

1. Federal laws apply to matters that have interstate connotations.

Examples in the health field are the inspection or certification of certain foods which are shipped interstate, such as meats, shellfish, and fruits or vegetables which may have been treated with insecticides, and the certification of drinking-water supplies for interstate carriers.

2. The Federal Constitution gives the states the right to exercise the police power in order to safeguard the health and welfare of their citizens. Their laws are known as statutes. Some deal directly with health matters. The states have also, however, by statutes or city charters delegated some of their police powers to the cities and also to the counties. Counties, however, usually depend upon the statutes. State laws affecting health presumably apply to the whole state. Examples of statutes concerning health are a sanitary code for the whole state; laws prohibiting pollution of streams; and the requirement that all cities having a given population or more provide plumbing inspection.

3. The city is the creation of the state and is totally subservient to the state. Cities, therefore, exercise the health-protective powers granted to them by the state. They do this by means of local laws passed by the cities' legislative bodies known as ordinances. These ordinances may not conflict with statutes; they may be more exacting, but they must not be more lenient. Examples are milk-quality-control ordinances, food-establishment-control ordinances, and city housing codes.

4. Regulations may be written by administrative officials to supplement or "fill out" the statutes or ordinances. For example, a statute or ordinance may require "adequate cleansing and disinfection of all multiuse utensils used in food service." The regulations would specify the methods that would be approved by the inspecting authority, such as wash-water temperature, holding or contact times, and chemical disinfectants that might be used. Regulations must be authorized by the legislative bodies, and they must be adopted and amended by authorized procedures. They have several important advantages. They can embody the technical knowledge necessary to attain the law's ends, and they can readily be amended should knowledge of sanitary procedures and experience warrant change.

5. Under the Federal Constitution and state constitutions, legislative and executive actions are subject to review by the courts. Statutes, ordinances, and regulations may be challenged as to their constitutionality and reasonableness.

6. Administrative acts under statutes, ordinances, and regulations may be subjected to court action or review. For example, a health officer, for certain reasons, revokes a permit to operate a food-service establishment, refuses a permit, or refuses to reissue a suspended permit, and the aggrieved person applies to a court for an injunction or court order. The court will be guided by the facts in the case, as they are presented to it, and possibly also by precedents. The administrative

officer, therefore, should have the facts well in hand and see that they are clearly presented.

Laws or ordinances may authorize administrative officers to condemn and destroy property that is dangerous to the public health, or acts may be authorized that will result in property damage. The state or city itself would be immune from damage suits resulting from public health activities, but the administrative officer might be personally held liable, even though he had obviously acted in good faith. Successful defense of such a case would require convincing a jury that a dangerous health hazard had existed. This might be difficult, and a jury's sympathy for the property owner might affect its judgment.

Inspectors on duty may enter private property that is in public use, such as restaurants, motels, privately owned public swimming pools, etc. The right of entry to residential property, however, is uncertain. Therefore, the inspector who wishes to inspect residential property for rodent- or mosquito-control purposes and who is confronted by an uncooperative and bellicose householder should consult the city attorney for advice as to his procedure.

Health Organizations

20-11. The World Health Organization. The World Health Organization came into existence Apr. 7, 1948, when the necessary 26 nations had notified the Secretary General of the United Nations that the constitution of the proposed organization had been ratified. Its organization includes a Health Assembly made up of delegates representing the member countries. Countries that are not members of the United Nations may join the Organization. The Health Assembly appoints an Executive Board and a Director General, who is the chief technical and administrative officer of the Organization. The functions of the Organization as given in its constitution are:

(*a*) to act as the directing and co-ordinating authority on international health work;

(*b*) to establish and maintain effective collaboration with the United Nations, specialized agencies, governmental health administrations, professional groups and such other organizations as may be deemed appropriate;

(*c*) to assist governments, upon request, in strengthening health services;

(*d*) to furnish appropriate technical assistance and, in emergencies, necessary aid upon the request or acceptance of governments;

(*e*) to provide or assist in providing, upon the request of the United Nations, health services and facilities to special groups, such as the peoples of trust territories;

(f) to establish and maintain such administrative and technical services as may be required, including epidemiological and statistical services;

(g) to stimulate and advance work to eradicate epidemic, endemic and other diseases;

(h) to promote, in co-operation with other specialized agencies where necessary, the prevention of accidental injuries;

(i) to promote, in co-operation with other specialized agencies where necessary, the improvement of nutrition, housing, sanitation, recreation, economic or working conditions and other aspects of environmental hygiene;

(j) to promote co-operation among scientific and professional groups which contribute to the advancement of health;

(k) to propose conventions, agreements and regulations, and make recommendations with respect to international health matters and to perform such duties as may be assigned thereby to the Organization and are consistent with its objective;

(l) to promote maternal and child health and welfare and to foster the ability to live harmoniously in a changing total environment;

(m) to foster activities in the field of mental health, especially those affecting the harmony of human relations;

(n) to promote and conduct research in the field of health;

(o) to promote improved standards of teaching and training in the health, medical and related professions;

(p) to study and report on, in co-operation with other specialized agencies where necessary, administrative and social techniques affecting public health and medical care from preventive and curative points of view, including hospital services and social security;

(q) to provide information, counsel and assistance in the field of health;

(r) to assist in developing an informed public opinion among all peoples on matters of health;

(s) to establish and revise as necessary international nomenclatures of diseases, of causes of death and of public health practices;

(t) to standardize diagnostic procedures as necessary;

(u) to develop, establish and promote international standards with respect to food, biological, pharmaceutical and similar products;

(v) generally to take all necessary action to attain the objective of the Organization.

At the 1948 meeting of the Organization permanent headquarters were set up in Geneva, the Director General and Executive Board were appointed, and a program was adopted. Top priority was given to six major problems: malaria, maternal and child health, tuberculosis, venereal diseases, environmental health, and nutrition. For these, funds were set up for staffs and travel costs in order to give expert advice and to provide demonstration teams and training programs. Second priority was given to four problems: public health nursing, parasitic diseases, virus diseases, and mental health. To each of these were assigned a staff member and a small committee of experts.

Funds for the World Health Organization are derived from the member countries. An annual budget is prepared by the Director General and presented to the Executive Board, which submits it to the Health Assembly with any recommendations it cares to make. The Assembly, after reviewing and approving the budget, apportions the expenses according to some plan adopted by the Assembly. Six geographic divisions were set up to be served by regional offices.

20-12. U.S. Department of Health, Education, and Welfare. This is the principal agency of the national government which is concerned with health. Of its various operating agencies two, the Public Health Service and the Food and Drug Administration, carry on health activities. The Public Health Service is headed by a Surgeon General, and it is staffed in part by a corps of commissioned officers, including physicians, engineers, and other professional employees, who hold corresponding rank to officers in the armed services. In the space available here it is difficult to do justice to its contributions to public health in the United States. The scope of its services is indicated in Fig. 20-1, and the functions of its bureaus and other subdivisions will be given very briefly.

The Bureau of State Services administers Federal-state and interstate health programs, including interstate quarantine. It administers programs assisting and supplementing state and local activities in the areas of (1) community health, including accident prevention, chronic and communicable diseases, dental public health, hospital and other care facilities, medical facilities and resources, nursing, and community health practice, and (2) environmental health, including air pollution; protection of milk, shellfish, and other foods; occupational health; radiological health; and water-supply and pollution control. It also administers grants programs, such as monetary assistance to cities for construction of sewage treatment plants. Much of the work of the Bureau is carried out through its regional offices, which have directors and professional specialists to represent the Service in its relationship with the state and local authorities and private agencies in connection with grants-in-aid; provide consultation services to state and other agencies on public health; and coordinate Public Health Service civil defense activities within the region. Mention should also be made of the Communicable Disease Center, located at Atlanta, Ga., which provides epidemiological services when and where needed, studies vector-borne diseases, and gives training in vector and rodent control. The Robert A. Taft Sanitary Engineering Center conducts studies of air and water pollution and remedial measures and also of radiological health. It conducts training courses in those fields. The results of studies of the Service are available in many official publications.

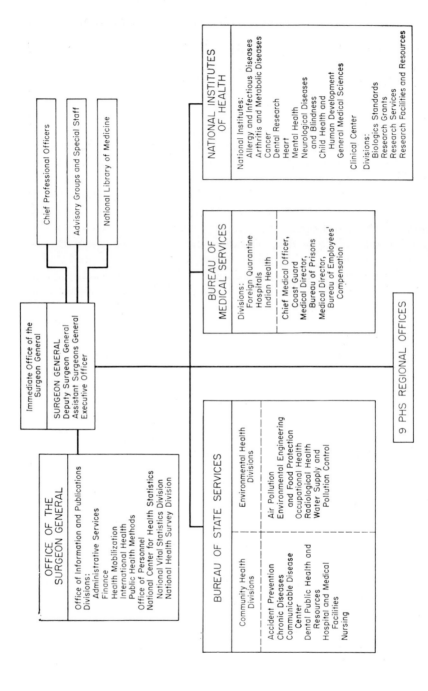

FIGURE 20-1 Organization chart of the Public Health Service, U.S. Department of Health, Education, and Welfare, 1963.

The National Institutes of Health conduct research on the diseases shown in Fig. 20-1 and also make grants for research and training.

The work of the Bureau of Medical Services is also outlined in the figure. Its most conspicuous activity is the quarantine service applied at entry ports to all types of transportation arriving from foreign countries. It includes examination of persons and fumigation of ships and other conveyances when considered necessary. It also administers the Public Health Service hospitals and clinics and the health service for Indians and Alaskan natives.

The National Center for Health Statistics develops programs of health, demographic, and related statistics; collects and compiles such statistics from governmental sources, from health surveys of the population, and from special studies of health subjects; and analyzes and publishes such statistics.

The Food and Drug Administration, which is not a part of the Public Health Service, enforces the Federal Food, Drug, and Cosmetic Act. It provides the premarketing safety clearances required for new drugs, pesticides, and additives to foods through its laboratory work. Field investigations and enforcement are carried out by district offices.

20-13. Other Health Agencies of the National Government. There are other agencies of the national government which are concerned to a greater or lesser degree with health matters. Of these, only the more important can be mentioned here.

The Department of Agriculture includes the Bureau of Animal Industry, which studies animal diseases, including eradication of tuberculosis and brucellosis in dairy cattle. The Meat Inspection Division carries on inspection of meat and meat products that will be shipped interstate. The Biological Survey cooperates in the eradication of rodents. The Bureau of Entomology studies insects which affect the health of man and is also concerned with insecticides. The Department also enforces the Federal Insecticide, Fungicide, and Rodenticide Act.

The National Bureau of Standards of the Department of Commerce and the Atomic Energy Commission study, correlate, and publish information on radiological health hazards and protection and the disposal of radioactive wastes.

In the Department of the Interior, the Bureau of Mines cooperates with the Public Health Service in the investigation of health hazards in mining and industry, smoke prevention, and methods of ventilation.

The Labor Department maintains a Children's Bureau, which investigates infant mortality and diseases of children and administers maternity and infancy laws; a Women's Bureau, which is concerned with the health of women in industry; and a Bureau of Labor Statistics, which studies problems of industrial hygiene.

The Civil Defense Administration is charged with the development of a nationwide plan for the defense of civilians in the event of an emergency. It has also given much attention to protection from radioactive fallout and has issued many informative bulletins on preparedness.

The Labor Department and many other Federal agencies are interested in certain phases of health and sanitation. The Labor Department carries on certain studies in the field of health in industry.

The work of the Housing and Home Finance Agency has been discussed in Chap. 14.

Since all the above bureaus or divisions publish pamphlets and bulletins giving the results of their investigations, anyone interested in these fields has valuable mines of information available on request from the agency concerned.

20-14. State Health Departments. The health departments of the states vary considerably in their organizations and powers. In general they are given control over the health work of the states and enforce the health laws enacted by the state legislatures. The laws generally cover such matters as the control of communicable disease, reporting of diseases, registration of births and deaths, control of the quality and sanitation of foods, child and maternal hygiene, and prevention and investigation of stream pollution. They usually require the submission and approval of plans for sewerage and waterworks before construction by a municipality or private agency.

In some cases, a somewhat centralized control of health matters with decentralization of the state organization has been obtained through the division of the state into districts and the placing of a state official or district health officer in each. See Fig. 20-2. In general, however, the formation of local health departments in the individual cities and counties and their assumption of responsibility are encouraged, and the state cooperates with these local departments, advises them, and gives aid in emergencies. Where no local department is functioning, the state renders the only health service which such an unfortunate community receives.

The organization of a state health department is prescribed by the state law. Invariably the chief officer, generally known as the state health officer or the commissioner of public health, is required to be a physician; preferably he should be trained and experienced in public health work, although this requirement is not the rule as yet. Generally also there is a state board of health which acts in an advisory capacity to the state health officer but exercises no executive functions. In most cases the health officer and the state board of health are appointed by the governor, although the practice of having the state board choose the health officer is currently followed in some states and advocated in others. In this case the board is rotating, two of six members, for instance, being replaced every 2 years. This arrangement makes for continuity of policy and tends to take the health department out of politics.

As mentioned before, the state health activities are very largely advisory and cooperative, although they follow closely the lines described in the first section of this chapter. The communicable disease division keeps records of communicable diseases so that it may recognize emergencies. It aids local health departments and communities without health departments to overcome epidemics and keeps on hand supplies of vaccine, antitoxin, and other immunizing agents for use and distribution where needed.

The division of vital statistics is the final repository of birth and death certificates and furnishes copies of them when requested. Tabulations and analyses are or should be made.

The division of child hygiene functions very largely through nurses who work in districts where local departments are nonexistent or weak.

The food and drug division administers the food and drug laws and maintains a force of inspectors. These inspectors, in addition to making special investigations, make routine inspections of food-handling establishments, such as restaurants, groceries, meat markets, slaughterhouses, creameries, and dairies, particularly in those sections where local health departments are not functioning. Attention is also given to the larger food-manufacturing establishments doing a statewide trade. Samples are collected for laboratory examination.

The division of sanitary engineering or environmental health is called upon to approve all plans for sewer systems, sewage treatment plants, water distribution systems, and water treatment plants and also for major alterations to them. This requirement is to ensure protection to the citizens and is a service to the smaller cities, which may otherwise sink money in worthless projects. Inspections are made of existing sewage treatment and water treatment plants. This division also administers stream-pollution laws and makes investigations as to the effects upon streams of sewage, effluents from sewage treatment plants, and industrial wastes. Engineering advice is given to other divisions, particularly to the division of communicable diseases in connection with epidemics, and like service is rendered to local health departments requiring it. Other duties of this division include making sanitary surveys and organizing and carrying out demonstration campaigns against mosquitoes, rats, and flies. This division is also concerned with milk sanitation (in some states, particularly pasteurization), industrial hygiene, air pollution, and radiological health, and it does research along the varied lines of sanitation.

The other divisions vary in number and character according to the state laws and local problems. If housing is controlled by state law, there may be a division accordingly, or it may be administered by the

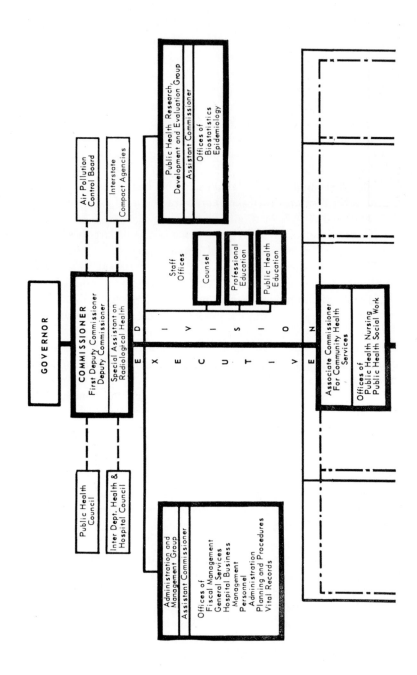

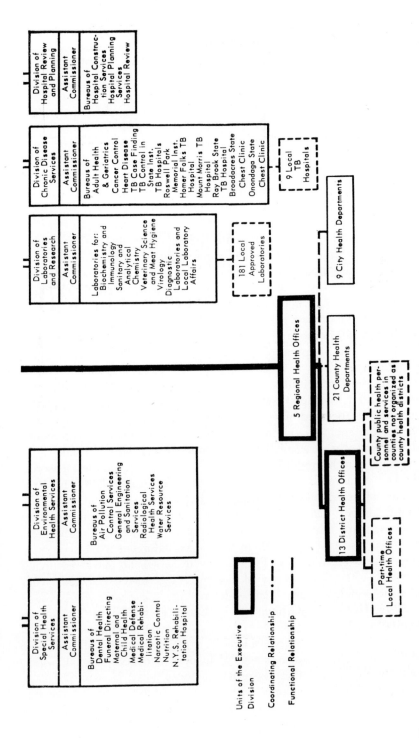

FIGURE 20-2 Organization chart of the New York State Health Department.

593

sanitary engineering division. The division of local health services is mainly concerned with the stimulation of local health work and the formation of local health departments. A division of public health nursing furnishes to the other divisions the required number of nurses, thus allowing flexibility.

As mentioned before, the state health officer is invariably a physician. The chiefs of bureaus or divisions are also physicians, with some exceptions. The division of food and drugs is sometimes headed by a chemist. The chief of the division of sanitary engineering is in all cases an engineer versed in environmental health techniques. His assistants are, in general, engineers also, with sanitarians and inspectors used for special purposes. Milk sanitation is frequently carried on by veterinarians and sometimes by sanitarians.

20-15. City Health Departments. While the state health department performs important duties in supervising, standardizing, and cooperating in state health work as a whole, it is the local health department which must serve the average citizen in the matters which touch him closely. In a city it is the municipal health department or the city health officer who must solve the local problems and do the detailed work. This need, in the large cities, necessitates an organization differing but little in form from that of the state but showing differences in duties and personnel.

In the smaller cities the problem of obtaining effective local health work is still far from solution. Most states require health officers (usually they must be licensed physicians) for each county and incorporated city. But the compensation of such officers is left to the city or county and is frequently so small that the incumbent can afford to take little or no time from his regular practice to attend to public duties. Theoretically he is required by the state to enforce the control, isolation, placarding, etc., of communicable diseases and report them to the state. The authority of city health officers is also enlarged by city ordinances to include sanitary inspection and abatement of nuisances. But the part-time official is at a disadvantage here since enforcement of such ordinances makes enemies, and the practice by which he makes his living may suffer. The possibilities of accomplishing effective health work under such conditions are discussed later.

20-16. Health Department of a Large City. Figure 20-3 is an organization chart suggested for a city of 100,000 population. It would also serve for a city of considerably greater size with the possible addition of such divisions as mental hygiene and occupational health. It will be noted that there is provision for a board of health. This is advisory and deliberative only, without executive duties, though possibly with the power to formulate a sanitary code. The health officer or director of public health is head of the department; he should be a full-

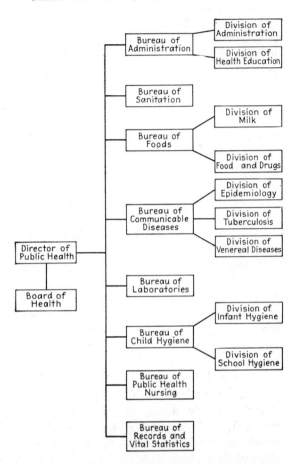

FIGURE 20-3 Organization chart of a health department for a city of 100,000 population, as recommended by the Committee on Municipal Health Department Practice of the American Public Health Association.

time employee and should be specially trained and experienced in public health work. The duties and personnel of the various bureaus and divisions are briefly given below.

The bureau of administration is directly under the supervision of the health officer and includes the divisions of administration and education. The former handles the routine office business of the department, and the latter performs the work described in Art. 20-9. The educational division should include a man or woman experienced in writing who can obtain and put into popular form the technical matter furnished by the other bureaus.

The bureau of sanitation or environmental health for a city of

100,000 should be in the charge of a sanitary engineer whose technical advice is available to the other bureaus and also to other city departments in connection with plumbing, housing, refuse collection, school sanitation, milk pasteurization, and water treatment. The force under him should consist of four inspectors with such additional help and labor as may be needed for mosquito control or other special measures. The routine work would include inspection of privies and of fly breeding conditions and possibly also of ratproofing and rat extermination; investigation of complaints; and remedying of nuisances. The sanitation of "fringe areas" of the city which do not have water or sewers requires much attention. The supervision of housing conditions should also be placed within the jurisdiction of this bureau. To further its activities there should be comprehensive ordinances and regulations.

The bureau of foods should have as its head a technically trained man, perhaps a veterinarian, whose time is divided between the two divisions—milk, and food and drugs. In some instances this work is placed under the sanitary engineer. Each division requires two inspectors. The milk division should carry out the work as outlined in Chap. 6, modified by the particular milk ordinance of the city in question. The food and drugs division inspects all food-processing and food-serving establishments and enforces state laws and ordinances regulating the quality and handling of food. Both divisions of this bureau are greatly strengthened by ordinances requiring the licensing of, or holding of permits by, all food establishments, including dairies, hotels, restaurants, bakeries, candy stores, groceries, markets, slaughterhouses (including poultry), soda fountains, ice-cream stands, bars, and fruit stands. Provision should be made for inspection of meats not examined by Federal inspectors. This may be cared for by a part-time veterinarian aided by lay inspectors.

The bureau of communicable diseases is divided into the three divisions of epidemiology, tuberculosis, and venereal diseases. The work of this bureau is outlined in Art. 20-4. Each division is in the charge of a full-time physician who should be an expert in his line. The division of epidemiology also requires the services of a nurse. The tuberculosis division requires, in addition to the director, a part-time physician to assist in the work at the clinic or dispensary. Half of the time of a social worker could profitably be used to visit the homes of patients, and the services of four nurses are essential. The venereal diseases division needs a part-time physician to assist at the clinic and could use the other half of the time of the social worker. For assistance at the clinic and home visiting, two nurses are needed.

The bureau of child hygiene is composed of two divisions: infant hygiene, which is concerned with the health of mothers and young children, and school hygiene, which deals with the health of children of school age. The activities of these divisions are briefly given in Art. 20-5. A clinic is required for infant hygiene and necessitates the use of part-time physicians who are specialists in infant and maternal care. The chief of the bureau divides his time between the two divisions, being assisted in the inspection of schoolchildren by five part-time medical inspectors, two dentists, and five dental hygienists. The nursing service would be required to furnish 15 nurses for infant hygiene and eight for school hygiene. The work of the division of school hygiene is frequently done by the schools themselves, although there are advantages in having all health work centralized in the health department.

The bureau of public health nursing should furnish the nurses for the various activities previously mentioned. A force of 30 nurses is needed under such an arrangement. If provision for care of the sick in their homes is also to be made, 10 to 20 more nurses are required, making a total of 50, with six supervisors, the latter to be specialists in the various branches of the work. The head of this bureau should be a nurse with special qualifications for the position. It has been suggested that the home nursing work be done by agencies other than the city health department, such as the schools and various private charitable organizations.

The work of the laboratory has been described elsewhere. Its director should be a bacteriologist with a trained assistant, preferably a chemist who is able to assist in bacteriological work. A helper with no special training may also be required.

The activities of the bureau of records and vital statistics have already been described. The chief should be a person trained in health work with special study in statistics. A combination clerk and draftsman would also be useful.

In some cities welfare work is placed under the director of public health, the combined department being called "public health and welfare." Welfare work includes free care of the diseased, dependent, and defective and includes treatment of indigent persons in hospitals. By some authorities this has been considered charitable work and not a part of health work, which is preventive medicine and not curative medicine. There are advantages, however, in having hospitals closely related to the health department, and accordingly there is some disposition on the part of health officers to encourage placing of publicly supported hospitals in the county or city health departments.

20-17. Health Department of a Medium-sized City. The health department of a city of 50,000 population is, of course, considerably modified over that of the large city, although the activities are along the same lines. Figure 20-4 is a chart of the health department organization recommended to a city of this size by the American Public Health Association. It illustrates very well the combination of functions

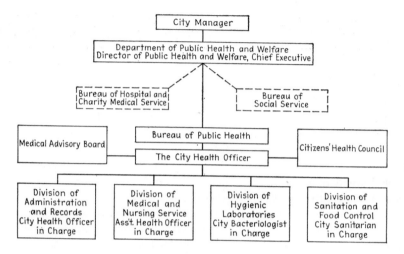

FIGURE 20-4 Proposed organization of a health department for a city with a population of 50,000.

and duties necessitated by the smaller number of personnel. In the proposed organization the director of public health and welfare is also the city health officer and in addition is in direct charge of the division of administration and records. This division also includes educational work. The division of medical and nursing service, with an assistant health officer in charge, combines communicable disease control, child hygiene, and nursing. All the work of sanitation, including milk and food sanitation, is concentrated in one division, with a sanitarian, or sanitary engineer, in charge.

The medical advisory board and citizens' health council replace the old-fashioned board of health. As usually constituted, the medical advisory board consists of four or five physicians and a dentist, the members to be as agreed upon or appointed jointly by the local medical and dental societies and by the city council, mayor, or city manager. The citizens' health council consists of representatives of the chamber of commerce and other civic organizations, the members to be appointed by agreement. Since the health department must cooperate with physicians, dentists, and the public, the value of advisory boards of this sort, with the possibility of getting various viewpoints on health problems or emergencies, is very apparent. Such boards serve without pay.

The personnel aside from the chiefs required to carry on the necessary activities of a department of this size are somewhat as follows: division of administration and records—one clerical assistant or secretary; division of medical and nursing service—a dentist for the schools, 10 nurses and a supervising nurse, a quarantine officer, and a clerical assistant; division of sanitation—a meat inspector who is a veterinarian, a dairy inspector, three or at least two sanitary inspectors, and extra labor when required.

20-18. Health Department of a Small City. Health work in many of the small cities, those having populations of 5,000 or less, and frequently in those having 15,000 to 20,000, is practically nonexistent. The state health department may inspect the water supply and require the sewage to be properly treated, but the local health work in general is sadly neglected. This is due in part to lack of recognition of the need for health work by the city councils and in part to the system of part-time health officers. The laws of many states require that a health officer be appointed, usually a physician. He must necessarily work part time in the small cities, and generally, since at best he can do but little, his salary is nominal, and the work that he does is commensurate.

In a city of 5,000, it may be taken for granted that with school examinations and other work a public health nurse would find herself a busy woman. There is also sufficient sanitary work to take the full time of a sanitary inspector. It is better still to obtain a sanitarian with sufficient knowledge to do routine bacteriological testing of water and milk. It is also necessary in most cases to satisfy the state requirement of a medical health officer, and in any event the services of a physician are necessary in connection with the isolation of communicable diseases. He may, therefore, be retained on part time.

This organization may easily be expanded for larger cities and the costs varied to meet the local conditions, but to meet the needs of smaller communities is more difficult. It may be possible in very small towns to cooperate with the county in obtaining the services of a nurse and sanitary inspector on a part-time basis. A small city may also cut down expenses by employing a lower salaried inspector or by requiring the city marshal or policeman to give to sanitation the attention it deserves. Little will be gained, however, unless the inspector or policeman has been given some instruction or training. Such training, in some states, may be obtained through the state health department. A better solution is the combined city-county health department, which is discussed in the following article.

20-19. County Health Department. Of the 3,072 counties in the United States, 2,425 are recognized by the states as providing public health services [3]. Of these, 902 are organized as single counties, and the others are in multicounty health districts or in state health districts. There are 647 counties, with 5.6 per cent of the total population of the country, not reported as receiving health services.

The services rendered by state districts are inadequate in many instances. Yet rural communities are in need of health service as much as municipalities are. The county health department is a local health agency and, in addition to providing basic services, frequently carries

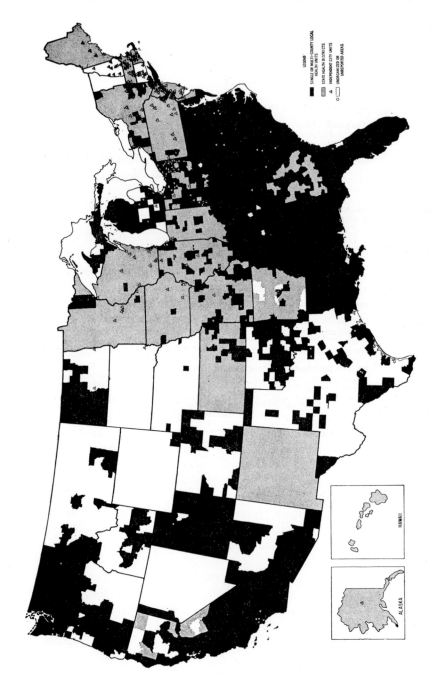

FIGURE 20-5 Areas organized for local health services. *(From Organization and Staffing for Local Health Service, Public Health Service Pub. 628, rev. 1961.)*

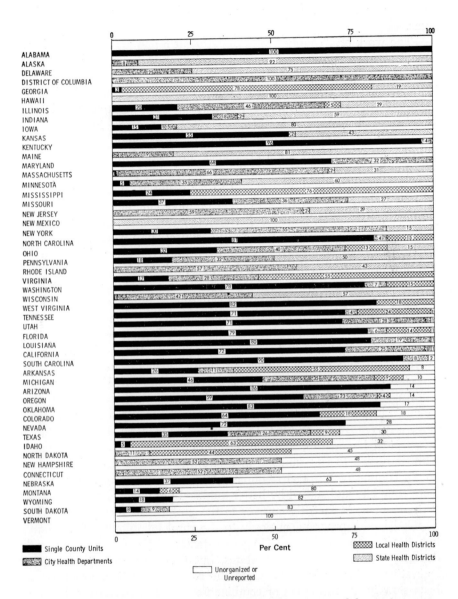

FIGURE 20-6 Per cent of each state's total population covered by various types of health organizations. (*From Organization and Staffing for Local Health Service, Public Health Service Pub. 628, rev. 1961.*)

on activities to control special health problems not common in other areas.

The work of a county health department follows closely that of the city. A rural program may be summarized as including the following activities: keeping of records and vital statistics; isolation, quarantine, immunization, and bedside instruction to prevent the spread of communicable disease; discovery and instruction as to treatment and care of tuberculosis cases and incipient cases; child hygiene, including prenatal care, infant hygiene, care of the preschool child, examination of schoolchildren, and sanitation of schools; instruction of midwives; safeguarding of water supplies of villages and farms; provision for proper excreta disposal to prevent soil and water pollution and fly carriage of disease; food sanitation by inspection of food-handling establishments, dairies, and slaughterhouses and examination of food handlers; control of insects and rodents, if necessary; educational measures through lectures, motion pictures, demonstrations, printed matter, formation of clubs for instruction in hygiene, and physical training.

In most cases rural health work on a county basis has resulted through the cooperation of state and county governments, with financial assistance from the Federal government allotted by the Public Health Service. The last-named agency may start work in a county with the understanding that it will be continued with funds contributed jointly by the state and county. Following several demonstration years, it is expected that the county will assume a greater share of the budget.

An economical arrangement, which also encourages greater efficiency in health work, is the formation of city-county health departments. Obviously epidemics and health problems in general are not limited by political boundaries, and the health department which can operate without regard to city limits is in a stronger position than if it cannot do so. Pooling of financial resources also allows an organization that is more complete and staffed by better-qualified personnel. The city-county department is, in fact, the answer to the problem of furnishing a well-rounded health program, not only to the rural inhabitants of a county, but also to the small towns. Legal obstacles to the formation of such departments are met in some states, but these can be eliminated by legislative action or amendment to the state constitution. Progress has been slow in the formation of combination health departments, but it is probably safe to predict that they will become more numerous as time goes on.

20-20. District Organization. In some states, state health work has been decentralized to a considerable extent. The state is subdivided into districts, and a district health officer, with assisting personnel, is placed in each area. This arrangement is defended by some as permitting closer state supervision over sections which may otherwise be neglected and also for its usefulness in giving health service to those areas where economic conditions or lack of interest has operated to prevent establishment of city and county health organizations. The following considerations enter into any discussion of this subject.

The solution of local health problems is primarily a responsibility of local authorities. Only where emergencies exist and other communities are endangered or the lives of people are threatened through gross local neglect should the state assume responsibility and control. This conforms to the American idea that local self-government is desirable and even necessary. In populous areas, when public sentiment for adequate health work arises, it is provided, and the state should contribute to the crystallization of that sentiment.

Recognition should also be given to the fact that there are many areas in some states, such as the sparsely settled sections of the poorer agricultural districts, where it is a practical certainty that sufficient local funds will never be available for health protection. Here the district organization, created by the state, can mobilize and employ all available financial resources, Federal, state, and local, for the required protection. It should be recognized, however, that where the district plan is widely adopted a closely integrated system results which, at a whim of the state legislature, may be swept away entirely. On the other hand, county health units, while tending to be unstable individually, permit gains to be made slowly with less danger of complete disappearance.

20-21. Private Health Organizations. The work of the public health agencies is supplemented by many private organizations. In fact, many of the most important of the present-day functions of public health departments were first developed by private agencies and later taken over by governmental departments. A few of the more important organizations are mentioned below.

The International Health Board of the Rockefeller Foundation has done work both in the United States and abroad in the control of hookworm, malaria, and yellow fever. It has also aided in the organization of rural health work and conducted studies leading to the bettering of public health organizations. The policy of the board in general is to work in cooperation with governmental agencies, and its assistance has been welcomed by the Public Health Service, states, counties, municipalities, and foreign countries whose funds for adequate health work have been limited.

The American Public Health Association has a membership of over 13,000 persons who are engaged or interested in health work. It publishes the *American Journal of Public Health* and conducts meetings and section meetings at which there are valuable interchanges of ideas. The association is divided into sections corresponding to the various lines of health work. These are health officers, public health engineering, epidemiology, laboratory, vital statistics, industrial hygiene, health education, food and nutrition, public health nursing, and child hygiene. It has also made surveys and evaluations of the health work of individual cities. The committee reports and other publications of the association have been very influential and useful in advancing and standardizing practice in all public health fields.

The American National Red Cross, in addition to its military and emergency work, also performs community service. This consists in the formation and instruction of classes in nursing hygiene and nutrition.

In addition to the above there are the National Tuberculosis Association, the American Social Hygiene Association, the Council on Health and Public Instruction of the American Medical Association, the Russell Sage Foundation, the National Physical Education Service, the Milbank Foundation, the Commonwealth Foundation, and the Kellogg, Hogg, and Cullen Foundations and others. Much work is also done by state public health associations, state tuberculosis associations, and similar bodies which are organized on a city or county basis.

Bibliography

1. Tobey, J. A.: "Public Health Law," 3d ed., Commonwealth Fund, New York, 1947.
2. Peck, C. J.: "Public Health and Sanitation Law," Sanitarian's Desk Manual, National Association of Sanitarians, Denver, Colo.
3. Organization and Staffing for Local Health Service, *Public Health Service Pub.* 682, rev. 1961.
4. Confrey, E. A. (ed.): "Administration of Community Health Services," International City Managers Association, Chicago, 1961.
5. Smillie, W. G., and E. K. Kilbourne: "Preventive Medicine and Public Health," 3d ed., The Macmillan Company, New York, 1963.
6. Blum, H. L., and A. R. Leonard: "Public Administration: A Public Health Viewpoint," The Macmillan Company, New York, 1963.

21

ENVIRONMENTAL ENGINEERING PLANNING

21-1. Readers of the preceding chapters will have noted that many of the problems discussed are closely concerned with the community and require community action for solutions. The problems are provision of safe water in adequate amounts; collection and disposal of sewage; collection and disposal of solid refuse of various types; prevention of atmospheric pollution; housing and urban renewal; and control of ionizing radiation.

Man controls his own environment. He adversely affects it by his waste products, which include those resulting from his living processes, his industries, and his other activities. As air, water, and soil reach their limits in absorbing these wastes, he must use his knowledge and abilities to aid nature. He must depend upon community organization and planning for the application of science to maintain his environment in a reasonably satisfactory condition as far as his health, safety, comfort, and convenience are concerned. Obviously the greater the concentration of people within a relatively small area, the more serious the problem of maintaining a wholesome environment in that area becomes.

Communities can be classified as follows: village or rural type; town or city, with variations as to size and type, *i.e.*, industrial or residential; suburban; fringe areas contiguous to a city; or metropolitan areas. Small cities in the metropolitan area surrounding a large core city are sometimes called satellite cities.

21-2. Population Trends. The term "population explosion" has seen much use, and it is important that its relationship to environmental health problems be understood. From 1950 to 1960, the total population of the United States increased from 151,326,000 to 179,323,000, an increase of 18.5 per cent. Since 1960 it is estimated to be increasing at the rate of about 2,800,000 per year.

The urban population increased from 96,847,000 to 125,269,000 in the same decade, an increase of 29.3 per cent. Of the urban population, 29,420,000 live outside the highly urbanized areas but in rather densely settled fringe areas, incorporated or unincorporated, around the larger cities. These areas have many of the problems of the growing communities without, in many cases, a community organization to care for them.

Highly important as environmental planning problems are the Standard Metropolitan Statistical Areas (SMSA's)[1] of which there were 212 in 1962. The total population of the SMSA's in 1950 was 89,317,000; in 1960 it was 112,885,000, a growth of 26.4 per cent. About 63 per cent of the total population of the country in 1960 lived in the SMSA's. The population of the central cities of the SMSA's grew in the same decade from 52,386,000 to 58,004,000, an increase of 10.7 per cent, while in the areas outside the central cities the population grew from 36,931,000 to 54,881,000, an increase of 48.6 per cent. This population increase outside the central cities is extremely significant to the environmental engineer.

[1] A Standard Metropolitan Statistical Area as defined by the Census Bureau, except in New England, is a county or group of contiguous counties containing at least one city of 50,000 population or more or two cities having contiguous boundaries with a combined population of at least 50,000. If two or more adjacent counties each have a city of 50,000 inhabitants or more and the cities are within 20 miles of each other, they are included in the same metropolitan area. The counties must be essentially metropolitan in character and socially and economically integrated with the central city. In New England, SMSA's are defined on a town rather than a county basis [6].

The 1960 census classified a population of 54,054,000 as rural. It should be recognized that the Census Bureau classifies as rural towns of less than 2,500 population if they are not within SMSA's or otherwise in the classified urban areas.

It will be seen that population growth and movements in the immediate past have been toward concentrations that have created environmental problems, many still unsolved, and that, if the trend continues those problems will grow in magnitude and complexity. These new concentrations may result in very large metropolitan areas. Some foresee a single metropolitan complex extending from Boston southward into Virginia, another in the states south of the Great Lakes, and another in California extending from San Francisco to Los Angeles.

21-3. Planning. Planning by competent professionals is necessary to remedy existing environmental problems and to prevent those looming in the immediate future and those which may be expected in the foreseeable future, say, 20 years. The problems will be difficult, and solutions will require much effort and money; but with community willingness and, in some cases, intercommunity cooperation, difficulties can usually be overcome.

The engineer, unfortunately, has little influence in initiating community efforts. His attempts are likely to be met by apathy, defeatism, or even the charge that he is "looking for a job." Of these attitudes apathy is likely to be based upon ignorance of the present and future needs. Defeatism may be based upon the obstacles frequently encountered in the initiation of community efforts—lack of funds or political difficulties. The answer to these difficulties is to enlist the efforts of community leaders. This will be discussed later.

Community planning may be considered to fall into three categories: city planning, regional or metropolitan planning, and, what is of special interest to the sanitarian and sanitary engineer, environmental planning as it is applicable to the individual city or to a metropolitan area. They will be discussed separately.

21-4. City Planning. City planning is recognized as a necessity by many cities, and much good work has been done by professional planners. A city plan covers such matters as the street system; transportation facilities such as airfields and railway and bus terminals, etc.; parks, parkways, and recreation centers; location of public buildings, including schools; and zoning, or regulation of land as to type of use, such as residential, commercial, or industrial, and as to height and bulk of buildings constructed. A criticism sometimes made of city planning is that civil engineers and environmental engineers are frequently not consulted in the formulation of the plan. The consequences are sometimes serious. Industrial areas may be located where topographical conditions cause air movements that result in atmospheric hazards to residential areas or to schools. No consideration may be given to sites for refuse incinerators, landfills, or sewage treatment plants.

21-5. Metropolitan or Regional Planning. If metropolitan planning is considered city planning on a larger scale, it will cover the following features: an arterial highway plan, provision of transport facilities, provision of parks and recreation areas, and zoning, or regulation of land use. It should, however, cover other ubiquitous regional problems: adequate and safe water supplies, collection and disposal of liquid wastes, collection and disposal of solid wastes, atmospheric pollution, and control of ionizing radiation, a problem which will become more important in the future.

Less has been accomplished in regional planning than in city planning. The foremost difficulty is lack of political integration. A metropolitan area will probably include several counties. It may be crossed by state boundaries, and in addition to the core city, there may be smaller incorporated cities and a number of school districts, park districts, water districts, etc., all autonomous in their own fields and all, as indicated in Art. 21-2, experiencing population increases.

Among the schemes that have been proposed and put into effect to the end that united action can be obtained are:

1. Annexation, which is the acquisition by a governmental agency of territory outside of, and usually contiguous to, its boundary.

2. Establishment of special districts, agencies, or authorities as independent administrative units with specified governmental authority to provide a certain service or services. Instances are school districts, park districts, water districts, drainage districts, and sanitary sewerage districts.

3. Mutual cooperation—informal working arrangements among people in different political subdivisions to solve common problems.

4. Extending city services by contractual arrangements between a municipality and adjacent territories to provide for the use of the municipal services and facilities according to a regional plan. For example, the core city of a region may have developed a large water supply and the only one available to the region. A regional distribution plan is made, and the core city sells water to other municipalities of the region.

5. City-county consolidation. This implies combination of functions of the core city with the county. The county retains some of its identity, and the incorporated cities remain independent for local purposes, such as policing and fire protection.

6. City-county separation. This is the creation of a city-county in the core city and a new county to cover the outlying areas.

7. Federation. This implies the establishment of a new level of government with responsibility for certain regional and area-wide functional services. The machinery of this plan is a commission or council made up of representatives of the various governmental units of the area and having authority to adopt plans and raise funds to carry out their specified aims, which may be regional water supply, sewerage, etc.

8. Functional transfer. This is the transfer of a service or function by one governmental unit to another existing governmental unit.

9. Consolidation of smaller municipal service corporations.

The above expedients have been successful in some areas, and in others they have not. Which is most applicable to a specific area will depend largely upon local political behavior and traditions.

The formation of special districts is probably the most popular method, but the multiplication of single-purpose governmental units is confusing to the voter and can be wasteful of money and effort. Federation for a broader coverage of regional problems is more promising and will allow focusing of public attention on the merits and accomplishments of a single governing body.

Establishment of any type of metropolitan governmental scheme is difficult. In most types an affirmative popular vote is required. The voter tends to be conservative and even suspicious of matters that he does not understand. Therefore, much educative work is required.

Movement for a regional plan for any purpose and the necessary authority to implement that plan must originate with the community leaders. The engineer may make representations to them directly or through his local professional organization. Civic organizations may then become interested. Much publicity will be needed. The services of former mayors and other former officials will be valuable since they are aware of the difficulties arising from governmental fragmentation in the area.

21-6. Environmental Planning in General. Some environmental planning requirements and procedures are applicable to either individual cities or metropolitan areas, and these will be mentioned in this article.

Each appropriate governmental unit should have the following:

1. An adequate staff of environmental engineers in its health department. The health department, in general, should be strong and active. It can have a great influence upon the development of comprehensive planning.

2. A modern and comprehensive sanitary code that will include control of air and water pollution, sewage disposal, ionizing radiation, refuse collection and disposal, water supply, milk and food supplies, realty developments, rural and resort sanitation, etc.

3. Authority to control real estate subdivisions. Preferably this should be conferred by a state law designed to protect the public health and prevent the installation of substandard water and sewerage facilities and inadequate surface drainage.

4. A zoning ordinance which recognizes not only major highways, convenient industrial sites, and commercial areas, but also such features as topography, drainage and possible flooding, prevailing winds, and soil conditions.

5. A housing ordinance which sets up minimum standards as to dwelling

occupancy, facilities supplied, and maintenance and which also considers neighborhood living environment.

6. A modern building code with sections on plumbing, heating, electrical requirements, ventilation, fire prevention, and structural requirements.

COMPREHENSIVE PLANS. Plans for improvements should always be long-term solutions and not temporary abatements. In the fields of water and sewerage particularly, long-term plans are necessary for an orderly development that will meet the ever-increasing demands for service. Long-term plans for water-service, for example, based upon expected population increase and other trends should probably be made for about 20 years in the future but should be subject to a searching review and modification every 5 years. Obviously the existence of a city plan or regional plan will be helpful. The city or regional plan and the long-term plan for water, sewerage, and other public works will allow the acquisition of sites for water and sewage treatment plants, reservoirs, incinerators, and sanitary landfill before land values have risen.

CAPITAL BUDGETING. Public works require much capital, which must be obtained from revenues derived from services and/or taxation. Borrowing by means of bond issues to be paid off by revenues will be necessary in many instances. A careful analysis of the amount and date of capital needs and the revenues that will be collected will allow the formulation of an orderly plan of borrowing and repayment for the community. Such a plan will inspire confidence in the authorities among the more thoughtful citizens.

21-7. Environmental Planning for the City. In addition to the needs outlined in Art. 21-6, the city's principal problem is the control of real estate subdivisions. In the present era of urban growth, this has become further complicated by the development of fringe areas beyond the city's boundary, inhabited in many cases by persons who have listened to the real estate salesman's song, "city conveniences without city taxes." Later these areas are likely to be annexed, and a variety of troubles may result.

Some states permit cities to control real estate subdivision for some stated distance beyond the city limits. In some cases this applies only to cities having a city plan, and compliance with it can then be required.

If possible, the zoning should also extend beyond the city limits. In addition, the real estate developer should be required not only to make the street system comply with the city street plan but to make the water distribution system and the sewer system comply also. The city which has a long-term comprehensive plan for water and sewerage works is in a position to require such compliance. In any case, the developer should pay for the improvements, with reimbursement made for any extra costs necessary to conform to the city's over-all plan.

In some developments water is available, but the city will be unable to extend sewers until some future time. Development should not be permitted unless the soil is favorable to septic tanks and disposal fields or perhaps seepage pits. In this case the developer may be required to put in sewers and cap or plug the house sewers at the property line. When city sewers are extended to the subdivision, the house connection is completed. This procedure will protect the homeowner from a large and perhaps unexpected payment for sewer installation.

21-8. Environmental Planning for the Metropolitan Area. If it is assumed that the area has a regional plan and has otherwise complied with requirements mentioned in the preceding articles, control of real estate development is again the principal subject in need of discussion.

A metropolitan area will probably include land ranging from rural to suburban to fringe areas near municipal boundaries. Uncontrolled subdivision development has resulted in health hazards, use of periodically flooded areas for residential purposes, and trouble and expense for homeowners. Cesspools and tile disposal fields have endangered wells and have caused sewage to overflow on the ground surface near homes or to appear at some distance on lower ground. Where unfavorable soil conditions prevail, subdivision should not be permitted until sewerage is available.

Lot sizes may be used to guide the character of development. Small lots may be permitted in areas with public water supply and sewerage. In rural areas with private wells, septic tanks, and tile disposal fields, large lots, 1.0 to 2.5 acres, will be useful in preventing fringe-area sanitation problems.

"Spatter" and "ribbon" developments, which are likely to spring up along major highways, should be discouraged. They are often expensive and difficult to supply with water and, even more so, with sewerage service. Control can be exercised by requiring that sewage be treated in plants that will produce an effluent satisfactory at all times to the state and local health authorities.

An areal plan for sewage treatment and disposal can be efficient and economical and can avoid nuisances and health hazards. The plan would be adapted to the topography and natural drainage of the area. It would include the following features: In the early stages the core city and the satellite cities would be served by existing sewage treatment plants if adequate. Newly developing communities would be served by small sewage treatment plants, possibly of the "package" type (Art. 4-26). The plan would also include future intercepting sewers that would be constructed and extended into the area as it developed. As sewage volumes increased the small treatment plants would be abandoned, and the sewage would be conveyed by an intercepting sewer, either to the plant of the core city or to another plant somewhere in the area. The result would be the concentration of the sewage in a few large treatment plants. These would be carefully operated, and there would be none of the stream-pollution dangers that are often noted where there is no comprehensive plan. With careful capital budgeting of revenues derived from sewer-service charges, the plan can be followed without undue financial burdens on the area.

Bibliography

1. Environmental Health in Community Growth (reprint), *Am. J. Public Health,* vol. 53, no. 5, May, 1963.
2. Environmental Health Planning Guide, *Public Health Service Pub.* 823, 1962.
3. Logan, J. A., *et al.* (ed.): "Environmental Engineering and Metropolitan Planning," Northwestern University Press, Evanston, Ill., 1962.
4. "Man and His Environment," Second National Congress on Environmental Health, School of Public Health, University of Michigan, Ann Arbor, Mich., 1961.
5. Estrada, A. A., and R. P. Heurich: County Develops Master Plan for Water Supply and Sewerage, *Public Works,* vol. 92, no. 10, October, 1961.
6. "Population of Standard Metropolitan Statistical Areas: 1960 and 1950," Supplementary Report, 1960 Census of Population.

APPENDIX A

Classification of Illnesses Attributable to Foods

A. FOOD INFECTIONS (BACTERIAL)

Illness	Causative agent	Foods usually involved	Other modes of transmission	Incubation period	Signs and symptoms	Measures to prevent spread by food
1. Bacillary dysentery (shigellosis)	Members of the genus *Shigella*	Moist prepared foods and milk or other dairy products contaminated with excreta	Direct or indirect contact with case or carrier, or contaminated water	Usually 2–3 days; extremes, 12 hr to 7 days	Diarrhea, bloody stools; fever in severe cases	Strict personal cleanliness in food preparation; refrigeration of moist foods during storage periods; cooking of foods prior to serving; elimination of flies
2. Brucellosis (undulant fever or Bang's disease)	*Brucella abortus, Brucella melitensis, Brucella suis*	Raw contaminated milk; dairy products made from raw contaminated milk	Contact with fresh tissues or discharges of infected animals	3–21 days; may be several months in some cases	Insidious onset, fever, chills, sweats, weakness, malaise, headache, muscle and joint pains, loss of weight	Eradication of brucellosis from livestock; pasteurization of milk and other dairy products

Classifcation of Illnesses Attributable to Foods (Continued)

Illness	Causative agent	Foods usually involved	Other modes of transmission	Incubation period	Signs and symptoms	Measures to prevent spread by food
3. Diphtheria	Corynebacterium diphtheriae	Milk contaminated from human sources	Direct or indirect contact with case or carrier	Usually 3–5 days; extremes, 2–7 days	Insidious onset; inflammation of throat and nose	Pasteurization of milk; search for, and isolation of, carriers
4. Hemolytic streptococcal infections (scarlet fever or septic sore throat)	Certain strains of beta hemolytic streptococci	Foods contaminated with nasal or oral discharges from case or carrier; milk from cows having udder infections caused by these organisms	Direct contact with case or carrier	Usually about 3 days; extremes, 1–7 days	Fever, sore throat; rash occasionally	Pasteurization of milk and other dairy products; excluding persons with known streptococcal infections from handling food; isolation of carriers; prophylactic antibiotic treatment of contacts of known cases
5. Streptococcal food infection	Enterococcus group S. fecalis (Lancefield group D.); pyogenic group S. pyogenes (Lancefield group A)	Food products contaminated with excreta; foods contaminated by respiratory discharges of case or carrier	Contact with contaminated persons or fomites; wound infection or contact with discharges of infected wounds	2–18 hr	Nausea; sometimes vomiting, colicky pains, and diarrhea; usually milder than staphylococcal food poisoning	Cooking of food thoroughly; refrigeration of moist foods during storage periods

6. Salmonellosis (a) Typhoid fever	Salmonella typhosa	Any milk, shellfish, or other food product contaminated with excreta from human case or carrier	Water polluted by human excreta	Usually 7–21 days; extremes, 3–38 days	Insidious onset with malaise, lack of appetite, headache, fever, diarrhea; in children, onset may simulate early pneumonia	Pasteurization of milk and other dairy products; certification of shellfish; chlorination of water; prohibiting of carriers from handling food; elimination of flies; examination of stools of food handlers who have history of having had typhoid fever
(b) Paratyphoid A	S. paratyphi A	Same as for typhoid fever	Contact with unrecognized case or carrier	Usually a few days; extremes, 1–10 days	Fever, malaise; may resemble mild typhoid	Same as typhoid fever
(c) Other types	Members of the genus Salmonella, e.g., S. typhimurium, newport, oranienburg, montevideo, newington, enteritidis, choleraesuis, pullorum, and others, including Arizona group	Meat and poultry salads; eggs and egg products	Direct or indirect contact with human or animal carriers	Usually 12–24 hr; extremes, 5–72 hr	Abdominal pain, diarrhea, chills, fever; frequent vomiting, prostration	Cooking of food thoroughly; strict sanitation in food preparation; refrigeration of moist foods during storage periods; frequent washing of hands; protection of foods from animal excreta

Classification of Illnesses Attributable to Foods (*Continued*)

Illness	Causative agent	Foods usually involved	Other modes of transmission	Incubation period	Signs and symptoms	Measures to prevent spread by food
7. Tuberculosis (extrapulmonary)	*Mycobacterium tuberculosis* (human and bovine types)	Raw contaminated milk or other contaminated dairy products	Contact with infected animals and humans	Variable	Depends upon part of body affected	Eradication of tuberculosis from cattle; pasteurization of milk and other dairy products
8. Tularemia	*Pasteurella tularensis*	Meat of wild rabbits, squirrels, and similar animals	Dressing or handling infected animals; bites of infected ticks and deerflies	Usually about 3 days; extremes, 1–10 days	Sudden onset with headache, chills, body pains, vomiting and fever; swollen lymph glands	Use of rubber gloves and care when handling wild rabbits and squirrels; cooking the meat thoroughly; arthropod-suppressive measures

B. FOOD INTOXICATIONS (BACTERIAL)

Illness	Causative agent	Foods usually involved	Incubation period	Signs and symptoms	Measures to prevent spread by food
1. Botulism	Toxins	Home-processed foods; contaminated canned foods with pH over 3.5	Usually 12–36 hr; extremes, 2 hr to 6 days	Dizziness; lassitude; double vision; loss of reflex to light; muscular weakness; difficulty in swallowing, speech, and respiration; frequently fatal	Thorough cooking of foods before serving (boil 15 min with stirring to ensure heating of all parts, or pressure-cook)
2. Staphylococcal food poisoning (intoxication)	Enterotoxin-producing staphylococcus (preformed enterotoxin)	Cooked ham or other meats; cream-filled or custard pastries and other dairy products; bread puddings; potato salad and other salads of protein foods; Hollandaise sauce; "warmed over" foods	Usually 2–6 hr; extremes, 1–11 hr	Nausea, vomiting, diarrhea, and acute prostration; abdominal cramps	Exclusion from food handling of persons with nasal discharges or purulent local skin infections; thorough cooking of foods; refrigeration of moist foods during storage; reheating of custard pastries; frequent washing of hands
3. *C. welchii* poisoning	*Clostridium welchii* (Type A)	Meat which has been boiled, steamed, braised, stewed, or insufficiently roasted and allowed to cool slowly and served the next day, either cold or reheated	8–22 hr	Acute abdominal pain and diarrhea; nausea and vomiting rare; fever, shivering, and headache seldom seen	Exclusion from food handling of known carriers; cooking of meat immediately before consumption or rapid cooking and refrigeration between cooking and use

Classification of Illnesses Attributable to Foods (Continued)

C. PARASITIC INFECTIONS (NONBACTERIAL)

Illness	Causative agent	Foods usually involved	Incubation period	Signs and symptoms	Measures to prevent spread by food
1. Amoebic dysentery (Amoebiasis)	*Endamoeba histolytica*	Water contaminated with sewage; moist food contaminated with human feces	Several days to 4 weeks	Diarrhea of varying severity; fatalities not uncommon	Protection of water supplies; cleanliness in food preparation; ensuring proper disposal of human excreta
2. Beef tapeworm (Taeniasis saginata)	*Taenia saginata*	Raw or insufficiently cooked beef containing live larvae	Several weeks	Abdominal pain, hungry feeling, vague discomfort	Use of meat processed under veterinary inspection; thorough cooking of beef
3. Fish tapeworm (Diphyllobothriasis)	*Diphyllobothrium latum*	Raw or insufficiently cooked fish containing live larvae	3–6 weeks	Usually none; anemia in heavy infections	Thorough cooking of fish; avoidance of raw smoked fish
4. Pork tapeworm (Taeniasis solium)	*Taenia solium*	Raw or insufficiently cooked pork containing live larvae	Several weeks	Varies from a mild chronic digestive disorder to severe malaise with encephalitis; may be fatal	Use of meat processed under veterinary inspection; thorough cooking of pork

618

Illness	Causative agent	Foods usually involved	Incubation period	Signs and symptoms	Measures to prevent spread by food
5. Trichinosis	*Trichinella spiralis*	Raw or insufficiently cooked pork and pork products; whale, seal, bear, or walrus meat containing live larvae	Usually 9 days, but may vary from 2 to 28 days; in heavy infections, 24 hr	Nausea, vomiting, diarrhea, muscular pains, fever, labored breathing, swelling of eyelids; occasionally fatal	Thorough cooking of pork and pork products; freezing pork at 5°F for 30 days, at −10°F for 20 days, or at −20°F for 12 days; cooking garbage fed to swine; elimination of rats from hog lots

D. CHEMICALS

Illness	Causative agent	Foods usually involved	Incubation period	Signs and symptoms	Measures to prevent spread by food
1. Antimony poisoning	Enamelware (gray) containing antimony	Any foods contaminated by leaching of container by acid foods	Few minutes to hours	Vomiting, abdominal pains, spasms, collapse; occasionally fatal	Discontinuing use of utensils with antimony in finish
2. Arsenic poisoning	Insecticides and rodenticides	Any food accidentally contaminated	1 hr or less	Vomiting, diarrhea; occasionally fatal	Use of colored pesticides and proper storage of same
3. Cadmium poisoning	Plating metal	Any food contaminated by leaching of containers and trays by acid foods, including fruit juices	½ hr or less	Nausea, vomiting, cramps; often fatal	Discontinuing use of cadmium-plated utensils as food containers

Classification of Illnesses Attributable to Foods (Continued)

Illness	Causative agent	Foods usually involved	Incubation period	Signs and symptoms	Measures to prevent spread by food
4. Copper poisoning	Copper food-contact surfaces	Any acid food contaminated by leaching of copper surfaces by such food	1 hr or less	Vomiting; no specific symptoms	Preventing acid foods or liquids or carbonated liquids from contacting exposed copper
5. Cyanide poisoning	Silver polish containing cyanide	Any food accidentally contaminated	½ to 6 hr	Nausea, vomiting, diarrhea, cold perspiration, exhaustion; often fatal	Discontinuing use of cyanide silver polishes or exercising care in their use
6. Fluoride poisoning	Insecticides containing sodium fluoride	Any food accidentally contaminated	1 hr or less	Vomiting, retching, cramps, pallor, collapse; often fatal	Discontinuing use in food establishments of pesticides containing fluorides
7. Lead poisoning	Pesticides	Any food accidentally contaminated	½ hr or longer	Abdominal pains, vomiting; may be fatal	Use of colored pesticides and proper storage of same
8. Zinc poisoning	Galvanized ware	Any food accidentally contaminated; leaching of galvanized containers by acid foods	1 hr or less	Diarrhea, astringent taste	Education of persons preparing food

E. POISONOUS PLANTS AND ANIMALS

Illness	Causative agent	Foods usually involved	Incubation period	Signs and symptoms	Measures to prevent spread by food
1. Castor bean poisoning	Ricin (a toxin in the castor bean)	Castor bean	Few minutes to several hours	Colic, thirst, vomiting, diarrhea, cold sweat, collapse	Not eating castor beans
2. Ergotism	Parasitic fungus of rye (*Claviceps purpurea*)	Rye meal or bread	Gradual, usually after several meals of diseased rye in meal or bread	Gangrene involving limbs, especially fingers and toes, and occasionally ears and nose; convulsive depression, weakness and drowsiness, headache, giddiness, painful cramps in limbs, itching of skin	Using only rye products made from rye that is free of the parasitic fungus
3. Favism	Bean (*Vicia fava*) or inhalation of pollen from blossoming plant	The bean, *Vicia fava*	Few minutes to several hours	Dizziness and collapse; headache, malaise, nausea, yawning, vomiting, chills, pallor	Education of persons preparing food

Classification of Illnesses Attributable to Foods (Continued)

Illness	Causative agent	Foods usually involved	Incubation period	Signs and symptoms	Measures to prevent spread by food
4. Mushroom poisoning	Toxins (phalloidine and other alkaloids) of certain species of mushrooms	Poisonous mushrooms (usually *Amanita phalloides* and *A. muscaria*)	15 min to 15 hr	Salivation; sudden severe abdominal pain; intense thirst; nausea, retching; vomiting; profuse watery stools; excessive perspiration; a flow of tears; often fatal	Eating only mushrooms known to be of non-poisonous species; education of persons preparing food
5. Rhubarb leaf poisoning	Oxalic acid	Rhubarb leaves	2–12 hr	Diarrhea, vomiting, thirst	Education of persons preparing food
6. Selenium poisoning	Selenium	Milk, eggs, meat, vegetables, and cereal grains produced in seleniferous regions	Unknown	Dermatitis, skin rash, fatigue, dizziness, sleepiness, depression, dullness, jaundice	Withdrawing areas known to produce toxic grain from cultivation of food plants

7. Shellfish poisoning	A thermostable alkaloid contained in plankton (*Gonyaulax*) consumed by shellfish	Mussels and clams (especially during certain seasons of the year)	5 to 30 min or longer	Respiratory paralysis; milder symptoms consist of trembling lips to complete loss of power in muscles of extremities and neck	Control of harvesting of shellfish from toxic areas; avoiding clams or mussels of unknown quality
8. Snakeroot poisoning	Tremetol from snakeroot (*Eupatorium urticaefolium*)	Milk from cows pastured on snakeroot	Variable period; after repeated use of milk from cows pastured in an area in which snakeroot is present	Weakness or prostration; vomiting; severe constipation; stomach pain	Preventing milk cows from grazing in pastures where snakeroot is present
9. Solanine poisoning	*Solanum tuberosum*	Green or sunburned potatoes, wild celery	Few hours	Vomiting, diarrhea, headache, abdominal pains, prostration	Not using sprouts or peel of green potatoes, sunburned potatoes, or wild celery
10. Water hemlock poisoning	Cicutoxin or resin from water hemlock (*Cicuta maculata*)	Leaves and root of water hemlock	1–2 hr	Nausea, vomiting, convulsions	Not eating any part of the water hemlock plant

623

Classification of Illnesses Attributable to Foods (Continued)

F. PHYSICAL

Illness	Causative agent	Foods usually involved	Incubation period	Signs and symptoms	Measures to prevent spread by food
Radiation poisoning	Ionizing radiations	Any food exposed to contamination from radioactive materials	Variable over lifetime, depending on degree and type of contamination	Excessive radio-activity of body discharges; variable signs and symptoms depending upon dosage and parts of body exposed	Removal of source of exposure; monitoring of foods suspected of being contaminated and destruction of contaminated foods

NOTE: While carbon monoxide poisoning is not attributable to food, it sometimes causes illness that may be confused with food intoxication. This should be considered when illnesses suspected of being food-borne are investigated.

SOURCE: "Procedure for the Investigation of Foodborne Disease Outbreaks," International Association of Milk and Food Sanitarians, Inc., Shelbyville, Ind.

APPENDIX B

Threshold Limit Values of Industrial Atmospheric Contaminants for 1963

Adopted at the 25th Annual Meeting of the American Conference of Governmental Industrial Hygienists, Cincinnati, Ohio, May 6, 7, 1963.

[*Reprinted by permission of the American Conference of Governmental Industrial Hygienists*]

These values should be used as guides in the control of health hazards and should not be regarded as fine lines between safe and dangerous concentrations. They represent conditions under which it is believed that nearly all workers may be repeatedly exposed, day after day, without adverse effect. The values listed refer to time-weighted average concentrations for a normal workday. The amount by which these figures may be exceeded for short periods without injury to health depends upon a number of factors such as the nature of the contaminant, whether very high concentrations even for short periods produce acute poisoning, whether the effects are cumulative, the frequency with which high concentrations occur, and the duration of such periods. All must be taken into consideration in arriving at a decision as to whether a hazardous situation exists. Because it has been recognized that the threshold limits of certain acutely-acting substances may not provide a safety factor comparable to that of chronically-acting substances for which a time-weighted average applies, a "C" designation or "ceiling" has been affixed to such values indicating that the Threshold Limit Value should not be exceeded. The bases for the "C" listing is given in Supplement 3.

Special consideration should be given to the application of these values in assessing the health hazards which may be associated with exposure to mixtures of two or more substances. A brief discussion of basic considerations involved in developing threshold limit values for mixtures, and methods for their development, amplified by specific examples are given in Supplement 2.

Threshold limits are based on the best available information from industrial experience, from experimental studies, and, when possible, from a combination of the two. These values are based on various criteria of toxic effects or on marked discomfort; thus, they should not be used as a common denominator of toxicity, nor should they be considered as the sole criterion in proving or disproving diagnosis of suspected occupational disease.

These limits are intended for use in the field of industrial hygiene and should be interpreted and applied only by persons trained in this field. They

625

are not intended for use, or for modification for use, (1) as a relative index of toxicity, by making a ratio of two limits, or (2) in the evaluation or control of community air pollution or air pollution nuisances, or (3) in estimating the toxic potential of continuous uninterrupted exposures.

These values are reviewed annually by the Committee on Threshold Limits for revisions, or additions, as further information becomes available. The Committee welcomes the suggestion of substances to be added to the list and also comments, references, or reports of experience with these materials.

Recommended Values

(IN ALPHABETICAL ORDER)

Substance	ppm*	Mg/M³**
Acetaldehyde	200	360
Acetic acid	10	25
Acetic anhydride	5	20
Acetone	1,000	2,400
Acetonitrile	40	70
Acetylene tetrabromide	1	14
† Acrolein	0.1	0.25
Acrylonitrile—Skin	20	45
Aldrin (1,2,3,4,10,10-hexachloro-1,4,4a,5,8,8a-hexa-hydro-1,4,5,8-dimethano-naphthalene)—Skin	—	0.25
† Allyl alcohol—Skin	2	5
Allyl chloride	1	3
C Allyl glycidyl ether (AGE)	10	45
Allyl propyl disulfide	2	12
† Ammonia	50	35
Ammonium sulfamate (Ammate)	—	15
† Amyl acetate	100	525
Amyl alcohol (isoamyl alcohol)	100	360
Aniline—Skin	5	19
Antimony	—	0.5
ANTU (alpha naphthyl thiourea)	—	0.3
Arsenic	—	0.5
Arsine	0.05	0.2
Barium (soluble compounds)	—	0.5
C Benzene (benzol)—Skin	25	80
Benzidine	—	A¹
Benzyl chloride	1	5
Beryllium	—	0.002
Boron oxide	—	15
C Boron trifluoride	1	3
Bromine	0.1	0.7
Butadiene (1,3-butadiene)	1,000	2,200
2-Butanone (methyl ethyl ketone)	200	590

Recommended Values (Continued)

Substance	ppm*	Mg/M³**
2-Butoxy ethanol (Butyl Cellosolve)	50	240
Butyl acetate (n-butyl acetate).	200	950
Butyl alcohol.	100	300
tert. Butyl Alcohol	100	300
C Butylamine	5	15
n-Butyl glycidyl ether (BGE)	50	270
Butyl mercaptan.	10	35
p-tert. Butyltoluene.	10	60
Cadmium oxide fume	—	0.1
Calcium arsenate.	—	1
Carbon dioxide	5,000	9,000
Carbon disulfide—Skin.	20	60
Carbon monoxide	100	110
Carbon tetrachloride—Skin.	10	65
Chlordane (1,2,4,5,6,7,8,8-octachloro-3a,4,7,7a-tetra-hydro-4,7-methanoindene)	—	0.5
Chlorinated camphene, 60%	—	0.5
Chlorinated diphenyl oxide.	—	0.5
Chlorine	1	3
Chlorine dioxide.	0.1	0.3
C Chlorine trifluoride	0.1	0.4
C Chloroacetaldehyde.	1	3
Chlorobenzene (monochlorobenzene)	75	350
Chlorobromomethane	200	1,050
Chlorodiphenyl (42% Chlorine)—Skin	—	1
Chlorodiphenyl (54% Chlorine)—Skin	—	0.5
C Chloroform (trichloromethane).	50	240
1-Chloro-1-nitropropane.	20	100
Chloropicrin.	0.1	0.7
Chloroprene (2-chloro-1,3-butadiene).	25	90
Chromic acid and chromates (as CrO₃)	—	0.1
Cobalt.	—	0.5
Crag (R) herbicide (sodium 2-[2,4-dichlorophenoxy]ethanol hydrogen sulfate).	—	15
Cresol (all isomers)—Skin	5	22
Cyanide (as CN)—Skin.	—	5
Cyclohexane.	400	1,400
Cyclohexanol.	50	200
Cyclohexanone	50	200
Cyclohexene	400	1,350
2,4-D (2,4-dichlorophenoxyacetic acid)	—	10
DDT (2,2-bis [p-chlorophenyl]-1,1,1-trichloroethane)—Skin	—	1
Decaborane—Skin	0.05	0.3

Recommended Values (Continued)

Substance	ppm*	Mg/M³**
Diacetone alcohol (4-hydroxy-4-methyl-2-pentanone)	50	240
Diborane	0.1	0.1
1,2-Dibromoethane (Ethylene dibromide)	25	190
o-Dichlorobenzene	50	300
p-Dichlorobenzene	75	450
Dichlorodifluoromethane	1,000	4,950
1,1-Dichloroethane	100	400
1,2-Dichloroethane (ethylene dichloride)	50	200
1,2-Dichloroethylene	200	790
C Dichloroethyl ether	15	90
Dichloromonofluoromethane	1,000	4,200
C 1,1-Dichloro-1-nitroethane	10	60
Dichlorotetrafluoroethane	1,000	7,000
Dieldrin (1,2,3,4,10,10-hexachloro-6,7-epoxy-1,4,4a,5, 6,7,8,8a-octahydro-1,4,5,8-dimethanonaphthalene) —Skin	—	0.25
Diethylamine	25	75
Difluorodibromomethane	100	860
†C Diglycidyl ether (DGE)	0.5	2.8
Diisobutyl ketone	50	290
Dimethyl acetamide—Skin	10	35
Dimethylaniline (N-dimethylaniline)—Skin	5	25
Dimethylformamide	20	60
1,1-Dimethylhydrazine—Skin	0.5	1
Dimethylsulfate—Skin	1	5
Dinitrobenzene—Skin	—	1
Dinitrotoluene—Skin	—	1.5
Dinitro-o-cresol—Skin	—	0.2
Dioxane (diethylene dioxide)	100	360
Dipropylene glycol methyl ether	100	600
EPN (O-ethyl O-p-nitrophenyl thionobenzenephos- phonate)—Skin	—	0.5
Ethyl acetate	400	1,400
Ethyl acrylate—Skin	25	100
Ethyl alcohol (ethanol)	1,000	1,900
Ethylamine	25	45
C Ethylbenzene	200	870
Ethyl bromide	200	890
Ethyl chloride	1,000	2,600
Ethyl ether	400	1,200
Ethyl formate	100	300
†C Ethyl mercaptan	20	52
Ethyl silicate	100	850
Ethylene chlorohydrin—Skin	5	16

Recommended Values (Continued)

Substance	ppm*	Mg/M³**
Ethylenediamine	10	30
Ethylene glycol dinitrate (combined EGDN + NG) —Skin	0.2	1.2
Ethylene imine—Skin	5	9
Ethylene oxide	50	90
2-Ethoxyethanol (Cellosolve)	200	740
2-Ethoxyethylacetate (Cellosolve Acetate)	100	540
Ferbam (ferric dimethyl dithiocarbamate)	—	15
Ferrovanadium dust	—	1
Fluoride (as F)	—	2.5
Fluorine	0.1	0.2
Fluorotrichloromethane	1,000	5,600
C Formaldehyde	5	6
Furfural	5	20
Furfuryl alcohol	50	200
Gasoline	500	2,000
Glycidol (2,3-Epoxy-1-propanol)	50	150
Heptane (n-heptane)	500	2,000
Hexane (n-hexane)	500	1,800
Hexanone (methyl butyl ketone)	100	410
† sec-Hexyl acetate	50	295
Hexone (methyl isobutyl ketone)	100	410
C Hydrazine—Skin	1	1.3
Hydrogen bromide	3	10
C Hydrogen chloride	5	7
Hydrogen cyanide—Skin	10	11
Hydrogen fluoride	3	2
Hydrogen peroxide, 90%	1	1.4
Hydrogen selenide	0.05	0.2
C Hydrogen sulfide	20	30
Hydroquinone	—	2
C Iodine	0.1	1
Iron oxide fume	—	15
Isophorone	25	140
Isopropylamine	5	12
Isopropyl glycidyl ether (IGE)	50	240
Ketene	0.5	0.9
Lead	—	0.2
Lead arsenate	—	0.15
Lindane (hexachlorocyclohexane, gamma isomer)	—	0.5
Lithium hydride	—	0.025
Magnesium oxide fume	—	15
Malathion (o,o-dimethyl dithiophosphate of diethyl mercaptosuccinate)—Skin	—	15

Recommended Values (*Continued*)

Substance	ppm*	Mg/M³**
C Manganese	—	5
Mercury—Skin	—	0.1
Mercury (organic compounds)—Skin	—	0.01
Mesityl oxide	25	100
Methoxychlor (2,2-di-*p*-methoxyphenyl-1,1,1-tri-chloroethane)	—	15
Methyl acetate	200	610
Methyl acetylene	1,000	1,650
Methyl acrylate—Skin	10	35
Methylal (dimethoxymethane)	1,000	3,100
Methyl alcohol (methanol)	200	260
C Methyl bromide—Skin	20	80
Methyl cellosolve (2-methoxyethanol)—Skin	25	80
Methyl cellosolve acetate (ethylene glycol monomethyl ether acetate)	25	120
C Methyl chloride	100	210
† Methyl chloroform (1,1,1-trichloroethane)	350	1,900
Methylcyclohexane	500	2,000
Methylcyclohexanol	100	470
Methylcyclohexanone	100	460
Methyl formate	100	250
Methyl isobutyl carbinol (methyl amyl alcohol)	25	100
†C Methyl mercaptan	20	40
α Methyl styrene	100	480
Methylene chloride (dichloromethane)	500	1,750
Monomethyl aniline—Skin	2	9
Molybdenum		
(soluble compounds)	—	5
(insoluble compounds)	—	15
Naphtha (coal tar)	200	800
Naphtha (petroleum)	500	2,000
β-Naphthylamine	—	A²
Nickel carbonyl	0.001	0.007
Nicotine—Skin	—	0.5
Nitric acid	10	25
p-Nitroaniline—Skin	1	6
Nitrobenzene—Skin	1	5
Nitroethane	100	310
C Nitrogen dioxide	5	9
C Nitroglycerin (combined EGDN + NG)—Skin	0.2	2
Nitromethane	100	250
1-Nitropropane	25	90
2-Nitropropane	25	90

Recommended Values (*Continued*)

Substance	ppm*	Mg/M³**
N-Nitrosodimethylamine (Dimethylnitrosamine)—Skin	A^3	—
Nitrotoluene—Skin	5	30
Octane	500	2,350
Osmium tetroxide	—	0.002
Ozone	0.1	0.2
Parathion (O, O, diethyl-O-*p*-nitrophenyl thiophosphate)—Skin	—	0.1
Pentaborane	0.005	0.01
Pentachloronaphthalene—Skin	—	0.5
Pentachlorophenol—Skin	—	0.5
Pentanone (methyl propyl ketone)	200	700
Pentane	1,000	2,950
Perchloroethylene (tetrachloroethylene)	100	670
Perchloromethyl mercaptan	0.1	0.8
Perchloryl fluoride	3	13.5
Phenol—Skin	5	19
Phenyl glycidyl ether (PGE)	50	310
Phenylhydrazine—Skin	5	22
Phosdrin (2-carbomethoxy-1-methyl vinyl dimethyl phosphate)	—	0.1
Phosgene (carbonyl chloride)	1	4
† Phosphine	0.3	0.4
Phosphoric acid	—	1
Phosphorus (yellow)	—	0.1
Phosphorus pentachloride	—	1
Phosphorus pentasulfide	—	1
Phosphorus trichloride	0.5	3
Picric acid—Skin	—	0.1
Platinum (Soluble Salts)	—	0.002
Propyl acetate	200	840
Propyl alcohol (isopropyl alcohol)	400	980
Propyl ether (isopropyl ether)	500	2,100
n-Propyl nitrate	25	110
Propylene dichloride (1,2-dichloropropane)	75	350
Propylene imine—Skin	25	60
Propylene oxide	100	240
Pyrethrum	—	5
Pyridine	5	15
Quinone	0.1	0.4
Rotenone (commercial)	—	5
Selenium compounds (as Se)	—	0.1
Sodium fluoroacetate (1080)—Skin	—	0.05
Sodium hydroxide	—	2

Recommended Values (Continued)

Substance	ppm*	Mg/M³**
Stibine	0.1	0.5
Stoddard solvent	500	2,900
Strychnine	—	0.15
Styrene monomer (phenylethylene)	100	420
Sulfur dioxide	5	13
Sulfur hexafluoride	1,000	6,000
Sulfuric acid	—	1
Sulfur monochloride	1	6
Sulfur pentafluoride	0.025	0.25
Sulfuryl fluoride	5	20
2,4,5T (2,4,5-Trichlorophenoxyacetic acid)	—	10
TEDP (tetraethyl dithionopyrophosphate)—Skin	—	0.2
Teflon (R) decomposition products	—	A⁴
TEPP (tetraethyl pyrophosphate)—Skin	—	0.05
Tellurium	—	0.1
1,1,2,2-Tetrachloroethane—Skin	5	35
Tetrahydrofuran	200	590
Tetranitromethane	1	8
Tetryl (2,4,6-trinitrophenylmethylnitramine)—Skin	—	1.5
Thallium (soluble compounds)—Skin	—	0.1
Thiram (tetramethyl thiuram disulfide)	—	5
Titanium dioxide	—	15
C Toluene (toluol)	200	750
o-Toluidine—Skin	5	22
C Tolylene-2,4-diisocyanate	0.02	0.14
Trichloroethylene	100	520
Trichloronaphthalene—Skin	—	5
1,2,3-Trichloropropane	50	300
1,1,2-Trichloro 1,2,2-trifluoroethane	1,000	7,600
Triethylamine	25	100
Trifluoromonobromomethane	1,000	6,100
Trinitrotoluene—Skin	—	1.5
Triorthocresyl phosphate	—	0.1
Triphenyl phosphate	—	3
Turpentine	100	560
Uranium		
(soluble compounds)	—	0.05
(insoluble compounds)	—	0.25
Vanadium		
C (V₂O₅ dust)	—	0.5
(V₂O₅ fume)	—	0.1
C Vinyl chloride (chloroethylene)	500	1,300
Vinyl toulene	100	480
Warfarin (3[α acetonylbenzyl]-4-hydroxycoumarin)	—	0.1
Yttrium	—	5

Recommended Values (Continued)

Substance	ppm*	Mg/M³**
C Xylene (xylol)	200	870
Xylidene—Skin	5	25
Zinc oxide fume	—	5
Zirconium compounds (as Zr)	—	5

Radioactivity: For permissible concentrations of radio-isotopes in air, see U.S. Department of Commerce, National Bureau of Standards, Handbook 69, "Maximum Permissible Body Burdens and Maximum Permissible Concentrations of Radionuclides in Air and in Water for Occupational Exposure," June 5, 1959. Also, see U.S. Department of Commerce, National Bureau of Standards, Handbook 59, "Permissible Dose from External Sources of Ionizing Radiation," September 24, 1954, and addendum of April 15, 1958.

Note: The word "Skin" following a substance indicates that the substance can penetrate the skin to contribute to the exposure and threshold limit value should be reduced accordingly.

† 1963 Revision.

* Parts of vapor or gas per million parts of air by volume at 25°C and 760 mm. Hg pressure.

** Approximate milligrams of particulate per cubic meter of air.

A Numbers, See Supplement 1.

Mineral Dusts

Substance	mppcf§

SILICA

Crystalline

Quartz, Threshold Limit calculated from the formula. . . $\dfrac{250}{\%SiO_2\ddagger + 5}$

Cristobalite   "   "   "

Amorphous, including natural diatomaceous earth   20

SILICATES (less than 1% crystalline silica)

Asbestos.	5
Mica.	20
Soapstone	20
Talc	20
Portland Cement	50

Miscellaneous (less than 1% crystalline silica) 50

Conversion factors

mppcf × 35.3 = million particles per cubic meter
= particles per c.c.

§ Millions of particles per cubic foot of air, based on impinger samples counted by light-field technics.

‡ The percentage of crystalline silica in the formula is the amount determined from air-borne samples, except in those instances in which other methods have been shown to be applicable.

Tentative Values

Substance	ppm*	Mg/M³**
C tert. Butyl chromate (as CrO₃)—Skin	—	0.1
† Calcium oxide	—	5
Camphor	—	2
† Copper Fume	—	0.1
Dusts & Mists	—	1.0
DDVP (O, O-Dimethyl-2,2-dichlorovinyl phosphate)	—	1
† Demeton (R) (Systox)	—	0.1
Endrin (1,2,3,4,10,10-hexachloro-6,7-epoxy-1,4,4a, 5,6,7,8,8a-octa hydro 1,4-endo-5,8-dimethano-naphthalene)—Skin	—	0.1
Epichlorhydrin	5	19
Ethanolamine	3	6
† Graphite	—	15 mppcf
† Hafnium	—	0.5
Heptachlor (1,4,5,6,7,8,8a-heptachloro-3a,4,7,7a-tetrahydro-4,7-methanoindene)	—	0.5
† Methylamine	25	31
† Methyl Methacrylate	100	410
†C Methylene bis phenylisocyanate	0.02	0.2
† Mineral Wool (Fiberglas)	—	2
† Naphthalene	10	50
Oil (mineral)	—	5
† β-Propiolactone	—	A⁵
† Silver	—	0.05
† Tantalum	—	5
† 1,1,1,2-Tetrachloro-2,2-difluoroethane	1,000	8,340
† 1,1,2,2-Tetrachloro-1,2-difluroroethane	500	4,170
† Tetraethyl lead—Skin	—	0.075
† Tin		
(inorganic compounds)	—	2
(organic compounds as Sn)—Skin	—	0.1

† 1963 Additions.

* Parts of vapor or gas per million parts of air by volume at 25°C and 760 mm. Hg pressure.

** Approximate milligrams of particulate per cubic meter of air.

A numbers, See Supplement 1

SUPPLEMENT 1

A¹ **Benzidine.** Because of high incidence of bladder tumors in man, any exposure, including skin, is extremely hazardous.

A² **β-Naphthylamine.** Because of the extremely high incidence of bladder tumors in workers handling this compound, and the inability to control exposures,

β-naphthylamine has been prohibited from manufacture, use and other activities that involve human contact by the State of Pennsylvania.

A[3] N-Nitrosodimethylamine. Because of extremely high toxicity and presumed carcinogenic potential of this compound, contact by any route should not be permitted.

A[4] Teflon® decomposition products. At least one identified component of Teflon decomposition products is extremely toxic, but in the absence of more complete toxicity information and suitable analytic methods, a definite threshold limit value is not recommended at this time; but air concentrations should be minimal.

A[5] β-Propiolactone. Because of high acute toxicity and demonstrated skin tumor production in animals, contact by any route should be avoided.

SUPPLEMENT 2:   THRESHOLD LIMIT VALUES FOR MIXTURES

When two or more hazardous substances are present, their combined effect, rather than that of either individually, should be given primary consideration. **In the absence of information to the contrary, the effects of the different hazards should be considered as additive.** That is, if the sum of the following fractions,

$$\frac{C_1}{T_1} + \frac{C_2}{T_2} + \cdots \frac{Cn}{Tn}$$

exceeds unity, then the threshold limit of the mixture should be considered as being exceeded. C indicates the observed atmospheric concentration, and T_1 the corresponding threshold limit, (See Example 1A.a.).

Exceptions to the above rule may be made when there is good reason to believe that the chief effects of the different harmful substances are not in fact additive, but independent as when purely local effects on different organs of the body are produced by the various components of the mixture. In such cases the threshold limit ordinarily is exceeded only when at least one member of the series $\left(\frac{C_1}{T_1} \text{ or } \frac{C_2}{T_2} \text{ etc.}\right)$ itself has a value exceeding unity, (See Example 1A.b.).

Antagonistic action or potentiation may occur with some combinations of atmospheric contaminants. Such cases at present must be determined individually. Potentiating or antagonistic agents are not necessarily harmful by themselves. Potentiating effects of exposure to such agents by routes other than that of inhalation is also possible, e.g. imbibed alcohol and inhaled narcotic (trichlorethylene). Potentiation is characteristically exhibited at high concentrations, less probably at low.

When a given operation or process characteristically emits a number of harmful dusts, fumes, vapors or gases, it will frequently be only feasible to attempt to evaluate the hazard by measurement of a single substance. In such cases, the threshold limit used for this substance should be reduced by a **suitable** factor, the magnitude of which will depend on the number, toxicity and relative quantity of the other contaminants ordinarily present.

Examples of processes which are typically associated with two or more harmful atmospheric contaminants are welding, automobile repair, blasting, painting, lacquering, certain foundry operations, diesel exhausts, etc. (Example 2.)

THRESHOLD LIMIT VALUES FOR MIXTURES—EXAMPLES

1A. General case, where air is analyzed for each component.

    a. **ADDITIVE EFFECTS**

$$\frac{C_1}{T_1} + \frac{C_2}{T_2} + \frac{C_3}{T_3} + \cdots \frac{C_n}{T_n} = 1$$

Air contains 5 ppm of carbon tetrachloride (TLV, 10), 20 ppm of ethylene dichloride (TLV, 50) and 10 ppm of ethylene dibromide, (TLV, 25).

$$\frac{5}{10} + \frac{20}{50} + \frac{10}{25} = \frac{65}{50} = 1.3$$

Threshold limit is exceeded.

    b. **INDEPENDENT EFFECTS**

Air contains 0.15 mg/m³ of lead (TLV, 0.2) and 0.7 mg/m³ of sulfuric acid (TLV, 1).

$$\frac{0.15}{0.20} = 0.75; \frac{0.7}{1} = 0.7$$

Threshold limit is not exceeded.

1B. Special case when source of contaminant is a mixture and atmospheric composition is assumed similar to that of original material, i.e. vapor pressure of each component is the same at the observed temperature.

    a. **ADDITIVE EFFECTS,** approximate solution.

      1. A mixture of equal parts (1) trichloroethylene (TLV, 100), and (2) methyl chloroform (TLV, 350).

$$\frac{C_1}{100} + \frac{C_2}{350} = \frac{C_m}{T_m}$$ Solution applicable to "spot" solvent mixture usage, where all or nearly all, solvent evaporates.

$$C_1 = C_2 = \frac{1}{2} C_m$$

$$\frac{C_1}{100} + \frac{C_1}{350} = \frac{2C_1}{T_m}$$

$$\frac{7C_1}{700} + \frac{2C_1}{700} = \frac{2C_1}{T_m}$$

$$T_m = 700 \times \frac{2}{9} = 155 \text{ ppm}$$

1B.b. General Exact Solution for Mixtures of **N** Components With Additive Effects and Different Vapor Pressures.

    (1) $\frac{C_1}{T_1} + \frac{C_2}{T_2} + \cdots + \frac{C_n}{T_n} = 1;$

    (2) $C_1 + C_2 + \cdots + C_n = T;$

    (2.1) $\frac{C_1}{T} + \frac{C_2}{T} + \cdots + \frac{C_n}{T} = 1.$

By the Law of Partial Pressures,

    (3) $C_i = ap_i,$

And by Raoult's Law,

    (4) $p_i = F_i p_i^\circ.$

Combine (3) and (4) to obtain

(5) $C_i = aF_ip_i{}^\circ.$

Combining (1), (2.1), and (5), we obtain

(6) $\dfrac{F_1p_1{}^\circ}{T} + \dfrac{F_2p_2{}^\circ}{T} + \cdots + \dfrac{F_np_n{}^\circ}{T} = \dfrac{F_1p_1{}^\circ}{T_1} + \dfrac{F_2p_2{}^\circ}{T_2} + \cdots + \dfrac{F_np_n{}^\circ}{T_n}.$

and solving for T,

(6.1) $T = \dfrac{F_1p_1{}^\circ + F_2p_2{}^\circ + \cdots + F_np_n{}^\circ}{\dfrac{F_1p_1{}^\circ}{T_1} + \cdots + \dfrac{F_np_n{}^\circ}{T_n}}$

or

(6.2) $T = \dfrac{\sum\limits_{i=1}^{i=n} F_ip_i{}^\circ}{\sum\limits_{i=1}^{i=n} \dfrac{F_ip_i{}^\circ}{T_i}}$

T = Threshold limit value in ppm.
C = Vapor concentration in ppm.
p = Vapor pressure of component in solution.
p° = Vapor pressure of pure component.
F = Mol fraction of component in solution.
a = A constant of proportionality.
Subscripts 1, 2, . . . n relate the above quantities to components 1, 2, . . . n, respectively.
Subscript i refers to an arbitrary component from 1 to n.
Absence of subscript relates the quantity to the mixture.

Solution to be applied when there is a reservoir of the solvent mixture whose composition does not change appreciably by evaporation.

Exact Arithmetic Solution of Specific Mixture

	Mol. wt.	Density	T	p° at 25°C	Mol fraction in half-and-half solution by volume
Trichloro-ethylene (1)	131.4	1.46 g/ml	100	73mm Hg	0.527
Methylchloro-form (2)	133.42	1.33 g/ml	350	125mm Hg	0.473

$$F_1p_1{}^\circ = (0.527)(73) = 38.2$$
$$F_2p_2{}^\circ = (0.473)(125) = 59.2$$

$$T = \dfrac{38.2 + 59.2}{\dfrac{38.2}{100} + \dfrac{59.2}{350}} = \dfrac{(97.4)(350)}{133.8 + 59.2} = \dfrac{(97.4)(350)}{193.0} = 177$$

T = 177 ppm   (Note difference in T.L.V. when account is taken of vapor pressure and mol fraction in comparison with above example where such account is not taken.)

2. A mixture of one part of (1) parathion (TLV, 0.1) and two parts of (2) EPN (TLV, 0.5).

$$\frac{C_1}{0.1} + \frac{C_2}{0.5} = \frac{C_m}{T_m} \qquad C_2 = 2C_1$$

$$C_m = 3C_1$$

$$\frac{C_1}{0.1} + \frac{2C_1}{0.5} = \frac{3C_1}{T_m}$$

$$\frac{7C_1}{0.5} = \frac{3C_1}{T_m}$$

$$T_m = \frac{1.5}{7} = 0.21 \text{ mg/m}^3$$

1C. INDEPENDENT EFFECTS

1. From naphtha (TLV, 500) containing 10 mole per cent benzene (TLV, 25) the narcotic effects can be considered as approximately the same as that of benzene-free naphtha.

   The blood effects can be considered as due to the benzene alone.

   For **intermittent exposure,** a TLV of 500 ppm may be used as long as the **average** concentration does not exceed $25 \times \dfrac{100}{10} = 250$ ppm, the TLV based on the benzene content.

2. Diesel engine exhaust contains several irritants, one of which is nitrogen dioxide. A limit of 2 ppm NO_2 has been found to correlate fairly well with the beginning of subjective (irritation) effects from such gases, although no subjective effects are experienced from NO_2 alone at 5 ppm.

SUPPLEMENT 3:   BASES FOR ASSIGNING LIMITING "C" VALUES*

T.L.V. RANGE ppm* or mg/m³	Permitted Fluctuation Factor of T.L.V. for 5, 10 or 30 min.	Examples
0 to 1	3	Boron trifluoride (1 ppm) at 3 ppm if repeatedly encountered for periods of 5, 10, or 30 minutes, may lead to pneumonitis; a "C" listing recommended.
1+ to 10	2	
10+ to 100	1.5	Ethyl benzene (200 ppm) at 250 ppm if repeatedly encountered for periods of 5 or
100+ to 1000	1.25	10 minutes may prove intolerably irritating to the eyes; a "C" listing recommended.

* According to this limitation, the presently listed TLVs will or will not be candidates for a "C" (ceiling) listing. 1963 TLVs not coming within this limitation will bear a "C" before the substance name. Judgment is based on whether the excursions in concentration under the time limits stated may result in a) intolerable irritation, b) chronic or irreversible tissue change, or c) narcosis of sufficient degree to increase accident proneness or materially reduce work efficiency.

APPENDIX C

Glossary of Radiological Health Terms

absorption Transformation of radiant energy into other forms of energy when passing through a material substance.

alpha particles Charged particles emitted from the nuclei of some atoms and having a mass of four units and two-unit positive electric charges. They are composed of two neutrons and two protons.

atoms The chemical units of which all matter is made. The atom may be defined as the smallest particle of an element which is capable of entering into a chemical reaction.

atomic mass The mass of an atom of an element compared with one-sixteenth the mass of an oxygen 16 atom.

atomic number Number of protons in the nucleus, and hence the number of positive charges on the nucleus. Also the number of electrons outside the nucleus of a neutral atom. Symbol: Z.

atomic radiation Radiation produced by energy changes in atomic nuclei or atomic electron clouds: ionizing radiation.

background The counting rate or the ionizing radiation produced by cosmic radiation and naturally occurring trace amounts of radioactive elements.

beta particle Charged particle emitted from the nucleus and having a mass and charge equal in magnitude to those of the electron.

betatron A machine used to accelerate electrons.

binding energy The energy that holds the nucleus together; it is quantitatively related to the difference in mass of the separate component parts and the actual mass of the nucleus.

chain reaction Any chemical or nuclear process in which some of the products of the process are instrumental in the continuation or magnification of the process.

curie Standard measure of rate of radioactive decay; the quantity of any radioactive nuclide in which the number of disintegrations per second is 3.700×10^{10}.

critical In nuclear-science usage, a term used to specify the mass, arrangement, or condition of a quantity of fissionable material such that it can sustain a chain reaction, *e.g.*, a critical mass or a critical assembly. Prompt critical is capable of sustaining a chain reaction without the aid of delayed neutrons.

criticality The attainment of a self-sustaining fissionable reaction.

cyclotron A machine which accelerates charged particles by electric and magnetic forces.

decay Disintegration of the nucleus of an unstable element by the spontaneous emission of charged particles and/or photons.

decay time See *half-life*.

dose (dosage) According to current usage, the radiation delivered to a specified area or volume or to the whole body. Units for dose specifications are roentgens for X or gamma rays; also it is the amount of energy absorbed by tissue per unit mass at the site of interest (see *rad*).

dose, air X or gamma ray expressed in roentgens delivered at a point in free air. In radiologic practice it consists of radiation of the primary beam and that scattered from surrounding air.

dose, cumulative The total dose resulting from repeated exposures to radiation of the same region or of the whole body.

dose, exit Dose of radiation at surface of body opposite to that on which the beam is incident.

dose, integral (volume dose) A measure of the total energy absorbed by a patient or any body during exposure to radiation. According to British usage, the integral dose of gamma or X rays is expressed in gram-roentgens.

dose, maximum permissible Maximum dose of radiation which may be received by persons working with radiation.

dose, median lethal Dose of radiation required to kill, within a specified period, 50 per cent of the individuals in a large group of animals or organisms.

dose, permissible The amount of radiation which may be received by an individual within a specified period without expectation of significantly harmful results.

dose, skin Dose at center of irradiation field on skin.

dose, threshold The minimum dose that will produce a detectable degree of any given effect.

dosimeter Instrument used to detect and measure an accumulated dosage of radiation; usually a pocket electroscope.

electron Negatively charged particle which is a constituent of every atom. Unit of negative electricity equal to 4.80×10^{-10} electrostatic unit (esu). Its mass is about 1/2,000 of that of a proton.

electron cloud The group of electrons surrounding an atomic nucleus and, with it, forming the neutral atom.

electron volt Amount of energy gained by an electron in passing across a potential difference of one volt. Abbreviation: ev. One million electron volts is abbreviated Mev.

electroscope An instrument used to measure cumulative exposure to ionizing radiation.

element A substance consisting of atoms of the same atomic (Z) number.

equilibrium, radioactive Among members of a radioactive series, the state which prevails when the ratios between the amounts of successive members of the series remain constant.

erg Unit of work done by a force of one dyne acting through a distance of one centimeter. Unit of energy which can exert a force of one dyne through a distance of one centimeter.

excitation   The addition of energy to a system, thereby transferring it from the ground state to an excited state. Excitation of a nucleus, an atom, or a molecule can result from absorption of photons or from inelastic collisions with other particles. The ground state of a nucleus, atom, or molecule is that at which it has its lowest energy.

external radiation   Radiation entering the body from without.

film badge   Small piece of X-ray or similar photographic film enclosed in a lightproof paper usually crossed by lead or cadmium strips and carried in a small metal or plastic frame. The badge is used to estimate the amount of radiation to which an individual has been exposed.

fission, nuclear   A nuclear transformation characterized by the splitting of a nucleus into at least two other nuclei and the release of a relatively large amount of energy.

fusion, nuclear   Act of coalescing two or more atomic nuclei, with a reduction of mass and release of energy. It is supposed that this reaction occurs in the sun. Helium is synthesized by fusion of hydrogen atoms with a reduction in mass and an equivalent release of energy in the form of heat.

gamma ray   Electromagnetic radiation emitted from the nucleus of a radioactive atom.

Geiger-Müller (G-M) counter   Highly sensitive instrument for detecting radiation.

half-life   Time required for a radioactive substance to lose by decay 50 per cent of its activity.

half-thickness   Thickness of absorbing material necessary to reduce the intensity of radiation by one-half.

internal radiation   Radiation arising from inside the body, as from radioisotopes assimilated and contained within the tissues.

ion   Atomic particle, atom, or chemical radical (group of chemically combined atoms) bearing an electric charge, either positive or negative, caused by an excess or deficiency of electrons.

ionization   The process or result of any process by which a neutral atom or molecule acquires either a positive or a negative charge.

ionizing radiation   Radiation possessing sufficient energy to ionize the atoms or molecules absorbing it.

ion pair   Two particles of opposite charge, usually referring to the electron and positive atomic or molecular residue resulting after the interaction of ionizing radioaction with the orbital electrons of atoms.

isotope   One or two or more forms of an element having the same atomic number (nuclear charge) and hence occupying the same position in the periodic table. All isotopes are identical in chemical behavior but are distinguishable by small differences in atomic weight. The nuclei of all isotopes of a given element have the same number of protons but differ in the number of neutrons.

mass   Quantity of matter, popularly thought of as identical to "weight."

mass, critical   See *critical*.

mass number   The number of nucleons in the nucleus of an atom. Symbol: A.

mass unit (mu)   Unit of mass, one-sixteenth of the mass of an oxygen atom (0^{16}) taken as 16.00000.

maximum permissible body burden   The total body content of a radioisotope which, if maintained, will not deliver to any critical organ a dose greater than the maximum permissible.

maximum permissible concentration   The concentration of a radioisotope in air, water, milk, etc., which will deliver not more than the maximum permissible dose to a critical organ when breathed or consumed at a normal rate.

Mev   Abbreviation for one million electron volts. See *electron volt.*

microcurie   A millionth of a curie (37,000 disintegrations per second) or 10^{-6} curie.

micromicrocurie   A millionth of a microcurie or 10^{-12} curie.

millicurie   A thousandth of a curie.

molecule   Orderly group of atoms joined together by chemical bonds. Some molecules are small and simple, such as water (H_2O); others are large and complex, such as chlorophyll ($C_{55}H_{72}O_5N_4Mg$).

neutron   A nuclear particle with a mass approximately the same as that of a proton and electrically neutral; a constituent of the atomic nucleus. Its mass is 1.00893 mu. Neutrons are classified as slow or thermal if of less than 100 ev; fast if over 0.1 Mev; and intermediate if between.

neutron flux   A term used to express the intensity of neutron radiation. The number of neutrons passing through a unit area in unit time. For neutrons of a given energy, the product of neutron density and speed.

nuclear energy   The energy released by fission or fusion of atomic nuclei.

nuclear fission   A special type of nuclear transformation characterized by the splitting of a nucleus into at least two other nuclei and the release of a relatively large amount of energy.

nuclear fusion   Act of coalescing two or more nuclei.

nuclear reactor   A device or machine for producing energy by fission or fusion of atomic nuclei.

nucleon   Generic name for the constituent parts of the nucleus. At present applied to protons and neutrons, but will include any other particle found to exist in the nucleus.

nucleus   Heavy central part of an atom in which most of the mass and the total positive electric charge are concentrated.

nuclide   A general term referring to any nuclear species of the chemical elements capable of existing for a measurable time.

photon   A quantity of energy emitted in the form of electromagnetic radiations, such as radio waves, light, X rays, and gamma rays.

picocurie   Synonym for microcurie.

positron   Nuclear particle equal in mass to the electron and having an equal but opposite charge. Its mass is 0.000548 mu.

potential difference   Difference in potential between any two points in a circuit; work required to carry a unit positive charge from one point to another.

proportional counter   Gas-filled radiation detection tube in which the pulse produced is proportional to the number of ions formed in the gas by the primary ionizing particle.

proton   Nuclear particle with a positive electric charge equal numerically to the charge of the electron and having a mass of 1.007575 mu.

rad   One hundred ergs of absorbed energy per gram of absorbing material.

radiation   Propagation of energy through space; an electromagnetic wave or rapidly moving atomic or subatomic particle.

radiation sickness   The group of symptoms developed consequent to an overexposure to ionizing radiation; symptoms include weakness, nausea, vomiting, diarrhea, leukocytopenia, anemia, and spontaneous bleeding.

radioactivity   Process whereby unstable nuclei undergo spontaneous atomic disintegration with liberation of energy, generally resulting in the formation of new elements. The process is accompanied by the emission of one or more types of radiation, such as alpha particles, beta particles, and gamma radiation.

radioisotope   A radioactive isotope.

radiological health   The public health aspects of the use of ionizing radiation.

relative biological effectiveness (RBE)   The ratio of gamma- or X-ray dose to the dose that is required to produce the same biological effect by the radiation in question.

rem   See *roentgen equivalent man.*

roentgen   Standard unit of absorption of X and gamma radiation; quantity of X or gamma radiation such that the associated corpuscular emission per 0.0012038 g of air (dry and at standard temperatures and pressure) produces, in air, ions carrying one electrostatic unit of quantity of electricity of either sign.

roentgen equivalent man (rem)   That quantity of radiation of any type which when absorbed by man produces a biological effect equivalent to that produced by the absorption of one roentgen of X or gamma radiation.

roentgen equivalent physical (rep)   That amount of ionizing radiation which in tissue produces the same amount of ionization as that produced by one roentgen in air; the dose of radiation (other than that covered by the definition of the roentgen) which produces energy absorption of 93 ergs per gram of tissue. This unit is now obsolete.

Van de Graaff accelerator   A machine using static electricity to accelerate charged particles.

X ray   A penetrating electromagnetic radiation similar to gamma radiation. This radiation is produced as a result of sudden decrease in electron energy.

INDEX